Reproductive and Developmental Toxicity of Metals

Reproductive and Developmental Toxicity of Metals

Edited by

Thomas W. Clarkson

University of Rochester School of Medicine
Rochester, New York

Gunnar F. Nordberg

University of Umea
Umea, Sweden

and

Polly R. Sager

University of Rochester School of Medicine
Rochester, New York

Plenum Press • New York and London

Library of Congress Cataloging in Publication Data

Main entry under title:

Reproductive and developmental toxicity of metals.

"Proceedings of a joint meeting organized by the Division of Toxicology, University of Rochester, and the Scientific Committee on the Toxicology of Metals of the Permanent Commission and the International Association on Occupational Health, and cospon- sored by the World Health Organization, held May 24–27, 1982, in Rochester, New York"—Verso t.p.

Includes bibliographical references and indexes.

1. Metals—Toxicology—Congresses. 2. Generative organs—Diseases—Congresses. 3. Reproduction—Congresses. 4. Abnormalities, Human—Etiology—Congresses. I. Clarkson, Thomas W. II. Nordberg, Gunnar. III. Sager, Polly R. IV. University of Rochester. Division of Toxicology. V. Permanent Commission and the International Association on Occupational Health. Scientific Committee on the Toxicology of Metals. VI. World Health Organization. [DNLM: 1. Metals—Adverse effects—Congresses. 2. Metals—Metabolism—Congresses. 3. Reproduction—Congresses. 4. Growth-Congresses. QV 290 R425 1982]

RA1231.M52R46 1983	615.9′253	83-11112

ISBN-13: 978-1-4615-9348-5   e-ISBN-13: 978-1-4615-9346-1
DOI: 10.1007/978-1-4615-9346-1

Proceedings of a joint meeting organized by the Division of Toxicology, University of Rochester, and the Scientific Committee on the Toxicology of Metals of the Permanent Commission and the International Association on Occupational Health and cosponsored by the World Health Organization, held May 24–27, 1982, in Rochester, New York

© 1983 Plenum Press, New York
Softcover reprint of the hardcover 1st edition 1983
A Division of Plenum Publishing Corporation
233 Spring Street, New York, N.Y. 10013

A PROCEEDINGS PUBLICATION:

Rochester International Conference on Environmental Toxicity
Series Editors: T.W. Clarkson, M.W. Miller

Scientific Committee on the Toxicology of Metals of the
Permanent Commission and International Association of
Occupational Health (PCIAOH)

UNEP/ILO/WHO
International Programme on Chemical Safety
IPCS Joint Symposia 2

EDITORS:

*T.W. Clarkson   Division of Toxicology
                      Department of Radiation Biology and Biophysics
                      University of Rochester School of Medicine
                      Rochester, New York

*G.F. Nordberg   Department of Environmental Medicine
                      University of Umea
                      Umea, Sweden

*P.R. Sager   Division of Toxicology
                      Department of Radiation Biology and Biophysics
                      University of Rochester School of Medicine
                      Rochester, New York

PREFACE

The Permanent Commission and International Association on Occupational Health (PCIAOH) established in 1969 a Subcommittee on the Toxicology of Metals under the chairmanship of Lars Friberg. This committee, which later was named the Scientific Committee on the Toxicology of Metals, has organized a number of previous meetings that have led to publications in three major areas of metal toxicology: a preliminary meeting in Slanchev Bryag, Bulgaria in 1971, followed by a meeting in 1972 in Buenos Aires, Argentina which produced two reports (Dukes and Friberg, 1971; Task Group on Metal Accumulation, 1973), that discussed the metabolism of metals with special reference to absorption, excretion and biological half-times. The effects and dose-response relationships of toxic metals, including a discussion of general principles, was the second major topic addressed by the Scientific Committee at a meeting in Tokyo in 1974 (Nordberg, 1976). The philosophy of this conference, as well as the previous one in Buenos Aires, was based on the concept of a "threshold dose" for the occurrence of adverse effects. In a conference held in Atlanta, USA in 1980, the scope of discussion on metal effects was broadened to include the role of metals in carcinogenesis. Thus, for the first time, the Scientific Committee took under consideration the possibility of non-threshold relationships (Belman and Nordberg, 1981). In addition, the Scientific Committee on the Toxicology of Metals organized a workshop on metal interactions in Stockholm 1977 (Nordberg et al., 1978) as well as meetings on specific metals which were jointly organized with other institutions. A conference on arsenic was held in Ft. Lauderdale, 1977 (Fowler, 1977) and another conference on cadmium held in Bethesda, Maryland, 1978 (Fowler, 1979) and a workshop on permissible limits for lead held in Amsterdam, 1977 (Zielhuis, 1977).

To this point, the deliberations of the Scientific Committee had been almost exclusively restricted to the toxicology of metals in the mature organism. Consequently, it was decided in Atlanta to hold the next meeting on the Reproductive and Developmental Toxicity of Metals. This topic is important because of the potential for greater sensitivity of the conceptus or the newborn to metal toxicity and because it brings with it the possibility of delayed developmental defects. Such a topic involves both philosophies of threshold and non-threshold effects and it was, therefore, an appropriate follow-up to the two previous meetings.

The Scientific Committee accepted an invitation from the University of Rochester to hold a joint meeting along with the Annual Rochester Conference on Environmental Toxicology. This meeting, which also received co-sponsorship from the World Health Organization, was held in Rochester, New York from May 24-27, 1982. Dr. Gunnar Nordberg, representing the Scientific Committee, and Dr. Thomas W. Clarkson, representing the University of Rochester, were co-chairpersons of the conference. Opening remarks were given by Dr. Clarkson on behalf of the Division of Toxicology, by Dr. Lars Friberg, Chairman of the Scientific Committee, and by Dr. Jiri Parizek, from the World Health Organization, representing the International Programme on Chemical Safety.

Scientists from nine countries participated in the Conference, including chairpersons of individual sessions, invited speakers, those presenting posters and a number of invited discussants. A full list of participants is included elsewhere. The conference combined the "working group" approach used at previous Scientific Committee meetings with the "invited paper-discussion format" of previous Rochester meetings.

The invited papers were presented in six formal sessions as follows:

EFFECTS OF METALS

1. The Reproductive System - Male

    Session Chairperson: Maths Berlin, University of Lund
    Co-chairperson: Lonnie D. Russell, Southern Illinois University

2. The Reproductive System - Female

    Session Chairperson: Donald R. Mattison, Pregnancy Research
                          Branch, NIH
    Co-chairperson: Allen H. Gates, University of Rochester

3. Birth Defects and Perinatal Toxicity

    Session Chairperson: N. Karle Mottet, University of Washington
    Co-chairperson: Bruce Fowler, NIEHS

4. The Developing Nervous System

    Session Chairperson: Patricia Rodier, University of Rochester
    Co-chairperson: J. Julian Chisolm, Johns Hopkins School of
                     Medicine

METABOLISM OF METALS

1. Prenatal Aspects

    Session Chairperson: Richard K. Miller, University of Rochester
    Co-chairperson: Zahir A. Shaikh, University of Rochester

2. Postnatal Aspects

    Session Chairperson: Harold Sandstead, U.S. Department of
                          Agriculture, Agricultural Research Service
    Co-chairperson: Richard A. Doherty, University of Rochester

     A Poster Session was held on Tuesday evening with Dr. Bruce
Kelman, Battelle Pacific Laboratories, and Dr. Curtis Klaassen,
University of Kansas, as chairpersons. Abstracts of their Poster
Session have been published elsewhere (Klaassen, C. and Kelman, B.,
1982, Teratology, 26(1):45A-51A).

     Subsequent to the conference, the session chairpersons arranged
for peer review of the invited papers and each prepared a "review
chapter" based on the deliberations of the working group.
Scientific editors met at Rochester during the week of October 24-30
to make preparation for the final editorial board meeting. A draft
of the overview section was circulated to the entire Editorial
Board, to members of the Scientific Committee, and to additional
reviewers prior to an Editorial Board meeting which was held in
Caracas, Venezuela on the 8th and 9th December 1982. At this
meeting the Editorial Board gave a final review of the material
presented in this book. However, only the authors themselves are
responsible for their views, statements and opinions in the invited
papers and session review chapters.

ACKNOWLEDGEMENTS

     On the 10th and 11th December, the Editorial Board shared a
joint meeting on perinatal toxicity with the Red Nacional
Toxicologica de Venezuela. Dr. Arellano Parra acted as co-organizer
with Drs. Clarkson and Nordberg representing the University of
Rochester and the Scientific Committee on the Toxicology of Metals,
respectively. Co-sponsorship was received from the World Health
Organization and the Pan American Health Organization.

     We wish to thank the following agencies for their financial
support: the Swedish Work Environment Fund, the Swedish Coal Health
Environment Project, U.S. Department of Energy, Electric Power and
Research Institute, Environmental Protection Agency, the National
Institute of Environmental Health Sciences, Varian Instrument Group
and Mobil Oil Company.

The Editorial Board wishes to express its appreciation to Laszlo Magos for reviewing the overview chapter and to members of the staff of the Division of Toxicology, including Muriel Bank Klein and Joyce Morgan, for their untiring efforts in supplying logistic support to the conference. A special thank you is also in order to Nancy Scott and the staff of the Word Processing Center for their contribution in the preparation of this work. The arduous task of indexing was skillfully done by Jean Clarkson. In addition, the Board gratefully acknowledges the cooperation of the staff of the Red Nacional Toxicologica de Venezuela and those of the Division of Toxicology, including Elsa and Omar Cernichiari and Michael Terry, in making arrangements for the joint meeting on perinatal toxicity in Caracas.

The Editors and the Editorial Board wish to thank each contributor for her/his work and cooperation in completing the document.

On behalf of the Editorial Board,

                                          Tom Clarkson
                                          Gunnar Nordberg
                                          Polly Sager

PREVIOUS ANNUAL PUBLICATIONS FROM ROCHESTER INTERNATIONAL
CONFERENCES IN ENVIRONMENTAL TOXICITY

1968 Conference: Chemical Fallout: Current Research on Persistent Pesticides (eds. Miller and Berg), Charles C. Thomas Publishers, Inc., 1969.

1969 Conference: Effects of Metals on Cells, Subcellular Elements, and Macromolecules (eds. Maniloff, Coleman, and Miller), Charles C. Thomas Publishers, Inc., 1970.

1970 Conference: Assessment of Airborne Particles (eds. Mercer, Morrow, and Stoeber), Charles C. Thomas Publishers, Inc., 1971.

1971 Conference: Mercury, Mercurials and Mercaptans (eds. Miller and Clarkson), Charles C. Thomas Publishers, Inc., 1973.

1972 Conference: Behavioral Toxicology (eds. Weiss and Laties), Plenum Press, 1975.

1973 Conference: Molecular and Environmental Aspects of Mutagenesis (eds. Prakash, Sherman, Miller, Lawrence, and Taber), Charles C. Thomas Publishers, Inc., 1973.

1974 Conference: Fundamental and Applied Aspects of Non-Ionizing Radiation (eds. Michaelson, Miller, Magin and Carstensen), Plenum Press, 1975.

1975 Conference: Environmental Toxicity of Aquatic Radionuclides: Models and Mechanisms (eds. Miller and Stannard), Ann Arbor Science Publications, 1976.

1976 Conference: Membrane Toxicity (eds. Miller and Shamoo), Plenum Press, 1977.

1977 Conference: Environmental Pollutants: Detection and
                   Measurement (eds. Toribara, Coleman, Dahneke, and
                   Feldman), Plenum Press, 1978.

1978 Conference: Neurotoxicity of the Visual System (eds. Merigan
                   and Weiss), Raven Press, 1980.

1979 Conference: Polluted Rain (eds. Toribara, Miller, and
                   Morrow), Plenum Press, 1980.

1980 Conference: Measurement of Risks (eds. Berg and Maillie),
                   Plenum Press, 1981.

1981 Conference: Induced Mutagenesis: Molecular Mechanisms and
                   their Implications for Environmental Protection.
                   (ed. Lawrence), Plenum Press, 1983.

1982 Conference: Reproductive and Developmental Toxicity of Metals
                   (eds. Clarkson, Nordberg, and Sager), Plenum
                   Press, 1983.

PREVIOUS PUBLICATIONS OF THE SCIENTIFIC COMMITTEE
ON THE TOXICOLOGY OF METALS

Absorption and excretion of toxic metals. Report from a meeting at Slanchev Briag, Bulgaria (eds. Dukes and Friberg), September 10-24, 1971. Nord. Hyg. Tidskr. 52: 70-104, 1971.

Accumulation of toxic metals with special reference to their absorption, excretion and biological half-times (ed. Nordberg). Task Group on Metal Accumulation. Environ. Physiol. Biochem. 3: 65-107, 1973.

Effects and Dose-Response Relationships of Toxic Metals (ed. Nordberg). Elsevier, Amsterdam, 1976.

Proceedings of the International Conference on Environmental Arsenic, Fort Lauderdale, Florida, October 5-8, 1976 (ed. Fowler). Environ. Health Perspect. 19: 1-242.

Second International Workshop on Permissible Levels for Occupational Exposure to Inorganic Lead, September 21-23, 1976, Colonel Laboratory, Faculty of Medicine, University of Amsterdam (ed. Zielhuis). Int. Arch. Occup. Environ. Health 39: 59-72, 1977.

Factors influencing metabolism and toxicity of metals: A consensus report by the Task Group on Metal Interactions (ed. Nordberg). Environ. Health Perspect. 25: 3-41, 1978.

Metallothionein. Proceedings of the "First International Meeting on Metallothionein and other Low Molecular Weight Metal-Binding Proteins." Zurich, July 17-22, 1978 (eds. Kagi and Nordberg). Birkhauser Verlag, Basel, 1979.

Proceedings of an International Conference on Environmental Cadmium, Bethesda, Maryland, June 7-9, 1978 (ed. Fowler). Environ. Health Perspect. 28: 1-300, 1979.

Workshop Conference on the role of metals in carcinogenesis (ed. Belman). Environ. Health Perspect. 40: 3-42, 1981.

Reproductive and Developmental Toxicity of Metals (eds. Clarkson, Nordberg, and Sager). Plenum Publishing Corp., New York, in press.

CONTENTS

SPECIAL TOPIC PAPERS

AN OVERVIEW OF THE REPRODUCTIVE AND DEVELOPMENTAL TOXICITY OF METALS

Authors: *The Editorial Board*

Working Group: Arthur Furst, Myron Mehlman, J. Vostal

Overview Contents:

AN OVERVIEW OF THE REPRODUCTIVE AND DEVELOPMENTAL TOXICITY OF METALS

T.W. Clarkson, G.F. Nordberg, and P.R. Sager;
M. Berlin, L. Friberg, D.R. Mattison, R.K. Miller, N.K.
Mottet, N. Nelson, J. Parizek, P.M. Rodier and
H. Sandstead

INTRODUCTION

The field of metal toxicology has received much interest over the past few years. In this volume, the emphasis has been focused on the effects of metals on reproduction and development for several reasons. First, damage to reproduction and development is more likely to have irreversible consequences than damage to most other bodily functions. Indeed, under certain circumstances damage may be passed on to subsequent generations. Irreversible damage sustained before birth may have adverse consequences throughout the entire life span representing a continued burden both to the individual and to society. Second, occupational health and other standards have not always taken into account risks to reproductive and developing tissues. At best, risk to people of childbearing age or to the conceptus has been covered by an arbitrary safety factor; at worst, they have not been taken into account at all. Third, the current tendency in a number of countries is to delay parenthood to later years with the result that the preconception exposure period is increased. Fourth, the current public interest in occupational and environmental exposures during the reproductive years makes it very important to transfer the findings of laboratory, clinical, and epidemiological work to public health officials and administrators, to organized labor and management, and to the public at large.

In this context we have considered metal exposure of the male, the non-pregnant female, and the maternal-offspring unit. For the first two situations - male and non-pregnant female - the primary targets are the gonads, although gonadal effects may also be the result of action of metals on hormonal control. Within the mother-offspring unit, the mutual relationship is a constantly

3

changing one. This relationship starts with the fertilized ovum, moves through the growth of the embryo, during which the period of organogenesis provides a relatively short window for toxic disturbances resulting in terata, and finally through the fetal and perinatal stages. During this period of development the central nervous system is especially vulnerable. In parallel, the placenta itself undergoes both metabolic and morphological changes especially in the very early stages of pregnancy. Either the placenta or the offspring may be the primary target of the insult, resulting in a developmental aberration.

Well defined teratogenic effects have been found as a result of exposure of humans to a number of exogenous chemicals. There is also a wealth of information, from experimentation in animal species, that maternal exposure to metallic compounds during organogenesis may give rise to fetal anomalies. Such effects are specific with regard to both the type of anomaly and the species of metallic compound. These effects are the result of relatively high doses; their relevance to possible human risk is wholly unknown.

For humans, there are indications that metals may cause abortions and other effects on the conceptus although the specific metal compounds responsible have not been defined since the exposures were to a mixture of compounds. There is also evidence of effects on the CNS as a result of metal exposure both in utero and in the suckling infant. Methylmercury gives rise to a range of irreversible effects on the CNS in the human fetus as a result of oral maternal exposure. These effects on the developing CNS are believed to occur at doses lower than those associated with effects on the mature CNS. Although reported effects of lead and arsenic on the developing CNS in children are related mainly to postnatal exposure during infancy and early childhood, there is reason to believe that some effects may also occur as a result of prenatal exposure, based mainly on experience in animals. In addition to these effects related to the mother-offspring unit, certain metal compounds have been shown to influence both male and female reproductive competence.

A number of effects related to reproduction and development have thus been demonstrated in connection with exposures to certain metals in experimental animals and it was considered of importance during this conference to:

1. Examine the reported effects of metallic compounds in relation to present knowledge about the biology of reproduction and development, in order to arrive at indications about mechanisms that lie behind observed effects;

2.   Evaluate present evidence concerning reproductive and developmental effects of metals in relation to their possible impact from a public health perspective; and

3.   Identify the most urgent research needs related to these two main areas of concern.

The products of these efforts are brought together in this book which is thus intended to 1) evaluate and summarize our present state of knowledge for scientists in this field, and 2) serve as an introductory source for those wishing to acquaint themselves with the field, and to lead the reader through the bibliographies towards more detailed sources. Although this book may provide a source of background information for those involved in the development of control or regulatory procedures, it is not intended to reach final judgments on human health effects.

At previous meetings organized by the Scientific Committee on the Toxicology of Metals, a conceptual framework had been worked out that related biological effects at various levels of observation (cell, tissue, organ or whole organism) to their possible significance from a public health point of view. These concepts have been useful when discussing systemic effects of metals and an attempt will be made in the present overview to apply some of these concepts to developmental and reproductive effects.

For a discussion of effects on the adult male and female reproductive system it is of importance to recognize that these effects may be due 1) to an alteration of hormonal balance, which may be reversible should the causative agent be removed, 2) to an influence on the ovum or spermatazoon that is unrelated to the genetic material, or 3) to a mutagenic or clastogenic effect. The first two categories of effects, while giving rise to infertility, usually do not have irreversible effects in the offspring; such a possibility exists for the third category.

The three categories mentioned above would be applicable to both the male and the female system; however, there are definite differences between the two systems. The ovum is present in the female and held in meiotic arrest from birth until just prior to ovulation. It may suffer adverse influence of various types during the whole of this period, whereas the spermatozoa are formed only during the relatively short period of spermatogenesis.

When evaluating the influence of metal exposures on the developing organism, it is of particular concern that the response is often both qualitatively and quantitatively different than that seen in an adult organism. A greater sensitivity of the developing organism is especially important. A classical example is offered by methylmercury. Mothers without overt signs of poisoning gave birth to children with developmental defects. In many of these cases, the extent of damage was not evident until some time (even years) after birth. Such differential sensitivity might arise either from preferential distribution of the metal to the offspring or from a higher sensitivity of the immature versus adult tissue.

Development involves many processes which are special to this period. Proliferation is one of these basic processes; agents that disrupt mitosis directly may give rise to fetal abnormalities, but agents influencing proliferation by other mechanisms (e.g., inhibition of DNA replication) may also give rise to such anomalies.

The concept of a "critical period" or "window" when the conceptus is particularly sensitive to insult is a special feature of developmental effects. This concept has long been accepted in classical teratology. Since the duration and timing of the critical period for specific effects varies among species and agents, exposure to the metal in question should be related to the critical period. This may cause considerable difficulties in the interpretation of many epidemiological studies. Partly for this reason, only few such studies can provide useful data on dose-response relationships of developmental effects.

In evaluating reports of developmental effects, it is also important to recognize that there may exist both a true and an apparent latency period before the effect can be demonstrated. An apparent latency period may be related to the functional reserve capacity that exists for many organs.

It is recognized in other fields of toxicology that manifestations originating from mutagenic or clastogenic effects are often irreversible; such is also the case for similarly induced effects on reproduction and development. However, during development other mechanisms of damage also may give rise to irreversible defects. It is necessary, therefore, to develop the concepts of "critical effect" and "critical concentration" further in order to accommodate the different situations that are presented when discussing reproductive and developmental effects. Such a discussion is included in the section on "Effects and Dose-Response Relationships."

The identification and quantitation of the risks associated with metal exposures require that the special tissue sensitivity parameters be taken into account. For example, those which have been alluded to in the foregoing text for reproductive and developmental effects. It is also of fundamental importance that the dose to the target tissue be assessed in a precise manner. The following overview, therefore, will first consider the factors that are related to the metabolism of metallic compounds and to the analysis of such compounds and then go on to discuss effects and dose-response relationships.

METABOLIC FACTORS DETERMINING DOSE TO TARGET TISSUE AND BIOCHEMICAL UNIT

The biological responses to metals and their compounds are determined by the interplay of the chemical nature of the metal compounds, their alteration and transport within the organism, and the specific responses of the tissue or biochemical unit. The nature of the metal compound is generally all-important for its entry, excretion, and movement through the organism. Thus, methylmercury is efficiently absorbed and transported, easily crossing the placenta and blood-brain barrier and may lead to severe damage to the developing nervous system. Other mercury compounds have very different patterns of absorption, transport, and tissue accumulation. Also involved are the valence state of the metal as well as the anion or complex with which it is associated. Thus, the cation chromium VI can enter the cell whereas chromium III cannot. These factors may be decisive in determining the target organs and the nature of the effects.

For reproductive effects, the extent of the biological response in the gonad will be influenced by metabolic and pharmacokinetic factors which determine the dosage to the gonad. However, in the case of the mother-offspring unit, new sets of considerations enter wherein the metabolic processes of the placenta, embryo, fetus or suckling infant are now important in determining dosage. In the case of methylmercury, fetal blood concentrations are actually higher than the maternal blood concentrations.

During breast feeding, movement of the agent into the milk may be the critical factor determining infant dosage. The placenta during the in utero period is, in some cases, a barrier, while in other cases it is an easy route for the entry of the metal compound into the embryo or into the fetus. Indeed, the rate of transplacental movement of the metal may vary during gestation as the placenta and the extraembryonic membranes mature. In some instances, e.g., with cadmium, the placenta itself is the target organ.

Indicator Media

A major challenge in studies of the reproductive and developmental toxicity of metals is how to define the dose. Without an appropriate definition of dose, it is difficult to extrapolate from experimental work on animals and infer risks in humans. In previous reports of the Scientific Committee dealing with the systemic toxicity of metals, dose is defined in terms of the average metal concentration in the critical organ or tissue.

In many experimental studies, the target tissues themselves are accessible for analysis. In human studies and some experimental studies, more accessible media such as urine, blood or hair are analyzed. The relative value of these indicator media depends on the agent and our knowledge of its metabolism and distribution. Indicator media have been established which correlate with critical tissue concentrations of some metals in adults. For example, with some arsenic compounds, urinalysis is useful; with lead, blood is far more informative than urine; in the case of methylmercury, both blood and hair are good indices of exposure, while urine is not a good indicator.

The application of indicator media in a reproductive or developmental model clearly depends upon establishing a metabolic model for each metal whereby quantitative correlations may be developed between the concentration of metal in the appropriate medium and the concentration in the critical tissue. Unfortunately, metabolic data for reproductive organs or the maternal-offspring unit are lacking. Methylmercury is one of the few examples where indicator media (maternal hair and blood) are apparently a valid estimate of dose to the fetal nervous system and a predictor of adverse developmental effects.

Analytical Aspects and Quality Control

Accurate analysis of metals in indicator media or other tissues is essential for both experimental and epidemiological studies. Modern sophisticated instrumentation, including atomic absorption, spectrophotometers using electrothermal atomization, and anodic stripping voltametry may be employed for the analysis of various metals. However, with such equipment, possibilities for gross systematic errors due, for example, to the nature of the supporting medium, are large. Added to this are possibilities for contamination which may become critical when analyzing trace metals in the parts per billion range.

The need for a rigid quality assurance program accompanying actual monitoring data has become obvious as a result of several interlaboratory comparisons and from recently documented quality assurance studies. Reference is made to a report from UNEP/WHO global monitoring project on lead and cadmium (Friberg, this volume). Indeed, even in well experienced laboratories large, sysetmatic errors can occur which may invalidate the results.

It has, unfortunately, been more the exception than the rule in the past that published reports are accompanied by valid quality assurance data. This makes it necessary to exercise great caution when evaluating actual data on the relationship between exposure and dose.

There is a need to prepare standard reference materials for different tissues, metals and concentrations. Thus, through the establishment of reference samples via national and international bodies, and by organizing regular interlaboratory comparisons, badly needed progress may be made in quality control assurance. Such activities are now underway for cadmium, nickel, selenium, and chromium under the auspices of the International Union of Pure and Applied Chemistry (IUPAC). In addition, several national and international agencies have developed biological reference materials. These include urine and bovine liver, but there are no reference materials for blood. One drawback is that only very few concentrations, and always officially published concentrations, are available.

Further needs should be considered for reference standards for biological materials that are certified for a number of metals. Protocols for obtaining certification have been established, for instance, by the National Bureau of Standards. Therefore, it is emphasized that biological standards for blood and other tissues are needed, especially for low concentrations of metals.

EFFECTS OF METALS ON REPRODUCTION AND DEVELOPMENT

Many metals such as arsenic, cadmium, lead and mercury are potent systemic toxicants in animals and man. Thus, systemic toxicity may indirectly affect reproductive function via toxicity to the mother, resulting in retarded growth and development of the fetus and the suckling animal. It is therefore important to distinguish between direct and indirect effects of metals on reproduction and development, and to identify those metals that affect reproduction and development directly at levels lower than those which cause systemic toxicity.

In consideration of the systemic toxicity in mature organisms, the Scientific Committee identified the "critical effects" of certain metals. The critical effect often occurs at an early stage of intoxication and, if prevented, may guard against more serious effects. For example, in cadmium exposure the critical effect is probably a defect in renal tubular reabsorption as evidenced by the excretion of low molecular weight proteins. If prevented, more serious effects, such as a Fanconi-like syndrome or impaired lung function (emphysema), will be avoided. However, in some cases, there are or there may be no detectable early warning or herald signs related to possible later injury, e.g., cancer.

The question arises in the case of certain metals or certain compounds of the same metal, that a reproductive or developmental effect may constitute the critical effect. Interference with normal development of the central nervous system probably represents the

critical effect for methylmercury, and possibly for other
short-chain alkyl mercurials and mercury vapor.

The identification of the critical effect is of interest from a
public health point of view for the reasons given above, i.e., the
prevention of this effect implies prevention against other more
serious effects. In the earlier workshops organized by the
Scientific Committee on the Toxicology of Metals, critical effects
were discussed only in relation to effects other than cancer and
genetic alteration. The present workshop and the one held on metal
carcinogenesis made it necessary to discuss critical effects that
are serious in nature and may occur at low exposure levels even if
they occur only in a low incidence.

Obviously it is not possible to discuss whether a certain
effect on the reproductive system or on the conceptus should be
regarded as a critical effect without some knowledge about the
relationship between dose and response for effects that may be
caused by the toxic metal in question. The shape of the dose-
response curve for the various effects will be of importance.
Effects which are of a threshold type (s-shaped dose-response
curves) are less likely to dominate in the low dose range, whereas
effects which have a linear dose-response relationship with a
shallow slope will be more likely to dominate at low doses.

In the following text, a brief overview will be given
concerning various effects that can be caused by metallic compounds
on reproductive tissues and on the embryo-fetus. Comments on the
nature of the target, the nature of the dose-response relationship
and an evaluation of whether the respective effects may be regarded
as a "critical effect" will be given whenever possible.

Effects on Reproductive Tissues

Effects of metals on the reproductive system of the male or
female may involve any one of a number of organs and tissues either
in the adult or during development. Effects that may occur during
development of reproductive tissues are similar to those that may
occur in other tissues and include effects on the genetic material
in the cell as well as on other biochemical targets.

There is evidence for effects on the developing female
reproductive system in experimental animals from metals such as
cadmium, mercury, selenium and arsenic, and on effects on sexual
maturation from lead, cadmium and mercury. Effects of the sexually
mature female reproductive system include possible effects on the
hypothalamus or pituitary, the ovary or the uterus. With regard to
possible effects on hormone production in these tissues, effects in
the experimental animal have been reported for lead, inorganic

mercury, and nickel. Hormone production depends on a complex series of biochemical events and, in the absence of actual data, it is difficult to express an opinion as to whether or not the interaction between metallic compounds and sensitive biochemical steps of hormone production would be of a threshold type.

Certain compounds of lead, cadmium, nickel, lithium, and copper affect germ cells in female animals. The molecular mechanisms are not yet known, but may include both genetic and nongenetic targets. Effects on fertilization and implantation have been documented in experimental animals for lead and appear to be related to biochemical changes in the endometrium. Also, cadmium, chromium, nickel, selenium, lithium, and copper have been reported to affect the preimplantation embryo or to give rise to resorptions, but the mechanisms are not known.

For obvious reasons, it is much more difficult to obtain detailed information concerning effects on the reproductive system in humans than in animals. Epidemiological evidence concerning effects is limited to studies of fertility and spontaneous abortions. Lead has been used an abortifacient and occupational exposure in the past has been associated with an increased risk of abortion. There are also some indications of such effects as a result of community exposures although the data is very uncertain.

Two studies of women smelter workers exposed to a mixture of metallic compounds (arsenic, lead, zinc, cadmium) have suggested an increased frequency of spontaneous abortion. Infertility in women exposed to lead has been reported in the past. In the general population, chromosomal abnormalities are found in a large proportion of fetuses aborted spontaneously; however, a variety of other mechanisms (including hormonal imbalances) may also be involved. In the case of lead and possibly other metals, the mechanisms underlying the abortions are unknown.

Like the situation in the female, effects on the male reproductive system can theoretically occur during development although there are no data. Effects on the mature male reproductive system may be at the level of the hypothalamus, pituitary, or the testes, including gametogenesis or hormone production by the interstitial cells (Leydig cells). Information on the effects of metals on hormone production is sparse although such effects are conceivable on the basis of distribution patterns. Effects on testosterone production by Leydig cells may result from deficient pituitary function, from a vascular effect giving rise to insufficient blood supply to the interstitial tissue, or from a direct interference with hormone production in the Leydig cells. The most thoroughly investigated effects of metallic compounds on these systems are those exerted by acute or long term cadmium exposure in various experimental animal models. These effects after chronic exposure are modified by the induction of metallothionein synthesis.

Effects of inorganic mercuric mercury as well as methylmercury have been reported on DNA, RNA and protein synthesis of spermatogonia. Manganese chloride may arrest spermatogenesis and cause enzymatic alterations in semeniferous tubules of rabbits. Observations on lead exposed workers suggest the possibility of an effect of lead on the maturation process of the sperm which may be related either to an effect on the epididymis or a direct effect on the spermatozoa.

In animals, the effects on male fertility have been reported for lead and methylmercury. Oral administration of lead to male animals has also given rise to decreased litter size, reduced survival rate and diminished growth rate of offspring. In humans, there is evidence from the older literature that effects on the progeny may result from male lead exposure.

Effects on Embryo-Fetal Development

As pointed out in the introduction, there are several aspects that are special features of development and which should be taken into account when evaluating effects.

Developmental Processes

The remarkable rate at which cell proliferation and differentiation take place during the early development of the zygote (fertilized egg) to the fetus makes it likely that this period is extremely sensitive to injury. This embryonic period of proliferation also involves cell differentiation; cells become committed to form placental or embryonic tissue, and then to form the germ layers from which various tissues arise. The formation of tissues and organs is achieved by a limited number of cellular morphogenic actions. Influence on either the genetic instruction for morphogenesis or the metabolism of cells established to perform the genetic instructions may give rise to developmental abnormalities.

Influence on the genetic instructions for cell differentiation can occur at any point from the beginning of gametogenesis to maturation of the offspring. In the case of metals which tend to accumulate in tissues, exposure of either parent prior to conception may be important. In theory, certain alterations in the genetic instructions (e.g., point mutations) may give rise to irreversible changes in the offspring some of which may be inheritable. The dose-response curves for such genetic effects are assumed by some to be of a non-threshold type.

Differentiation may also be affected by alterations in chromosomal structure (e.g., breakage) or number (e.g., trisomy). Such effects can be produced by damage to nongenetic targets, for example the mitotic spindle, and may exhibit dose-response relationships of the threshold type. Indeed, chromosomal abnormalities are not uncommon, as indicated by the fact that a large proportion of spontaneously aborted embryos have chromosomal abnormalities.

Mechanisms of morphogenesis that may be influenced include: cell proliferation, migration, differentiation, cell-cell interaction, and programmed cell death. Proliferation is one of the most basic processes in development. Most tissues retain some proliferative capacity in their adult state. However, the CNS represents the extreme case where proliferation of neuronal cells is restricted to the period of development. Therefore, agents which disrupt mitosis in neurons can act by this mechanism in the immature, not in the adult, CNS. Methylmercury, for example, appears to affect mitosis in proliferating cells of the cerebellum.

Cell migration is reported to be affected in at least one specific instance; that is, the disruption of neuronal migration after human exposure to methylmercury. Cell loss also has a unique role in development, where programmed cell death is necessary for proper differentiation and maturation in some areas. Two examples are the programmed cell death in spinal cord and the cell loss necessary for proper digit formation in limb buds. Malformations may arise if the timing or extent of this cell death is disrupted. Cell death might, in theory, be accelerated by certain metals known to be cytotoxic such as lead, methylmercury, arsenic, and cadmium.

Critical Periods

The concept of a critical period or "window" when the embryo is particularly sensitive to insult has long been accepted in the production of classical terata. The duration and timing of the window of susceptibility vary among species for a particular effect and agent. The concept of insult during a critical period may be applied not only to specific effects occurring over a short interval, but also to effects arising from those processes occurring over extended time periods and to those agents that persist in developing tissues for a long time. For example, if one considers a functional disturbance which results from interference with a maturational process, the critical period may extend from the end of organogenesis until birth or later.

The integration of sequential processes over time is more complex for the CNS than for other organs - e.g., liver, lung, or kidney. In a system such as the CNS, the possibility arises that agents may act by different molecular or cellular mechanisms - for example, inhibition of proliferation or by direct cytotoxicity - to produce the same result of reduced cellularity. On the other hand, the metal producing injury may act by one mechanism to produce different effects within the same tissue. For example, disruption of cellular microtubules may be manifested as decreased cell production, failure of cells to migrate, or as a defect in extension of cellular processes such as axons and dendrites. Which manifestation appears will depend on the developmental stage of that particular area of the CNS at the time of exposure. Indeed, by examining several areas of the brain, one may find several effects arising from the same agent through a common mechanism.

Differentiation and Plasticity

As cells differentiate, they lose their plasticity to various degrees depending on the cell type. Some tissues retain the capacity to generate new cells and to undergo differentiation long after organogenesis. Although production of neurons does not occur in CNS after rather narrow, prescribed periods in development, its functional plasticity may be rather high. Although a lower neuron population, either by reduced production or by direct cytotoxicity, is permanent, alternate circuits can develop from other neurons, leading to replacement of function. In other tissues, certain functions can be performed only by certain cells. After selective damage of those cells, others cannot assume lost functions unless the cells undergo a new cycle of differentiation.

Functional Reserve Capacity and Latency

In research on CNS effects during development, much attention has been focused on functional measures of damage - for example, behavior and neurotransmitter levels. Few attempts have been made to correlate these effects with morphologic alterations even though much is known about the histological development of the brain. The opposite situation exists for non-nervous tissue where data consist primarily of morphologically defined damage with only rare measurements of functional parameters. It may be this contrast in approach that has encouraged the separation of CNS effects from other effects, although the mechanisms of damage are not likely to be unique.

While manifestations of some damage during development are observable soon after insult, others do not apear until some time after exposure has occurred. Interference with organogenesis produces identifiable anomalies; however, maturational processes are susceptible to damage which may not appear until some later stage. Behavioral effects are a prime example of this both in humans and in experimental animals. Delays in sensory-motor or cognitive development may not appear until a considerable time after exposure when the organisms are required to display new behaviors. The mechanisms underlying these phenomena are not clear. It may be related to a reduced functional reserve capacity of the tissue, which is revealed only under certain conditions. Alternatively, delayed effects may result from subtle alterations in maturational processes - below limits of current detection - which are manifest only after a certain interval following injury. The CNS is likely to exhibit this second type of latent effect since its functional maturation can occur over a period of years.

FACTORS AFFECTING REPRODUCTIVE AND DEVELOPMENTAL TOXICITY OF METALS

Species and Strain Differences

        Species and strain differences are very important in the reproductive and developmental toxicology of metals. Basic species differences in anatomy and physiology of the reproductive system and of the developmental processes underlie many of the substantial species differences seen in both the metabolism and toxicity of metals. The reproductive toxicity of cadmium may exhibit differences even within strains of the same species. The sensitivity of certain inbred strains of mice to testicular damage from cadmium appears to be regulated through the expression of a single gene. Species and strain differences also play a dominant role in determining both the nature and severity of specific embryopathic or teratogenic lesions for a given metal or chemical species of that metal. Strain and species differences greatly complicate the problem of interference of human health risks from experimental results in animals.

Dietary Factors

        Reproductive and developmental processes may be indirectly affected by diet via effects on the health and well-being of the animal as a whole. Most non-specific effects may be anticipated because of the well known potential in adult animals for metals to interact with other metals and trace elements, as previously described by the Scientific Committee. Thus, the reproductive and developmental toxicity of any given metal may be affected by simultaneous body burdens of other metals and trace elements. A dramatic example is the protection against cadmium-induced testicular atrophy by the administration of an equimolar dose of selenium. The selenium content of the diet might well be important in affecting the metabolism and toxicity of a number of metals. Pre-existing body burdens of metals that are capable of inducing the synthesis of the metal binding protein, metallothionein, or other metal binding proteins, might well influence the action of other metals. Thus in both experimental and epidemiological investigations, a knowledge of dietary factors is of great importance.

A new and interesting example of dietary interaction is reported in this volume. The fecal excretion of methylmercury occurs at a low rate in suckling animals but switches to the much higher adult rate at the end of the suckling period. Intestinal microflora are known to convert methylmercury to inorganic mercury in adult animals. The inorganic form is preferentially excreted whereas methylmercury is reabsorbed into the blood stream. It is of interest that the change from a milk to a solid diet at the termination of suckling is accompanied by a change in intestinal microflora to organisms capable of breaking down methylmercury to inorganic mercury.

Environmental Factors

In addition to diet, other less well defined environmental factors must be considered. For example, experimental studies on primates have indicated that isolation of young animals, typical in the laboratory setting, may indirectly influence the extent of CNS injury.

In human populations, factors related to life style may affect the outcome of pre- and perinatal exposure to metals.

CONCLUSIONS AND RECOMMENDATIONS FOR SPECIFIC METALS

In recent years, we have observed a growing interest in the effects of metals related to reproduction and prenatal and/or postnatal development. Exposure of pregnant women to methylmercury can result in permanent brain damage of fetuses and the effects of methylmercury on the developing central nervous system represent the critical effect occurring at levels of exposure even lower than the neurotoxic effects associated with methylmercury exposure in adults. The feto- and embryotoxic effects of methylmercury certainly deserve the highest attention both from the scientific point of view and from the point of protection of this critical segment of the population.

The neurotoxic effects of lead exposure during development are another area of highest priority, where the concerns of research groups and regulatory agencies are well supported by the existing experience from humans. In addition, there is evidence of gonadal effects of lead exposure in human males. Arsenic is another case where studies on humans provide direct evidence of hazard associated with exposure during development.

It should be recognized that the well known constraints on human studies and the power of epidemiological methods limit considerably the possibility of obtaining direct evidence of reproductive and developmental effects of metals. Thus, in predicting the risk in humans, we must rely on animal experiments, taking into account the conditions and levels of exposure as well as other variables, including species differences.

A separate category represents studies in which cadmium salts were given to experimental animals by parenteral administration where the primary aim of research has not been focused on the assessment of the risk in humans. For this reason these studies have been a stimulus for further research to indicate site or mechanism of action even though they may not be considered as direct indication of human hazard. The same may apply to studies on teratogenic effects of administration of high doses of certain metals during specific critical periods of pregnancy.

Knowledge concerning reproductive and developmental toxicity of other metals is more limited. It is clear that more research is needed to determine if some of these metals could have specific effects on reproduction and development and/or if such effects could occur under conditions comparable to human exposure.

These and other findings are summarized in the following discussion for four of the metals - arsenic, cadmium, lead, and mercury. While material on other metals appears throughout this volume, these four metals were selected because we felt enough data were available to warrant general conclusions and specific recommendations. Further details and additional recommendations for these and other metals are included in the Review Chapters.

Arsenic

Human beings may be exposed to arsenic occupationally or through food, drinking water and ambient air. Food contains both inorganic and organic forms of arsenic. There is evidence in four animal species that arsenic is essential for normal growth and development; arsenic deficiency can cause fetal deaths. Considerable concentrations of arsenic in the form of an arseno-lipid (mol wt ~ 400) occurs naturally in seafood from marine waters. Although no toxic effects of this form of arsenic have been reported, and this substance is excreted rapidly like other organic forms of arsenic, no extensive investigations have been carried out with modern techniques.

The main forms of inorganic arsenic are the tri- and pentavalent forms. With the exception of arsine gas (AsH_3) which is a potent hemolytic agent, it has been difficult in the past to make clear distinctions between exposure to and toxic manifestations of the tri- and pentavalent forms due to the environment and in vivo interconversions that take place. A distinction between the mentioned inorganic compounds and methylated arsenic compounds, e.g., cacodylic acid (dimethylarsinic acid) is also sometimes made difficult because inorganic arsenic compounds are methylated in vivo.

In mature animals both the tri- and pentavalent forms of inorganic arsenic and organic arsenicals are well absorbed after dietary intake or after inhalation. Whole body retention is about three times longer after trivalent than after pentavalent arsenic. The trivalent form is accumulated in the liver and excreted in bile more so than the pentavalent form. Both forms of arsenic accumulate in skin, hair and in the squamous epithelia of the oral cavity, esophagus and esophageal cavity of the stomach consistent with the well known affinity of arsenic for keratin. Finally, after exposure to either oxidation state, arsenic accumulates slowly but selectively in the thyroid gland, the epididymis and the ocular lens. Furthermore, penta- but not trivalent arsenic accumulates rapidly in calcified areas of the skeleton probably due to similarities between arsenate and phosphate anions. Concentrations of arsenic in the ovaries and uterus in autopsy studies were unremarkable.

The fetal uptake of either oxidation state is similar except that the pentavalent form accumulates in the skeleton in late gestation. Both forms freely pass into the fetus throughout gestation. In monkeys, trivalent arsenic attained high fetal levels and distribution was similar to that observed in the mother. Little arsenic crossed the blood-brain barrier of the fetus.

Dimethyl arsenic differs in tissue distribution from inorganic arsenic in mature animals. No specific uptake is seen in skin, squamous epithelia or skeleton. Dimethyl arsenic, in experimental animals, is transferred to the fetus and accumulates in the fetal ocular lens.

Surprisingly few observations are available on the effect of arsenic compounds on the female reproductive system or on developing mammals. Treatment of pregnant experimental animals with high doses of inorganic arsenic produces fetal reabsorptions as well as genitourinary defects among surviving offspring.

Adverse effects have been observed in young children in an episode of arsenic poisoning in Japan. Several thousand infants became ill and over 100 died. Evidence up to now suggests that arsenic trioxide in amounts sufficient to produce clinical effects in infancy may cause subsequent appearance of permanent neurobehavioral deficits.

In view of the paucity of data nothing can be said concerning the likelihood of reproductive and developmental effects being critical effects. Because of the widespread occurrence of arsenic and its compounds and the potential danger it represents, it is important to encourage experimental research as well as epidemiological studies on human populations exposed to arsenic under natural conditions in drinking water or as a result of industrial or agricultural exposure.

Recommendations

1. In view of the suggestion of an increase in spontaneous abortions in studies of female smelter employees exposed to arsenic and other metals, it is recommended that population groups with arsenic exposure, for example, through drinking water, should be monitored for effects on reproductive endpoints.

2. Follow-up studies should continue on those populations of adults who have been exposed to arsenite compounds in milk during infancy. Special attention should be given to reproductive performance.

3. Studies on arsenic toxicity are difficult to evaluate due to significant species differences in metabolism. Accordingly, a search for appropriate animal models should be conducted and the mechanisms underlying these differences elucidated.

4. The toxicity of the organic forms of arsenic in shellfish and other seafood needs to be carefully evaluated with modern toxicologic techniques.

Cadmium

Previous meetings of the Scientific Committee on the Toxicology of Metals discussed the uptake of cadmium from air (10-50 percent) and food (3-20 percent) in adult animals and humans. Cadmium is taken up in reproductive tissues such as the gonads and uterus. Gastrointestinal uptake of cadmium in the newborn (up to 55 percent) is higher than in the adult and remains high in the suckling period. The concentration of cadmium in the mother's milk, however, is low and exposure of the infant by this route probably is of limited significance. While maternal and cord blood levels of cadmium may be nearly equal, there is considerable accumulation of cadmium in the placenta itself.

Parenteral administration of a single dose of cadmium salts produces, in various animal species, acute hemorrhagic necrosis in the testes, hemorrhages and necrosis in non-ovulating ovaries and destruction of placentae during the last third of pregnancy with specific lethal changes in the mother. Testicular necrosis is not produced when cadmium is administered bound to metallothionein; this should explain why these testicular changes are not observed with chronic exposure. Metallothionein binding has also been found to protect against the acute effects of cadmium in the placenta. Zinc or selenium can also protect against the reproductive toxic effects of cadmium. Acute cadmium dosing also blocks embryonic implantation in sexually mature rats. Such effects, although documented in a large number of animal species, have not been reported in humans.

Chronic treatment with cadmium causes thickening of the walls of the small blood vessels in the uterus and the ovaries of rats, and may also lead to ovarian atrophy. Cadmium has not been identified as a human teratogen either in clinical case reports or in epidemiological studies. In one report, occupationally exposed women had offspring with lower birth weights than in controls.

Damage to reproductive tissue is considered the critical effect after acute parenteral doses. Although there are some indications that effects of cadmium on placental blood vessels might take place at low level cadmium exposure, present evidence is insufficient to consider this effect the critical effect of cadmium exposure. These and other effects of cadmium on reproductive tissues observed in animals have not been seen in humans.

Recommendations

Both experimental and epidemiological studies should be continued into the possible effects of chronic low doses of cadmium on placental structure and function, e.g., effects on placental vasculature.

Lead

The exposure to lead for the general population differs in different countries. In some non-industrialized areas of the world, blood values are as low as 5 μg/100 ml. In industrialized areas median values of 10-20 μg/100 ml are often seen and 90 percentile values of between 30-40 μg/100 ml may be found. The reasons for such high values are not known in detail, but with all probability the use of high concentrations of lead in gasoline is a major contributor. Other sources of lead for the general population are food (particularly canned food) and wine. In addition, there may also be occupational exposure, which may be considerably higher than that from general environmental sources.

Organic and inorganic forms of lead are absorbed after inhalation or after oral exposure in adult animals or humans and may be found in reproductive tissues such as the gonads and uterus. Organic lead compounds are also absorbed to a significant extent through the skin. The maternal/fetal blood concentration ratio has been measured in humans at term and is near unity, which demonstrates that the placenta constitutes a very poor barrier to lead. It is interesting that an epidemiological survey in the United States found that cord blood concentrations of lead have decreased in recent years. At earlier gestational periods, the transfer may be lower as indicated in animal experiments. The distribution in fetal tissues resembles qualitatively the pattern in adults. Concentration in mother's milk may lead to continued exposure of the offspring. The percentage of dietary lead absorbed in the newborn is considerably greater than in the adult as demonstrated by observations in both humans and experimental animals. This may be related partly to the immature state of the intestinal mucosa and partly to differences in the dietary content of nutrients and trace metals.

Historically, stillbirths and spontaneous abortions have been reported in heavily exposed women. More recent epidemiological evidence also suggests that women are susceptible to adverse reproductive effects including decreased fertility and increased risk for spontaneous abortion from lead exposure. In female experimental animals, lead alters pubertal progression and multiple reproductive endpoints along the hypothalamic-pituitary-ovarian-uterine axis in sexually mature female experimental animals.

Lead may also affect the male reproductive system. Effects on the prostate have been reported in experimental animals although neither the mechanism for this effect nor its significance to the human situation has been established. Decreased litter size, reduced survival rate and diminished growth of offsrping have been demonstrated after male experimental animals were exposed to lead. Testosterone levels have not been altered in persons with blood lead concentrations of 23-35 µg/100 ml, although infertility related to oligospermia, teratospermia and asternospermia has been reported. In another study, no similar effects could be documented in workers with blood lead concentrations of 40-62 µg/100 ml.

Congenital malformations (caudal vertebral column and tail defects) can be induced in animals injected with lead compounds. Decreased birth weights have been observed in infants whose mothers were exposed to high concentrations of lead. In monkeys exposed to lead from birth with average blood values of 55 µg/100 ml, which fell to average steady state blood levels of 33 µg/100 ml, an impairment of selected behavioral parameters has been observed. Some investigators have reported data which might indicate effects at lower levels. In humans, postnatal exposure to lead through lead-containing drinking water, food and dust may give rise to high blood lead concentrations in young children which have been associated with neurological and neurobehavioral effects (blood lead concentrations above 30-40 µg/100 ml).

Although there is evidence implicating lead in a number of effects on reproductive function both in the male and the female, it is not possible at present to state whether these effects should be regarded as the critical effect of lead exposure. Experimental studies in animals suggest that they are not. At previous meetings organized by the Scientific Committee, effects on heme intermediates such as increased levels of free erythrocytic protoporphyrin, including zinc protoporphyrin, and/or increased aminolevulinic acid excretion in urine were considered to be the most sensitive adverse effects (critical effects) of lead exposure. It is not possible to establish with certainty whether reproductive damage in mature adults or effects on the developing CNS or neurobehavioral effects in children can occur at blood lead levels lower than those causing adverse effects on heme-synthesis. The results of ongoing prospective studies concerning behavioral effects in childhood lead poisoning are likely to be of great value in making a more precise evaluation of these effects.

Recommendations

1. Ongoing studies relating behavioral effects (intelligence and learning ability) in children to lead exposure should continue. However, these studies may require re-examination to see if different biological endpoints and new methods for measuring cumulative lead exposure will be required in order to define dose-response relationships.

2. In countries where exposure to lead is exceptionally high or in the event that occupational exposure to lead occurs:

    a)   females should be monitored for reproductive performance, and

    b)   prenatally exposed children should be carefully evaluated for adverse effects such as impaired functional development.

Pre-conception paternal exposure and continued postnatal exposure of the child to lead should also be taken into account as possible confounding variables.

3. In the event that exposure to lead occurs, prospective studies both in males and females are needed in order to define at

what lead levels effects on reproductive endpoints can occur. Determination of blood lead levels and other appropriate methodologies for monitoring exposure should be considered. Such information would provide a useful basis to evaluate whether these effects should be regarded as the most sensitive or critical effects of lead.

    4. Information concerning current lead concentrations in fetal and perinatal brains for populations with different lead exposures is lacking; such information should be obtained.

    5. The development of better techniques to assess the body burden of lead is needed, with special attention to the new non-invasive techniques.

    6. Our understanding of the mechanisms underlying pre- and postnatal effects of lead on CNS development is inadequate. More basic research is needed particularly on the mechanisms of damage at low doses.

Mercury

    No information is available on the accumulation and retention of mercury by reproductive tissues in man. Studies in mice indicate that methylmercury is taken up by the testes four times faster than inorganic mercury (Hg^{++}). Uptake of methylmercury is greater in the testes than in seminal vesicles or epididymides. Mercury was accumulated to the same extent in the testes after exposure to mercury vapor (Hg°) as after an equivalent dose of inorganic mercury. However, retention was longer in the testes than in the whole body for both Hg° and Hg^{++}. Elimination from the testes is much more rapid for methylmercury (half-time 34 days) than for inorganic mercury (half-time 56 days).

    Various forms of mercury accumulate in ovarian tissue. Inorganic mercury is concentrated in the granulosa cells of the graefian follicles whereas metallic mercury (Hg°) accumulates in the corpora lutea in mice. Experimental data on methylmercury accumulation in ovarian tissue does not seem to have been published.

    Information on mercury metabolism in extragonadal tissue is sparse. Methylmercury is known to accumulate in the CNS and areas related to control of reproductive function, such as the hypothalamus.

    The transport of mercury across the placenta was discussed at a previous Scientific Committee meeting. Subsequent data reported in this book have confirmed the main features. Methylmercury and inhaled mercury vapor readily cross the placenta whereas inorganic mercury is transported less rapidly but accumulated more avidly. Selenium, at least in animal studies, has been shown to further decrease placental transport and augment accumulation of inorganic mercury. Clinical and epidemiological studies have shown that methylmercury in umbilical cord blood was present at concentrations in a similar range (but about 30 percent higher) as maternal blood. The placenta has not been widely used as an indicator tissue but may be useful for inorganic mercury in view of its ability to accumulate this form of mercury.

Methylmercury, according to experimental studies, reaches somewhat higher concentrations in the fetus than those found in maternal tissues. Thus, maternal blood or hair concentrations are useful indicators of minimal fetal levels. As in the mature animal, methylmercury distributes to all tissues in the fetus including the developing central nervous system. Concentrations in amniotic fluid are very low. Elemental mercury accumulation in the fetus is increased about four-fold by prior administration of high doses of ethanol to the mother. Furthermore, ethanol leads to a selective increase in fetal liver levels and to a more uniform distribution within this tissue.

Secretion of mercury in milk was also discussed at the Scientific Committee meeting in Argentina. Subsequent data have not changed the main conclusions: human milk contains mercury at a level of about 5 percent of maternal blood levels after either short-term (months) or long-term (years). Epidemiological studies of the Iraqi outbreak of methylmercury poisoning have revealed that exposure of infants solely via suckling may give rise to hazardous levels in the infant if the mother has been heavily exposed. Levels in milk roughly paralleled levels in maternal blood and hair. No human data are available on levels in milk after exposure to mercuric or elemental mercury, although animal data indicate inorganic mercury is accumulated in the mammary gland.

Information on the metabolism of mercury in the suckling infant or lactating mother is sparse. The lactating mother generally has a significantly shorter half-time (about 40 days) in blood than the non-lactating female (half-time about 50 days). Experimental studies indicate that the suckling infant excretes mercury at a very low rate after exposure to methyl or inorganic mercury. Methylmercury is almost completely absorbed from the gut of suckling animals and inorganic mercury is more efficiently reabsorbed (about 50 percent) as compared to adult humans (about 8 percent).

Adverse effects of mercury compounds on human reproductive function have not been unequivocally established. Work on experimental animals has indicated a remarkable sensitivity of spermatogenesis to methylmercury. This form of mercury produced

significant antifertility effects at doses at least one order of
magnitude lower than those causing damage to the nervous system in
mice. These findings indicate the need to include fertility
assessment in future epidemiological studies on methylmercury
exposed human populations.

No experimental findings on effects on female fertility have
been reported.

Adverse effects on the developing CNS in humans appear to be
the critical effect based on recent dose-response studies in the
Iraqi outbreak. Methylmercury in maternal hair during pregnancy
appears to be a valid prediction of adverse developmental and
neurological deficits in the offspring. Mild neurological and
developmental delays have been reported in infants exposed to
methylmercury in their mothers' milk. However, these effects appear
at higher blood levels than those which produce effects after
prenatal exposure.

Recommendations

1. There should be prospective studies of children with
defined prenatal and early postnatal exposure to methylmercury in
fish-eating populations. These studies should include correlations
of effects with maternal exposure by use of indicator media such as
maternal hair and blood and offspring blood. Effects measured
should include reproductive loss, as well as developmental,
neuropsychological and encephalographic measurements in the
offspring.

A thorough clinical (including neurologic) assessment of the
mother is also desirable, both to compare relative sensitivity of
the fetus versus that of the mother as well as to guard against
overlooking secondary effects on the fetus due to illness in the
mother.

2. Parallel studies in appropriate animal models should be
undertaken to identify the mechanisms of prenatal damage
particularly in the nervous system.

3. Studies of specific mercury species concentrations in human
reproductive tissues and products of conception should be undertaken
in populations with defined exposure. These may include both
surgical and autopsy material.

4. Considering the large number of female dental technicians
exposed to mercury vapor, the effects of such exposure should be
evaluated urgently by epidemiological and experimental studies.

REVIEW ARTICLES

EFFECTS OF METALS ON MALE REPRODUCTION

Maths Berlin, Insu P. Lee and Lonnie D. Russell

Working Group: Maths Berlin, Insu P. Lee, Lonnie D. Russell

Review Article Contents:

EFFECTS OF METALS ON MALE REPRODUCTION

Maths Berlin,[1] Insu P. Lee,[2] and Lonnie D. Russell[3]

[1]Institute of Environmental Health, University of Lund,
Lund, Sweden
[2]National Institute of Environmental Health Sciences
Research Triangle Park, North Carolina
[3]Southern Illinois University School of Medicine
Carbondale, Illinois

INTRODUCTION

This chapter aims to summarize what is known to members of the conference on the effect of environmental metal exposure on human male reproductive function. The increasing tendency to alter the natural environment and to replace it with a man-made artificial environment will give rise to changes in environmental exposure to trace elements such as essential or non-essential metals. It has been our experience that such changes can affect health adversely due to toxic effects or to the lack of essential micronutrients. Such effects may also involve the male reproductive system. In reviewing what is known to conference members about such effects, we will discuss the theoretical basis for expected toxic effects.

An attempt will be made to point out those areas where, although effects of metal exposure may be expected, our knowledge is lacking or insufficient. In cases of known effects, dose-response relationships and the health significance of observed effects will be discussed. When discussing specific effects, reference will, if possible, be given to suitable or recommended methods to assess such effects.

Interaction of metals with the male reproductive function may cause effects of varying health significance. Metals, through interference with potency or ejaculatory ability, may affect the ability of the individual to enjoy a normal sex life. They may cause sterility without affecting virility and finally, they may provoke changes in the progeny e.g., through mutations. This latter possibility is potentially the most serious health hazard as it affects future generations. Male reproductive organs are under complex neuroendocrine and hormonal control and any of these processes may be affected by metals or metal compounds.

The precise regulatory control of male reproductive organ functions remains unknown, but some of the target sites which have been identified will be discussed below. Direct effects on the reproductive organs will be discussed separately from indirect effects brought about through interference with the regulatory system of the male reproductive organs.

Indirect Effects of Metals on Male Reproductive Organs

The coordination of male reproductive function by extra-gonadal hormones is accomplished mainly by endocrine secretions from the hypothalamus and the pituitary gland. Hypophysial gonadotropins, FSH and LH are essential to maintain spermatogenesis. Prolactin may also play an important role, as does the pineal antigonadotropin factor which appears to have a special effect on spermatogenesis during the prepubertal period of sexual development. The release of gonadotropins is regulated by the hypothalamic-gonadotropin-releasing hormone (GnRH). It is conceivable that metals and metal compounds might interfere with the synthesis, release, transport, metabolism and binding of these hormones at their respective receptors. However, little information is available on such effects. For example, from autoradiographic studies in animals (Berlin and Ullberg, 1963a), cadmium is known to accumulate in the pituitary gland and in the adrenals. At the present time, there is no information available on either the significance of this observation or on the studies of pituitary function and plasma levels of FSH, LH or prolactin in cadmium poisoning. Plasma FSH and LH levels after subchronic exposure to cadmium showed no significant changes although plasma LH levels appeared to increase but were not statistically significant (Dixon et al., 1976). Methylmercury and inorganic mercury are known to accumulate in the central nervous system and in the hypothalamic area. No information is available on the effects of mercury intoxication on the hypothalamic-pituitary testicular axis. In the case of lead exposure, a number of reports are available concerning effects on pituitary function.

Lancranjan et al. (1975) studied gonadotropin levels in the urine of 20 battery-factory workers exposed to toxic levels of lead and they found no difference in gonadotropin levels between exposed and non-exposed workers. Molinini et al. (1981) obtained similar results in a study on moderately exposed battery-factory workers. Braunstein (1978), however, found a decrease in serum LH levels after stimulation with gonadotropin-releasing hormones when compared to non-intoxicated lead-exposed workers, suggesting an effect of lead intoxication on pituitary function.

Several metals such as lead, mercury and manganese have been shown to interfere with nervous function (Friberg et al., 1979) at the level of release and action of transmitter (Bondy et al., 1979). The extent to which exposure to such metals interferes with the nervous regulation of male reproductive organs remains unknown. In the case of lead, lead colic has been suggested to be due to interference with autonomous nerve control of peristaltic movement in the gastrointestinal tract. Similar effects may be anticipated in the case of nervous control of erection and ejaculation. A clinical report (Lancranjan et al., 1975) indicates interference with ejaculation and erection in lead-poisoned workers. However, no experimental evidence of or details on the mechanisms behind such effects has been reported previously.

Direct Effects on Male Reproductive Organs

When discussing the effects of metals on male reproductive organs, a number of specific targets must be considered. Metals can interfere with the supply of blood nutrients to the gonads by interfering, for example, with the complicated blood-testis barrier similar to that of blood-brain barrier. Sertoli cells are mainly responsible for nursing various stages of spermiogenic cells, sperm release, androgen metabolism, and secretion of retetestis fluid, a specific milieu in the lumen of the seminiferous tubules (Waites and Glandwell, 1982).

Metals could interfere directly with the endocrine function of Leydig cells and with the different steps of spermatogenesis. When considering interference with the spermatogenesis, one must take into account differences between the response of target cells such as spermatogonia or spermatocytes and of the spermatids or the spermatozoa. Metals could inhibit spermatogonial cell divisions or meiosis of spermatocytes. They may interfere with either the maturation of spermatozoa, by changing the function of the epididymis, or with the functions of accessory glands. Finally, metals may affect spermatozoa directly in the semen, if excreted by the accessory glands. All these effects may result in reduced fertility, or more importantly, with mutated spermatozoa associated with pregnancy wastage, congenital malformation and/or heritable genetic disease.

Effects of Metals on Blood-testis Barrier, Leydig Cells and Testicular Blood Vessels

A number of metals have in animal experiments been observed histochemically or autoradiographically to accumulate in the interstitial tissue of the testis. This is the case of lead (Timm and Schultz, 1966), cadmium (Berlin and Ullberg, 1963a), mercury,

inorganic mercury and methylmercury (Berlin and Ullberg, 1963b),
polonium (Soremark and Hunt, 1966), plutonium (Ullberg et al.,
1962), selenium (Jacobsson and Hansson, 1965), cesium (Nelson et
al., 1961), vanadium (Scharma et al., 1980), ruthenium (Nelson et
al., 1962), and americium (Hammarstrom and Nilsson, 1970).
Information concerning the functional consequences of this
observation is limited, however. In the case of cadmium, a single
toxic dose causes, in many laboratory species, damage to the
vascular bed of the testis, with deficiency of Leydig cell
testosterone production, necrosis of Sertoli cells and inhibition of
spermatogenesis. However, if metallothionein is induced with small
chronic doses of cadmium, the testis is protected from damage
(Nordberg, 1972). Among experimental animals, there are large
species differences in testis sensitivity to cadmium. Long-term
cadmium exposure in the mouse has resulted in decreased testosterone
activity (Nordberg, 1975). In man, cadmium-induced testicular
dysfunction has not yet been reported.

    Lead has been demonstrated in rats to accumulate in the
endothelial cells of the vascular capillaries and arterioles of the
testis (Timm and Schultz, 1966), but the functional significance of
this remains obscure. In poisoned animals, lead has been identified
inside the seminiferous tubules (Tarabayeva, 1959). Whether this is
a result of the breakdown of the blood-testis barrier constituted by
the Sertoli cells, or whether lead normally passes this barrier is
presently unknown. Burton and Meikle (1980) observed decreased
testosterone in serum of methylmercury-treated rats, indicating an
impaired Leydig cell function. For other metals, information
concerning the consequences of accumulation in testes and
interstitial tissue, their effects on vascular bed, Sertoli cells or
Leydig cells is not available.

Effects of Metals on Spermatogonia and Primary Spermatocytes

    Any direct effect of metals on spermatogonia and primary
spermatocytes requires the metal to be transported into these
cells. Detailed information on the extent to which metals can
penetrate spermatogonia and spermatocytes is very limited. In
animals, divalent mercury has been observed to accumulate in
spermatogonia and spermatocytes (Lee and Dixon, 1975) and to inhibit
DNA, RNA and protein synthesis, demonstrated by reduced uptake of
thymidine, uridine, and L-leucine in mouse spermatogenic cells.
Methylmercury penetrates the seminiferous tubules of the mouse more
easily than does inorganic mercury and causes mercury concentrations
in spermatogonial cells approximately three times higher than those
of inorganic mercury at corresponding dose levels (Lee and Dixon,
1975). The inhibiting effect of methylmercury on DNA, RNA, and
protein synthesis in spermatogonial cells of mice is also more
pronounced, as seen by inhibition of thymidine uptake.

Although lead has been demonstrated autoradiographically in the seminiferous tubules in animal experiments (Tarabayeva, 1959) and spermatogenic cell arrest has been observed in rats after oral dosing of lead (Hilderbrand et al., 1973), it remains uncertain that lead affects the spermatogonia and primary spermatocytes directly. In mice, selenium has been observed to be distributed in testicular tubuli and epithelial cells (Jacobsson and Hansson, 1965). The toxicological significance of this observation has not been studied.

Intravenous administration of manganese chloride to rabbits has been shown to arrest spermatogenesis and inhibit succinic dehydrogenase activity in seminiferous tubule cells but which cells of the spermatogenesis that are actually affected is not known (Imam and Chandra, 1975). Nelson et al. (1961) reported that cesium administered intravenously to the mouse is distributed in all testicular cells.

Some of the plutonium accumulated in mouse testes after intravenous injection is located within the seminiferous tubules. The toxic consequences of this is unknown, although the radiological hazard involved is obvious (Beechey et al., 1975; Ashe and Parker, 1978).

Effects of Metals on Secondary Spermatocytes, Spermatids, Spermatozoa, and Accessory Glands

Information concerning direct effect of metals on spermatids is extremely limited. Lee and Dixon (1975) observed in mouse testes (by serial mating) an effect of methylmercury on early spermatids. Specific information concerning other metals is not avavilable. It might be predicted that toxic effects of metals are directed either to the excurrent duct system of the male or to the accessory sex glands.

The caput and corpus epididymis are the sites of biochemical and morphological maturation of sperm (Bedford, 1975) and are occasionally the target of specific agents (a-chlorohydrin, Gomes, 1977). Also, metals may affect this part of the epididymis. Another potential site for the action of toxic metals is the cauda epididymis, where sperm are stored.

Studies on lead-exposed workers suggest an effect of lead on the maturation process (Wildt et al., this volume). It is unclear whether this is an effect of the epididymis or a direct effect on the spermatids or spermatozoa. Arsenic accumulates in the epididymis of rodents (Lindgren et al., 1982). The toxicological significance of this observation is, however, unknown. The prostate and seminal vesicles secrete prostatic and seminal fluid to form major portions of semen. These accessory organs may be affected by

metals (e.g., cadmium accumulation in the prostate, Berlin and
Ullberg, 1963a). The functional significance of this is unknown at
the present time. In animals, lead has been observed to cause
hyperplasia of the prostate (Fahim and Khare, 1980). Whether this
has a direct effect on the prostate or an indirect effect via the
endocrine system is unknown. It cannot be excluded that lead,
cadmium and other metals may be secreted by the prostate or seminal
vesicles, and that metals in the semen may affect the functionality
of spermatozoa. In vitro studies have shown that sperm are
sensitive to a number of metals such as lead, copper, mercury,
manganese, iron (Fe^{2+}) and cadmium (White, 1955).

Effects of Metals on Semen, Fertility and Progeny

The endpoints of metal interference with male reproductive
function are: abnormal semen, infertility, spontaneous abortion --
early fetal loss and late fetal loss, stillbirth, prematurity, birth
defects, low birth-weight for gestational age, postmaturity,
increased childhood morbidity, and childhood malignancies. These
effects and endpoints can be studied in experimental animals with
well established tests (Galbraith et al., 1982) or by
epidemiological studies assessing the effects on exposed male
populations. As mentioned above, changes in semen quality have been
observed in animal experiments after exposure to lead, inorganic
mercury, methylmercury and manganese. The ejaculate is amenable to
analysis in humans. A thorough semen analysis would be the most
practical means to assess toxic effects of metals on the testis and
in the male reproductive tract. To evaluate semen quality, the
semen sample can be analyzed for volume, metal content, key
substances content, sperm motility, sperm quantity (count), sperm
quality (general morphology) and sperm function (fertilization).
The reader is referred to a comprehensive review on this subject by
Mann and Lutwak-Mann, 1981. The semen sample can be used to further
test sperm function by heterologous human sperm-hamster egg
penetration test (Hall, 1981; Yanagimachi et al., 1976). Moreover,
the effects of metals can be assessed by introducing them into such
in vitro fertilization test systems.

Reports on semen analyses from human populations exposed to
metals are scarce. Information concerning metal concentrations in
semen is also lacking. In the case of lead exposure, a few reports
are available which indicate hypospermia and teratospermia under
conditions of clinically manifest poisoning (Lancranjan, 1975). The
occupational lead exposure data which is available suggests some
interference of lead with the maturation process of sperm and
accessory gland function (Wildt et al., this volume; Molinini et
al., 1981). Plechaty et al. (1977) reported that lead concentration
in semen from men who were not specifically exposed to lead was less
than that in whole blood but more than that in serum. Semen quality

or metal concentrations in semen after exposure to other metals is not known. Although human semen determinations are extremely important indicators of reproductive perturbations, certain considerations must be taken into account in the planning phase of studies on semen quality. First, one must consider the willingness of the individuals (workers) to donate semen. Cultural and sociological reasons, as well as lack of complete information and the question of what is to be done with the information obtained, hamper investigators' attempts to obtain semen samples. For similar reasons, union and management are often uncooperative in such attempts. These obstacles can be overcome only by supplying proper and adequate information to involved parties well in advance of undertaking such studies. Proper controls require age-matched semen samples and samples prior to exposure to metals.

In non-human studies, there appear to be no particular species assumed to be ideal models for the study of effects of metals on male reproduction. Rodent species may be acceptable for evaluation of the testis but accessory glands in these species are functionally not homologous with those of man.

Fertility tests and studies of progeny in non-human animals are a major endpoint in assessing the male reproductive function. The importance of fertility tests should not be underestimated since it represents the ultimate expression of the functionality of male reproductive organs. Other reports of important tests for the quality of sperm are teratological and dominant lethal assays. Dominant lethality studies of paternal effects of environmental metals are very few and inconclusive (Sutter, 1975).

Oral administration of lead to male animals has resulted in decreased fertility, decreased litter size, reduction in birth rate of progeny and reduction in survival rate and growth rate. This has been observed in rats (Stowe and Goyer, 1971), in rabbits (Cole and Bachhuber, 1914) and in guinea pigs (Weller, 1915). Lee and Dixon (1975) demonstrated reduced fertility in the mouse after administration of methylmercury and mercury chloride (Lee, this volume). Large doses of boron in drinking water to rats resulted in impaired fertility, associated with germinal aplasia and elevated FSH (Lee et al., 1978).

Increased abortion rate, stillbirth, reduced body weight and impaired development, as well as increased rates of malformations in humans, can be detected only by epidemiological methods. As most of these effects are rare events, it takes a large population for study and/or very pronounced effects to detect changes in the normal prevalence (Cohen, 1977). This is probably the reason that very few epidemiological studies are available regarding evidence of adverse effects on progeny, due to paternal exposure to metals. Those studies available refer to occupational exposure to high levels of

lead. Some of the reports have been summarized by Oliver (1911) and
by Weller (1915). According to these old clinical reports,
increased abortion and stillbirth rates, and decreased survival time
of children were observed in couples in which the man had been a
lead worker. These reports precipitated the animal experiments
cited above, confirming in several species the observations made in
man. The scientific validity of such clinical studies is always
questionable; however, one should not completely dismiss such
observations since some of the experimental data appear to support
such clinical observations. It seems, however, that the number of
persons exposed to high levels of lead in different parts of the
industrial world is still large enough to permit a useful
epidemiological study in order to elucidate the effects of paternal
lead exposure and consequent risk to their progeny. Considering our
present ability to assess exposure reliably by determination of
blood-lead concentrations, dose-response relations for such effects
should be possible to assess.

Conclusions, based on discussions of the working group.

1. Metals do accumulate in male reproductive organs such as the
    testicle and prostate.
2. Animal experiments indicate that certain metals e.g., such as
    lead and methylmercury can cause toxic injuries and can
    interfere with male reproductive function.
3. Data on the effects of metal exposure on male reproductive
    function in man are scarce and insufficient to allow
    conclusions as to the risk of adverse effects on male
    reproductivity. In the case of lead, data show that toxic
    exposure interferes with male reproductive function. Effects
    like hypospermia and impaired fertility have been reported.
4. Genetic effects on male germ cells cannot at present be
    excluded although no current epidemiological data indicate such
    effects.
5. Metals, with the possible exception of lead, have not been
    clearly identified in the scientific literature as
    environmental agents, such as dibromochloropropane,
    a-chlorohydrin, that are known to cause adverse effects on male
    reproductive function.
6. There are valid methods available for studying the specific
    effect of metal exposure on male reproductive function in
    exposed populations. However, these methods have so far not
    been used extensively.
7. Experimental designs for past studies have generally reflected
    parenteral route of administration, acute experiments and
    unusually high dosages which make it difficult to extrapolate
    to human metal exposure. A major problem with experimental
    reproductive studies and their interpretation is how to define
    dose.

Recommendations, based on discussions of the working group.

1. Identify areas for further study (e.g., molecular biology, biochemistry, endocrinology, and male reproductive physiology, etc.) and further develop improved and validated testing methods to assess male reproductive toxicity.
2. Identify the factors modifying toxic effects on male reproductive organs.
3. Comprehensive studies in experimental animals with well designed protocols are necessary to optimize extrapolation to human data. Appropriate experimental protocols include considerations directed toward determining:
    1. Appropriate fluid (blood) and tissue (including semen) levels of the metal under consideration.
    2. Use of chronic studies.
    3. Consideration of and testing for genetic factor.
4. Information concerning potential toxic-metal concentration in human male reproductive organs is needed.
5. Studies of the male reproductive function in human populations exposed to metals are needed and should be performed.
6. Special efforts should be made to develop procedures in order to facilitate the cooperation of workers and people subject to metal exposure to take part in studies and to provide semen samples. Procedures should also be worked out to enhance investigator and management cooperation. Comprehensive studies in humans should also be well designed and should include:
    1. Metal levels in semen and blood.
    2. Fertility.
    3. Teratology.
    4. Possible biopsy.
    5. Semen analysis.
    6. Statistical analysis.

It is stressed that studies must be carefully controlled regarding age, exposure time, sampling prior to exposure and other factors.

REFERENCES

Ashe, P. and Parker T., 1978, The ultrastructure of mouse testicular interstitial tissue containing plutonium-239 and its significance in explaining the observed distribution of plutonium in the testis, Int. J. Radiat. Biol. 74:523-536.
Bedford, J.M., 1975, Maturation, transport, and fate of spermatozoa in the epididymis, in: "Handbook of Physiology", Vol. V, D.W. Hamilton and R.O. Greep, eds., pp. 303-317, American Physiological Society, Washington, DC.
Beechey, C.D., Green, D., Humphreys, E.R. and Searle, A.G., 1975, Cytogenic effects of plutonium-239 in male mice, Nature 256:577-578.

Berlin, M. and Ullberg, S., 1963a, The fate of Cd^{109} in the mouse. An autoradiographic study after a single intravenous injection of $Cd^{109}Cl_2$, Arch. Environ. Health 7:686-693.

Berlin, M. and Ullberg, S., 1963b, Accumulation and retention of mercury in the mouse. I-III, Arch. Environ. Health 6:589-616.

Bondy, S.C., Anderson, C.L., Harrington, M.E. and Prasad, K.N., 1979, The effects of organic and inorganic lead and mercury on neurotransmitter high-affinity transport and release mechanisms, Environ. Res. 19:102-111.

Braunstein, G.D., Dahlgren, J. and Loriaux, D.L., 1978, Hypogonadism in chronically lead-poisoned men, Infertility 1:33-51.

Burton, G.V. and Meikle, A.W., 1980, Acute and chronic methylmercury poisoning impairs rat adrenal and testicular function, J. Tox. Environ. Health 6:597-606.

Cohen, J., 1977, "Statistical Power Analysis for Behavioral Sciences", Academic Press, New York.

Cole, L.J. and Bachhuber, L.J., 1914, The effect of lead on the germ cells of the male rabbit and fowl as indicated by their progeny, Proc. Soc. Exp. Biol. Med. 12:24-29.

Dixon, R.L. and Lee, I.P., 1976, Methods to assess reproductive effects of environmental chemicals: Studies of cadmium and boron administration orally, Environ. Health Persp. 13:59-67, 1976.

Fahim, M.S. and Khare, N.K., 1980, Effects of subtoxic levels of lead and cadmium on urogenital organs of male rats, Arch. Androl. 4:357-362.

Friberg, L., Nordberg, G.F. and Vouk, V.B., 1979, "Handbook on the Toxicology of Metals", Elsevier/North Holland Biomedical Press, Amsterdam, New York, Oxford.

Galbraith, W.M., Voytek, P. and Ryon, M.G., 1982, Assessment of Risks to Human Reproduction and to Development of the Human Conceptus from Exposure to Environmental Substances. Proc. of U.S. Environmental Protection Agency Sponsored Conferences: Oct 1-3, 1980, Atlanta, Georgia, and Dec. 7-10, 1980, St. Louis, Missouri. Oak Ridge National Laboratory, Oak Ridge, Tennessee.

Gomes, W.R., 1977, Pharmacological agents and male fertility, in: "The Testis", Vol. IV., A.D. Johnson and W.R. Gomes, eds., pp. 605-628, Academic Press, New York.

Hall, J.L., 1981, Relationship between semen quality and human sperm penetration of zona-free hamster ova, Fertil. Steril. 35(4):457-463.

Hammarstrom, L. and Nilsson, A, 1970, Radiopathology of americium 241. I. Distribution of americium in adult mice, Acta Radiol. 9:433-442.

Hilderbrand, D.C., Der R., Briffin, W.T. and Fahim, M., 1973, Effect of lead acetate on reproduction, Amer. J. Obstet. Gynecol. 115:1058-1061.

Imam, Z. and Chandra, S.V., 1975, Histochemical alterations in rabbit testis produced by manganese chloride, Toxicol. Appl. Pharmacol. 32:534-544.

Jacobsson, S.O. and Hansson, E., 1965, Distribution of selenium in mice studied by whole-body autoradiography after injection of Se^{75}-sodium selenite, Acta Vet. Scand. 6:287-298.

Lancranjan, I., Popescu, H.I., Gavanescu, O., Klepsch, I. and Serbanescu, M., 1975, Reproductive ability of workmen occupationally exposed to lead, Arch. Environ. Health 30:396-401.

Lee, I.P. and Dixon, R.L., 1975, Effects of mercury on spermatogenesis studied by velocity sedimentation cell separation and serial mating, J. Pharmacol. Exp. Ther. 193:171-181.

Lee, I.P., Sherins, R.J. and Dixon, R.L., 1978, Evidence for induction of germinal aplasia in male rats by environmental exposure to boron, Toxicol. Appl. Pharmacol. 45:577-590.

Lindgren, A., Vather, M. and Dencker, L., 1982, Autoradiographic studies on the distribution of arsenic in mice and hamsters, administered ^{74}As-arsenite and -arsenate, Acta Pharmacol. Toxicol. 51:253-365.

Mann, T. and Lutwak-Mann, C., 1981, "Male Reproductive Function and Semen. Themes and Trends in Physiology, Biochemistry and Investigative Andrology", Springer Verlag, Berlin, Heidelberg, New York.

Molinini, R., Assennato, G., Altamura, M., Gagliano Candela, R., Gagliardi, T. and Paci, C., 1981, Lead effects on male fertility in battery workers. Proceedings of the Tenth International Congress on Occupational Health, Cairo, Sept. 25-Oct. 1.

Nelson, A., Ullberg, S., Kristoffersson, H. and Ronnback, C., 1961, Distribution of radiocesium in mice, Acta Radiol. 55:374-384.

Nelson, A., Ullberg, S., Kristoffersson, H. and Ronnback, C., 1962, Distribution of radioruthenium in mice, Acta Radiol. 58:335-360.

Nordberg, G., 1972, Cadmium metabolism and toxicity - experimental studies on mice with special reference to the possible protective effects of metallothionein, Environ. Physiol. Biochem. 2:7-36.

Nordberg, G., 1975, Effects of longterm cadmium exposure on the seminal vesicles of mice, J. Reprod. Fert. 45:165-167.

Oliver, T., 1911, Lead poisoning and the race, Brit. Med. J. 1:1096-1098.

Plechaty, M.M., Noll, B. and Sunderman, Jr., F.W., 1977, Lead concentrations in semen of healthy men without occupational exposure to lead, Ann. Clin. Lab. Sci. 7:515-518.

Scharma, R.P., Oberg, S.G. and Parker, R.D.R., 1980, Vanadium retention in rat tissues following acute exposures to different dose levels, J. Toxicol. Environ. Health 6:45-54.

Stowe, H.D. and Goyer, R.A., 1971, The reproductive ability and progeny of F_1 lead-toxic rats, Fertil. Steril. 22:755-760.

Sutter, K.E., 1975, Studies on the dominant-lethal and fertility effects of the heavy metal compounds methylmercuric hydroxide, mercuric chloride, and cadmium chloride in male and female mice, Mutation Res. 30:365-374.

Soremark, R. and Hunt, V.R., 1966, Autoradiographic studies of the distribution of polonium-210 in mice after a single intravenous injection, Int. J. Radiat. Biol. 11:43-50.

Tarabayeva, G.I., 1959, Distribution of radioactive lead in the sexual organs of animals, 1959, Izv Adad Nauk Kaz SSR, ser Med I Fiziol 2:5.

Timm, F. and Schulz, G., 1966, Hoden und Schwermetalle, Histochemie 7:15-21.

Ullberg, S., Nelson, A., Kristoffersson, H. and Engstrom, A., 1962, Distribution of plutonium in mice, Acta Radiol. 459-471.

Waites, G.M.H. and Glandwell, R.T., 1982, Physiological significance of fluid secretion in the testis and blood-testis barrier, Physiol. Rev. 62:624-671.

Weller, C.V., 1915, The blastophthoric effect of chronic lead poisoning, J. Med. Res. 33:271-293.

White, I.G., 1955, The toxicity of heavy metals to mammalian spermatozoa, Austral. J. Exp. Biol. 33;359-366.

Wildt, K., Eliasson, R. and Berlin, M., 1983, Effects of occupational exposure to lead on sperm and semen, in: "Reproductive and Developmental Toxicity of Metals", T. Clarkson, G. Nordberg, and P. Sager, eds., Plenum Press, New York. This volume.

Yanagimachi, R.H., Yanagimachi, H. and Rogers, B.J., 1976, The use of zona-free animal ova as a test system for the assessment of the fertilizing capacity of human spermatozoa, Biol. Reprod. 15:471-476.

REPRODUCTIVE AND DEVELOPMENTAL TOXICITY OF METALS:

FEMALE REPRODUCTIVE SYSTEM

Donald R. Mattison

Working Group: Allen H. Gates, Alain Leonard, Mariann Wide,
Kari Hemminki, J.H.J. Copius Peereboom-Stegeman,
Donald R. Mattison, Helene Gardner

Review Article Contents:

REPRODUCTIVE AND DEVELOPMENTAL TOXICITY OF METALS:

FEMALE REPRODUCTIVE SYSTEM

Donald R. Mattison,[1] Allen H. Gates,[2] Alain Leonard,[3]
Mariann Wide,[4] Karri Hemminki[5] and
J.H.J. Copius Peereboom-Stegeman[6]

[1]Pregnancy Research Branch
National Institute of Child Health and Human Development
Bethesda, Maryland
[2]Division of Genetics and Toxicology
University of Rochester, Rochester, New York
[3]Department of Radiation Biology
C.E.N.-S.C.K.
[4]Institute of Zoology
University of Uppsala, Uppsala, Sweden
[5]Institute of Occupational Health
Helsinki, Finland
[6]Laboratory of Histology and Cell Biology
University of Amsterdam, Amsterdam, Holland

INTRODUCTION

In the female, reproduction is a continuous process beginning
with the development of the reproductive organs prenatally,
continuing through sexual maturation and extending to the time of
reproductive scenescence. In this chapter we will briefly outline
the prenatal development of the female reproductive system, and
sexual maturation, as well as the integrated function of the sexually
mature female reproductive system. This discussion will serve as a
prelude to our consideration of the site and mechanism of action of
metals which have been reported to alter the development, maturation
or function of the female reproductive system. Finally, we will
present a series of conclusions and recommendations derived from our
consideration of these data.

DEVELOPMENT AND FUNCTION OF THE FEMALE REPRODUCTIVE SYSTEM

Development of the Female Reproductive System

In mammalian species in general the development of the reproductive system begins and is completed prenatally. Maturation of the reproductive system and integrated function of the hypothalamus, pituitary, ovary, uterus, and accessory sexual tissue occurs postnatally.

Some aspects of gametogenesis, the development of spermatocytes or oocytes are similar in males and females. These similarities, however, tend to be confined to the early stages of gonadal development (Gondos, 1978). Late in gestation and postnatally the function and morphology of the testis and ovary are considerably different. These differences in structure and function are important because, although prenatal exposures may produce similar disruption in the development of the male or female reproductive systems, the manifestations in the weanling, maturing or sexually mature animal may be different. This difference may also have a profound influence on the toxicology of the sexually mature reproductive system. An example of the importance of this difference is derived from consideration of men or women with galactosemia, an inherited disorder of carbohydrate metabolism. Women with galactosemia experience premature ovarian failure (menopause), typically before the age of 30. Men with galactosemia, however, apppear to have normal reproductive function (Kaufman et al., 1981).

Ovarian development. Ovarian development requires the cooperation of embryonic and extraembryonic tissues (Baker, 1972). Primordial germ cells, the precursors of the oocytes, are formed in an extraembryonic region near the yolk sac (Langman, 1981; Balinsky, 1970). An estimated 1700 of these cells then migrate into the region of the urogenital ridge on the mesonephros, the site of the developing gonad. During migration and after arriving at the genital ridge, these cells proliferate, and then differentiate into oogonia, stem cells of the oocytes. Meiosis, integral with these processes, will be considered later.

After arrival of the primordial germ cells in the genital ridge, at about one month gestational age in humans, oogonia are formed and begin to proliferate. Oogonial proliferation is similar to spermatogonial proliferation in that a group of gonial cells develops together, connected by cytoplasmic bridges. During the development of the ovary, a cohort of oogonial cells connected by cytoplasmic bridges will cease proliferation, enter meiosis, lose their cytoplasmic interconnections, and begin to recruit ovarian stromal cells to form follicles. The follicle or follicle complex is the minimal functional unit of the ovary. A follicle complex consists of an oocyte, its surrounding granulosa cells, a basement membrane, and associated thecal cells arranged adjacent to the basement membrane (Harrison and Weir, 1977). The oocyte depends on the follicle complex for support, and in the absence of an oocyte a follicle complex degenerates, or functions in a very abnormal fashion.

After the onset of meiosis, oocytes unable to recruit granulosa cells will degenerate; additionally, some oocytes may be physically extruded from the surface of the ovary. Loss of oocytes during the formation of follicles accounts for the initial large decrease in oocyte number during the latter part of gestation. The human ovaries contain approximately 7 million oocytes at 4 months gestational age, approximately 1 million oocytes at birth, and less than 200,000 at puberty. From birth to approximately age 50 the number of oocytes decreases from 1 million to essentially zero. From this large number of oocytes only about 400 oocytes are ovulated; the remainder are lost to an ill-defined process called atresia (Weir and Rowlands, 1977). The average number of ova resulting in live births is only about one millionth of the maximum number of oocytes present during fetal life.

This rapid loss of oocytes suggests that pre- or postnatal alterations in oocyte number produced either by toxins or developmental abnormalities may have a profound effect on the reproductive lifespan. Actually, clinical and experimental evidence as well as theoretical considerations suggest that the duration of ovarian competence is only weakly dependent on oocyte number. Unfortunately, atresia, a process which is poorly understood appears to have the major impact on the duration of ovarian function. Diseases (e.g., chromosomal abnormalities, autoimmune disorders) or toxic exposures (e.g., alkylating agents, ionizing radiation, cigarette smoking) which increase the rate of atresia appear to have a profound impact on the functional lifespan of the ovary (Mattison, 1982; Baker, 1973; Sieber and Adamson, 1975; Ash, 1980).

At birth, the developed ovary contains a large number of small or resting follicles. The resting follicle consists of an oocyte, several surrounding granulosa cells, and a basement membrane. These oocytes, which represent more than 95 percent of the oocytes in the ovary, are generally found near the surface epithelium of the ovary. Throughout the life of the animal, a much smaller number of oocytes will be in the growing and preovulatory pools. The growing oocytes are those found in follicles which are larger than resting follicles, with many more granulosa cells. Once follicles leave the resting pool and enter the growing pool, they continue to grow and develop until they are ovulated, or they undergo atresia and degenerate. Those follicles and their enclosed oocytes selected to ovulate will continue to grow and ultimately develop a fluid filled cavity called the antrum, becoming preovulatory follicles.

Mullerian development. The Mullerian system includes the posterior portion of the vagina, cervix, body of the uterus and the fallopian tubes, structures which function with the ovaries for the expression of fertility. Because the development of the reproductive and excretory systems occurs anatomically and temporally in concert, it is necessary to consider them together (Villee and Dethier, 1976). The development of the ovary, discussed previously, occurs on the surface of the mesonephros, a rudimentary kidney which may function for a short period of time in the embryo. The developing reproductive system utilizes some of the tissues developed with the mesonephros to form the reproductive tract.

The embryonic mesonephric (Wolffian) duct is utilized in the male for the vas deferens; in the female this structure remains rudimentary. In the female the growth of the Mullerian duct is stimulated and the Wolffian duct regresses. The Mullerian duct forms the fallopian tubes bilaterally, then fuses in the midline to form the uterus (Balinsky, 1970). In rodents normally, and humans with developmental abnormalities, this fusion is not complete, resulting in two separate uterine structures. The solid mass of cells which comprises the ventral portion of the fused Mullerian tissue initially makes contact with, then penetrates the urogenital sinus which forms the ventral portion of the vagina (Langman, 1981). Ultimately, this solid Mullerian structure canalizes forming the posterior vagina, cervix, and uterus. Developmental disturbances acting on the Mullerian structures which alter the formation of the vagina, cervix, or uterus can have subtle effects on fertility. The best example is diethylstilbestrol (DES) which alters the formation of the uterus, cervix and vagina. These structural alterations in the uterus and cervix are thought to explain in part the decreased capability of DES offspring to carry pregnancies to term (Mattison, 1981).

Ovarian and Mullerian development, like most other developmental processes, requires a series of molecular and cellular events including: differentiation, differential tissue growth, cell-cell contact, chemotaxis and other cellular·processes for correct formation of the reproductive tract. These developmental events are susceptible to interruption by non-specific as well as specific toxins. For example, compounds which alter chemotaxis may influence population of the genital ridge by the primordial germ cells; another possible site of adverse effect by such an agent may be on the fusion of the Mullerian ducts or the interaction of the Mullerian duct with the urogenital sinus. In theory, metal ions or organometallic compounds may alter these developmental processes by general or specific toxicity. Generalized toxicity will probably also be reflected by an adverse effect on the size or weight of the fetus, while specific adverse effects may be subtle and difficult to recognize.

Sexual Maturation

Sexual maturation includes a series of endocrine-dependent and endocrine independent events (Reiter and Grumbach, 1982). The prepubertal individual has undeveloped secondary sexual characteristics (i.e., breasts, pubic and axillary hair, sex skin, etc.) as a result of low circulating levels of gonadal hormones (testosterone or estrogen). However, neither the accessory reproductive organs nor the gonads appear to control the onset of sexual maturation. In the primate, for example, treatment of a young monkey with pulses of the hypothalamic hormone, gonadotropin releasing hormone (GnRH), supports the development of complete ovarian function (Pohl and Knobil, 1982; Knobil, 1980). These data and other complementary experiments suggest that the onset of sexual maturation is controlled in the central nervous system through the hypothalamus (Reiter and Grumbach, 1982). Additional influences such as light/dark cycles, body weight, or exposure to compounds containing androgens or estrogens (i.e., phytoestrogens or xenobiotics with hormone agonist or antagonist properties) may alter the time course of maturation at the level of the accessory organs or the central nervous system (Bulger and Kupfer, 1983). Similarly, xenobiotic compounds which alter end organ response to the circulating gonadotropins or gonadal steroid hormones will appear to alter sexual maturation.

A series of experiments in rodents has demonstrated that the development and function of the hypothalamus may be altered by early treatment with xenobiotics which have estrogenic or androgenic properties. Although these animals demonstrated relatively normal reproductive function early in life, they quickly lost cyclic ovarian function, developed an anovulatory syndrome and became infertile (Gellert, 1978). Of interest is the observation that this syndrome appears to mimic a human anovulatory syndrome called polycystic ovary disease. Although the role of human hypothalamic function in control of the ovarian cycle is known to differ from that in rodents, a series of tantalizing epidemiological observations suggest that prenatal human exposure to estrogenic pesticides may increase the incidence of polycystic ovarian disease.

Organometallic compounds or metal ions which interact with gonadotropin or steroid hormone receptors may alter the time course of sexual maturation. Fortunately, the hypothalamus and pituitary of the primate appear more resistant to early exposure to androgens or estrogens than the rodent. Primate experiments in which prenatal androgen treatment has been given in doses sufficient to alter the development of the vagina, cervix and uterus and delay sexual maturation appear to have little effect on the functioning of the sexually mature hypothalamic-pituitary-ovarian (HPO) axis (Goy and Robinson, 1982). Similarly, it has been difficult to detect alterations in HPO function in sexually mature women exposed prenatally to DES (Mattison, 1981). These observations, however, do not preclude the possibility that primates may be more sensitive than rodents to an adverse reproductive effect of a xenobiotic compound acting at the level of the hypothalamus or pituitary (Smith, 1983). As a first assumption, however, it seems reasonable to assume that primates including humans are at least as sensitive to the adverse effects of metals or organometallic compounds on the developing HPO axis.

Integrated Function of the Mature Reproductive System

In the sexually mature individual fertility requires integration of the functions of the hypothalamus, pituitary, ovary, and uterus. This integration is controlled by protein or steroid hormones which link these diverse and separate tissues into an integrated organ system.

Hypothalamus and pituitary. A protein hormone, gonadotropin releasing hormone (GnRH), secreted by the hypothalamus into portal vessels which reach the pituitary appears to be responsible for stimulating the release of the two pituitary hormones, follicle stimulating hormone (FSH) and leutinizing hormone (LH) (Pohl and Knobil, 1982; Knobil, 1980). Although the exact mechanism is uncertain, present evidence suggests that pulsatile release of gonadotropin releasing hormone (GnRH) with a frequency of 60 to 90 minutes permits normal function of the HPO axis. This pulse frequency produces similar pulses of FSH, and to a lesser extent LH. These intermittent pulses of FSH circulate to the ovary where they support follicular growth.

As mentioned in the discussion of sexual maturation, the hypothalamus appears to be the tissue which matures during the peripubertal period. During this period the frequency and/or amplitude of GnRH pulses increases, this in turn increases the frequency and amplitude of FSH pulses in the circulation. The increasing levels of FSH supports follicular growth for longer periods of time and ultimately result in the support of follicular growth to the antral stage which allows ovulation. With sufficient levels of FSH, a cohort of follicles are stimulated to mature and produce estrogen. Estrogen provides first negative then positive feedback to the hypothalamus and pituitary, resulting in the midcycle surge of LH. The number of follicles chosen to ovulate depends on the species. Ovulation appears to depend on this surge of LH released in response to rising levels of estrogen secreted by the growing preovulatory follicles. This release of LH appears to be responsible for a cascade of events culminating in the breakdown of the follicle, release of the oocyte, as well as resumption of meiosis by the oocyte selected to ovulate.

At the present time, the role of the hypothalamus and pituitary appears to be permissive for ovarian function with the ovary assuming the dominant role in controlling interactions in part through hormonal production by growing follicles. The dependence on GnRH, FSH and LH, however, suggests that interruption of these permissive hormonal pathways by xenobiotics will disrupt reproductive function in the female (Smith, 1983).

Ovary. The role of the ovary throughout the life of the female is nurture of the oocytes and production of the steroid hormones necessary for integration of reproductive processes along the hypothalamic-pituitary-ovarian-uterine axis. As indicated previously, most of the follicles in the ovary are in the resting pool. At some point a cohort of these follicles will begin to grow, this initial period of growth to a pre-antral stage appears to be independent of gonadotropins (both FSH and LH). Growth into the preovulatory pool, that is the development of an antrum, and production of large amounts of circulating estrogen requires the support of FSH. If sufficient FSH is present, a cohort of follicles will grow and develop an antrum and secrete large amounts of estrogen which will ultimately produce a surge of LH. Following the LH surge the wall of the follicle(s) selected to ovulate will break down and release the oocyte, the basement membrane will degenerate and the previously avascular follicle will be penetrated by vessels (Harrison and Weir, 1977).

This change in the architecture of the follicle is also accompanied by changes in the morphology and secretory product of the granulosa cells. The initially round granulosa cells which produced increasing quantities of estrogen become polygonal in shape and begin to secrete progesterone. This increasing synthesis of progesterone is necessary to prepare the endometrium for implantation in the event of fertilization, and may also act on the fallopian tube to influence transport of the oocyte into the uterus. If pregnancy does not occur, the corpus luteum degenerates, the level of progesterone falls and the endometrium lining the uterine cavity is sloughed.

Xenobiotic compounds which alter the growth and development of the follicles (i.e., granulosa cell growth) will have a profound effect on reproductive function because of the central role of the ovary in reproduction. Xenobiotic compounds which destroy resting follicles may alter the reproductive lifespan of an individual; however, this ovarian toxicity may not be apparent until the ovary fails to function near the end of the reproductive lifespan (Mattison, 1980; Silbergeld and Mattison, 1983). Compounds which destroy growing or large preovulatory follicles may be recognized more readily because of their immediate effects on ovarian function, especially hormone production (Chapman, 1983). Xenobiotics which only affect growing or preovulatory follicles may be very difficult to identify and may require epidemiological investigations on early pregnancy loss, measure of inter-birth intervals, or duration of infertility (Wilcox, 1983).

Uterus. The uterus has two divergent functions in reproduction: to nurture and protect the conceptus during gestation, and then at the end of gestation when the fetus is capable of surviving in the extrauterine environment to expel this uterine passenger. The steroid hormones secreted by the ovary prepare the uterus to receive the conceptus if fertilization occurs (Noyes et al., 1950). Under the influence of estrogen during the follicular phase of the cycle the endometrium increases in thickness due to proliferation of endometrial stromal cells, endometrial vessels and endometrial glands.

Following ovulation, under the influence of progesterone secreted by the corpus luteum, the endometrial stroma becomes more cellular, the endometrial vascular supply increases and the endometrial cells discharge their secretory products into the lumen of the endometrial glands. These hormonally mediated changes appear necessary for support of the conceptus before, as well as after implantation. Diseases characterized by inadequate endometrial development in the luteal phase are associated with infertility, or abnormal placentation.

If fertilization does not occur, the corpus luteum will cease progesterone production. The blood supply to the endometrium will decrease as a result of increasing vascular spasm. As a result of decreasing vascular support the endometrium will become necrotic and slough. The basal layer of the endometrium remains attached to the myometrium and forms the stem cells for the next cycle of estrogen-stimulated endometrial proliferation.

If fertilization occurs, the conceptus secretes a hormonal signal (chorionic gonadotropin in primates) which "rescues" the corpus luteum, and stimulates further progesterone secretion. Failure to rescue the corpus luteum, or inadequate progesterone secretion prior to fertilization severely compromises the endometrium leading to failure of implantation, or early spontaneous abortion.

Oocyte Maturation, Fertilization and Implantation

Meiosis. General aspects: Oogenesis, the process leading to formation of mature ova, begins in fetal life and is completed in adulthood (Baker, 1973). An essential feature of oogenesis immediately prior to ovulation is accumulation of cytoplasmic components required for metabolism of the egg during the first few days after fertilization. Also during oogenesis there is an exchange of genetic information between the two "homologous" members in each of the 23 pairs of maternally and paternally derived chromosomes. Each oocyte undergoes two meiotic divisions characterized by the number of chromosomes being halved (to 23 singletons); at fertilization the spermatozoon contributes a matching set of 23 chromosomes, thus assuring that the normal "diploid" complement of 23 pairs is present in the newly formed embryo from the one-cell stage onward.

The first meiotic division begins in the three-month-old female fetus, when primary oocytes first form. After replication, each chromosome pairs, and exchanges segments with its homolog presumably at the microscopically visible sites referred to as chiasmata. Further chromosomal maturation is arrested in all oocytes of a newborn infant's ovary. A given oocyte does not resume maturation until years later. The mid-cycle surge of LH triggers resumption of meiosis in the oocyte destined for ovulation. The first meiotic division is completed just before ovulation, and the second division just after the fertilizing spermatozoon penetrates into the ovular cytoplasm.

Chromosomal Aspects: Chromosomal or cytogenetic errors during gametogenesis play a major role in human pregnancy loss. The frequency of pregnancy wastage is considerable; an estimated 31 percent of ova fail to reach the stage of uterine implantation, and cumulative losses total 69 percent by late gestation (Witschi, 1970; Wilcox, 1983). An abnormal number of chromosomes (aneuploidy) was observed in about 50 percent of clinically recognized spontaneous abortuses (Carr and Gedeon, 1977; Sankaranarayanan, 1982). Seventy-one percent of such anomalous conceptuses were characterized by fetal cells having one chromosome in excess (trisomy) or missing (monosomy) and 24 percent had multiple "polyploid" sets (triploid or tetraploid) of chromosomes (Boue and Boue, 1973). All polyploid and most trisomic fetuses fail to survive to early infancy. Monosomy is believed to occur as frequently among fertilized ova as its counterpart, trisomy, but since monosomy is rarely observed, it apparently is highly lethal during early embryogenesis.

Trisomy and monosomy are thought to be due primarily to the nondisjunction of chromosomes during meiosis. These two forms of aneuploidy are believed to originate more commonly during oogenesis than spermatogenesis (Langenbeck et al., 1976; Jacobs and Morton, 1977) and during the first, rather than the second, meiotic division (Niikawa et al., 1977). Triploidy may also be due largely to ovular factors: either halving of chromosome number fails to occur, or surface components (zona pellucida and/or vitelline membrane) fail to block the entry of an additional spermatozoon.

Nondisjunction has been induced experimentally in oocytes by the environmental agents such as heat, radiation and chemicals

(Grell, 1979). Maternal age is also highly correlated with
frequency of conceptuses which have trisomy resulting from
nondisjunction. Although there is some evidence for a prenatal,
oogenetic origin to the maternal age effect (Polani and Jagiello,
1976), environmental influences during the long period of meiotic
arrest in the primary oocyte may play an important synergistic role.

Gene and chromosome alterations both contribute significantly
to human illness. The actual estimates (UNSCEAR, 1979) of the
frequency of different kinds of genetic disorders per 100 liveborns
are: 1.0 autosomal dominants, 0.36 autosomal recessives and
disorders maintained by heterozygous advantage, 0.40 carriers of
chromosomal anomalies, and 9.00 congenital malformations giving a
total of 10.76.

Sperm - egg interaction. The ovaries of postnatal mammals
contain more than 90 percent primordial follicles surrounded by a
single layer of flattened or cuboidal granulosa-cells and 1-10
percent growing follicles some of which will become Graafian or
antral follicles. Irrespective of the stage of follicular growth,
the oocytes are at an arrested stage of meiosis until 12 to 48 hours
before ovulation (Baker, 1971,1972). Following the LH surge the
oocyte resumes meiosis at diakinesis and when ovulation occurs the
egg has reached metaphase of the second meiotic division which is
completed only after sperm entry.

Sperm penetration usually occurs when ovulated eggs have
reached the fallopian tube. Following penetration the female
pronucleus, formed by the resumption of the second meiotic division,
and the male pronucleus, originating from the nucleus of the sperm
head, lose their nuclear membrane. The two haploid sets of
chromosomes move together making a single group which resolves into
the metaphase plate of the first cleavage spindle. In the mouse,
the first division occurs 20-24 hours after fertilization (Table
1). The migration to the uterus occurs at the morula stage on the
4th day after fertilization.

Pre-implantation embryo and implantation. Soon after their
entry into a uterus prepared by estrogen, embryos differentiate into
blastocysts and lose their zona pellucida. This occurs in the mouse
on about day 5 of gestation (Swartz, 1983). Embryos undergo
important metabolic changes (activation) involving carbon dioxide
production, synthesis of RNA and proteins during this period (Dean,
1983). After differentiation into trophoblasts and embryoblasts
they become located at regular distances along the length of the
uterus in crypts of the uterine epithelium. Giant cells are formed
in the trophoblast which begin to invade luminal epithelium with
long thin processes. Carbon dioxide liberated by the embryo is
thought to provoke in the mucosa the formation of deciduous cells
with large nuclei and PAS-positive (glycogen rich) cytoplasm. The

Table 1   Temporal Sequences in Murine Pregnancy

Day 1 of pregnancy - day of observation of vaginal plug, 24 hours after fertilization - 1st cleavage.

Day 3 - embryos in <u>morula</u> stage.

Day 4 - embryos in <u>blastocyst</u> stage, zona pellucida intact.

Day 5 - lysis of zona pellucida (by proteolytic enzyme from uterine epithelium - one of the few proteins known to be synthesized as a response to estradiol; the others are receptors for estradiol and progesterone), and <u>attachment</u> to uterine epithelium, <u>closure</u> of uterine lumen. Early signs of <u>decidual reaction</u> (one is the leakage of serum into intercellular spaces of uterine stroma at the site of an attached blastocyst).

Late Day 5 - <u>invasion</u> of trophoblast cells into endometrium, maternal blood contact.

Day 6 - blastocyst completely embedded, surrounded by maternal <u>blood sinus</u>. Inner cell mass differentiated into <u>ectoderm</u> and <u>endoderm</u>.

Day 7 - primitive streak - mesoderm formation.

Day 8 - somite formation.

---

two phases of hormonal action during implantation: sensitization of the uterus by estrogens, and activation of the embryos which requires progesterone, slightly overlap. Table 1 summarizes the temporal sequences of early events in the murine pregnancy.

METALS AND FEMALE REPRODUCTION: EXPERIMENTAL ANIMALS

In this section we will review the reported effects of metals on female reproductive processes. As with the first section, this will also be a cryptic review. However, we have attempted to provide more extensive documentation for this discussion (see the table for each metal). In most instances we find it necessary to rely on experimental data gathered from subprimate species. Although certain physiological mechanisms may be different in rodents in comparison with primates, our working hypothesis is that the molecular mechanisms of reproduction and toxicity are similar

among different species. Therefore demonstration of an adverse
reproductive effect on one species is considered presumptive
evidence that the compound can also disrupt reproduction in another
species. Note that although the end points may not be the same in
different species, the molecular event affected presumably will be
similar.

Effects of Metals on the Development of the Reproductive System

Developing organisms are particularly susceptible to the action
of certain heavy metals. At all stages of development placental
function (gas and nutrient exchange), and maternal function
(physiological and immunological changes), play a role in adaptation
to pregnancy and support of the developing individual.

A few metal ions cross the placenta readily, but for the
majority the placenta modulates fetal exposure (see sections on
prenatal metabolism, this volume). Inorganic arsenic enters the
fetus easily. Cadmium does not cross the placenta of experimental
animals readily during the late stages of pregnancy, although it
apparently does so earlier in gestation. Cadmium has also been
reported to retard placental growth (Copius Peereboom-Stegeman et
al., 1983). Chromium passes the placenta in an organically bound
form. Lead crosses the placental barrier less readily than methyl
mercury but more than cadmium. Nickel reaches the embryos of mice
from day 5-8 of pregnancy but not before.

Several metals can provoke prenatal death (Table 2) which may
occur before or after implantation. The mechanism of early
pregnancy failure induced by metal exposure of experimental animals
has been studied in detail for lead (Wide, this volume; Leonard,
this volume).

In spite of the fact that only small amounts of xenobiotics
reach preimplantation embryos when treatment by feeding is started
at fertilization, isolation of embryos from females receiving a diet
containing increasing doses of lead showed that at 48 hours after
mating, the development of embryos is delayed as the dose of lead is
increased from 0.1 percent to 1 percent of the diet (Jacquet et al.,
1976; Streffer et al., 1978).

The transport of xenobiotics into the uterus and fallopian tube
may play a role in this early toxicity (McLachlan et al., 1976).
For example, adverse effects of lead on the mother are the decisive
factor in the action of lead on implantation in the rodent (Jacquet
et al., 1977a,b; Jacquet, 1978; Wide, this volume).

Studies on experimental animals have shown that administration
of certain metal salts (cadmium, mercury, selenium, arsenic) during

Table 2 Reported Effects of Metals on Development and Function of the Female Reproductive System in Experimental Animals and Humans

	Metal (Table Number*)								
	Lead (3)	Cadmium (4)	Mercury (5)	Chromium (6)	Nickel (7)	Selenium (8)	Lithium (9)	Copper (10)	Arsenic (11)
I. Effect in Experimental Animals									
A. Developing Reproductive System	+	+	+			+			+
B. Sexual Maturation	+	+	+						
C. Mature Reproductive System									
Hypothalamus	+	-	+		+				
Pituitary	+	-	+		+				
Ovary	+	+	μ						
Uterus	+	+	μ						
Other	+	μ(1)			+			+	+(2)
D. Oocyte Maturation, Fertilization and Implantation									
Female Germ Cells	+	+		+		+	+	+	
Preimplant embryo	+	+	+	+		+	+	+	
Implantation	+	+						-	
Resorption	+	+		+	+	+	+	+	
II. Epidemiologic Evidence in Humans									
Fertility	+	-(μ)				+(μ)			
Abortion	+	+							+

Legend: + = evidence suggestive of an effect; μ = effect or lack of effect uncertain; - = evidence suggestive of no effect; blank = no data available; *see the indicated table for reference citations used in constructing this overview; 1. mammary vessels; 2. vulvar carcinoma.

organogenesis can produce genitourinary defects (Nolen et al., 1972; Scharpf, 1972; Earl and Vish, 1980; Ferm et al., 1971). These effects on the developing reproductive system appear to represent generalized toxicity rather than a specific adverse effect on a given cell type or action by a particular mechanism. However, further experiments will be necessary to verify this assumption.

Effects of Metals on Sexual Maturation

As indicated previously, sexual maturation is thought to be mediated by the hypothalamus (Pohl and Knobil, 1982). In experimental animals, adverse effects on sexual maturation may be manifest by one of several parameters, including: age of vaginal opening, age of prepubertal gonadotropin elevation, age of first pregnancy.

As indicated in Table 2, three metals appear to alter sexual maturation. Lead appears to alter sexual maturation at the level of the hypothalamus or pituitary (Grant et al., 1976; Kimmel et al., 1980). Cadmium appears to have a different effect than lead in its effect on sexual maturation; the ovaries appear exquisitely sensitive to cadmium toxicity during this period (Der et al., 1977). After sexual maturation, however, the ovary appears relatively resistant to cadmium toxicity (Parizek et al., 1968). Several investigators have also suggested that mercury may alter hypothalamic function in developing rodents.

Effects of Metals on Reproductive Function in the Sexually Mature Female

Hypothalamus - pituitary. Lead, cadmium, mercury and nickel are thought to have an adverse effect on hypothalamic-pituitary function (Tables 2-5; Table 7). Lead may affect only developing rather than sexually mature rodents, although one study suggested that ovarian atrophy in sexually mature animals was the result of diminished FSH levels in lead treated animals (Vermande-Van Eck and Meigs, 1960).

Mercury may also have an adverse effect on the hypothalamus and pituitary (Lamperti and Niewenhuis, 1976; Lamperti and Printz, 1973,1974); however, most evidence suggests an effect on the ovary; latent, adverse effects on ovulation have been shown for mercuric compounds. Mercuric chloride injected daily during the estrous cycle (total, 3-4, mg/kg) caused a reduced ovulation rate by the third cycle in the hamster. The suggested mode of action was reduction in gonadotropin output because mercury was seen localized in the hypothalamic arcurate nucleus (Lamperti and Printz, 1974). A similar latent effect occurred also after acute treatment with 12.8 mg/kg mercuric chloride (Watanabe et al., 1979, 1982). In the rat,

mercuric chloride also prolonged diestrus following daily
injections, and there was evidence suggesting direct action on this
ovary (Stadnicka, 1980).

Ovary. Lead and cadmium are well documented to produce direct
ovarian toxicity (Vermande-Van Eck and Meigs, 1960; Der et al.,
1977). Although differential follicular counts have not been
performed, it is expected that the effects will be manifested on the
growing and preovulatory follicles. Inorganic mercury also appears
to alter on ovarian function in the sexually mature female rodent
Lach and Srebro, 1972).

Uterus. At the present time lead, copper, nickel and cadmium
appear to alter the function of the uterus. The effect of lead
appears to be specific for estrogen receptors, altering endometrial
response to ovarian estrogen creating an endometrial environment
hostile to preimplantation embryos (Wide, this volume). The effect
of cadmium on the uterus appears subtle; however, reports of altered
microcirculation suggest that cadmium may also alter uterine
responses to ovarian steroids (Copius Peereboom-Stegeman and
Jongstra-Spaapen, 1979,1981). The effect of copper appears to occur
only locally, when copper metal is inserted into the uterus (Zipper
et al., 1968; Chang et al., 1970).

The Effects of Metals on Oocyte Maturation, Fertilization and Implantation

Meiosis. Several organomercurials exhibit an oocyte
maturation-promoting capacity in an amphibian system in vitro.
These compounds simulate progesterone action in requiring calcium
ion presence, but differ by necessitating a longer period of action
(Brachet et al., 1975) Organomercurials act directly on the oocyte;
those which penetrate the oocyte readily cause toxicity, whereas
those which don't may promote meiotic maturation. A proposed
mechanism of action is as follows: sulfhydryl (-SH) groups in the
oocyte surface are known to prevent induction of maturation;
organomercurials may block -SH groups, thereby allowing nuclear
maturation to proceed (Pays et al., 1977). In mammals, it is not
known whether organomercurials have a similar progesterone-like,
meiosis-inducing action.

Can metals cause cytogenetic (i.e., chromosomal) alteration in
ova and thereby compromise reproduction and development? The
production of aneuploidy in cells of developing organisms could
explain the abortive and teratogenic properties of several metals.
The induction of aneuploidy in the germ cells of the fetal as well
as of the adult ovary could result in transmitted aneuploidy which
in humans is a major contribution to spontaneous abortion, to
genetically related mental retardation, and to some lethal birth

defects. The most evident effect of metals on chromosomal apparatus
appears, in fact, to be the production of c-mitosis in plant cells.
Mercury, lead and tin organocompounds also caused chromosomal
nondisjunction in an X-trisomy test using Drosophila larvae; and
methylmercury induced nondisjunction in female gametes, only, at the
first meiotic division (Ramel and Magnusson, 1979).

In mammals, adverse effects on chromosome number in secondary
oocytes have been claimed for cadmium chloride. Parenteral
treatment (1-4 mg/kg) within a few hours preceding ovulation in the
hamster resulted in a highly significant increase in frequency of
diploid oocytes which if fertilized would become triploid embryos
that do not survive to birth. The same treatment led to an increase
in hyperhaploid ova (Watanabe et al., 1979); if nondisjunction was
the mechanism, an equal frequency of hypoploidy would be expected,
and virtually all resultant embryos with nondisjunction of autosomal
chromosomes presumably would not survive to term. However, this
work requires confirmation, and the treated mother rather than the
exposed oocyte needs to be considered the experimental unit for
statistical analysis.

Negative findings were obtained in other studies involving
metal exposure in mouse germ cells. No increased nondisjunction
occurred from treatment of females about 6-12 hours before ovulation
with methylmercuric chloride, mercuric chloride, mercaptomerin or
mercuric acetate (Jagiello and Lin, 1973). The latter authors
suggested that access of mercury to the ovum nucleus or spindle
apparatus was prevented by a barrier, possibly residing in the zona
pellucida, the vitelline membrane or the follicular cells which
surround the ova. Reproductive toxicity tests after exposure to
methylmercuric oxide or mercuric chloride failed to provide evidence
for chromosomal aberration induction (commonly designated "dominant
lethal") in male mouse germ cells (Lee and Dixon, 1975). Cadmium
chloride also failed to induce dominant lethal effects in male mice
(Gilliavod and Leonard, 1975). Further discussions of metal
compound effects on male germ cells is presented in the review
chapters by Berlin et al.; Lee; and Leonard et al. (this volume).

Contradictory findings concerning the effect of metals on
chromosomal aberrations in humans have been reported with somatic
cell exposure to lead, cadmium and methylmercury (Gerber et al.,
1980; Degraeve, 1981; Skerfving et al., 1974). Chromosomal effects
on human female germ cells are virtually unknown due to the current
lack of appropriate experimental or epidemiological approaches. The
use of ovulation induction and laparoscopic harvesting of oocytes in
nonhuman primates may represent a useful model for exploring female
germ cell effects.

Although few metals have known aneuploidy-inducing properties
(e.g., nickel and chromium), a plausible mechanism exists for the

occurrence of such clastogenicity by other metals. Methylmercury is a known inhibitor of microtubules which function in meiotic pairing, chromosome contraction and spindle formation -- three events which are presumably pivotal to aneuploidy production (Onfelt and Ramel, 1979). Consequently, methylmercury would seem to be a likely causative agent for aneuploidy in germ cells. Unfortunately, aneuploid-sensitive stages of gametogenesis are poorly understood and may vary with the toxicant used (Russell, 1976).

Research is required to identify stages in the developing ovum that may be sensitive to induction of structural or numerical chromosomal aberrations by metals. Germ cells in the fetal as well as the adult ovary are potential targets for cytogenetic toxicity. Aneuploidy induction could possibly involve toxicant exposure at any of the three stages: 1) during early oogenesis causing reduced chiasmata frequencies; 2) during meiotic division leading to spindle damage; or 3) throughout oogenesis whenever the kinetochore is susceptible to damage (Russell, 1979).

The most frequently used test systems for chromosomal aberration induction by heavy metals provide only circumstantial evidence for ovum cytogenetic toxicity (e.g., somatic cell cytogenetics or sister-chromatid exchange assays). The more specific tests require very time-consuming procedures (e.g., direct cytogenetic screening in oocytes and early embryos) and may yield results which require cautious interpretation (Rohrborn et al., 1977; Adler and Brewen, 1982). Nevertheless, the use of these ovum tests for cytogenetic screening of metals seems justified by the serious hazard of aneuploidy to human reproduction and development.

Regarding possible metal mutagenicity, a review of the literature (Leonard et al., 1982) shows that many heavy metals react readily with DNA, affect RNA and protein synthesis as well as cell proliferation and may also modify transcription. Most metals, however, fail to induce gene mutations in microorganisms and gave negative results in the rec-assay with Bacillus subtilis. Furthermore, even if metals should prove to be mutagenic, the resultant impact on reproduction although difficult to predict, would be of great concern.

In evaluating current knowledge concerning the reproductive hazard of metals due to possible chromosomal damage in oocytes, two factors are noteworthy. First, the cytogenetic studies which reported the clastogenicity of cadmium chloride involved treatment during a very narrow developmental window; thus, in women the comparable time period would be the 24-hour period following the midcycle surge of LH. Second, past studies suggest that the dose required for chromosomal effects may be sufficiently great that general toxicity could occur and might either act as a deterrent to further long-term exposure, or produce recognized or unrecognized

spontaneous abortion. Although these factors suggest there could be
minimal chance of cytogenetic damage from metals, any risk of ovum
aneuploidy induction in humans is of major concern. Because of
this, we recommend that the potentially clastogenic organic metals
be tested more intensively for their aneuploidy-inducing capacity
particularly in mammalian systems and that such tests include
treatment at a variety of stages of oogenesis.

       Fertilization - implantation. Lead is the only metal which has
been studied extensively with respect to its effects on the
preimplantation embryo and on implantation. In the experiments of
Jacquet et al. (1975), mice treated with dietary lead (0.125 percent
or more) from the time of fertilization had a reduced number of
pregnancies, due probably to a toxic effect on the embryo producing
a delay in cell cleavage. Interference with implantation could also
be related to a hormonal imbalance of the mothers leading to an
early regression of the corpora lutea (Jacquet et al., 1976; 1977a),
or alteration in uterine steroid hormone receptors (Wide, this
volume). There is evidence suggesting that cadmium, mercury, copper
and lithium may have adverse effects on the preimplantation embryo
(Storeng and Jonsen, 1980a,b; Pedersen and Lin, 1977; Brinster and
Cross, 1972). Copper has been reported to alter both blastocyst
viability and blastocyst formation in vitro.

       Resorption. Early embryonic development and placentation
appears to be very sensitive to metals as indicated by increased
resorption reported after exposure to lead, cadmium, chromium,
nickel, selenium, lithium and copper (Gerber et al., 1980; Nolen et
al., 1972; Gale and Bunch, 1979; Sunderman et al., this volume).

METALS AND FEMALE REPRODUCTION: HUMAN EPIDEMIOLOGICAL DATA

       Endpoints for Monitoring: Spontaneous abortion is a frequent
event resulting in the termination of as many as 50 percent of human
pregnancies. Only 10-15 percent of pregnancies terminate in a
clinically manifest (late) spontaneous abortion, while most of the
early spontaneous abortions can only be recognized using hormonal
pregnancy determination (Wilcox, 1983). The early spontaneous
abortions contain chromosomal anomalies in a large percentage (more
than 50 percent) and thus originate from damage to the parental germ
cells. By contrast, late spontaneous abortions have fewer
chromosomally abnormal specimens, and are likely to be caused by
deleterious factors operating during pregnancy (e.g., placental,
fetal, endometrial or myometrial toxicity).

       Methods of monitoring late (clinically manifest) spontaneous
abortions may be recorded by interviews or by hospital records. For
routine monitoring, only hospital records can be used. Interview
studies are usually more sensitive in registering late spontaneous

abortions. Interview reporting is sensitive to factors such as
social status, knowledge of medicine, concern about harmful
environmental factors; it is thus very sensitive to bias. Hospital
records may also give biased information as the degree of
hospitalization or access to medical care varies by country, social
class or physician preference.

Early spontaneous abortions can only be recognized by
monitoring human chorionic gonadotropin levels in urine or blood
(Wehmann et al., 1981). Although the method appears to be sensitive
and reliable, it may be useful only in specific detailed studies
because of the need to collect vast numbers of urinary samples in an
orderly manner. Only minimal experience in monitoring early
spontaneous abortions has been reported; however, several prospective
studies are presently in progress (Miller et al., 1980; Wilcox,
1983).

Spontaneous Abortions and Metals: Historically, lead has been
used as an abortifacient (Paul, 1860; Aub et al., 1926; Rom, 1976).
Historical data is also available associating occupational exposure
to lead with a risk of spontaneous abortion (Rom, 1976). Community
exposure through food and drinking water has also been suspected as
a risk factor for spontaneous abortions in Australia and Glasgow,
and ingestion of fish contaminated with methylmercury has been
associated with an increased frequency of spontaneous abortions.
Exposure to a mixture of metals (arsenic, lead, cadmium, zinc, etc.)
and other industrial pollutants in a copper smelter has been
reported to be associated with an increased frequency of spontaneous
abortion in the working woman (Nordstrom et al., 1978a,b). Results
from a Finnish smelter provide some support to this observation,
although the number of spontaneous abortions recorded was small
(Hemminki et al., this volume).

Infertility Caused by Metals: Literature is available only on
lead, which has been associated with fertility problems through male
exposure (Berlin et al., this volume; Lee, this volume) and
historically through female exposure (Rom, 1976).

Infertility can be monitored through infertility clinics. The
patients seeking the clinics are, however, likely to be selected,
and provide a biased data base. No broad experience is available on
attempts to use such data to resolve the contribution of
environmental factors to infertility on a population basis. However,
at least one human reproductive toxin, dibromochloropropane, has
been identified by exposed workers seeking to understand their
collective infertility (Whorton et al., 1977; Torkelson et al., 1961;
Infante and Tsongas, 1983).

Infertility, another end point for reproductive effects
monitoring, is thought to affect between 10 and 15 percent of
couples attempting to conceive. The proportion of male, female and

both partners responsible for infertility is thought to be approximately 20 percent, 40 percent and 40 percent, respectively. Unfortunately, these data are soft and difficult to verify. More effort is needed to quantify the epidemiology of infertility, as well as occupational, racial, and environmental differences in infertility.

CONCLUSIONS AND RECOMMENDATIONS

Specific Metals

Arsenic (Table 3): Due to the large amounts of arsenic released in the environment by industrial processes and pesticides, as well as extremely high concentrations observed in drinking water in some areas, the metabolism and general toxicity of arsenic has been widely studied. While the trivalent form is associated with toxicity, the pentavalent form of arsenic is substantially less toxic. Arsenical insecticides have been implicated in vulvar carcinomas (Friedrich, 1972). Surprisingly, however, very few observations are available on the effect of this metal on the female reproductive system and on developing mammals. Because of the effects of arsenic on DNA synthesis and repair it may be expected to alter many proliferation-dependent events in the reproductive process and to be toxic to the germ cells. Arsenic is mutagenic and clastogenic in a variety of assays (Leonard et al., 1982). Treatment of pregnant experimental animals produces fetal resorptions as well as genitourinary defects among surviving offspring. The fetal toxicity of arsenic can be blocked by selenium (Ferm et al., 1971).

In view of the widespread occurrence of arsenic and of the potential danger it represents, it is important to encourage experimental animal research as well as epidemiological studies on human populations exposed to arsenic in drinking water or in industrial or working environments.

Cadmium (Table 4): Although we have no epidemiologic evidence in humans that cadmium affects fertility or the rate of spontaneous abortion, it is known to affect reproductive organs in laboratory animals (Parizek et al., 1968). Tracer experiments have demonstrated the localization of cadmium in ovarian follicles and corpus luteum as well as pituitary (Dencker, 1975). Cadmium has been reported to produce superovulation. It is not known if the effects of cadmium on the corpus luteum and microsomal monoxygenases also plays a role in fetal toxicity. Acute exposure will produce hemorrhage and necrosis in the developing uterus and ovaries as well as ovaries of rodents in constant estrus. Cadmium treatment also blocks embryonic implantation in sexually mature rats, although other studies have not demonstrated effects on implantation or resorption at doses up to 9 mg/kg during days 6-14. Cadmium does increase the resorption rate most likely as a result of placental and to a lesser extent decidual toxicity (Levin et al. this volume).

Table 3 Effect of Arsenic on Female Reproduction

Site of Action	Reference
I. Effect in Experimental Animals	
A. Developing reproductive system	Holmberg and Ferm (1969) Ferm et al. (1971)
B. Sexual maturation	None
C. Mature reproductive system	
1. Hypothalamus - pituitary	None
2. Ovary	Leonard and Lauwerys (1980)
3. Uterus	None
4. Oocyte maturation and preimplantation events	None
5. Implantation events	Schroeder and Mitchener (1971) Takeuchi (1979)
6. Resorption - embryonic death	James et al. (1966) Birge and Roberts (1976) Holmberg and Ferm (1969) Schroeder and Mitchener (1971) Ferm et al. (1971)
II. Epidemiologic Evidence in Humans: fertility and spontaneous abortion	Luego et al. (1969) Nordstrom et al. (1978a,b)

Chronic treatment with cadmium causes thickening of the wall of the small blood vessels in the uterus and the ovaries of rats, and may also lead to ovarian atrophy. Also of interest were observations that Itai-Itai disease (osteomalacia and renal damage) was most prevalent in postmenopausal women. Cadmium has been reported toxic to ovulated oocytes and to produce meiotic errors (Watanabe et al., 1977, 1979). Subacute treatment produces persistent diestrus and decreases the weight of the uterus, ovaries and pituitary. Because one common source of human exposure to cadmium is via smoking, decreasing cadmium content of tobacco will decrease cadmium exposure and therefore is desirable. Cessation of smoking will also provide additional health benefits.

Table 4 Effects of Cadmium on Female Reproduction

Site of Action	Reference
I. Effect in Experimental Animals	
A. Developing reproductive system	Nolen et al. (1972) Scharpf et al. (1972)
B. Sexual maturation	Der et al. (1977) Parizek et al. (1968)
C. Mature reproductive system	
1. Hypothalamus - pituitary	Der et al. (1977) Saksena and Dahlgren (1977)
2. Ovary	Parizek et al. (1968) Der et al. (1977) Watanabe et al. (1977) Kar et al. (1959) Degraeve (1981) Watanabe et al. (1979) Copius Peereboom-Stegeman and Jongstra-Spaapen (1979) Dencker (1975) Kaul and Ramaswami (1970) Unger and Claussen (1973) Gunn et al. (1963) Sutter (1975) Laskey et al. (1980) Henning et al. (1971)

Chromium (Table 5): Chromium is an essential element as its deficiency state is characterized by abnormal carbohydrate metabolism. The inorganic form of hexavalent chromium (Cr^{6+}) has been reported to pass the placenta and produce resorptions in experimental animals while the trivalent form is thought to be nontoxic, probably due to poor absorption (Gale, 1978; Iijina et al., 1975).

Exposure to doses sufficient to produce physiological or pathological changes appear to be restricted to high doses. In view of the relative absence of data on reproduction and the increasing industrial and agricultural use of chromium, additional experimental investigations and epidemiological surveys of occupationally exposed

Site of Action	Reference
3. Uterus	Copius Peereboom-Stegeman and Jongstra-Spaapen (1979) Der et al. (1977) Young et al. (1977) Dencker (1975) Copius Peereboom-Stegeman et al. (1981)
4. Oocyte maturation and preimplantation events	Storeng and Jonsen, (1980a,b) Gilliavod and Leonard (1975) Pedersen and Lin (1977) Giavini et al. (1980) Degraeve (1981)
5. Implantation events	Chiquoine (1965) Chang et al. (1980) Nolen et al. (1972) Zipper et al. (1968)
6. Resorption - embryonic death	Nolen et al. (1972) Scharpf et al. (1972) Ferm and Carpenter (1968)
II. Epidemiologic Evidence in Humans: fertility and spontaneous abortion	Marinova et al. (1973) Tsvetkova (1979)

populations appear necessary. This seems especially true because of
the toxicity and carcinogenicity of chromium in other organs as well
as its reported ability to alter the fidelity of DNA transcription
(Leonard et al., 1982).

Table 5   Effects of Chromium on Female Reproduction

Site of Action	Reference
I. Effect in Experimental Animals	
A. Developing reproductive system	None
B. Sexual maturation	None
C. Mature reproductive system	None
1. Hypothalamus - pituitary	None
2. Ovary	None
3. Uterus	None
4. Oocyte maturation and preimplantation events	None
5. Implantation events	None
6. Resorption - fetal death	Gale (1974) Gale (1978) Gale and Bunch (1979) Iijina et al. (1975)
II. Epidemiologic Evidence in Humans: fertility and spontaneous abortion	None

Copper (Table 6): Most information available concerning the
effects of copper on female reproduction has focused on implantation
and intrauterine events. Copper effectively blocks implantation and
for this reason is used in intrauterine contraceptive devices (IUD)
(Orlans, 1974). No metal toxicity on other reproductive endpoints
have been described as a result of this type of exposure.

In vitro experiments have revealed an interference with the
development of murine blastocysts. However, copper toxicity could be

modified by adding albumin to the medium (Van Winkle and Campione, 1982).

Review of reproductive performance of patients with disorders of copper metabolism such as Menkes or Wilson's Disease may represent useful models for studying the effects of copper on reproduction.

Table 6 Effects of Copper on Female Reproduction

Site of Action	Reference
I. Effect in Experimental Animals	
A. Developing reproductive system	None
B. Puberty	None
C. Mature reproductive system	
1. Hypothalamus - pituitary	Phatak and Patwardhan (1950) Fevold et al. (1936)
2. Ovary	Haukkman et al. (1974)
3. Uterus	Hagenfeldt (1972) Adaderoh and Dada (1973) Aedo and Zipper (1973) Ghosh et al. (1975) Tamaya et al. (1976)
4. Oocyte maturation and preimplantation events	Brinster and Cross (1972) Van Winkle and Campione (1982) Holland and Pike (1978) Naeslund (1972) Giavini et al. (1980) Suzuki and Bialy (1964) Chang et al. (1970)
5. Implantation events	Zipper et al. (1968) Orlans (1974) Chang et al. (1970)
6. Resorption - embryonic death	Ferm and Hanlon (1974b) James et al. (1966)
II. Epidemiologic Evidence in Humans: fertility and spontaneous abortion	Nordstrom et al. (1978a,b)

Table 7 Effects of Lead on Female Reproduction

Site of Action	Reference
I. Effect in Experimental Animals	
A. Developing reproductive system	Stowe and Goyer (1971)
B. Puberty	Grant et al. (1976) Maker et al (1975) Kimmel et al. (1980)
C. Mature reproductive system	
1. Hypothalamus - pituitary	Petrusz et al. (1979) Stowe and Goyer (1971) Vermande-Van Eck and Meigs (1960) Govoni et al. (1978)

Lead (Table 7): Lead alters pubertal progression and multiple reproductive endpoints along the hypothalamic-pituitary-ovarian-uterine axis in sexually mature female experimental animals (Grant et al., 1976;1980). Lead also appears to alter reproductive function of unexposed rats whose parents were exposed pre- and postnatally (Stowe and Goyer, 1971). Lead can delay the onset of vaginal opening in rats treated pre- and postnatally (Kimmel et al., 1980). Histochemical studies have demonstrated lead accumulation in the hypothalamus, an area of the brain necessary for normal pituitary function. Rodents and primates treated with lead have impaired ovarian function both before and after ovulation (Vermande-Van Eck and Meigs, 1960). However, it is not known if the effect is direct or indirect through alteration in secretion of gonadotropins. Additionally, the effect of organic or inorganic lead blocking implantation appears to be due to altered uterine responsiveness to endogenous ovarian steroids as well as decreased progesterone synthesis or secretion (Wide, this volume). Existing epidemiological evidence also suggests that women are susceptible to adverse reproductive effects including decreased fertility and increased risk for spontaneous abortion from lead exposure (Rom, 1976).

Because of this evidence implicating lead as a reproductive toxin in both female experimental animals and humans, industrial and environmental exposure to lead requires careful monitoring. Surveillance for adverse reproductive effects in women exposed to lead should be encouraged. Also, further detailed studies exploring the mechanism of action by which lead produces these adverse effects on female reproduction are necessary.

Site of Action	Reference
1. Hypothalamus - pituitary (continued)	Grant et al. (1980) Stumpf et al. (1980) Sandstead et al. (1970) Grant et al. (1976)
2. Ovary	Jacquet et al. (1977a) Vermande-Van Eck and Meigs (1960) Odenbro and Kihlstrom (1977) Lach and Srebro (1972) Hildebrand et al. (1973) Stowe and Goyer (1971) Jacquet et al. (1975) Schroeder and Mitchener (1971) Panova (1972)
3. Uterus	Wide (1980) Wide and Wide (1980)
4. Oocyte maturation and preimplantation events	Jacquet et al. (1975) Jacquet et al. (1976) Wide (1978) Jacquet et al. (1977a)
5. Implantation events	Jacquet et al. (1977b) Wide (1980) Gerber et al. (1980) Wide and Nilsson (1979) Odenbro and Kihlstrom (1977) Jacquet (1978) Wide and Nilsson (1979)
6. Resorption - embryonic death	Jacquet et al. (1975) James et al. (1966) Azar et al. (1972) Weller (1975) Gerber et al. (1980) Grant et al. (1980) Schroeder and Mitchener (1971)
II. Epidemiological Evidence in Humans: fertility and spontaneous abortion	Paul (1860) Oliver (1911)

(continued)

Table 7 Effects of Lead on Female Reproduction (continued)

Site of Action	Reference
II. Epidemiological Evidence in Humans: (continued)	Nogaki (1958) Hall (1905) Taussig (1936) Legge and Goadby (1912) Chang et al. (1980) Bourret and Mehl (1966) Pindberg (1945) Rom (1976) Nordstrom et al. (1978a,b)

Lithium (Table 8): We have no data concerning the effects of lithium on reproduction, although it is known to be teratogenic and fetotoxic. As the salts of this metal (lithium carbonate) are used to treat manic-depressive bipolar diseases, it is important to explore the effects of long-term treatment with lithium on reproductive function and outcome of laboratory animals. At present the evidence concerning the fetal toxicity or teratogenicity of lithium carbonate is uncertain, while some studies demonstrate effects and others are unable to see an effect. In rodents, lithium chloride appears to retard cellular proliferation in preimplantation embryos. Observations of the reproductive performance and pregnancy outcome of women treated with this drug are encouraged; a registry of patients treated during pregnancy is presently functioning (Weinstein and Goldfield, 1975a,b).

Table 8 Effects of Lithium on Female Reproduction

Site of Action	References
I. Effect in Experimental Animals	
A. Developing reproductive system	None
B. Sexual maturation	None
C. Mature reproductive system	
1. Hypothalamus - pituitary	None
2. Ovary	Trautner et al. (1958)

Table 8   Effects of Lithium on Female Reproduction (continued)

Site of Action	References
3. Uterus	None
4. Oocyte maturation and preimplantation events	None
5. Implantation events	None
6. Resorption - embryonic death	Bass et al. (1951) Izquierdo and Becker (1982)
II. Epidemiologic Evidence in Humans: fertility and spontaneous abortion	Dumont and Mignot (1980) Goldberg and DiMascio (1978) Weinstein and Goldfield (1975a,b)

Mercury (Table 9): Mercury has been shown to affect the developing reproductive system as well as puberty in experimental animals. In the sexually mature reproductive system, the hypothalamic-pituitary ovarian-uterine axis appears to be adversely affected by mercury. Both organic and inorganic mercury gain access to the hypothalamus where it is associated with morphological alterations, as well as the pituitary where it is associated with changes in LH and FSH content (Lamperti and Printz, 1973;1974).

For the ovary, there is evidence demonstrating an adverse effect on corpus luteum function and suggesting adverse effects on follicular growth and ovulation (Lach and Srebro, 1972). Mercury has been identified in human follicular fluid and in the walls of growing murine follicles (Stadnickey, 1980). There is at present no direct experimental toxicity data for the uterus as well as other structures in the sexually mature female reproductive system. Evidence demonstrating cytogenetic alterations in plant cell mitosis and meiosis in Drosphila and decreased fertility of mice treated with organic mercury compounds increases concern for adverse genetic effects of these compounds. Other investigators have demonstrated adverse effects of organic and inorganic mercury on murine oocyte meiosis in vitro but were unable to produce similar effects in vivo, suggesting that the compounds do not have access to the maturing or mature oocyte (Jagiello and Lin, 1975). Sea urchin eggs lost the post-fertilization block to polyspermy after treatment with mercurials. There is evidence suggesting that mercury can disturb implantation in experimental animals. Resorption of newly implanted embryos has also been reported following mercury treatment in experimental animals. Other studies utilizing methylmercury in rats between gestation days 6-14 (the peri- and post-implantation period) of doses as high as 4 mg/kg have not demonstrated alterations in number of implantations or resorptions. For the human, there is epidemiologic evidence of an increased frequency of abortions as a result of exposure to mercury (Skerfving et al., 1974).

More experimental work is needed to get information on the mechanisms of action of mercury in disturbing the development of the female reproductive system, puberty, function of the neuroendocrine system, implantation and early postimplantation development. Since there are no data on the effect of mercury on the function of the uterus or any of the other female accessory organs (i.e., mammary gland) further experimental investigation is necessary. Also, additional epidemiological data is needed to determine the effect of mercury on the fertility of exposed population.

Table 9 Effects of Mercury on Female Reproduction

Site of Action	Reference
I. Effect in Experimental Animals	
A. Developing reproductive system	Nolen et al. (1972) Scharpf et al. (1973) Chang and Sprecher (1976)
B. Sexual maturation	None
C. Mature reproductive system	None
1. Hypothalamus - pituitary	Lamperti and Niewenhuis (1976) Lamperti and Printz (1973, 1974) Chang and Hartmann (1972a,b) Berlin and Ullberg (1963) Kurland et al. (1969) Nordberg and Serenius (1969)
2. Ovary	Stadnicka (1980) Lamperti and Printz (1973, 1974) Lach and Srebro (1972) Brachet et al. (1975)

Table 9 Effects of Mercury on Female Reproduction (continued)

Site of Action	Reference
2. Ovary (continued)	Pays et al. (1977)
	Watanabe et al. (1982)
	Khayat and Dencker (1983
	Khayat and Dencker (1982)
	Von Kaulla et al. (1958)
	Ostlund (1979)
	Kazantzis and Lilly (1979)
	Runnstrom and Manelli (1964)
3. Uterus	Jensen et al. (1967)
4. Oocyte maturation and preimplantation events	Khera (1973)
	Jagiello and Lin (1973)
	Lee and Dixon (1975)
	Ramel and Magnusson (1979)
	Skerfving et al. (1974)
	Onfelt and Ramel (1979)
	Watanabe et al. (1979, 1982)
5. Implantation events	Nolen et al. (1972)
6. Resorption - embryonic death	Mottet (1974)
	Nolen et al. (1972)
	Piechoka (1968)
	Scharpf et al. (1973)
	Ramel (1967)
	Lofroth (1970)
	Khera (1973)
II. Epidemiologic Evidence in Humans: fertility and spontaneous abortion	Skerfving er al. (1974)

Nickel (Table 10): Nickel ingestion can alter the fertility of female mammals and has been shown to cross the placenta after implantation and produce preimplantation and postimplantation losses. Nickel also appears to interfere with interactions between the hypothalamus and pituitary glands of female mammals, and high concentrations of nickel have been identified in the hypothalamus and pituitary (La Bella et al., 1973a,b). In addition, nickel has been demonstrated to alter the metabolic activity of microsomal monoxygenase, some of which are essential for steroid metabolism.

The effects on implantation and embryonic development could result, therefore, from a direct action on the developing organism as well as an indirect effect via hormonal imbalance in the mother. Recent observations have demonstrated effects of nickel on uterine contractile activity, first increasing baseline tone, then at higher concentrations abolishing uterine contractions (Rubanyi and Balogh, 1982).

Table 10   Effects of Nickel on Female Reproduction

Site of Action	Reference
I. Effect in Experimental Animals	
A. Developing reproductive system	None
B. Sexual maturation	None
C. Mature reproductive system	
1. Hypothalamus - pituitary	LaBella et al (1973a, b)
2. Ovary	Phatak and Patwardhan (1950) Von Waltschewa et al. (1972)
3. Uterus	Rubanyi and Balogh (1982)
4. Oocyte maturation and preimplantation events	Storeng and Jonsen (1980a)
5. Implantation events	Chang et al. (1970)
6. Resorption - embryonic death	Schroeder and Mitchener (1971) Ambrose et al. (1976) Nadenko et al. (1979) Sunderman et al. (this volume)
II. Epidemiologic Evidence in Humans: fertility and spontaneous abortion	None

Although nickel is widely used in the metallurgical industry it is not released extensively into the environment. In addition, with the exception of nickel carbonyl, it is apparently only partly absorbed. Certain nickel compounds are known to be mutagens which can alter the fidelity of DNA transcription (Leonard et al., 1982). Additional information on the effect of nickel on female reproduction and the developing organism are required.

Selenium (Table 11): Selenium is reported to alter the development of the female reproductive system in experimental animals, and to increase the frequency of resorption in early gestation. Available evidence suggests that exposure to selenium may also increase the risk of spontaneous abortion in women (Robertson, 1970). At the present time, it is not known if selenium alters reproductive function in the mature human. However, chronic selenium treatment (7.5 ppm in drinking water) produces sterility in female rats and appears to interfere with ovarian function in swine (Rosenfeld and Beath, 1954; Wahlstrom and Olson, 1959).

Because little is known about the adverse reproductive effects of selenium in experimental animals, further experimental investigation is necessary. As existing epidemiological data suggest human hazard from selenium exposure, more detailed observations on populations exposed to this metal are necessary, particularly as selenium supplements are ingested by many people.

Table 11 Effect of Selenium on Female Reproduction

Site of Action	Reference
I. Effect in Experimental Animals	
A. Developing reproductive system	Earl and Vish (1980)
B. Sexual maturation	None
C. Mature reproductive system	
1. Hypothalamus - pituitary	None
2. Ovary	None
3. Uterus	Rosenfeld and Beath (1954) Wahlstrom and Olson (1959)

(continued)

Table 11 Effect of Selenium on Female Reproduction (continued)

Site of Action	Reference
4. Oocyte maturation and preimplantation events	None
5. Implantation events	None
6. Resorption - embryonic death	Schroeder and Mitchener (1971) Rosenfeld and Beath (1954) Wahlstrom and Olson (1959)
II. Epidemiologic Evidence in Humans: fertility and spontaneous abortion	Robertson (1970)

Miscellaneous Metals: There is as yet no evidence for reproductive toxicity following exposure to a number of other metals, e.g., beryllium or vanadium. However, in view of the potential widespread exposure of human populations to these metals, epidemiologic studies, but more especially, reproductive toxicological screening are warranted in experimental animals.

Overall Conclusions

1. Lead, cadmium and mercury have definite multiple adverse effects along the mature hypothalamic-pituitary-ovarian-uterine axis in experimental animals. In addition, cadmium, mercury, selenium and arsenic appear to alter the development of the reproductive system in experimental animals.

2. In spite of the adverse effects along the hypothalamic-pituitary-ovarian-uterine axis, and for the developing reproductive system noted above, there remain large gaps in our knowledge of the sensitivity of the female reproductive system to metals.

3. At the present time, it is not possible to rank the relative sensitivity of reproductive endpoints along the hypothalamic-pituitary-ovarian-uterine axis, or the developing female reproductive system. Because of this, it is necessary to consider all of these endpoints in studies exploring the reproductive toxicity of metals.

4. The available epidemiological techniques are adequate to begin to assess human hazards to reproduction from occupational accidents or environmental exposures. Indeed, delays in accumulation of data on human exposure and reproductive function will result in equivalent delays in our understanding of the sensitivity of the human reproductive system to toxic insult. However, groups for monitoring are frequently small, and existing endpoints may be limited and not completely understood.

Overall Recommendations

1. More extensive experimental exploration of the sensitivity of the female reproductive system to metals is necessary to fill the broad gaps in our present knowledge.

These studies should address the following issues:

a. strain and species differences in sensitivity to reproductive toxicity

b. demonstrations of dose-effect relationship

c. age-dependent differences in sensitivity

d. exposure during "critical periods" or sensitive windows of vulnerability and subsequent function

e. hormonal and/or gonadotropic dependent effects on reproductive toxicity; and

f. relationship between the reproductive endpoint and blood, tissue and/or local fluid levels need to be explored.

2. Additional directed epidemiological studies of exposed populations are needed to develop an understanding of human hazard and evaluate risk.

3. An International Clearinghouse for reproductive toxins for occupational, environmental or accidental exposures needs to be established to collect and evaluate worldwide data on reproductive toxicity.

a. As reproduction is a fundamental human need, this clearinghouse must have free access to data from all countries.

b. A permanent team of toxicologists, reproductive biologists and epidemiologists should be assembled to evaluate or collect data on a regular as well as an "as needed" basis in certain emergencies.

   c. An ongoing catalog of research projects in reproductive toxicology should be developed and published on a frequent basis. This should encourage international collaboration and a more efficient utilization of expensive scientific resources.

4. Worldwide educational programs should be developed to increase the awareness of health scientists and physicians to the potential for reproductive hazards.

5. Specific focused studies of occupationally exposed populations to measure early unrecognized pregnancy loss should be encouraged to evaluate the utility of this promising technique.

6. Regional differences in human and domestic animal reproductive endpoints with respect to exogenous food/or water contamination should be explored. This technique has been helpful in exploring environmental factors in carcinogenesis and in lead toxicity and may prove useful in reproductive toxicology.

7. Animal experiments should be designed to explore exposure to multiple agents as existing data indicates that interactions which increase or decrease the toxicity of metals are common.

Metals with increasing industrial use and environmental contamination should be flagged for characterization of effects on the female reproductive system (e.g., aluminum, cobalt, iron, lead, molybdenum, tungsten and vanadium).

REFERENCES

Adaderoh, B.K.M. and Dada, O.A., 1973, Effect of intrauterine copper on the uptake of estradiol 14-C by rat tissues, Fertil. Steril. 24:54-59.
Adler, I. and Brewen, J.G., 1982, Effects of chemicals on chromosome aberration production in male and female germ cells, in: "Chemical Mutagens. Principles and Methods for their Detection", Vol. 7, F.J. deSerres and A. Hollaender, eds., pp. 1-35, Plenum Press, New York.
Aedo, A.R. and Zipper, J. (1973), Effect of copper intrauterine devices on estrogen and progestrone uptake by the rat uterus, Fert. Steril. 24:345-348.

Ambrose, A.M., Larson, P.S., Borzelleca, J.F. and Hennigar, G.R., Jr., 1976, Long term toxicologic assessment of nickel in rats and dogs, J. Food Sci. Technol. 13:181-187.

Anonymous, 1982, Advice on limiting intake of bonemeal, FDA Drug Bulletin 12:5-6.

Aub, J.C., Fairhall, L.T., Minot, A.S. and Reznikoff, P., 1926, "Lead Poisoning", p. 158, Williams and Wilkins, Baltimore.

Austin, C.R. and Short, R.V., 1972, "Book 1, Germ Cells and Fertilization", Cambridge University Press, London.

Ash, P., 1980, The influence of radiation on fertility in man, Br. J. Radiol. 53:271-278.

Azar, A., Trochinowicz, H.J. and Mazfield, M.E., 1972. Review of lead studies in animals carried out at Haskell Laboratory; Two year feeding study and response to hemorrhage study, Proc. Lutern. Symp. Environm. Health Aspects of Lead 199-209, Amsterdam.

Baker, T.G., 1971, Comparative aspects of the effects of radiation during oogenesis, Mutation Res. 11:9-22.

Baker, T.G., 1972, Oogenesis and ovulation, in: "Reproduction in Mammals," Book 1. Germ Cells and Fertilization, C.R. Austin and R.V. Short, eds., pp. 14-45, Cambridge University Press, London.

Baker, T.G., 1973, The effects of ionizing radiation on the mammalian ovary with particular reference to oogenesis, in: "Handbook of Physiology", Section 7. Endocrinology, Vol. 2. The Female Reproductive System, Part I, R.O. Greep, ed., pp. 349-362, American Physiological Society, Washington, D.C.

Balinsky, B.I., ed., 1970, "An Introduction to Embryology", W.B. Saunders Co., Philadelphia, 3rd Edition.

Bass, A.D., Yatema, C.L., Hammond, W.S., and Frazer, M.L., 1951, Studies on the mechanisms by which sulfadiazine effects the survival of the mammalian embryo, Exp. Therap. 101:362-368.

Berlin, M., and Ullberg, S., 1963, Accumulation and retention of mercury in the mouse I. An autoradiographic study after a single intravenous injection of mercuric chloride, Arch. Environ. Health 6:589-601.

Biggers, J.D. and Schuetz, A.W., 1972, "Oogenesis", University Park Press, Baltimore.

Birge, W. and Roberts, O.W., 1976, Toxicity of metals to chick embryos, Bull. Environ. Contam. Toxicol. 16:319-324.

Boue, J. and Boue, A., 1973, Anomalies chromosomiques dans les avortements spontanes, in: "Les Accidents Chromosomiques de la Reproduction", A. Boue and C. Thibault, eds., pp. 29-55, I.N.S.E.R.M., Paris.

Bourret, J. and Mehl, J., 1966, Les aspects medicaux du travail feminin dans l'industrie, Arch. Mal. Prof. 27:1-29.

Brachet, J. and Baltus, E., DeSchutter-Pays, A., Hanocq-Quertier, J., Hubert, E. and Steinert, G., 1975, Induction of maturation (meiosis) in Xenopus laevis oocytes by three organomercurials, Proc. Nat. Acad. Sci. 72:1574-1578.

Brinster, R.L. and Cross, P.C., 1972, Effect of copper on the preimplantation mouse embryo, Nature 238:398-399.

Bulger, W.H. and Kupfer, D., 1983, Estrogen action of DDT analogs, in: "Reproductive Toxicology", D.R. Mattison, ed., pp. 163-174, Alan R. Liss, New York.

Carr, D.H. and Gedeon, M., 1977, Population cytogenetics of human abortuses, in: "Population Cytogenetics: Studies in Humans", E.B. Hook and I.H. Porter, eds., pp. 1-9, Academic Press, New York.

Chang, L.W. and Sprecher, J.A., 1976, Degenerative changes in the neonatal kidney following in utero exposure to methylmercury, Environ. Res. 11:392-406.

Chang, L.W. and Hartmann, H.A., 1972a, Electron microscopic histochemical study on the localization and distribution of mercury in the nervous system after mercury intoxication, Exp. Neurol. 55:489-501.

Chang, L.W. and Hartmann, H.A. 1972b, Blood-brain barrier dysfunction in experimental mercury intoxication, Acta Neuropathol. 21:179-184.

Chang, C.C., Tatum, H.J. and Kincl, F.A., 1970, The effect of intrauterine copper and other metals on implantation in rats and hamsters, Fertil. Steril. 21:274-278.

Chang, L.W., Wade, P.R., Pound, J.G. and Reuhl, K.R., 1980, Prenatal and neonatal toxicology and pathology of heavy metals, Adv. Pharmacol. Chemothera. 17:195-231.

Chapman, R., 1983, Gonadal injury resulting from chemotherapy, in: "Reproductive Toxicology", D.R. Mattison, ed., pp. 149-162, Alan R. Liss, New York.

Chiquoine, A.D., 1965, Effect of cadmium chloride on the pregnant albino mouse, J. Reprod. Fertil. 10:263-265.

Copius Peereboom-Stegeman, J.H.J. and Jongstra-Spaapen, E.J., 1979, The effect of a single sublethal administration of cadmium chloride on the microcirculation in the uterus of the rat, Toxicology 13:199-213.

Copius Peereboom, J.W. and Copius Peereboom-Stegeman, J.H.J., 1981, Exposure and health effects of cadmium, Part 2. Toxic effects of cadmium to animals and man, Toxicol. Environ. Chem. Revs. 4:67-187.

Copius Peereboom-Stegeman, J.H.J., Jongstra-Spaapen, E.J., Letschert, E.J. and Dessing, H., 1981, Effects of cadmium exposure on female reproductive organs, pp. 541-544, International Conference on Heavy Metals in the Environment, CEP Consultants, Ltd., London.

Copius Peereboom-Stegeman, J.H.J., van der Velde, W.J. and Dessing, J.W.M., 1983, Influence of cadmium on placental structure, in: "Ecotoxicology and Environmental Safety", in press.

Dean, J., 1983, Preimplantation development: Biology, genetics, and mutagenesis, in: "Reproductive Toxicology", D.R. Mattison, ed., pp. 32-50, Alan R. Liss, New York.

Degraeve, N., 1981, Carcinogenic, teratogenic and mutagenic effects of cadmium, Mutation Res. 86:115-135

Dencker, L., 1975, Possible mechanisms of cadmium fetotoxicity in golden hamsters and mice: Uptake by the embryo, placenta and ovary, J. Reprod. Fert. 44:461-471.

Der, R., Fahim, Z., Yousef, M. and Fahim, M., 1977, Effects of cadmium on growth, sexual development and metabolism in female rats, Res. Comm. Chem. Path. Pharmacol. 16:485-505.

Dumont, M. and Mignot, G., 1980, Lithium et grossesse, oui ou non, La Nouvelle Presse Medicale 9:3625.

Earl, F.L. and Vish, Th.J., 1980, Teratogenicity of heavy metals, in: "Toxicity of Heavy Metals in the Environment", F.W. Ochme, ed., pp. 617-639, Marcel Decker, Inc., New York.

Ferm, V.H., and Carpenter, S.J., 1967, Teratogenic effect of cadmium and its inhibition by zinc, Nature 216:1123.

Ferm, V.H. and Carpenter, S.J., 1968, The relationship of cadmium and zinc in experimental mammalian teratogenesis, Lab. Invest. 18:429-432.

Ferm, V.H. and Hanlon, D.P., 1974a, Placental transfer of zinc in the Syrian hamster during early embryogenesis, J. Reprod. Fert. 39:49-52.

Ferm, V.H. and Hanlon, D.P., 1974b, Copper toxicity in mammalian embryonic development, Biol. Reprod. 11:97-101.

Ferm, V.H., Saxon, A. and Smith, B.W., 1971, The teratogenic profile of sodium arsenate in the golden hamster, Arch. Environ. Health 22:557-560.

Fevold, H.L., Hisaw, P.L. and Greep R., 1936, Augmentation of the gonad-stimulating action of pituitary extracts by inorganic substances, particularly copper salts, Amer. J. Physiol. 117:68-70.

Friedrich, E.G., 1972, Vulvar carcinoma in situ in identical twins: An occupational hazard, Obstet. Gynec. 39:837-841.

Gale, T.F., 1974, Effects of chromium on the hamster embryo, Teratology 9:1917.

Gale, T.F., 1978, Embryotoxic effects of chromium trioxide in hamster, Environ. Res. 16:101-109.

Gale, T.F. and Bunch, J.D., 1979, The effects of the time of administration of chromium trioxide on the embryotoxic response in hamster, Teratology 19:81-86.

Gellert, R.J., 1978, Uterotrophic activity of polychlorinated biphenyls (PCB) and induction of precocious reproductive aging in neonatally treated female rats, Environ. Res. 16:123-130.

Gerber, G.B., Leonard, A. and Jacquet, P., 1980, Toxicity, mutagenicity, and teratogenicity of lead, Mutation Res. 76:115-141.

Ghosh, M., Roy, S.K. and Kar, A.B., 1975, Effect of copper intrauterine contraceptive device and nylon suture on the estradiol 17 β-6-H^3 and progesterone 1,2,-H^3 in the rat uterus, Contraception 11:45-51.

Gilliavod, N. and Leonard, A., 1975, Mutagenicity test with cadmium in the mouse, Toxicology 5:43-47.

Giavini, E., Prati, M. and Vismara, C., 1980, Effects of cadmium, lead and copper on rat preimplantation embryos, Bull. Environ. Comm. Toxicol. 25:702-705.

Goldberg, H.L. and DiMascio, A., 1978, Psychotropic drugs in pregnancy, in: "Psychopharmacology: A Generation of Progress", M.A. Lipton, A. DiMascio and K.F. Killan, eds., p. 1047, Raven Press, New York.

Gondos, B., 1978, Oogonia and oocytes in mammals, in: "The Vertebrate Ovary: Comparative Biology and Evolution", R.E. Jones, ed., pp. 83-120, Plenum Press, New York.

Govoni, S., Montefusco, O., Spano, P.F. and Trabucchi, M., 1978, Neurochemical correlates of chronic lead treatment in rat stratum and limbic areas, Abst. 78th Intl. Cong. Pharmacol. 765.

Goy, R.W. and Robinson, J.A., 1982, Prenatal exposure of rhesus monkeys to patent androgens: Behavioral and physiological consequences, in: "Environmental Factors in Human Growth and Development", V.R. Hunt, M.K. Smith, and D. Worth, eds., pp. 355-378, Cold Spring Harbor Laboratory, New York.

Grant, L.D., Kimmel, C.A., Martinez-Vargas, C.M. and West, G.L., 1976, Assessment of developmental toxicity associated with chronic lead exposure, Environ. Health Perspect. 17:290.

Grant, L.D., Kimmel, C.A., West, G.L., Martinez-Vargas, C.M. and Howard, J.L., 1980, Chronic low-level lead toxicity in the rat. II. Effects on postnatal physical and behavioral development, Toxicol. Appl. Pharmacol. 56:42-58.

Grell, R.F., 1979, Origin of meiotic nondisjunction in Drosophila females, Environ. Health Perspect. 31:33-39.

Gunn, S.A., Gould, T.C. and Anderson, W.A.D., 1963, The selective injurious response of testicular and epididymal blood vessels to cadmium and its prevention by zinc, Am. J. Path. 42:685-702.

Hagenfeldt, K., 1972, Intrauterine contraception with the copper device, Contraception 6:219-230.

Hagenfeldt, K., 1976, The modes of action of medicated intrauterine devices, J. Reprod. Fert. Suppl. 25:117-132.

Hall, A., 1905, Increasing use of leads as an abortifacient, Br. Med. J. 1:584-587.

Haukkman, M., Lukkainen, T. and Timonen, T., 1974, The effect of the copper-T 200 IUD on the lateral phase plasma progesterone concentration in the normal menstrual cycle, Ann. Clin. Res. 6:40-44.

Harrison, R.J. and Weir, B.J., 1977, Structure of the mammalian ovary, in: "The Ovary", Vol. I. General Aspects", S. Zuchiman and B.J. Weir, eds., pp. 113-218, Academic Press, New York, 2nd Edition.

Henning, A., Georgi, K. and Jerock, H., 1971, Arch. Exper. Vet. Med. 25:793.

Hilderbrand, D.C., Der, R., Griffin, W.T. and Fahim, M.S. 1973, Effect of lead acetate on reproduction, Amer. J. Obstet. Gynceol. 115:1058-1065.

Holland, M.K. and Pike, N., 1978, Albumen protection of mouse morulae and early blastocyts against the toxic effects of cuprons and curpic ions during development in vitro, J. Reprod. Fert. 53:335-339.

Holmberg, R.E. and Ferm, V.H., 1969, Interrelationships of selenium, cadmium and arsenic in mammalian teratogenesis, Arch. Environ. Health 18:873-877.

Iijina, S., Matsumoto, N., Lu, C.C. and Katsunuman, H., 1975, Placental transfer of CrCl$_3$ and its effects of foetal growth and development in mice, Teratology 12:198.

Infante, P.F. and Tsongas, T.A., 1983, Occupational reproductive hazards: Necessary steps to prevention, in: "Reproductive Toxicology", D.R. Mattison, ed., pp. 383-390, Alan R. Liss, New York.

Izquierdo, L. and Becker, M.I., 1982, Effects of Li$^+$ on preimplantation mouse embryos, J. Embryol. Exp. Morph. 67:51-58.

Jacobs, P.A. and Morton, N.E., 1977, Origin of human trisomics and polyploids, Hum. Hered. 27:59-72.

Jacquet, P., 1978, Influence de la progesterone et de l'estradiol exogenes sur le processus de l'implantation embryonnaine, chex souris femelle intoxiquell par le plomb, C.R. Soc. Biol. 172:1037-1040.

Jacquet, P., Leonard, A. and Gerber, G.B., 1975, Embryonic death in mouse due to lead exposure, Experientia 31:1312-1313.

Jacquet, P., Leonard, A. and Gerber, G.B., 1976, Action of lead on the early divisions of the mouse embryo, Toxicology 6:129-132.

Jacquet, P., Gerber, G.B., Leonard, A. and Maes, J., 1977a, Plasma hormone levels in normal and lead treated pregnant mice, Experientia 33:1375-1376.

Jacquet, P., Leonard, A. and Gerber, G.B., 1977b, Cytogenetic investigation on mice treated with lead, J. Toxicol. Environ. Health 2:619-624.

Jagiello, G. and Lin, J.S., 1973, An assessment of the effects of mercury on the meiosis of mouse ova, Mutation Res. 17:93-99.

James, L.F., Lazar, V.A. and Binns, F., 1966, Effects of sublethal doses of certain minerals on pregnant ewes and fetal development, Am. J. Vet. Res. 27:132-135.

Jensen, E.V., Hurst, D.H., De Sombre, E.R., and Jungblut, P.W., 1967, Sulfhydryl groups and estradiol receptor interaction, Science 158:385-387.

Kar, A.B., Das, R.P. and Karkun, J.N., 1959, Ovarian changes in prepubertral rats after treatment with cadmium chloride, Acta Biol. Med. Ger. 3:372-381.

Kaul, D.K. and Ramaswami, L.S., 1970, Effect of cadmium chloride on the ovary of the Indian desert gerbil Meriones hurricanae Jerdon, Indian J. Exp. Biol. 8:171-173.

Kaufman, F.R., Kogut, M.D., Donnell, G.N., Goebelsmann, U., March, C. and Koch, R., 1981, Hypergonadotropic hypogonadism in female patients with galactosemia, N. Eng. J. Med. 304:994-998.

Kazantzis, G. and Lilly, L.J., 1979, Mutagenic and carcinogenic
    effects of metals, in: "Handbook on the Toxicology of Metals",
    L. Friberg, G.F. Nordberg and V.B. Vouk, eds., pp. 237-272,
    Elsevier-North Holland Biomedical Press, Amsterdam.
Keino, H. and Yamamura, H., 1974, Effects of cadmium salts
    administered to pregnant mice on postnatal development of the
    offspring, Teratology 10:87.
Khayat, A. and Dencker, L., 1982, Fetal uptake and distribution of
    metallic mercury vapor in the mouse: Influence of ethanol and
    aminotriazole, Biol. Res. Preg. 3:38-46.
Khayat, A. and Dencker, L., 1983, Whole body and liver distribution
    of inhaled mercury vapor in the mouse: Influence of ethanol and
    aminotriazole measurement, J. Appl. Toxicol., in press.
Khera, K.S., 1973, Teratogenic effects of methyl mercury in the
    cat: Note on the use of this species as a model for
    teratogenicity studies, Teratology 8:293-304.
Kimmel, C.A., Grant, L.D., Sloan, C.S. and Gladen, B.C., 1980,
    Chronic low-level lead toxicity in the rat, Toxicol. Appl.
    Pharmacol. 56:28-41.
Knobil, E., 1980, The neuroendocrine control of gonadotropin
    secretion in the rhesus monkey, Recent Prog. Horm. Res. 36:53-88.
Kuhlmann, W., 1970, Cytology and timing of meiotic stages in female
    germ cells of mammals and man, in: "Chemical Mutagenesis in
    Mammals and Man", F. Vogel and G. Robertson, eds., pp. 180-193,
    Springer-Verlag, Berlin.
Kurland, L.T., Faro, S.N. and Siedler, H., 1969, Minimata disease,
    World Neurol. 1:370-395.
LaBella, F.S., Dular, R. and Leman, P., 1973a, Prolactin secretion
    is specifically inhibited by nickel, Nature 245:330-332.
LaBella, F.S., Dular, R. and Vivian, S., 1973b, Pituitary hormone
    releasing or inhibiting activity of metal ions present in
    hypothalamic extracts, Biochem. Biophys. Res. Comm. 786-791.
Lach, H. and Srebro, Z., 1972, The oestrus cycle of mice during lead
    and mercury poisoning, Arch. Biol. Crac. Sen. Zool. 15:121-191.
Lamperti, A.A. and Printz, R.H., 1973, Effects of mercuric chloride
    on the reproductive cycle of the female hamster, Biol. Reprod.
    8:373-387.
Lamperti, A.A. and Printz, R.H., 1974, Localization, accumulation,
    and toxic effects of mercuric chloride on the reproductive axis
    of the female hamster, Biol. Reprod. 11:180-186.
Lamperti, A.A. and Niewenhuis, R., 1976, The effects of mercury on
    the structure and function of the hypothalamo-pituitary axis of
    the hamster, Cell Tiss. Res. 170:315-324.
Langenbeck, U., Hansmann, I., Hinney, B. and Honig, V., 1976, On the
    origin of the supernumerary chromosome in autosomal trisomies -
    with special reference to Down's Syndrome, Hum. Genet. 33:89-102.
Lancranjan, I., Popescu, I.H., Gavanescu, O., Klepsch, I., and
    Serbvanescu, M., 1975, Reproductive ability of workmen
    occupationally exposed to lead, Arch. Environ. Health 30:396-401.

Langman, J., 1969, "Medical Embryology", Williams and Wilkins Co., Baltimore.

Langman, J., 1981, Chapt. 1. Gametogenesis, pp. 1-16, and Chapt. 2. Ovulation to Implantation, pp. 17-36, in: "Medical Embryology", Williams and Wilkins Co., Baltimore, 4th Edition.

Laskey, J.W., Rehnberg, G.L., Favor, M.J., Cahill, D.F. and Pietrazk-Flis, Z., 1980, Chronic ingestion of cadmium and/or tritium. II. Effects on growth development and reproductive function, Environ. Res. 22:466-475.

Lee, I.P. and Dixon, R.L., 1975, Effects of mercury on spermatogenesis studied by velocity sedimentation, cell separation and serial mating, J. Pharmacol. Exp. Ther. 193:171-181.

Legge, T.M. and Goadby, K.W., 1912, "Lead Poisoning and Lead Absorption", E. Arnold, ed., 308 p., London.

Leonard, A. and Lauwerys, R.R., 1980, Carcinogenicity, teratogenicity and mutagenicity of arsenic, Mutation Res. 75:49-62.

Leonard, A., Gerber, G.B., Jacquet, P. and Lauwerys, R.R., 1982, Carcinogenicity, mutagenicity, and teratogenicity of industrially used metals, in: "Carcinogenicity, Mutagenicity and Teratogenicity of Industrial Pollutants", M. Kirch-Volders, ed., Plenum Press, New York, in press.

Lofroth, G., 1970, Methylmercury: A review of health hazards and side effects associated with emission of mercury compounds into natural systems, Ecol. Res. Comm. Bull. 4:5-44.

Luego, G., Cassidy, G. and Palmisano, P., 1969, Acute maternal arsenic intoxication with neonatal death, Am. J. Dis. Child. 117:328-330.

Maker, H.S., Lehrer, G.M. and Silides, D.J., 1975, The effect of lead on mouse brain development, Environ. Res. 10:76-91.

Marinova, G., Osmankova, D., Dermendzhieva, L.L., Khadzhikolev, I., Chakirova, O. and Kaneva, Y.A., 1973, Professional injuries - Pesticides and their effects on the reproductive functions of women working with pesticides, Akush. Ginekol. 12:138-140, Sofia.

Mattison, D.R., 1980, Oocyte destruction by xenobiologic compounds, Contemporary Obs. Gyn. 15:157-169.

Mattison, D.R., 1981, Drugs, xenobiotics and the adolescent: Implications for reproduction, in: "Drug Metabolism in the Immature Human", L.F. Soyka and G.P. Redmond, eds., pp. 129-143, Raven Press, New York.

Mattison, D.R., 1982, The effects of smoking on fertility from gametogenesis to implantation, Environ. Res. 28:410-433.

McLachlan, J.A., Dames, N.M., Sieber, S.M. and Fabro, S., 1976, Accumulation of nicotine in the uterine fluid of the six-day pregnant rabbit, Fertil. Steril. 27:957-968.

Miller, J.F., Williamson, E., Glue, J., Gordon, Y.B., Grudziniskas, J.B. and Sykes, A., 1980, Fetal loss after implantation: A prospective study, Lancet ii:554-556.

Mottet, N.K., 1974, Effects of chronic low-dose exposure of rat fetuses to methylmercury hydroxide, Teratology 10:173-190.

Nadenko, V.G., Kenchenko, V.G., Azkhipenko, T.A., Saichenko, S.P., and Petrova, N.N., 1979, Embryotoxic effect of nickel ingested with drinking water, Gig. Sanit. 6:86-88.

Naeslund, G., 1972, Blastocytotoxic effect of copper in vitro, Contraception 6:281-285.

Niikawa, N., Merotto, E. and Kajii, T., 1977, Origin of acrocentric trisomies in spontaneous abortuses, Hum. Genet. 40:73-78.

Nogaki, K., 1958, On the action of lead on the body of refinery workers, particularly on the conception, pregnancy and parturition in the case of females and on the vitality of the new-born, Excerpta Med. 17:515-516.

Nolen, G.A., Buehler, E.V., Geil, R.G. and Goldenthal, E.I., 1972, Effects of trisodium nitrilotriacetate on cadmium and methylmercury toxicity and teratogenicity in rats, Toxicol. Appl. Pharmacol. 23:222-237.

Nordberg, G. and Serenius, F., 1969, Distribution of inorganic mercury in the guinea pig brain, Acta Pharmacol. et Toxicol. 27:269-283.

Nordstrom, S., Behrman, L. and Nordenson, I., 1978a, Occupational and environmental risks in and around a smelter in northern Sweden. I. Variations in birth weight, Hereditas 88:43-46.

Nordstrom, S., Behrman, L. and Nordenson, I., 1978b, Occupational and environmental risks in and around a smelter in northern Sweden. III. Frequencies of spontaneous abortion, Hereditas 88:51-54.

Noyes, R.W., Hertig, A.T., and Rock, J., 1950, Dating the endometrial biopsy, Fertil. Steril. 1:3-25.

Odenbro, A. and Kihlstrom, J.E., 1977, Frequency of pregnancy and ova implantation in triethyl lead-treated mice, Toxicol. Appl. Pharmacol. 39:359-363.

Oliver, T., 1914, Lead poisoning and the race, in: "Lead Poisoning", p. 192, H.K. Lewis, ed., London.

Onfelt, A. and Ramel, C., 1979, Some aspects of the organization of microfilaments and microtubes in relation to nondisjunction, Environ. Health Perspect. 31:45-52.

Orlans, B.F., 1974, Copper IUDs: A Review of the Literature, Contraception 10:543-559.

Ostlund, K., 1979, Studies on the metabolism of methyl and dimethyl mercury in mice, Toxicol. Appl. Pharmacol. 27(Suppl. 1):95.

Panova, A., 1972, Early changes in the ovarian function of women in occupational contact with inorganic lead, in: "Works of the United Research Institute of Hygiene and Industrial Safety", Sofia, Bulgaria.

Parizek, J., Ostadolova, I., Benes, I. and, Pitha, J, 1968, The effect of a subcutaneous injection of cadmium salts on the ovaries of adult rats in persistent oestrus, J. Reprod. Fert. 17:559-562.

Paul, C., 1860, Etude sur l'intoxication lente par des preparations de plomb; de son influence sur le produit de la conception, Arch. Gen. Med. 15:513-533.

Pays, A., Hubert, E. and Brachet, J., 1977, A comparison between organomercurial- and progesterone-induced maturation in amphibian oocytes, Differentiation 8:79-95.

Pedersen, R.A. and Lin, T.P., 1977, Effects of cadmium on early mouse embryo development, J. Cell Biol. 75:44a.

Phatak, S.S. and Patwardhan, V.N., 1950, Toxicity of nickel, J. Sci. Ind. Res. 96:70-76.

Petrusz, P., Weaver, C.M., Grant, L.D., Mushak, P. and Krigman, M.R., 1979, Lead poisoning and reproduction: Effects on pituitary and serum gonadotropins in neonatal rats, Environ. Res. 19:383-391.

Piechoka, J., 1968, Chemical and toxicological studies of the fungicide phenylmercuric acetate. Studies on the effect of food contaminated with fungitoxor on rats, Roczn. Panst. Zakl. Hig. 19:385.

Pindberg, S., 1945, On solverglod furgiftning i Danmark, Ugesfr. Laeg. 107:1-6.

Pohl, C.R. and Knobil, E., 1982, The role of the central nervous system in the control of ovarian function in higher primates, Ann. Rev. Physiol. 44:583-593.

Polani, P.E. and Jagiello, G.M., 1976, Chiasmata, meiotic univalents, and age in relation to aneuploid imbalance in mice, Cytogenet. Cell Genet. 16:505-529.

Ramel, C., 1967, Genetic effects of organic mercuric compounds, Hereditas 57:445-447.

Ramel, C. and Magnusson, J., 1979, Chemical induction of nondisjunction in Drosophila, Environ. Health Perspect. 31:59-66.

Reiter, E.O. and Grumbach, M.M., 1982, Neuroendocrine control mechanisms and the onset of puberty, Ann. Rev. Physiol. 44:596-613.

Robertson, D.S.F., 1970, Selenium, a possible teratogen, Lancet 1:518-519.

Rohrborn, G., Hansman, I. and Buckel, U., 1977, Cytogenetic analysis of pre- and postovulatory oocytes and preimplantation embryos in mutagenesis of mammals, in: "Handbook of Mutagenicity Test Procedures", B.J. Kilbey, M. Legator, W. Nichols, and C. Ramel, eds., pp. 301-310, Elsevier, Amsterdam.

Rom, W.N., 1976, Effects of lead on the female and reproduction: A review, Mt. Sinai J. Med. 43:542-552.

Rosenfeld, I. and Beath, O.A., 1954, Effects of selenium on reproduction in rats, Proc. Soc. Exp. Biol. Med. 87:295-298.

Rubanyi, G. and Balogh, I., 1982, Effect of nickel on uterine contraction and ultrastructure in the rat, Am. J. Obstet. Gynec. 142:1076-1020.

Runnstrom, J. and Manelli, H., 1964, Induction of polyspermy by treatment of sea-urchin eggs with mercurials, Exp. Cell Res. 35:157-193.

Russell, L.B., 1976, Numerical sex-chromosome anomalies in studies, in: "Chemical Mutagens. Principles and Methods for their Detection", Vol. 4, A. Hollaender, ed., pp. 55-91, Plenum Press, New York.

Russell, L.B., 1979, Meiotic nondisjunction in the mouse: Methodology for genetic testing and comparison with other methods, Environ. Health Perspect. 31:113-118.

Saksena, S.K. and Dahlgren, L., 1977, Reproductive and endocrinological features of male rats after treatment of cadmium chloride, Biol. Reprod. 16:609-613.

Sandstead, H.H., Orth, D.N. and Ate, K., 1970, Lead intoxication: Effect of pituitary and adrenal function in man, Clin. Res. 18:76.

Sankaranarayanan, K., 1982, "Genetic Effects of Ionizing Radiation in Multicellular Eukaryotes and the Assessment of Genetic Radiation Hazards in Man", Elsevier Biomedical Press, Amsterdam.

Scharpf, J.G. Jr., Hill, I.D., Wright, P.L., Plank, J.G., Keplinger, M.L. and Calandsa, J.C., 1972, Effect of sodium nitrilotriacetate on toxicity, teratogenicity, and tissue distribution of cadmium, Nature 239:231-233, London.

Scharpf, L.G. Jr., Hill, I.D., Wright, P.L. and Keplinger, M.L., 1973, Teratology studies on methylmercury hydroxide and nitrilotriacetate sodium in rats, Nature 241:461-463, London.

Schroeder, H.A. and Mitchener, M., 1971, Toxic effects of trace elements on the reproduction of mice and rats, Arch. Environ. Health 23:102-106.

Schroeder, H.A., Mitchener, M. and Nason, A.P., 1974, Long-term effects of nickel in rats: Survival, tumors, interactions with trace elements and tissue levels, J. Nutr. 104:239-243.

Sieber, S. and Adamson, R.H., 1975, Toxicity of antieoplastic agents in man: Chromosomal aberrations, antifertility effects, congenital malformations and carcinogenic potential, Adv. Cancer Res. 22:57-155.

Silbergeld, E.K. and Mattison, D.R., 1983, Effect of oocyte destruction by polycyclic aromatic hydrocarbons on fertility of DBA/ZN (2N), C57BL/6N (B6) and (D1xB6)F_1 mice. Abstract, Society for Gynecologic Investigation, Annual Meeting, Washington, D.C.

Skerfving, S., Hansson, K., Mangs, C., Lindsten, J. and Ryman, N., 1974, Methylmercury-induced chromosome damage in man, Environ. Res. 7:83-98.

Smith, C.G., 1983, Reproductive toxicity; hypothalamic pituitary mechanisms, in: "Reproductive Toxicology", D.R. Mattison, ed., pp. 107-112, Alan R. Liss, New York.

Stadnicka, A., 1980, Localization of mercury in the rat ovary after oral administration of mercuric chloride, Acta Histochem. Toxicol. 67:227-233.

Storeng, R. and Josen, J., 1980a, Effect of nickel chloride and cadmium acetate on the preimplantation mouse embryo in vitro, Toxicology 17:183-187.

Storeng, R. and Josen, J., 1980b, Nickel toxicity in early mammalian embryogenesis, Toxicol. Lett. 5:110.

Stowe, H.D. and Goyer, R.A., 1971, The reproductive ability and progeny of F_1 lead toxic rats, Fertil. Steril. 22:755-760.

Streffer, C., van Beuningen, D., Molls, M., Schulz, A.P. and
    Zamboglion, N., 1978, The in vitro culture of preimplanted mouse
    embryos. A model for studying combined effects, In: "Late
    Biological Effects of Ionizing Radiation, II", STI/PUP/489,
    IAEA, Vienna.
Stumpf, W.E., Sar, M. and Grant, L.D., 1980, Autoradiographic
    localization of ^{210}Pb and its decay products in rat forebrain,
    Neurotoxicol. 1:593-606.
Suzuki, M. and Bialy, H., 1964, Fertilizability of copper ovulated
    rabbit ova, Endocrinology 75:288-289.
Sutter, K., 1975, Studies on the dominant-lethal and fertility
    effects of the heavy metal compounds methylmercuric hydroxide,
    mercuric chloride and cadmium chloride in male and female mice,
    Mutat. Res. 30:365-374.
Swartz, W.J., 1983, Early mammalian embryonic development, in:
    "Reproductive Toxicology", D.R. Mattison, ed., pp. 51-62, Alan
    R. Liss, New York.
Takeuchi, I.K., 1979, Embryotoxicity of arsenic acid: Light and
    electron microscopy of its effects on neurulation-stage rat
    embryo, J. Tox. Sci. 4:405-416.
Tamaya, T., Nahata, Y., Ohno, Y., Nioka, S., Furuta, N. and Oksla,
    H., 1976, The mechanism of action of the copper intrauterine
    device, Fertil. Steril. 27:767-772.
Taussig, F.G., 1936, "Abortions, Spontaneous and Induced", Mosby,
    St. Louis.
Torkelson, T.R., Sadek, S.E., Rowe, V.K., Kodama, J.H., Anderson,
    H.H., Loquvam, G.S. and Hine, C.H., 1961, Toxicological
    investigation of 1,2-dibromo-3-chloropropane, Toxicol. Appl.
    Pharmacol. 3:545-559.
Trautner, E.M., Pennycuik, P.R., Morris, R.J.H., Gershon, S., and
    Shankley, K.H., 1958, The effects of prolonged sub-toxic lithium
    ingestion on pregnancy in rats, Aust. J. Reprod. Biol.
    36:305-309.
Tsvetkova, R.P., 1979, Materials concerning an investigation of the
    effect of cadmium compounds on the generative function, Gig. Tr.
    Prof. Zabol. 12:31-33.
Uebele-Kallahardt, B.-M., 1978, "Human Oocytes and Their Chromosomes",
    106 p., Springer-Verlag, Berlin.
Ullberg, S., Nelson, A., Kristoffersson, H. and Engstrom, A., 1963,
    Distribution of plutonium in mice. An autoradiographic study,
    Acta Radiologica Excerptum 6:457-471.
Unger, M. and Clausen, J., 1973, Liver cytochrome P-450 activity
    after intraperitoneal administration of cadmium salts in the
    mouse, Environ, Physiol. Biochem. 3:236-242.
UNSCEAR Report, 1979, Sources and Effects of Ionizing Radiation,
    Report of the United Nations Scientific Committee on the Effects
    of Atomic Radiation, 1977 Report, United Nations, New York.
Van Winkle, L.J. and Campione, A.L., 1982, Toxic effects of Zn^{++}
    and Cu^{++} on mouse blastocysts in vitro, Experientia 38:354-355.

Vermande-Van Eck, G.I. and Meigs, J.W., 1960, Changes in the ovary of the rhesus monkey after chronic lead intoxication, Fertil. Steril. 11:223-234.

Von Kaulla, K.N., Aikawa, J.K. and Pettigrew, J.D., 1958, Concentration in the human ovarian follicular fluid of radioactive tracers and drugs circulating in the blood, Nature 182:1238-1239.

Von Waltschewa, W., Slatema, M. and Michailow, I.W., 1972, Hodenveramderugen bei weissen Ratten durch chronische verabreichung von Nickelsulfat, Exper. Path. 6:116-120.

Villee, C.A. and Dethier, V.G., 1976, "Biological Principles and Processes", W.B. Saunders Co., Philadelphia.

Wahlstrom, R.C. and Olson, O.E., 1959, The effect of selenium on reproduction in swine, J. Anim. Sci. 18:141-145.

Watanabe, T., Shimada, T. and Endo, A., 1982, Effects of mercury compounds on ovulation and meiotic and mitotic chromosomes in female golden hamsters, Teratology 25:381-384.

Watanabe, T., Shimada, T. and Endo, A., 1977, Mutagenic effects of cadmium on the oocyte chromosomes of mice, Japanese J. Hygiene 32:472-481.

Watanabe, T., Shimada, T. and Endo, A., 1979, Mutagenic effects of cadmium on mammalian oocyte chromosomes, Mutat. Res. 67:349-356.

Wehmann, R.E., Harman, S.M., Birhen, S., Canfield, R.E. and Nisula, B.C., 1981, Convenient radioimmunoassay that measures urinary human choriogonadotropin in the presence of urinary human lutotropin, Clin. Chem. 27:1997-2001.

Weinstein, M.R. and Goldfield, M.D., 1975a, Cardiovascular malformations with lithium use during pregnancy, Am. J. Psychiat. 132:529-531.

Weinstein, M.R. and Goldfield, M.D., 1975b, Administration of lithium during pregnancy, in: "Lithium Research and Therapy", pp. 237-262, Academic Press, New York.

Weir, B.J. and Rowlands, I.W. 1977, Ovulation and atresia, in: "The Ovary, Vol. I. General Aspects", S. Zucherman and B.J. Weir, eds., pp. 265-302, Academic Press, New York, 2nd Edition.

Weller, V.C., 1975, The blastotrophic effects of chronic lead poisoning, J. Med. Res. 33:271-293.

Whorton, D., Krauss, R.M., Marshall, S. and Milby, T.H., 1977, Infertility in male pesticide workers, Lancet ii:1259-1261.

Wide, M., 1978, Effect of inorganic lead on the mouse blastocyst in vitro, Teratology 17:165-170.

Wide, M., 1980, Interference of lead with implantation in the mouse: effect of exogenous estradiol and progesterone, Teratology 21:187-191.

Wide, M. and Nilsson, B.O., 1977, Differential susceptibility of the embryo to inorganic lead during periimplantation in the mouse, Teratology 16:273-276.

Wide, M. and Nilsson, B.O., 1979, Interference of lead with implantation in the mouse: a study of the surface ultrastructure of blastocysts and endometrium, Teratology 20:101-114.

Wide, M. and Wide, L., 1980, Estradiol receptor activity in uteri of pregnant mice given lead before implantation, Fertil. Steril. 34:503-508.

Wilcox, A.J., 1983, Surveillance of pregnancy loss in human populations, in: "Reproductive Toxicology", D.R. Mattison, ed., pp. 285-292, Alan R., Liss, New York.

Witschi, E., 1970, Teratogenic effects from overripeness of the egg, in: "Congenital Malformation", F.C. Fraser and V.A. McKusick, eds., pp. 157-169, Excerpta Medica, Amsterdam.

Young, P.C.M., Cleary, R.E. and Ehrlich, C.E., 1977, Effect of metal ions on the binding of progesterone and estradiol by human endometrial cytosol, in: "Multiple Molecular Forms of Steroid Hormone Receptors", M.K. Agarwal, ed., pp. 215-228, Elsevier/North Holland Biomedical Press, Amsterdam.

Zipper, J., Medel, M. and Prager, R., 1968, Alterations in fertility induced by unilateral intrauterine instillation of cytoxic compounds in rats, Am. J. Obstet. Gynec. 102:971-978.

THE CONGENITAL TERATOGENICITY AND PERINATAL TOXICITY OF METALS

N. Karle Mottet and Vergil H. Ferm

Working Group: Robert Mermelstein, F. William Sunderman, Jr.
  Vergil H. Ferm, Laszlo Magos, N. Karle Mottet

Review Article Contents:

THE CONGENITAL TERATOGENICITY AND PERINATAL TOXICITY OF METALS

N.K. Mottet[1] and V.H. Ferm[2]

[1]University of Washington
 Seattle, Washington
[2]Dartmouth Medical School
 Hanover, New Hampshire

CONGENITAL AND PERINATAL TOXICITY CAUSED BY METALS

A.   Patterns of Normal Development of Structure and Function

The period in a person's lifespan which is most susceptible to
exogenous (environmental) injury is during the early stages of
development. During this period, proliferation and differentiation of
cells proceed at a remarkable rate, from the formation of the zygote
(fertilized egg) to the fetus. The human zygote is a sphere of
approximately 0.14 mm in diameter. By the end of the embryonic period
(55 days of gestation), it will have increased in volume approximately
27,000 times and have a crown-rump length of 30 mm. This increase in
volume is principally the result of cell proliferation. Throughout
the remaining fetal period (55th day gestation to birth), the body
volume increases about 40 times, and from birth to adulthood only
about 20 times. Thus proliferation occurs at an incredibly rapid rate
during the early phases of morphogenesis.

Not only does cell proliferation proceed rapidly during the
embryonic period, but differentiation also begins. It is during
this period that the basic body plan is established, including the
body axes -dorsal/ventral, left/right- and the extremities. The
three embryonic germ layers provide cells for organ rudiments and
organogenesis. During the fetal period, proliferation becomes a
less dominating factor; however, cell differentiation proceeds
continuously rate. The various organs and tissues increase the
biosynthetic activities characteristic of their specialized
functions. Enzyme systems particular to a biosynthetic function may
be established very early in morphogenesis; however, they do not
ordinarily achieve full expression of activity until late in fetal

development. Often the modulation to meet functional needs is not
accomplished until postnatal life. For example, Rutter et al.
(1968,1973) has shown that the secretion of pancreatic enzymes
begins early in morphogenesis when the cells of the pancreas are
first identifiable. There are two subsequent steps in which the
levels of enzyme secretion are enhanced during the fetal period; the
final level is controlled by the needs of the developing organism.

The establishment of this highly complex and specialized
integration of cells into an overall body plan consisting of various
tissues and organs is achieved by surprisingly few morphogenic
actions of a cell. The actions are normally exquisitely controlled
by both genetic and epigenetic mechanisms: 1) the genetic
instruction of morphogenesis, and 2) the unaltered metabolism of
cells established to carry out the genetic instructions (epigenetic
or morphogenic mechanisms). Environmental teratogenic chemical and
physical agents may injure either the genome or the cell metabolism
or both, and produce anomalies. In the processes of DNA/RNA
replication, transcription, translation, and protein biosynthesis,
any step in the chain of responses may be inhibited by metals
(Eichorn et al., 1981; Jacobson, 1966; Jacobson and Turner, 1980;
Sissoeff et al., 1976; Spiro, 1980). Irrespective of whether the
injury is to the genome or to the capacity of the cells to respond
to genetic instruction, the fundamental result is a biochemical
change affecting the intracellular integrity of the cell, which in
turn is reflected in altered activity of cells leading to anomalous
morphogenesis. Many of the details of the genetic mechanisms of
control have been described during the last two decades, and further
elaboration is not appropriate here. For example, the investigations
of Eichorn and Shin (1968) and of Zakour et al. (1981) reviewed the
various steps in the synthesis of DNA, and how metals may induce
infidelity in the reproduction of DNA. At least ten metals have
been shown to be mutagens as a result of incorrect base substitution
during DNA replication.

Epigenetic mechanisms of cell control can also be altered by
exposure to exogenous metals, resulting in deranged morphogenesis.
Genetic mutations have their principal effect on the male and female
germ cells, resulting in miscoding in the synthesis of the
macromolecules for the cells. Beyond the zygote stage, the effects
of mutation may be reflected in the somatic cell genetics of the
individual, but more likely the exogenous toxic chemical will result
in alterations of epigenetic processes, i.e., alteration of cell
action as a result of injury directly to its general chemical
processes.

Both genetic and epigenetic alteration of molecular activity
result in deranged organelle function, or alteration of the
morphogenic activity of the cell as a whole. Malformations
(anatomic defects) are the collective end result of molecular,
subcellular organelle, and cellular injury.

The general toxic potential of a metal in a species is also determined by the dose which is able to influence fertility, implantation, embryonic-fetal, or postnatal development. In relation to conception and the gestational period, there are changes both in the dose required to produce certain effects in a proportion of animals, quantified by the dose-response curve for a selected effect, and in the dose-effect relationship. For example, teratogenic effects may be produced only at a restricted period and by only a relatively low dose, while before or after this stage higher doses may be required to influence embryonic-fetal development. It is implicit in these changes in the dose-effect and dose-response relationships for the developing organism, that the mother may be affected at one stage of embryonic-fetal development and not at the other. Moreover, the sensitivity of the mother may change with different reproductive phases. Therefore it is essential to relate an abnormality in embryonic-fetal development not only to dose, but to the toxic effects in the maternal organism that may potentially occur.

Cellular Morphogenic Activities

Epigenetic kinds of molecular injury may result in at least six major derangements in cellular activities. These are: 1) altered rates of cell proliferation; 2) cell necrosis; 3) altered cell differentiation as characterized by anaplasia, metaplasia, or neoplasia; 4) altered cell biosynthesis; 5) altered cell-to-cell (or tissue-to-tissue) interactions; and 6) altered cell movements as demonstrated in migration, aggregation, and adhesion.

As noted above, metals can directly alter replication of the genome, but they also can, in an epigenetic manner, directly injure cells by attacking enzyme systems, organelles, and other cell components which may lead to altered cell activity, degeneration, or death. It is this altered molecular activity of cells during ontogenesis which can be reflected in altered morphogenesis of an organ or tissue (see Table 1).

Cell Number (Proliferation vs Loss)

Alteration of the rate of cell proliferation, and the time and rate of cell death are two mechanisms that affect the number of cells available for histogenesis and organogenesis. As pointed out by Ferm and Hanlon at this conference, most congenital malformations are "reductionist" in nature, i.e., there is a decreased or absent organ or tissue.

During the early phases of embryogenesis, the cells are dividing at a maximal rate, that is, about 8 to 9 hours for each cell cycle (Baserga, 1981; Kohler et al., 1972). Thus the pool of

Table 1 Cellular Mechanisms of Teratogenesis

Morphogenic Cellular Alteration	Mechanism	Altered by
Cell proliferation	Mitotic rate or index	Hg
Cell loss	Necrosis Exfoliation	Hg, Pb, As, Cd
Cell size	Hypertrophy Hypotrophy	Most metals
Cell location	Migration (chemoattractants)	Unknown Hg in CNS
	Aggregation	
	Delamination (decreased adhesion)	
Cell specialization	Differentiation	Hg
	Neoplasia	
	Metaplasia	
Cell interation	Induction	As

cells from which each organ differentiates is increased rapidly. One may reason a priori that the controls of the rate of proliferation involve extracellular as well as intracellular mechanisms (Goss, 1972). Rutter et al. (1973) have isolated a protein from connective tissues which is capable of stimulating the proliferation of epithelial cells such as the glandular exocrine portion of the pancreas by acting on the cell surfaces.

Epidermal growth factors, nerve growth factors, and many maternal humoral factors may influence the rate of cell proliferation in vitro (Baserga, 1981). Thyroxin produced by the mother's thyroid gland may have an overall stimulatory effect on fetal development as it does in oviparous embryos.

Brent and Jensh (1967) have reviewed the subject of intrauterine growth retardation and have listed many etiologic factors including various radiations, pharmaceutical agents, environmental chemicals, maternal endocrine and nutritional factors, and hypoxia. An additional growth-control mechanism may be self-inhibition. Experimental evidence suggests that as the population of cells enlarges, the density of the population may within itself diminish proliferation, depending in part on the availability of nutritional substances. Numerous growth factors are currently under investigation, among these the epithelial factor, the fibroblast growth factor, and the nerve growth factor. They apparently affect the surface membrane receptors as a signal to rates of self-proliferation.

In assessing the effects of a teratogenic agent on proliferating cells, one must consider not only the proportion of cells that are undergoing mitosis at a given time, i.e., the mitotic index, but also the rate at which cells that are dividing proceed through the various states of the cell cycle. These features of the cell cycle have recently been reviewed (Baserga, 1981). Most, if not all, toxic-metal exposures in the developing fetus, both viviparous and oviparous, result in offspring of decreased size (Mottet, 1981). There are several possible mechanisms for this effect. For most metals, the mechanism remains unknown. Some data now have been developed for the effects of methylmercury on the developing fetus. Continuous prenatal congenital exposure to methylmercury has been shown to produce offspring which are smaller, owing to decreased rate of cell proliferation in organs during the fetal period (Chen et al., 1979; Mottet, 1974). Necrosis may also contribute to the decreased number of cells per organ, especially at higher doses.

On the molecular level some recent interesting data presented by Sager at this conference suggest a possible mechanism. She has shown under in vitro conditions methylmercury, in a dose range similar to in vivo levels, impedes the assembly of microtubules, a principal element of the mitotic spindle. Vogel has further evidence indicating that the mercury binds to the sulfhydryl groups in the microtubule protein (Vogel et al, 1982 and unpublished). This alteration in the cell organelle interferes with the assembly of the microtubules into tubulin. This in turn is associated with a decrease in the cellular proliferative rate, and thus may alter the development of individual organs or, as in this case, the total weight of the offspring. Although an engaging concept, one must be mindful that other possibilities exist. As noted earlier, mercury compounds bind to the base of DNA, thus destabilizing the molecule, and may impede DNA synthesis by interfering with nuclear enzyme activities. Mercury may also alter mitochondrial energy production (Fowler, this volume; Southard et al., 1974; Fowler and Woods, 1977), lysosome function or plasma membranes (Ballan-Dufrancais et al., 1980; Fowler et al., 1975; Jeantet et al., 1980; Sternleib and Goldfischer, 1976; Verity and Reith, 1967), which in turn may alter cellular proliferative rate (Lauwerys and Buchet, 1972).

Cell death (and its end stage, necrosis) also diminishes the number of cells available for morphogenesis (Madsen and Christiansen, 1978). Following injury to a cell, a sequence of functional and structural modifications ensues which, if sufficiently severe and prolonged, may lead to the death and disintegration of cells. Some agents such as trauma, thermal burns, or corrosive chemicals may lead to immediate cell death and destruction, whereas others such as formaldehyde may lead to cell death immediately on contact but minimally alter the cell structure. However, usually the injurious agents act by depressing or otherwise altering essential cell functions such as energy metabolism or biosynthetic activities, resulting in recognizable changes in cell morphology. The changes may first be recognizable at the ultrastructural level within a few minutes of injury, whereas they may become visible by light microscopy after a longer period following the insult. Mild changes are usually reversible, and the cell will recover with restoration of normal function.

The distinction between mild cell injury and normal physiologic modulations cannot be precisely delineated. Injury may be defined as any perturbation that upsets cellular homeostasis sufficient to interfere with its functional role in the economy of the body. Toxicologists express this concept as "limits of tolerance." In the developing embryo and fetus, these limits change in the course of development, and different cells, tissues, and organs may become exceptionally sensitive to injury at different times. One must bear in mind that the features of injury will vary depending on the nature of the agent, the dose and rate of exposure, and the particular cells or tissues involved.

Necrosis can occur as a normal developmental event in many sites in the body and appears to have a role in the shaping of organs (Glucksmann, 1951). Individual necrotic cells or small patches of cell necrosis can be seen throughout the developing embryo, and the significance of these changes remains to be determined. They may represent a spurious cell development that is nonviable, or they may represent a programmed type of cell destruction that enables the shaping and formation of the pool of cells that gives rise to a particular organ.

The presence of selective spontaneous cell necrosis with distinctive features within the developing limb buds of the chick embryo has been reported (Mottet and Hammar, 1972). The cells appear to be destined to die long before there is ultrastructural evidence of degeneration and necrosis (Saunders, 1966). Several stages prior to the appearance of necrotic changes, the cells have been "determined" to die. For example, transplanting this region at stage 17 to a different region of the body of the embryo results in cell death in the usual manner. However, with transplantation at a prior stage the cells do not undergo necrosis.

Many cytotoxic agents, including metals, have been shown to produce necrosis in the developing embryo. Some have a selective effect, inducing necrosis in some cells but not harming adjacent cells. The explanation for this phenomenon is unknown. Some have speculated that the difference in cytotoxic effect may arise from the amount of the agent transported to the cell. Factors such as the differential permeability of the cell membrane to the agent, or the amount of intracellular or extracellular binding, might vary the sensitivity and resistance of different cell types.

Although decreased proliferation and necrosis are associated with malformations, the precise mechanism is not as yet understood. It is presumed that the diminished pool of cells available for the formation of an organ may result in a deficient critical mass. Above a minimal number of cells, a smaller but functional organ may be produced, whereas excessive diminution of the pool may produce a completely malformed organ. In other instances the diminution of the cell mass may interfere with other secondary mechanisms related to cell activity, such as the inductive interaction between different cell types. The arsenic effect on renal agenesis (vide infra) is an example of the latter.

Cell Size

Alteration in cell size is another mechanism associated with teratogenesis. The alterations in size can result in an increase in volume of cells (hypertrophy), or a decrease (hypotrophy). These changes are produced by altered biosynthetic activities of the cells. Biosynthesis is the central activity of all living cells, and the extent of its activity is carefully regulated. The products of the biosynthetic activity are macromolecules such as DNA, RNA, and proteins. This synthesis in turn is dependent upon the availability of precursors and adenosine triphosphate (ATP), which supplies the energy needed to synthesize the macromolecules. During the period of fetal development, particularly in the later periods of organogenesis, the embryo is especially vulnerable to alteration of normal biosynthetic activity. The products of the biosynthetic activity may be retained within the cell as part of the cellular structure and divided among daughter cells, or may be liberated into the cell environment, producing such components of interstitial tissues as collagen, elastin, and mucoprotein. The biosynthetic inhibition may involve the synthesis of DNA and/or RNA, and also the production of proteins in the cell. Thus any step along the replication, transcription, or translation of the genetic code may be inhibited by cytotoxic agents. Inhibition of DNA synthesis is virtually always teratogenic. In contrast, many inhibitors of protein synthesis have little or no teratogenic effect unless the inhibition is extreme. Some cytotoxic agents may induce teratogenesis by inhibiting cellular energy production. Cellular energy is stored in organic compounds such as glucose, which is utilized by a process of glycolytic respiration and of the terminal electron transport system to make ATP. ATP in turn provides the energy for the biosynthesis of macromolecules necessary for membrane integrity and energy for cell movement, osmotic regulation, etc. Thus anything that reduces the ATP level can be expected to markedly alter the development of an embryo. The report by Fowler (this volume) details how some metals can interfere with the energy metabolism of cells.

Generally, differentiated cells are recognized by their specialized biosynthetic products. Some cells retain their biosynthetic product in their cytoplasm, e.g., keratin in squamous cells, whereas others liberate the product into the surrounding milieu, e.g., fibroblasts and interstitial collagen. In other instances, the specialized product may be recognized both intracellularly and extracellularly, e.g., mucin on and in columnar epithelial cells.

Cell Differentiation

Information on the epigenetic effects of metals on cell differentiation is incomplete. The effects of fluoride on the deposition of bone minerals in tooth enamel is well-established; manganese deficiency is associated with a failure of otoliths to differentiate in the inner ear; and copper deficiency has been associated with defective myelination of the nervous system in experimental animals.

One type of alteration of cell differentiation is its misdirection by transplacental carcinogens. The concept that exposure of pregnant women to carcinogens can lead to the development of neoplasia in the offspring has existed for many years (Rice, 1973). Whether metals are transplacental carcinogens, either initiators or promotors, is unknown.

Morphogenic Cell Movements

Throughout the period of embryonic development many types of cells undergo carefully coordinated active and passive movement from one region of the embryo to another, participating in the formation of organs and tissues. The developmental events associated with cell movements are migration, aggregation, cavitation, delamination, and folding of tissues. Many cells in the developing embryo undergo active movement by ameboid activity from one site in the body to another. Major examples of these are the migration of germ cells (oogonia, spermatogonia) from their original location outside the developing embryo in the yolk sac into the developing gonad.

Similarly, the epithelium-derived neural crest cells adjacent to the neural tube of the early embryo migrate to many distant sites in the body. They give rise to a variety of cells, including pigment-forming cells (melanoblasts), autonomic nerve ganglia, and others. Similarly, portions of cells such as the developing axons of neurons migrate and pursue a path through the connective tissues of the body extending to distal sites, where they establish contact with muscle fibers or sensory end organs.

Cells may migrate singly or in groups. Two types of subcellular structures, microfilaments and microtubules, appear to be essential for cell movement. Intermediate filaments such as neurofilaments and tonofilaments may also be involved. The microfilaments appear similar in size and function to actin found in muscles, and appear to have a similar function within the cells. Using energy provided by ATP, the microfilaments react with myosin to produce a contractile activity in the cell structure in a manner analogous to that seen in muscle cells. However, the way in which these contractile proteins interact to produce directional cell movement is still unknown. It appears that the cytoplasmic actin and myosin are associated with regions of the plasma membrane, and that contraction by a sliding-filament mechanism similar to that in muscle, pulls selective portions of the cell membrane together, resulting in the production of a pseudopod such as is seen in ameboid movement.

In addition to their role in cell proliferation as part of the spindle, microtubules also appear to provide structural support for cellular shapes other than a simple globular shape. Microtubules (polymers of tubulin and associated proteins) are larger than microfilaments and intermediate filaments, and appear hollow when seen in cross-section. Cell migration has been most extensively studied using fibroblasts. As the cell undergoes ameboid movement in vitro, one can see bundles of microfilaments parallel to the lower surface of the cell and a network of fibers immediately under the plasma membrane. Microtubules form a network throughout the cytoplasm which is less dense at the periphery. The microfilaments are most prominent in those portions of the cell periphery most active in forming pseudopodia for movement, and in the leading ruffled membranes. The rays of parallel microfilament form a sheath along the bottom and dorsal surface of the cell. Some of these microfilaments appear to insert on the plasma membrane, where the cell is adhering to the substratum or to other cells. Disruption of the microfilaments by chemical agents such as cytochalasin B causes a cessation of movement.

Not only is the migratory movement of cells important in embryogenesis, but the ability of the internal skeleton of the cell to maintain diverse rearrangements of shape to produce folding, delamination, and cavitation appears to involve similar activities of the filaments and tubular subskeleton of the cell. For example,

epithelium may give rise to an organ rudiment by infoldings or
outpouchings. Under electron microscopy, bands of microfilaments
can be seen in the regions of the folds, suggesting that they may be
involved in the folding process. This has been shown to be true in
lower forms of marine life. In mammalian species, for example, the
pancreatic and lung buds arise as outpouchings from the primitive
embryonic gut. The formation of the pancreatic rudiment is the
product of changes in the shape of relative position of a few cells
in the epithelium of the duct. Microfilament bundles are abundant
at the apical end of such cells, and appear to be involved in shape
changes.

The control mechanisms of morphogenetic movements are poorly
understood. During early embryogenesis, migratory activity is much
more extensive than it is in late embryogenesis, and in turn much
less active in adult mature cells.

One important dimension of cell movement is cell aggregation.
Once cells have migrated to a new site, they must in some way
recognize the new environment and establish relationships there with
similar or other stromal cell types. The organization of the human
embryo into tissues and organs depends on the ability of individual
cells to be linked in very specific orientation to other appropriate
cells. These multicellular patterns arise in the course of embryonic
development and differentiation. The mechanisms that direct the
assembly of cells into tissues are dependent on genetic as well as
environmental factors that control embryonic development. As we
have seen, many cells leave their place of origin and move
individually or in groups to new sites by migrating through tissues,
between tissue layers and cells, or into the bloodstream, to be
transported to specific new sites distant from their origin. The
cells reassemble and reassociate with each other and with local
cells to form new structural entities within which differentiation,
histogenesis, and organogenesis occur.

Much of our knowledge of how cells associate following the
migratory pattern has been developed by Moscona (1973,1974).
Moscona reasoned that following the process of migration, cells must
have an affinity for similar types of cells (contact selectivity)
which enables them to select and establish their new residence
site. The surface of embryonic cells undergoes various changes in
structure, composition, and function in the course of embryonic
development and differentiation. These changes are reflected in
alterations in the selective adhesivity of cells, their movements
and migrations, and different changes in metabolism, intercellular
communication, etc. Among the properties of the cell surface that
appear to be very important in the process of cell migration and the
subsequent assembly of like cells into tissues and organs, is the
development of mutual adhesiveness of cells, and the major
characteristic of this developing adhesiveness is its selectivity.

The cells have a capacity to recognize and identify other cells of a similar nature, and accordingly adhere and interact developmentally. The recognition process not only involves self-recognition, but also recognition among different although functionally matching or complementary types. Cells that have been fully committed to specialized biosynthetic processes are less capable or even incapable of effectively regenerating the histologic association. The specific details of the mechanism of cell recognition remain to be discovered. It appears that the glycoprotein coat of the cell surface is an important factor which links adjacent cells by interaction of complementary sites. The effects of metals on these processes are unknown.

Tissue Interactions

Inductive cell-to-cell or tissue-to-tissue interactions are of utmost importance in determining the differentiation and morphogenesis throughout gestation. Since the early work of Spemann (1938), these interactions have been known as embryonic induction. Most, if not all, of the tissues of embryonic and later stages of development are engaged in these interactions, functioning either as inductors or as reactors, or in both capacities in some instances (Jacobson, 1966). Some of the better-known examples of these interactions have been more extensively investigated, such as the epithelial-mesenchymal interaction as identified by McLoughlin (1961), and the influence of the peripheral innervated field on neuron differentiation by Mottet (1952), who showed that motor neuroblasts differentiate into neurons in the embryo as a result of an interaction (induction) between the neuroblasts and the tissue being innervated. These observations contradicted the prevailing view at the time (Hamburger, 1958), namely, that neurons differentiated independently. Subsequent experiments have confirmed and extended our understanding of mechanisms of neural tissue interaction. A nerve growth factor, produced in vitro by fibroblasts derived from several sources in the body, has been demonstrated (Young et al., 1975). Further confirmation of this growth factor was recently provided using monoclonal antibody methods (Warren et al., 1980). A hybrid cell line has been developed which secretes an antibody capable of inhibiting the nerve growth factor by blocking its cell membrane receptor sites. A promising line of investigation is the study of the effects of toxic metals on cell membrane receptors as a possible mechanism of nervous system teratogenesis.

One model of alteration of an inductive interaction by a metal is kidney morphogenesis. Grobstein (1964,1967) has shown that the differentiation of the metanephric blastema into the definitive kidney in higher mammals does not ensue unless an interaction is carried out with the developing ureteric bud derived from the mesonephric duct. In his experiments, when the analogues of these

two structures were cultured in vitro in contact with one another,
the differentiation of the blastema ensued. However, if they were
cultured a short distance from one another in the same vessel, no
differentiation resulted. If the two primordia are separated by a
thin impermeable membrane, then again no differentiation is seen.
However, if the two primordia are separated by a permeable membrane,
then differentiation ensues, implying that there is a transfer of a
stimulus from the ureteric bud to the blastema leading to tubal and
nephron formation.

Ferm et al. (1971) have shown that administration of relatively
high doses of sodium arsenate at a critical period during
organogenesis in the rat resulted in defective renal formation or
complete renal agenesis (Ferm and Hanlon, this volume). Beaudoin
and Burk (1974; 1977) have confirmed Ferm's observation, and have
shown that the renal agenesis is caused by a failure of ureteric bud
formation; thus arsenic interferes with the inductive interaction by
impeding or destroying the formation of the ureteric bud. When the
ureteric bud was partially formed, the resultant kidney was also
partially formed, or if the ureteric bud formed unilaterally, the
nephrogenesis was unilateral as well.

Another potentially significant aspect of this demonstration of
interference by environmental agents with inductive interaction was
the observation by Ferm and Kilham (1977) that if the dose of sodium
arsenate was decreased by one-half, normal morphogenesis ensued.
If, however, at this dose level the animals were exposed to
hyperthermia during the sensitive period, then renal agenesis would
result. Hyperthermia alone at subteratogenic levels did not cause
the agenesis. This may be a model of how two or more agents could
act synergistically to produce an anomaly, when the dose level of
each individual agent was insufficient to produce anomalies.

B. Experimental Aspects of Metal Teratogenesis and Perinatal
    Toxicity

The design for experimental investigation of the teratogenic
and perinatal effects of metals must be carefully considered,
because the interpretation and significance of the results hinge
directly on it. The design variables can be readily divided into
three groups pertaining to the selection of a) animal or in vitro
models, b) the species of the metal, and c) treatment schedule. The
reports by Ferm and Hanlon (this volume), Sunderman et al. (this
volume), Magos and Webb (this volume), and Fowler (this volume)
clearly illustrate these parameters. The direct transposition of
laboratory animal results to humans is hazardous at best without
confirmation of the findings in human or subhuman primates. Even
the latter have some differences from humans in their biological
responses to metals. The laboratory production of malformations

makes it possible to study directly the mechanisms of abnormal
development. In addition, experimental models are an essential
method for screening agents for possible teratogenicity. Among the
major considerations for animal experimentation are species and
strain specificity. One cannot reliably predict from one species
the teratogenic effects in another. For example, the time necessary
for a rat to eliminate half a dose of methylmerury is 10-25 days,
whereas in the human and subhuman primate the half-time is 40-60
days. Therefore, rats are more tolerant to a given dose of mercury,
and the dosage must be increased to maintain a blood level
comparable to that of human exposure.

Another important species variable is the structure and
function of the placenta. One section of this conference
(Metabolism of Metals) deals in detail with this variable. Of
special import are the posters presented by Danielsson et al. and
the report by Copius Peereboom-Stegeman. Danielsson et al. (1982)
illustrated the role of the placenta in chromium transport in
cartilage formation. Copius Peereboom-Stegeman et al. (1982)
demonstrated the effects of chronic cadmium exposure on blood vessel
basal lamina formation in the placenta of pregnant rats. Two series
of experiments were performed in which the average wall thickness of
microcirculatory blood vessels in the myometrium of the uteri of
rats was studied qualitatively and quantitatively. In group 1, a
semichronic experiment, Wistar rats (females) of about 180 g
received subcutaneously 0.5 mg $CdCl_2$/kg body weight. The
injections were given every 2 days for a period of 29 weeks
maximally. In group 2, a chronic experiment, the animals received
doses of 0.036 mg or 0.18 mg $CdCl_2$/kg bodyweight. The injections
were given every 2 days for a period of 80 weeks maximally. In both
experiments the injection site was between the scapulae; control
animals received the same volume of saline or no treatment at all.

Quantitatively, an increase in thickness of the media could be
demonstrated in all exposed animals. Qualitative inventory revealed
that only half of the vessels reacted, the others looking normal.
This inventory gave an indication of the start of the early cadmium
effects, with percentage of affected vessels rising sharply at the
0.5 mg level from the 8-9th week onward, and at the 0.18-0.16 mg
level from the 24-37th week onward.

Many teratogenic agents appear to produce their effect on the
fetus indirectly by altering maternal metabolism or the maternal-
fetal exchange of metabolic substances. Development of our
knowledge in this important area of teratology has been delayed
because the placentas of most readily available experimental animals
are not structurally or functionally comparable to the human or
subhuman primate placenta (Shultz, 1970; Beck, 1976; Juchau, 1980a,
1980b; Waddell and Marlowe, 1981). Of the species that have
chorioallantoic placenta, the structural features are markedly

different from the human. For example, in laboratory rats and mice,
a yolk-sac placenta is a structure that persists throughout much of
the early stages of gestation and is at least as important during
organogenesis as the subsequent chorioallantoic placenta. A large
inverted yolk sac surrounds the rodent fetus and provides direct
contact with the uterine tissue. The cells lining the yolk sac are
continuous with those that form the feta gut. The yolk sac may be
viewed as an outpouching from the midgut. The eipthelial surface of
the yolk sac closely resembles the epithelium of the intestine and
kidney, and thus apparently is well-adapted for both abosorption and
excretory function. Studies based on observation of the
chorioallantoic placenta transport at term can yield erroneous
tertogenic information because the yolk-sac placenta is the important
one during the early phases of gestation when the fetus is most
susceptible to injury by many agents. Whereas the transport of
materials from the mother to the fetus in the human and subhuman
primates involves its movement across the vascular endothelium,
connective tissue, and trophoblastic epithelium of the fetal cell
layers, the laboratory rodents generally have only the endothelium
and connective tissue layers in their placental villi. The guinea
pig has only the endothelial layer. These laboratory species have
hemoendothelial placentas, whereas the humans and monkeys have
hemochorial placentas. Although these anatomic barriers differ, this
does not fully represent the functional differences among these
different types of placentas. One must keep in mind that not only
the structural but the functional capacities of these placentas vary
with the age and gestation.

        During early gestation, the yolk-sac placenta is usually the
predominant organ for transfer of material between mother and fetus
in the rodents and rabbits. The importance of the comparative
placental histology can be seen readily as one compares the
significant features of fetal and placental development in laboratory
animals compared with the human. In the rat, implantation occurs at
5-1/2 days following fertilization, which is 3 days before the
beginning of gastrulation. Throughout this period the nutrition of
the developing embryo is largely histiotrophic. By the stage of
gastrulation, the yolk-sac placenta develops, and at this stage the
embryonic nutrition is largely associated with the ability of the
extra embryoic endoderm of the yolk sac to degrade macromolecules.
The histiotrophic nutrition appears to come from maternal blood
serum, secretion of uterine glands, and the destruction of
endometrial cells by the trophoblastic layer of the developing
blastocyst. At about the 20-somite stage, the chorioallantoic
placenta develops as a result of the fusion of the allantois with the
chorion. This third phase of nutrition in the rat begins at 11 days
of gestation. However, the yolk-sac endoderm and yolk-sac placenta
continue to be active until full term. For example, the yolk-sac
placenta is able to take up radioactive iodine-labeled bovine serum
albumin and digest it, and is able to ingest and degrade horseradish

peroxidase at 17-18 days of gestation.

The human and primate placental systems differ markedly from that of the rat. Implantation begins at about 7-1/2 days, and a small hillock of trophoblasts is formed at the point of penetration. Histiotrophic nutrition begins by digestion of endometrial tissue and endometrial secretions, and within 4 to 5 days the blastocyst becomes completely buried in the compact layers of the endometrium. Circulation through these evolving placental structures begins at about 13 days of gestation, and within 3 days gastrulation begins. Nutrition of the developing embryo is still principally histiotrophic. About a week after the beginning of gastrulation, circulation is established through the chorionic ville, and the embryonic nutrition becomes hemotrophic. In contrast to the rodents, one can see that the human chorionic vesicle begins to develop rapidly following a brief period of histiotrophic nutrition, and soon the precocious development of the circulatory system results in hemotrophic nutrition through a hemochorial placenta at the 5-somite stage.

Old World monkeys follow a similar course of placental differentiation. As with the human, the cardiovascular system develops rapidly within two days of gastrulation, and the hemotrophic nutrition is established early at about the 5-somite stage of development. Thus the subhuman primates most nearly approximate the human in placental development and functions, and represent the best available model for the study of placental function and effects of noxious agents.

The placenta, being an organ derived from fetal cells, has the same genome as the fetus. The various cell layers of the placenta are derived from the developing embryo. The trophoblastic layer of cells is derived from the inner cell mass, and evidence strongly supports the idea that the connective tissue cells of the villous blood vessels, yolk sac, etc., are all derived from cells emanating from the endometrial stroma of the mother.

Age of the animals is another important variable in experimental design. The number and size of fetuses and the anomaly rate varies with the age of the dams; therefore, valid teratogenic studies must have animals of uniform age and parity. Many enzyme-dependent processes vary with the age of the experimental animals, as was described earlier in this chapter. This is especially true during the embryonic, fetal, and neonatal periods. The activity of an enzyme may be minimal during early development, subsequently increasing to higher levels during differentiation, and reaching high physiologically modulated levels following infancy. If a given dose of an agent is administered during early embryogenesis, its effect may be different from the same dose at a later stage of development.

Nutrition, seasonal variation, and physical environment of the laboratory are also important variables to consider. The mineral content of the food should be uniform and known, because of the well-established synergistic and antagonistic effects of trace metals. Diets developed to maximize body growth are not necessarily optimal for the study of health hazards. Diets must be adequate and uniform in all known nutritional groups, and trace mineral content should be known and standardized. Excessive loading with known wholesome elements should be avoided. Crowding and extremes in temperature are among factors which may stress the animals and alter their reproductive performance.

In recent years, cell and organ culture has replaced the use of animals in some teratogenic experiments because of low cost, opportunity to produce standard and uniform replicate conditions of experimentation, and the opportunity to investigate stages of development (preimplantation and early embryogenesis) that are difficult to study in vivo. While offering some advantages, the in vitro methods are associated with the introduction of major variables; the rate of differentation and proliferation of embryonic tissues may often be altered.

The chemical species of metal employed in experimentation is also a significant variable. Ionic mercury (Hg^+), for example, does not pass through the placenta, whereas methylmercury ($MeHg^+$) readily does. Nickel carbonyl is teratogenic, whereas many other nickel compounds are not. AsIII and AsIV have markedly different biological effects.

Similarly, the route of exposure is an important experimental variable. Oral, respiratory, and transcutaneous are the usual portals of entry for toxic metals. Experiments that utilize intravenous, peritoneal, or subcutaneous injections may significantly modify the effects of the toxic metal.

The manifestations of toxicological action depends upon the blood level of the agent; this in turn often depends upon the route of administration. The highest blood level is obtained when a soluble agent is administered intravenously. Subcutaneous and intramuscular routes also result in high blood levels. When the oral route is used, the relative rate and degree of absorption determine the blood level.

A sparingly soluble compound given orally may not produce a toxic effect, but if the same compound is administered by the endotracheal technique, the lung fluids may solubilize it readily. Many "insoluble" metals are also readily solubilized if administered intramuscularly.

If any attempt is made to extrapolate the teratological effects of a metal or its compounds to the human experience, the route of administration should if possible mimic the manner of human exposure.

Time of exposure is also an important parameter. Toxic agents generally affect a specific morphogenic event as noted above. Exposure to a toxic agent at the time the morphogenic event occurs is most likely to alter the developmental process. This is called the period of sensitivity, or critical stage. Since most visceral organ rudiments are actually formed during days 8 and 9 of development in rodents, this is referred to as the period of organogenesis or critical period.

Divalent metals may disturb these functions by acting as agonists or antagonists of calcium ions at binding sites. The potency at each site would then depend on the relative affinities of the site for calcium and of the competing metal ion.

Another class of toxic effects depends on the high affinity of metal ions to sulfhydryl groups at active site of membrane receptors, carriers, and enzymes. Again, the effects may be either activating or inhibitory at the lowest effective doses. At higher doses, and with a higher proportion of sulfhydryl groups bound by the metal, inhibition is the general effect of metals on all SH-dependent catalytic functions. This underscores the need for in vivo tests of realistic titers of metals.

Treatment schedules present another major group of variables. A single bolus of metal at high dose at a sensitive period of organogenesis is often used by teratologists to maximize the production of anomalous development. This approach, while highly useful in defining teratogenic potential, should not be assumed to provide information on teratogenic risk from environmental exposure. The latter is usually continuous throughout gestation at lower dose levels, and may yield markedly different results.

The pattern of exposure to a toxic metal is important to the developmental injury observed. Many teratogenesis experiments use a single-dose (usually high) exposure at a sensitive period of morphogenesis. Although an excellent probe to investigate morphogenic mechanisms and events, this seldom compares with the usual pattern of environmental exposure, namely, continuous chronic exposure throughout gestation. Often the latter provides markedly different results from the former.

Implicit in the above is the time of exposure. "Period of sensitivity" is a term used by teratologists to define the period of development when there is maximum effect of a teratogenic agent. Various sections of this conference deal with effects on the male and female reproductive organs, zygote, implantation, embryogenesis, fetogenesis, and perinatal stages of development. The effects vary depending on the metal and time of exposure.

The site of action of a teratogen may influence the method selected for quantitating the end point. The experiments of Magos and Webb (this volume) clearly demonstrate profound physiologic changes in the maternal organism during gestation produced by metal exposure. These changes can result in anomalous development of the fetus. Similarly, a metal may alter maternal nutrition, blood circulation, or placental function, indirectly producing maldevelopment.

In its broadest sense, the teratology of metals is a study of the adverse effects of metals on the developmental system. It includes all influences external to the developing individual, that is, amniotic fluid, placenta, uterus, maternal body, and the surrounding external physical and chemical environment. Temporally viewed, the toxic metal may affect the gonads of the paternal or maternal organism, resulting in genetic injury to the germ cells prior to fertilization, or the injurious interaction can occur between the event of fertilization and the implantation of the zygote in the uterine wall. Following implantation, the injurious agent may be transported through the maternal bloodstream to enter the developing embryo or fetus by passage through the yolk sac and/or placenta, resulting in injury at any time during embryonic or fetal development, or in the early postnatal period.

A list of possible sites of action follows:

1. Maternal/embryo-fetal relationships

2. Placenta effects

3. Direct embryofetal actions
    a. Inherent tissue sensitivity
    b. Cell-to-cell interactions
    c. Cell-organelles
        1) Cell membrane
        2) Nuclear/genetic
        3) Organelle (ER/mitochondria, etc)
        4) Embryovascular
    d. Molecular
        1) Morphogenic signals
        2) Energy supply
        3) Osmoregulation
        4) Biosynthetic capability

The extent of toxic action also depends on the effective concentration at the site of damage. For some compounds this can be estimated from the concentration in maternal blood. For others the blood level is not a good indicator. The toxicity of mercuric oxide (Berg and Smith, 1982) to pregnant mice is ample reminder that the species of a compound can modify the biologic effect observed.

Conference Reports on Congenital and Perinatal Toxicity

The foregoing provides a conceptual backgound with which the congenital defects and perinatal toxicity may be viewed.

The report by Ferm and Hanlon (this volume) on metal-induced congenital malformations is an excellent example of a classical teratogenesis experiment. Their objective is to reveal any teratogenic potential of the metals studied by maximizing the possibility of maldevelopment. They selected the hamster because of its short gestation period, accuracy of timed matings, brief and well-defined critical periods of organogenesis, and large litter size. By dosing the animals with one or two high-dose injections of a common salt of a metal at the critical period, the likelihood of an effect is maximal. Once an effect is revealed, then it is subject for further experiments designed to mimic actual environmental exposure conditions: portal of entry, dose, continuous exposure, etc. A common mistake is to assume that the classical teratogenic experimental results are transposable into environmental risk assessment. The experiments are not designed for that purpose.

Ferm and Hanlon (this volume) have reviewed the literature on metal-induced teratogenesis and observed that each metal causes a characteristic response in the form of a particular pattern of fetal anomalies. In general, the placenta is a partial barrier to the metals studied, and this suggests that maternal and placental mechanisms may be involved in the teratogenesis. Subsequent reports in this conference further defined some of these variables. Most of the abnormalities created by metal ions are reductive in nature, a decrease in developmental processes. Their experiments with arsenic teratogenesis represent a model of the way a subteratogenic dose of arsenic coupled with another factor (hyperthermia) can combine to be teratogenic. Further, this experiment is an excellent example of interference by a metal with cell-cell interactions resulting in an anomaly (renal agenesis).

The other major anomaly produced by congenital arsenic exposure is anencephaly or exencephaly, another reductionist effect. In the metabolism section of this conference, Dencker et al. (this volume) presented the results of their careful and precise whole-body embryo radioautography for a variety of metals throughout gestation. Their experiments on arsenic revealed high concentrations in the forebrain region. Morrissey and Mottet (this volume) have shown in a transmission and scanning electron microscopy study that there is

increased neuroepithelial cell necrosis in the forebrain at the time
of closure. It is tempting to presume that the high arsenic dose
leads to some necrosis in the forebrain, a reductionist effect,
leading to a failure of closure of the anterior neuropore and thus
anencephaly.

The embryotoxicity and teratogenicity of nickel compounds
reported by Sunderman et al. (this volume) utilize rats and a
similar experimental design, but with two major differences. They
studied the potential of several nickel compounds and found $Ni(CO_4)$
to be the most teratogenic. In addition to describing the fetal
malformations, they pursued the mechanisms on the cellular and
molecular levels, and the effects of intravenous versus oral
administration. Administration of $Ni(CO_4)$ to pregnant Fisher rat
dams by intravenous injection (11 µg/kg) on day 7 of gestation caused
increased fetal mortality, diminished body weight of live pups, and
16 percent incidence of fetal malformations, including anophthalmia,
microphthalmia, cystic lungs, and hydronephrosis. In the second
experiment, a dominant lethal mutation test in male rats,
administration of $Ni(CO_4)$ by inhalation (0.05 mg/Ni/liter/15 min)
2 to 6 weeks prior to breeding did not impair fertilization rates or
reproductive yields; under the same conditions, administration of
$Ni(CO_4)$ by intravenous injection (22 µg/kg) diminished the number
of live pups in litters sired during the fifth week, consistent with
chromosomal damage during the meiotic stage of spermatogenesis. In
the third experiment, administration of Ni_3S_2 to female rats by
intrarenal (IR) injection (30 µg/Ni/kg) one week prior to breeding
produced intense erythrocytosis in the dams but did not cause
erythrocytosis in the pups; on the contrary, pups from Ni_3S_2-
treated dams had diminished hematocrits at 2 weeks postpartum. In
the light of previous reports that Ni_3S_2-induced erythrocytosis
is mediated by increased renal production of erythropoietin, the
present observations suggest that increased erythropoietin activity
in maternal serum does not stimulate erythropoiesis in the fetus.

Whereas teratogenesis is the end point, in vivo experiments
such as the above do not ordinarily identify whether the metal is
acting on the maternal metabolism, placenta, or fetus, or a
combination of sites. Other sections of the conference describe
male and female reproductive effects prior to or during zygote
formation. The careful investigations of Magos and Webb (this
volume) clearly demonstrate the effects of physiologic and weight
changes in the maternal organism during pregnancy and lactation, and
the effects of these changes on the toxicity of mercury and cadmium.
Several often overlooked variables are clearly defined in their
investigation.

Weight and other physiological changes during pregnancy and
lactation may alter a) the target organ, b) the elimination rate,
and c) the whole-body concentration of a toxic metal, and also
disturb the use of weight loss as a toxic response.

Such changes and interactions are illustrated by the toxic effects of cadmium, mercury, and methylmercury. Thus at the end of pregnancy the target organ for cadmium is changed and acute toxicity is increased. The change in the toxicity of cadmium in late pregnancy can be related at least partly to an increase in the placental accumulation of this metal (Miller and Shaikh, this volume).

Lactation accelerates the elimination of methylmercury from the whole body and improves the clinical condition of lactating female rats without a decline either in the brain concentration of methylmercury or in cerebellar damage.

When weight loss is used as a response against dose, nonpregnant animals seem to be more sensitive to the toxic effect of methylmercury than pregnant ones because the toxic effect on weight (e.g., on food consumption) is imposed on very different weight curves. However, when coordination disorders are used against the body concentration of methylmercury, in virgin rats which lose more body weight and thus concentrate their body burden in a smaller body volume, coordination disorders occur at higher body concentrations than in pregnant rats.

Based on the above review, metal-induced teratogenesis has been well-studied in a number of animal models, and deleterious effects characterized at both organ and tissue levels of biological organization. The mechanisms underlying these changes in organ morphogenesis have received much less attention, but it seems clear that primary effects of metal-teratogens must be initially manifested on the molecular level. A description of teratogens is hence not complete without some discussion of the possible relationships between metal-induced biochemical dysfunction and tissue development.

There are at present relatively few intracellular studies concerning either the ultrastructural or biochemical effects of toxic elements on developing organelle systems. Ultrastructural studies which show cellular vesiculation, mitochondrial damage, and cellular necrosis have been reported for lead and arsenate. Ultrastructural and biochemical data are available for the effects of methylmercury on fetal organisms (Fowler and Woods, 1977; Fowler, this volume). These studies show cellular vesiculation of hepatocytes, decreased mitochondrial protein associated with inhibition of mitochondrial biogenesis, and decreased respiratory function. Other studies by Mottet (1974) and Chen et al. (1979) have also demonstrated reduced DNA synthesis in fetal rats, which suggests that a number of biochemical dysfunctions may be operating in concert to produce the observed effects. One, or a combination of these effects, appears to be responsible for the known reduction in fetal size at doses of methylmercury below which overt teratogenic or maternal toxicity are observed.

The ease of placental transport alters the site of injury for different metals. For example, 1) cadmium exposure during pregnancy and lactation may cause increased risk of adverse responses in the mother due to cadmium accumulation in maternal tissues (Ferm and Hanlon, this volume), whereas 2) lead exposure during pregnancy and lactation might first influence the fetus and neonate by ready transfer of lead to the fetus (Bridbord, 1978; Rom, 1980).

The influence of pregnancy and lactation on gastrointestinal absorption of cadmium and lead reveals a striking contrast between the two metals. Cadmium absorption in the dam during lactation is increased 2- to 3-fold over that in nonpregnant mice. Cadmium taken up by the dam during lactation is almost entirely retained by her own tissues (mainly kidney and liver); very little is passed on to the pups via milk or excreted via urine. Striking increases in cadmium retention by the kidney (5-fold), duodenum (12-fold), and mammary tissue (11-fold) of the dam occur during gestation and lactation.

As noted previously, the onset of prenatal enzyme activity may alter the prenatal toxicity of a metal. This applies to the perinatal period as well. A very interesting poster on ontogenic changes in the biliary secretion of methylmercury and glutathione, by Ballatori and Clarkson (1982), revealed that neonatal rats treated with methylmercury excrete only a small fraction of the administered dose of mercury, when compared to adults. At 16 to 18 days of age, there is an abrupt increase in mercury excretion, reaching adult rates of elimination. Bile is an important route for the elimination of methylmercury, which is present in bile mainly as a complex with glutathione. The rate at which the 14-day-old rat secretes methylmercury in bile is one-tenth that of the 28-day-old rat. Development of the ability to secrete methylmercury in bile parallels the development of the ability to secrete glutathione in bile. The immaturity of this biliary transport system in the neonate may explain the long biological half-time for methylmercury in suckling rats.

Berg and Smith (1982) presented a poster on the toxicity of mercuric oxide to pregnant mice and the mechanism of resistance of prenatally exposed litters. Single doses of mercuric oxide were administered by gavage to BALB/c mice at times ranging from day 4 through day 12 of gestation, at dosages ranging from 25 μg to 125 mg HgO/g (LD6 through LD55). Litters examined 17.5 days post impregnation showed only minor damages. Dose-dependent increases in late resorptions and decreases in fetal weights accounted for only 30 percent of weight deficits found in poisoned dams. Terata occurred more frequently in exposed litters than in sham-treated controls (35 in 202 litters compared to 5 in 77, single-tail, $p < 0.05$), frequency was not correlated with dose.

Elimination data fit a three-compartment model ($t_{1/2}$ respectively, 9 hours, 2 days, and 15 days) with rate constants 8 times faster than previously reported in rats. One hundred percent of dose was recovered in feces and urine in a 9:1 ratio. Highest organ concentrations were in maternal kidneys, liver, and placentae, lowest in maternal brains and fetuses; rates of loss were fastest from digestive tract and liver, slowest from brains and fetuses. Concentrations in neonates were several-fold lower than in delivered mothers.

HUMAN CLINICAL AND EPIDEMIOLOGICAL STUDIES

Numerous well-documented clinical and epidemiological studies on adults of the toxic effects of the metals discussed in this conference have been reported. Reports of congenital exposure and teratogenic or perinatal effects, either clinical or epidemiological, are scanty. Population exposure and congenital exposure to industrial effluents containing a mixture of metals have been reported (Milham, 1977; Pershagen et al., 1977). Hemminki's report (this volume) on spontaneous abortions using Finland's nation-wide registry illustrates the difficulty of identification of the offending agent. Female metalworkers and welders were identified as a high-risk population, but the specific agent or continuation periods of exposure remain elusive.

Congenital exposure to methylmercury in the human has been well-reported as collections of clinical cases (Piotrowski and Inskip, 1981). Harada (1968) discussed the findings of the 22 cases (including 2 deaths) of congenital exposure to mercury in the Minamata Bay episode. Most were breastfed; therefore they also had neonatal exposure to methylmercury. Twenty of the infants were below normal in size, and six had microcephal. All had "mental disturbances," with alteration of coordination, gait, and speech. The effects of mercury exposure on vision were not well-tested.

A report of one case of congenital exposure to alkyl mercury in Sweden (Engelson and Herner, 1952) revealed mental retardation. Amin-Zaki et al. (1979) reported follow-up studies of 15 mother-infant pairs from Iraq. Six of the fifteen infants showed gross motor incoordination, mental retardation, and cerebral palsy, with deafness and blindness in four cases. One case of congenital alkyl mercury exposure from the United States revealed grossly tremulous movements during the first few days of life. Myoclonic convulsions subsequently developed, and the child could not sit up at 1 year of age (Pierce et al., 1972).

Regretfully, pathologic studies of neonatal deaths are virtually absent; thus, other than microencephaly, virtually nothing is known of the nature of the malformations involved.

Lead effects on human reproduction have also been reported. Severe exposure of pregnant human females to high levels of lead has resulted in stillbirths or abortion (Rom, 1980). Following excessive industrial exposure of women with no neurologic symptoms, the offspring frequently have both an intrauterine and postnatal growth retardation, but no malformations have been documented.

Excessive intake of arsenic has been associated with a variety of disease processes in the adult human (Pershagen et al., 1977), and its toxic manifestations as a suicidal and homicidal agent have long been known. That arsenic compounds in the pregnant woman can be transported to the developing fetus has also long been known, since organic arsenicals were used as antisyphilitic agents long before the development of antibiotics (Eastman, 1931). The organic arsenicals are stored within the fetus and placenta (Underhill and Amatruda, 1923), and are slowly released into the fetal circulation. At the clinical doses used to treat syphilis there was no apparent induction of arsenic congenital malformations. A case of maternal human inorganic arsenic poisoning during pregnancy with subsequent fetal death was reported by Lugo et al. (1969). However, no unusual pathologic changes were seen in the fetus other than hyaline membrane disease, a very common cause of neonatal death.

Cadmium has not been identified as a human teratogen either in clinical case reports or in epidemiological studies. However, one report from the U.S.S.R. (Cvetkova, 1979) recorded that offspring of cadmium-exposed women had lower birth weights than controls.

Chronic exposure to excessive copper does not represent a major toxicological problem in human medicine, although occasionally it may occur in infants as a result of excessive intake. Women with Wilson's Disease (a genetically determined trait characterized by massive accumulation of copper in tissues, especially the liver and brain) have children without evidence of copper-induced anomalies. There is some evidence that these women have increased numbers of fetal deaths (Milham, 1977).

One might surmise that an excess or deficiency of copper might be significant in the developing embryo because copper plays an essential role in the activity of several enzymes, including tryosinase, uricase, and butyryl coenzyme-A-dehydrogenase. Also, copper occurs bound to proteins as a metalloprotein, and is an essential component of monoamine oxidase. In spite of the significant enzymatic activities for copper, only one of the experimental observations on the teratogenicity of copper is the study by Di Carlo (1980) on copper-induced cardiac malformations.

Nickel is an essential trace element in mammalian nutrition, but its functional role is not well-understood. Alteration of nickel metabolism is associated with several human diseases. These

include acute pneumonitis from inhalation of nickel aerosols,
increased incidence of cancers of the nasal cavities and lungs in
nickel workers, and a dermatitis and hypersensitivity reaction from
cutaneous exposures to nickel alloys. Although there are not
reports of embryotoxicity of nickel in the human, the teratogenic
effects of nickel carbonyl and subsulfide toxicity to embryos and
fetuses in experimental animals was presented by Sunderman et al.
(this volume).

The significance of manganese excess in producing toxicity to
the developing embryo and fetus remains largely unknown. Some
experiments indicate that the embryocidal levels of manganese in the
Golden hamster are relatively high; no teratogenic threat has been
demonstrated.

CONCLUSIONS AND RESEARCH NEEDS

The reports presented at this conference and the discussions
that followed amply demonstrated the need for further research on
the effects of metals on fertility, and on embryo/fetal and neonatal
development. It is one of the most pressing needs of industrial
society. Whether a human thrives, or indeed survives, is dependent
on undamaged maturation of the male and female germ cells, their
union to form a zygote, and its optimal prenatal and postnatal
development into a normal human. Some metals pose a potential risk
to that process.

It is clear that adverse effects in the maternal organism of
experimental animals produced by exposure to some metals may play a
role in altering normal embryonic/fetal developmental patterns, but
the molecular mechanisms by which these effects are produced are
incompletely known. Thus our knowledge is far short of predictive
value. Animal experiments, while valuable in identifying potential
problems, often cannot be directly transposed to the human. Animal
studies on prenatal exposure to lead, mercury, arsenic, and cadmium
are woefully inadequate.

Research Need No. 1. Further research is needed to elucidate
the various possible mechanisms of metal-induced alterations of
normal maternal-embryonic/fetal relationships which produce
developmental anomalies.

As revealed by the report of Magos and Webb (this volume),
physiological changes in dam during pregnancy and lactation may ater
the whole body concentration and elimination rate of a toxic metal.
Relative organ burdens may vary depending on dose, day of gestation
for administration, and dosage schedule (single large dose versus
repeated smaller doses). These important maternal changes need to
be defined in several species.

Research Need No. 2.   There is currently a paucity of data
concerning dose-response relationships between single high dose and
continuous low dose parental exposure to metals, and developmental
abnormalities, so that improvements may be made in interpretation
and extrapolation of experimental results.

The report of Ferm and Hanlon (this volume) amply demonstrates
the importance of dose as well as selection of species, time of
exposure (day of gestation) and route of administration when
malformations are most likely to be produced. When optimizing the
above conditions, they were able to show that mercury, copper,
arsenic, lead, cadmium, and indium were associated with specific
malformations. Others have shown that continuous low level exposure
throughout gestation may be less likely to produce specific
anomalies, but nevertheless, significant development defects. In
humans and in non-human primates, methylmercury and lead have been
shown to alter the development of the nervous system resulting in
probable behavioral changes. The effects of nickel, cadmium,
arsenic, and copper on human development lack specific
documentation. Further investigations, such as human epidemiologic
and non-human primate studies, are needed to determine the
significance of exposure to these metals to humans.

Research Need No. 3.   Different toxic trace elements and
chemical species of these elements have different embryopathic
effects, depending upon dose level and schedule before and during
pregnancy. Interactive factors such as dietary composition,
species, and strain differences appear to play an important role in
determining both the nature and severity of specific embryopathic/
teratogenic lesions for a given metal or chemical species of that
metal. Further studies are needed to delineate the most important
of these factors with respect to a specific given embryopathic end
point, and to evaluate the relationship between these interactive
factors and a given lesion.

Research Need No. 4.   The critical interactive factors
influencing the direct effects of metals on the target tissues of
the placental-embryofetal unit are diverse, and special attention
should be directed toward basic mechanisms of action. Further
studies at the cellular/molecular levels are needed to elucidate the
mechanisms by which interactive factors modify the direct critical
effects of metals on the parental-embryo/fetal unit.

As demonstrated by the experiments of Sunderman et al. (this
volume) reviewed in this volume, different routes of administration
as well as different compounds of nickel ($Ni(CO_4)$ versus
Ni_3S_2) profoundly alter the developmental effects observed. The
former produces several anatomic malformations whereas the latter
induces erythrocytosis in the rat dams but did not in the pups. The
dams had increased erythropoietin activity but this did not induce

erythropoietin in the pups. This is another example of the
importance of considering the maternal-embryo/fetal unit and the
importance of investigating the effects at the molecular level.

In a similar manner, Fowler (this volume) showed the value of
investigations on the subcellular and molecular level if one is to
develop a mechanistic explanation of toxic metal teratogenesis.
This may further serve to explain species and dose differences and
lead towards a more unified concept of mechanism.

Research Need No. 5. In vitro studies are needed to understand
mechanisms of direct metal action on embryonic/fetal tissues and to
develop test systems for screening potential teratogens.

There presently exists no logical basis for comparison of
effects of agents on non-human species to effects on humans.
Current testing protocols do not fill this need.

In vitro screening tests for evaluating teratogenic potential
have not been developed as they have for potential carcinogens.
Such tests would be useful for both mechanistic and screening
studies. Metals may provide useful probes in developing simple and
rapid screening tools for assessing teratogenic potential.

Viewing Research Needs 4 and 5 together, it becomes apparent
that much more extensive investigation of the mechanisms of action
on the subcellular and molecular levels are needed if one is to
ultimately evolve practical, valid in vitro tests for teratogenic
risks of toxic elements and their various chemical species.

Research Need No. 6. Investigations of basic mechanisms of
teratogenesis should be emphasized over screening protocols now in
use to allow intepretation of the way in which teratogenesis in
animals relates to humans. Carefully defined epidemiological
studies of human cogenital exposure are needed. The latter provide
guidance toward the most fruitful avenues of investigation.

REFERENCES

Amin-Zaki, L., Majeed, M.A., Elhassani, S.B., Clarkson, T.W.,
    Greenwood, M.R. and Doherty, R.A., 1979, Prenatal methylmercury
    poisoning: clinical observation over five years, Am. J. Dis.
    Child. 133:172-177.
Ballan-Dufrancais, C., Ruste, J. and Jeantet, A.Y., 1980,
    Quantitative electron probe microanalysis on insects exposed to
    mercury. I. Methods. An approach on the molecular form of the
    stored mercury. Possible occurrence of metallothionein-like
    proteins, Biol. Cellulaire 39:317-324.

Ballatori, N. and Clarkson, T.W., 1982, Ontogenic changes in the biliary secretion of methylmercury and glutathione, Teratology 26:46A.

Baserga, R., 1981, The cell cycle, N. Engl. J. Med. 304:453-459.

Beaudoin, A.R., 1974, Teratogenicity of sodium arsenate in rats, Teratology 10:153-158.

Beck, F., 1976, Comparative placental morphology and function, Env. Health Persp. 18:5-12.

Berg, G.G. and Smith, B.S., 1982, Toxicity of mercuric oxide to pregnant mice and the mechanism of resistance of prenatally exposed litters, Teratology 26:46A.

Brent, R.L. and Jensh, R.P., 1967, Intrauterine growth retardation, Adv. in Teratology 2:139-227.

Bridbord, K., 1978, Occupational lead exposure and women, Prev. Med. 7:311-321.

Burk, D. and Beaudoin, A.R., 1977, Arsenate-induced renal agenesis in rats, Teratology 16:247-260.

Chen, W.J., Body, R.L. and Mottet, N.K., 1979, Some effects of continuous low dose congenital exposure to methylmercury on organ growth in the rat fetus, Teratology 20:31-36.

Copius Peereboom-Stegeman, J.H.J., Jongstra-Spaapen, E. and Oosting, J., 1982, Effect of chronic cadmium exposure on blood vessels in the uterus of the rat, Teratology 26:50A.

Cvetkova, R.P., 1979, referred to in "Handbook of Toxic Metals", L. Friberg, G. Norberg, and V.B. Vouk, eds., p. 372, Elsevier/ North Holland, Amsterdam.

Danielsson, B., Hassoun, E. and Dencker, L., 1982, Placental transport of chromium (Cr) and its effects on cartilage formation, Teratology 26:47A.

Di Carlo, F.J., 1980, Syndromes of cardiovascular malformations induced by copper citrate in hamsters, Teratology 21:89-101.

Eastman, N.J., 1931, The arsenic content of the human placenta following arsphenamine therapy, Am. J. Obstet. Gynecol. 21:60-64.

Eichhorn, G.L. and Shin, Y.Y., 1968, Interaction of metal ions with polynucleotides and related compounds, Jour. Am. Chem. Soc. 90:7323-7328.

Eichhorn, G.L. and Marzilli, L., eds., 1981, "Metal Ions in Genetic Information Transfer", Elsevier/North Holland, New York.

Engelson, G. and Herner, T., 1952, Alkyl mercury poisoning, Acta Paed. Scand. 41:289-294.

Ferm, V.H. and Kilham, L., 1977, Synergistic teratogenic effects of arsenic and hyperthermia in hamsters, Env. Res. 14:483-486.

Ferm, V.H., Saxon, A. and Smith, B.M., 1971, The teratogenic profile of sodium arsenate in the Golden hamster, Arch. Env. Health 22:557-560.

Fowler, B.A. and Woods, J.S., 1977, The transplacental toxicity of methylmercury to fetal rat liver mitochondria: Morphometric and biochemical studies, Lab. Invest. 36:122-130.

Fowler, B.A., Brown, H.W., Lucier, G.W. and Krigman, M.R., 1975, The effects of chronic oral methylmercury exposure on the lysosome system of rat kidney. Morphometric and biochemical studies, Lab. Invest. 32:313-322.

Glucksmann, A., 1951, Cell death in normal vertebrate ontogeny, Biol. Rev. 26:59-85.

Goss, R.J., 1972, Theories of growth regulation, in: "Regulation of Organ and Tissue Growth", Chap. 1, R.J. Goss, ed., Academic Press, New York.

Grobstein, C., 1964, Cytodifferentiation and its control, Science 243:643-650.

Grobstein, C., 1967, Mechanisms of organogenetic tissue interaction, Nat. Cancer Inst. Monograph No. 26.

Hamburger, V., 1958, Regression versus peripheral control of differentiation and hypoplasia, Am. J. Anat. 102:365-409.

Harada, Y., 1968, Minamata disease, in: "Clinical Investigations on Minamata Disease", Chap. 3, Kumamoto Medical School Press, Kumamoto, Japan.

Jacobson, A.G., 1966, Inductive processes in embryonic development, Science 152:25-34.

Jacobson, B.J. and Turner, J.E., 1980, The interaction of cadmium and certain other metal ions with proteins and nucleic acids, Toxicology 16:1-37.

Jeantet, A.Y., Ballan-Dufrancais, C. and Ruste, J., 1980, Quantitative electron probe microanalysis on insects exposed to mercury. II. Involvement of the lysosomal system in detoxification processes, Biol. Cellulaire 39:325-334.

Juchau, M., 1980a, Drug biotransformation in the placenta, Pharm. Ther. 8:501-524.

Juchau, M., 1980b, "The Biochemical Basis of Chemical Teratogenesis", Elsevier/North Holland, New York.

Kohler, E., Merker, H.J., Ehmke, W. and Wojnorwicz, F., 1972, Growth kinetics of mammalian embryos during stages of differentiation, Naunyn-Schmiedebergs Arch. Pharmacol. 272:169-181.

Lauwerys, R. and Buchet, J-P., 1972, Study on the mechanism of lysosome labilization by inorganic mercury in utero, Eur. J. Biochem. 26:535-542.

Lugo, G., Cassady, G. and Palmiseno, P., 1969, Acute maternal arsenic intoxication with neonatal death, Am. J. Dis. Child 117:328-330.

Madsen, K.M and Christensen, E.I., 1978, Effects of mercury on lysosomal protein digestion in the kidney proximal tubule, Lab. Invest. 38:165-174.

McLoughlin, C.B., 1961, The importance of mesenchymal factors in the differentiation of chick epidermis, J. Embryol. Exper. Morph. 9:370-409.

Milham, S., 1977, Studies of morbidity near a copper smelter, Env. Health Persp. 19:131-133.

Morrissey, R.E. and Mottet, N.K., 1983, Arsenic-induced exencephaly in mice: Studies on lesions occurring during neurulation, Teratology, in press.

124   N. K. MOTTET AND V. H. FERM

Moscona, A.A., 1973, Cell aggregation, in: "Cell Biology in
    Medicine", E.E. Bittar, ed., pp. 571-591, John Wiley and Sons,
    New York.
Moscona, A.A., 1974, The cell surface development, in: "Surface
    Specification of Embryonic Cells: Receptors, Cell Recognition,
    and Specific Cell Ligands", Chap. 5, John Wiley and Sons, New
    York.
Mottet, N.K., 1952, The effect of the removal of somatopleure on the
    development of motor and sensory neurons in the spinal cord and
    ganglia, J. Comp. Neurol. 96:519-553.
Mottet, N.K., 1974, Effects of chronic low dose exposure of rat
    fetuses to methylmercury hydroxide, Teratology 10:173-189.
Mottet, N.K., 1981, Biochemical mechanisms of trace element
    teratogenesis, in "The Biochemical Basis of Chemical
    Teratogenesis", M. Juchau, ed., Chap. 7, Elsevier/North
    Holland, New York.
Mottet, N.K. and Hammar, S.P., 1972, Ribosome crystals in
    necrotizing cells from the posterior necrotic zone of the
    developing chick limb, J. Cell Sci. 11:403-411.
Pershagen, G., Elinder, C-G. and Bolander, A.M., 1977, Mortality in
    a region surrounding an arsenic emitting smelter, Env. Health
    Persp. 19:133-137.
Pierce, P.E., Thompson, J.F., Likosky, W.H., Nickey, L.N., Barthel,
    W.F. and Hinman, A.R., 1972, Alkylmercury poisoning in humans,
    JAMA 220:1439-1442.
Piotrowski, J.K. and Inskip, M.J., 1981, Health effects of
    methylmercury, MARC Technical Report No. 24, Chelsea College,
    London.
Rice, J.M., 1973, An overview of transplacental carcinogenesis,
    Teratology 8:113-126.
Rom, W.N., 1980, Effects of lead on reproduction, in "A Workshop on
    Methodology for Assessing Reproductive Hazards in the
    Workplace", P.F. Infante and M.S. Legator, eds., NIOSH,
    Cincinnati, Ohio.
Rutter, W.J., Clark, W.R., Kemp, J.D., Bradshaw, W.S., Sanders, T.G.
    and Ball, W.D., 1968, Multiphasic regulation in
    cytodifferentiation, in "Epithelial-Mesenchymal Interactions",
    R. Fleischmajer and R.E. Billingham, eds., Chap. 7, Williams
    and Wilkins Co., Baltimore.
Rutter, W.J., Pictet, R.L. and Morris, T.W., 1973, Toward molecular
    mechanisms of developmental processes, Ann. Rev. Biochem.
    42:601-621.
Sager, P.R., Doherty, R.A. and Rodier, P.M., 1982, Effect of
    methylmercury on developing cerebellar cortex, Teratology
    26:49A.
Saunders, J.W., Jr., 1966, Death in embryonic systems, Science
    15:604-612.
Schultz, R.L., 1970, Placental transport: A review, Obst. and
    Gynecol. Survey 25:979-1020.

Sissoeff, I., Grisvard, J., and Guille, E., 1976, Studies on metal
    ions-DNA interactions: Specific behavior of reiterative DNA
    sequences, Prog. Biophys. Molec. Biol. 31:1-34.
Southard, J., Nitisewojo, P., and Green, E.E., 1974, Mercurial
    toxicity and perturbation of the mitochondrial control system,
    Fed. Proc. 33:2147-2153.
Spemann, H., 1938, Embryonic development and induction, Yale
    University Press.
Spiro, T.G., ed., 1980, "Nucleic Acid-Metal Ion Interactions", John
    Wiley and Sons, New York.
Sternlieb, I., and Goldfischer, S., 1976, Heavy metals and
    lysosomes, in: "Lysosomes in Biology and Pathology", J.T.
    Dingle and R.T. Dean, eds., Vol. V, pp. 185-200, Elsevier/North
    Holland, Amsterdam.
Underhill, F.P. and Amatruda, F.G., 1923, The transmission of
    arsenic from mother to fetus, JAMA 81:2009-2012.
Verity, M.A. and Reith, A., 1967, Effect of mercurial compounds of
    structure-linked latency of lysosome hydrolases, Biochem. J.
    105:685-690.
Vogel, D.G., Margolis, R.L. and Mottet, N.K., 1982, The effects of
    methylmercury binding to microtubules, The Toxicologist 2:5.
Waddell, W.J. and Marlowe, C., 1981, Biochemical regulation of the
    accessibility of teratogens to the developing embryo, in: "The
    Biochemical Basis of Chemical Teratogenesis", M.R. Jachau, ed.,
    Elsevier/North Holland, New York.
Warren, S.L., Fanger, M. and Neet, K.E., 1980, Inhibition of
    biological activity of mouse β-nerve growth factor by
    monoclonal antibody, Science 210:910-912.
Young, M., Oger, J., Blanchard, M.H., Amos, H. and Arnason, B.G.W.,
    1975, Secretion of a nerve growth factor by primary chick
    fibroblast cultures, Science 187:361-362.
Zakour, R.A., Tkeshelashvili, L.K., Shearman, C.W., Koplitz, R.M.,
    and Loeb, L.A., 1981, Metal induced infidelity of DNA
    synthesis, J. Cancer Res. Clin. Oncol. 99:187-196.

EFFECTS OF METALS: THE DEVELOPING CENTRAL NERVOUS SYSTEM

Patricia M. Rodier

Working Group: J. Julian Chisolm, Jr., Ben H. Choi,
   Carol Kellogg, Nellie Laughlin, Deborah Rice, Tore Syversen,
   Patricia M. Rodier, Steve Gilbert, Robert Infurna, Helen Tryphonas

Review Article Contents:

EFFECTS OF METALS: THE DEVELOPING CENTRAL NERVOUS SYSTEM

Patricia M. Rodier

Department of Anatomy
University of Rochester School of Medicine
Rochester, New York

INTRODUCTION

There are many recent reviews of special aspects of lead or
mercury toxicity, and most focus on the effects of metal compounds on
the CNS. Most do not, however, address the question central to this
conference -- "Are the effects of metals on developing organisms
different from the effects on adults?" The purpose of this chapter
is to summarize the known effects very briefly, referring the reader
to more comprehensive sources, to highlight data suggestive of
distinctive developmental injuries, and to point out the kinds of
information still lacking.

The EPA Lead Standard (1977) references most of the lead
toxicity literature and a new standard, still in preparation, will
provide an update on the recent literature. Two excellent books have
appeared, "Lead Toxicity" by Singhal and Thomas (1980) and "Low Level
Lead Exposure: The Clinical Implications of Current Research" by
Needleman (1980). Many chapters from these volumes deal with
functional or biochemical effects of lead on the CNS and are cited
throughout this chapter. Each review has features of great value.
For example, Jason and Kellogg (1980) supply a section which helps
the reader estimate blood levels from treatments described as percent
of diet. The same chapter has an interesting discussion of the
behavioral tests which seem most sensitive to early lead exposure
effects. The companion clinical and animal model articles by
Bornschein et al. (1981) describe many important lead experiments in
some detail, and suggest some explanations of apparent contradictions
among the different studies. Rutter's (1980) review of the clinical
literature emphasizes the methodological difficulties that have
plagued the field, but also points out some consistent findings
across many studies.

The literature on mercury has been reviewed less extensively than that on lead, but several volumes are available. "Mercury, Mercurials and Mercaptans" (Miller and Clarkson, 1973) does not emphasize neurological effects, but provides background on the chemical and biologic properties of these metals. "Minimata Disease" (Tsubaki and Irukayama, 1977) is a compilation of papers based on the Japanese epidemic. A recent review by Clarkson (1983) discusses possible mechanisms of methylmercury action on developing nervous systems and a review by Chang et al. (1980) emphasizes effects on developing organisms. Chisholm and Thomas' review (this volume) was used in developing the part of this chapter on dose-response relationships.

PATTERNS OF DEVELOPMENT OF NORMAL STRUCTURE AND FUNCTION

The nervous system has long been a favorite subject of embryologists and so the literature on the development of its form and function is massive. Yet, because the nervous system offers so many developmental processes to be studied, and so many cell types and cell interactions to be described, the information toxicologists need to understand the reactions of developing neural tissue to toxic agents is often unavailable or at least, not easily accessible. The most comprehensive text on developmental neurobiology is Jacobson's (1978) superb monograph, which captures both the excitement and the frustrations of the field, and introduces many of the questions that have absorbed generations of investigators. What controls the number of neurons produced and the number which survive? How do neurons find their targets? How do they find their final locations? When do neurons lose their flexibility and become determined to differentiate along particular lines? To what extent do the characteristics of a neuron depend on internal versus external influences? To what extent are developmental "mistakes" reflected in function? What degree of deviation from normal form is necessary to produce functional differences? The questions seem endless and the answers to them may not be the same for different neurons or different groups of neurons.

As with many body systems, our knowledge of development of the human nervous system is particularly weak. In some regards, all the mammals studied appear to be similar. For example, the order in which different cell types form appears to be the same. But some aspects of the nervous system differ greatly from species to species, and we cannot expect development to be the same when even final form is different. For example, the projection of catecholamine neurons to hypothalamic nuclei (reviewed by Hoffman et al., 1976) appears to differ substantially among the rhesus monkey, squirrel monkey, cat, and rat. Lacking this kind of information for much of the brain, it is often difficult to know when we can extrapolate between species and when we cannot. We can hope that mechanisms of toxic action are similar, at least for similar cell types, in which case the ideal species for some studies may be any species about which we have good information on normal structure and function in the region of interest.

For the purpose of this chapter, we can ignore species differences in placental transport, metabolism of metals, etc., for if brain level is used as the dose indicator, we can study effects on developing brain without regard for issues of uptake, retention, etc. However, the selection of appropriate test species still remains a difficult problem. Small rodents have several advantages. The development of the CNS has been studied more extensively in mice and rats than in other species. On the other hand, some aspects of development are best known in other species. For example, cats have been the species of choice for many investigators of visual development, and the nocturnal rodents are poor choices for detailed studies of vision. Because rodents have been popular subjects for behavioral studies, there is a large literature on rodent behavior and how it is altered by experimental manipulations of the nervous system. However, the behaviors most easily investigated in rodents are not necessarily those in which clinical problems have been noted in humans exposed to metals, and it is sometimes difficult to find analogous behaviors for testing. In this regard, primates, with their more extensive behavioral repertoires, are surely the best species for many functional studies. The primate nervous system is the most similar to the human in structure, as well, and knowledge of its development is more extensive than that for many species. The major problems with the use of primates arise from the expenses of purchasing, housing, and testing these animals, which dictate the use of very small numbers of subjects. As several chapters in this volume point out, individual differences in functional responses to metal exposure are often great, and this makes results from small groups difficult to to interpret. The problems of small Ns are particularly difficult in studies of early injuries, because prenatal or neonatal exposure precludes the possibility of using each animal as its own control. That is, one cannot compare an animal's performance before and after exposure, as is commonly done in studies of adult toxicity. Thus, the issue of species choice for functional measures often comes down to using sensitive measures, analogous to those used in humans, on a small number of primates, or using less sensitive, less analogous measures on large numbers of rodents. Given such a decision, investigators may base their choice of one species over another on other features of their experiments. For example, if long-term chronic exposure is of interest, primates, with their long gestation period and preweaning period may be favored. Conversely, experiments involving repeated measures of brain levels of a compound after an acute exposure would almost necessitate the use of small mammals.

This discussion has been restricted to mammals, because few toxicologists or teratologists use non-mammalian species, but research in nervous system development has often employed amphibians and birds, so it is not inconceivable that these animals might prove useful in the future. However, recent studies in pigeons (Barthalmus et al., 1977, and Deitz et al., 1979) are not very promising for the use of this species. In these reports, the variability in behavioral response to lead was as great as that seen in mammals. Thus, there is no evidence as yet that pigeons offer an advantage by virtue of their behavioral characteristics. The ability of pigeon blood to bind lead, (Barthalmus et al., 1977), so that the bird can survive bood levels 100 times as great as those lethal to mammals, is a major drawback for the use of the species in many kinds of studies. Of course, rats also differ from humans in their brain/blood ratios (in the case of methylmercury, by a factor of 10 or 20 [Magos and Butler, 1976]) so this problem is not unique to the avian model.

EXPERIMENTAL ASPECTS OF METAL ACTION ON DEVELOPING TISSUE

To those unfamiliar with the nervous system the literature on metal effects may seem strange in that there is an issue of "tissue of choice," as well as "species of choice." Because various regions of the nervous system have such different cytoarchitecture and chemical features, it is crucial that pathologic comparisons be made from precisely the same tissue in controls and treated animals. Few studies involve attempts to survey the whole brain. Rather, investigators often restrict their attention to a few regions. These may be selected on the basis of previous demonstrations that an area is sensitive to the test agent or on some other basis, such as convenience for quantification or special developmental features. The cerebral cortex has been reported to be affected by both lead and methylmercury (Averill and Needleman, 1980; Choi et al., 1978). The corpus striatum has been used to demonstrate lead effects on synaptogenesis (Krigman et al., 1978), partly because it is more homogeneous in structure than many regions, and thus provides good samples for EM studies. The cerebellum has been the site for the majority of investigations of methylmercury, because: 1) It was implicated both structurally and functionally by the earliest reports of mercury poisoning, (Hunter and Russell, 1954; Harada, 1968); 2) It has a distinctive architecture, with cells of contrasting size, which can be separated (Syversen, 1981); 3) Its cell types form at different times, so that the various neurons can be exposed selectively by manipulating the time of treatment (Sager et al., 1982a,b); 4) Many of its neurons form postnatally in rodents, allowing split-litter designs for studies assessing developing cerebellum, while studies of comparable stages of many other brain regions would have to be carried out in utero.

As will be discussed below, different brain regions and cell types do seem to be differentially affected by metal exposure. This makes it imperative for structural and biochemical experiments to be designed to sample many parts of the nervous system, or to include a region already shown to be sensitive to injury by the test compound. Otherwise negative results become completely uninterpretable.

THE IMPORTANCE OF TIME OF TREATMENT

Both lead and mercury compounds are toxic to the mature nervous system. If the endpoint measured is the LD_{50}, or obvious neurological impairment, it is clear that they are even more injurious to the developing nervous system. However, few studies have made direct comparisons of any measure in adult and developing subjects similarly exposed to metals. For example, children appear to exhibit lead encephalopathy[1] far more frequently than adults, but children are usually exposed by ingestion and adults by other routes, such as inhalation. Does the difference in encephalopathy indicate a difference in response at different stages of brain development or a difference in exposure routes Studies of adults have emphasized neuromuscular effects of lead, such as slowing of maximal nerve conduction rates (Seppalainin and Hernberg, 1972). Such effects may occur in children also. For example, Landrigan et al. (1976) found a significant negative correlation between blood lead levels and nerve conduction velocities in children living near a lead smelter. However, most studies of childhood lead exposure have assessed cognitive effects, rather than neuromuscular effects. "Asymptomatic" lead exposure in children has been associated with a variety of behavioral abnormalities, such as I.Q. deficits (Albert et al., 1974; de la Burde and Choate, 1975) and hyperactivity (David et al., 1972), which have not been the focus of evaluations of adult toxicity. It is natural for experimenters to investigate school-related behaviors in children and work related behaviors in occupationally-exposed adults, but the result over many studies is that the data collected for subjects with different exposure periods are rarely comparable.

In animal studies it should be easy to make direct comparisons of the same treatment given at different stages of development. Yet few such experiments have been reported. One rare example is a study of fixed ratio responding after exposure to lead acetate (Padich and Zenick, 1976). Rats were exposed to a 750 mg/kg daily dose. A pre-weaning group of offspring came from dams exposed for 70 - 80 days before conception, and throughout gestation and

---

[1]The term encephalopathy should be reserved for an acute, often fatal condition characterized by a breakdown of the vascular system and swelling of the brain. Some authors apply the term to any overt neurological syndrome induced by lead.

nursing. A post-weaning group received the lead regimen directly, starting at weaning and continuing through testing. A third group was exposed through the mother and then after weaning as well. Only the latter group differed significantly from the controls, showing fewer reinforcements/minute. The simplest summary of the results is that repeated dosing over a long period is more injurious than shorter exposure, a conclusion which is not surprising. On the other hand, the outcome does indicate that both early and late exposure are toxic. The data do not allow any conclusions regarding possible differences between early and late exposures. Indeed, since the post-weaning treatment continued through testing, if the postweaning group had differed from controls and preweaning animals, it would not be known whether exposure at different stages of development has different effects, or whether exposure during testing was the critical variable. Thus, while this study clearly supports the idea that lead exposure can alter behavior, it does not answer our question regarding sensitive periods for exposure. More data are needed to make a case that time of exposure is important in lead effects on the CNS, and the necessary data are unlikely to come from studies not designed expressly for the purpose of comparing treatment times.

     In the case of methylmercury, the evidence for a special effect on developing CNS is stronger. Although experimental comparisons with age as an independent variable are lacking, the epidemic poisonings in Japan and Iraq provide clear evidence of a difference in level of effect (Harada, 1977; Amin-Zaki et al., 1974), and there are several lines of research, such as studies of cell proliferation and migration, that suggest mercury mechanisms of action specific to developing tissue (Rodier, this volume; Choi, this volume).

     Just as there are few data by which to compare different exposure periods, there are few by which to compare different metals. Clinical cases have most frequently come from those chronically exposed to lead or those acutely exposed to mercury. The animal literature tends to reproduce the human stituation, for the sake of relevance, but this makes comparisons between metals difficult. Similarly, the measures favored by most investigators have differed between the two metals. For example, a large literature has developed on the effects of lead on neurotransmitters (see reviews by Silbergeld and Hruska, 1980 and Hrdina et al., 1980) while few investigations of mercurial compounds have addressed the question of whether early exposure affects neurotransmitter levels or turnover. When brain biochemistry has been studied, results have been positive, to the extent that methylmercury exposure causes at least a transient effect on monamine systems (Taylor and DiStefano, 1976; Sabotka et al., 1974). Conversely, many known effects of methylmercury, such as interference with cell migration and protein synthesis have not been the subject of investigation in lead studies.

THE IMPORTANCE OF THE CNS MEASURES TAKEN

While problems of comparability like those just described exist in judging sensitivity of tissues and functions, we have more information in this area. For example, many investigations of behavior involve assessment of several tasks in the same animals, so that some true comparisons of different functions can be made. Jason and Kellogg (1981) concluded that maze-learning and simple discrimination tasks have been less sensitive measures of lead-induced CNS disturbances than tasks involving reversals or delays, and that tasks involving adversive stimuli may be more sensitive than those involving positive reinforcers. Active tasks have yielded more positive results than passive tasks. Cory-Slechta (1982) has pointed out several other differences in sensitivity of particular tasks. For example, performance on fixed interval schedules of reinforcement is more affected than performance on fixed ratio schedules, and brightness discriminations seem more sensitive than pattern discriminations.

Methylmercury toxicity in adults is associated with a progression of functional symptoms (reviewed by Clarkson, 1982), beginning with parasthesias and progressing to incoordination and visual constriction. Studies of prenatally-exposed children suggest that motor effects may be the ones occurring at the lowest levels of exposure, but there has been little research on the possible effects of methylmercury on cognitive functions, so it is not clear whether the gross intellectual impairment seen with high doses (Amin-Zaki et al., 1974; Takeuchi and Eto, 1977) has correlaries at lower doses, in such apical measures as I.Q. Data from primates chronically exposed to methylmercury may be interpreted to be suggestive of some cognitive or perceptual effects but some of the same animals had gross motor impairment and sensory effects (Rice, this volume), so these results do not contradict the hypothesis that sensory and motor disturbances may be the most sensitive indicators of methylmercury poisoning.

There appears to be a difference between lead and methylmercury in the sensory modalities most affected by exposure. Clinical reports of symptoms of mercury toxicity emphasize visual changes whereas lead toxicity is more strongly associated with auditory impairment (Repko et al., 1978). Although motor effects occur with both metals, reports of mercury poisoning have focused on coordination deficits, while lead is reported to cause weakness, tremors, and increased response latencies.

In regard to differential sensitivity to metals of cells or tissues in the nervous system, again, studies directly comparing several cell types or several tissues are rare. The early findings of cerebellar pathology in mercury-exposed subjects (Harada et al., 1968) along with the clinical symptoms of cerebellar injury have prompted many investigations of that structure (Chang and Hartman, 1972), usually to the exclusion of other brain regions. Within the adult rodent cerebellum, several investigators have noted granule cells to be more sensitive to mercury than the large Purkinje cells. It has been suggested that cell size may be a determining feature of the differential effect (Jacobs et al., 1977). Syversen (1977) has suggested a further explanation of differential sensitivity. He found that mercury interfered with protein synthesis in mature Purkinje cells as much as in granule cells, but that the former showed more recovery from the interference. Similarly, large neurons from cerebral cortex showed more recovery than granule cells. According to this author, cell size may be correlated with the recovery potential of cells, rather than the sensitivity of cells to initial injury. Whether differential recovery is characteristic of various cell types during development is not known. It would be valuable to have more data on response to methylmercury from a variety of cell types. For example, all postnatally-forming neurons are small, so their size is coupled with their age at the time of treatment. It would be interesting to study some small neurons that form early. Very little is known about differential sensitivity of different cell types during early development. For example, one might ask whether methylmercury's effects on mitosis occur in all neurons or only special types, whether the same effect can be demonstrated in non-neuronal tissue, etc.

From the work of Choi and others, we have suggestions that some regions of the young human brain exhibit methylmercury pathology more than others, but the number of cases is so small that one cannot be certain whether such differences are always characteristic of the toxic agent or whether they depend on the particular exposure history of the individuals examined. Further observations of regional differences in pathology have been reported in primates (Garman et al., 1975). These do not match the human findings, and the authors concluded that their squirrel monkeys and macque groups differed from one another, as well. As with the human autopsy cases, the observation of dieing cells in these brains is difficult to interpret. Even a small percentage of dying cells would deplete the brain of normal cells very rapidly, because dieing cells and cell debris are visible for such a short period. For example, in CNS regions that lose large proportions of their neurons naturally during development, a 50 percent reduction over less than a week is represented by peak levels of pyknotic nuclei of less than 5 percent (Harris-Flanagan, 1969). Thus, reports of dieing cells in methylmercury-exposed brains cannot mean that such loss was ongoing over weeks or months of exposure. Otherwise, the tissue would be virtually destroyed. Garman et al. (1975) found some areas of cortex, particularly visual cortex, to be depleted of neurons, but many other areas seemed to show cell death without massive loss of tissue. It is possible that cell death began just prior to death in the human victims, in which case this symptom may be related to their general illness, rather than a direct action of methylmercury on neurons and glia, but it would be a strange coincidence if cell death began only a few days before death in the primate studies, especially since the sacrifice times varied. A possible explanation of the findings is that the dieing cells do not represent direct methylmercury toxicity, but were injured by hypoxia between sacrifice and fixation. Regional differences then might represent areas of tenuous blood supply. Such regions could occur naturally or be induced by vascular injury associated with treatment.

Results of regional brain analyses of neurotransmitter levels after early lead exposure have not always been consistent from one study to another, but a few effects have been reported in several independent investigations. For example, decreased turnover in DA in the corpus stratum has been reported by many authors (Jason and Kellogg, 1981; Govoni et al., 1978; Lucchi et al, 1981). Carroll et al. (1977) have reported reductions in ACh release after lead exposure, Modak et al. (1975) have reported decreaed AChE in the midbrain, while Shih and Hanin (1978) have observed reductions in ACh turnover in several brain regions.

A common finding has been the elevation of a transmitter's activity in one brain region accompanied by a reduction of activity in another region. For example, Govoni et al. (1980) found a significant increase in GABA-specific binding in cerebellum and a significant decrease in the same measure in the striatum. Thus, there is substantial evidence that neurons differ in their response to lead exposure and that the difference is specific to particular transmitter systems and particular brain regions. There is, as yet, no clear correlation between these observations and the functional observations on early lead exposure. However, some recent studies may be relevant. Lucchi et al. (1981) found that the hyperactivity exhibited by rats exposed to lead during development could be alleviated temporarily with a drug treatment (sulpiride) which blocks one dopamine receptor. The same treatment did not alter activity in controls. Thus, the results argue for a specific pharmacologic effect on the abnormal brain, and support the hypothesis that DA abnormalities play a role in lead's effect on activity.

METAL SPECIATION, ROUTE OF EXPOSURE AND TIMING AND DURATION OF DOSE

The chemical form of metals is of great importance in their toxic effects on the CNS. Inorganic mercury has some teratogenic potential (Ferm and Hanlon, this volume), but methylmercury is considerably more hazardous, and has been the subject of most studies of mercury toxicity. A wide variety of lead compounds has been investigated and all seem to be toxic to the CNS. Whether they differ substantially in their effects is not clear. It would be helpful to have data on tissue levels of metal for a given dose for the various compounds, for it is possible that any differences observed are due to tissue levels rather than tissue sensitivity -- this is certainly a factor in the differences between inorganic and organic mercury. Little is known about the significance of different routes of exposure metals partly because exposure routes tend to be confounded with many other variables in clincial studies. For example, several authors (Rutter, 1980; Jason and Kellogg, 1980), have pointed out that the ingestion of lead in children with pica may itself be a symptom of underlying CNS difficulties, making it difficult to ascribe behavioral deficits reported in such children to lead injury. This is an important point, for it is true that these children probably represent a special group, whose proper controls would be children with pica but with no elevation of blood lead levels. The idea that particular exposure routes may be correlated with other factors influencing CNS function may be important for other metals also. For example, some of the Indian populations under study because of their intake of fish high in methylmercury, may be characterized by high intake of other toxic agents, such as selenium, alcohol, etc. That is, whenever we select a population for one variable (e.g., high intake of local fish), we may be selecting inadvertantly for other characteristics, which could be the cause of any differences observed.

Another problem in comparing exposure routes is that, outside the laboratory, the route of exposure may be difficult to determine. A particularly interesting study is that of Roels et al. (1980). The authors found high correlations between children's blood lead levels and proximity to a smelter. Not surprisingly, blood lead was highly correlated with lead levels in air and with lead levels in school-playground dust. Levels in air and dust were strongly related also. Lead on children's hands was significantly related to all the other measures. Partial correlations revealed that the major determinant of blood levels was, in fact, hand lead, rather than airborne lead, suggesting that ingestion of lead was critical to the elevated blood levels near the smelter. Thus, while it is often assumed that the route of exposure around smelters, or in other occupational settings, is by inhalation, and the high correlations between air levels and blood levels support this assumption, one must be cautious in concluding that the most obvious route of exposure is the major route. A more careful examination of the situation may reveal alternative explanations, as in this study.

INDICATORS MEDIA, STRAIN AND SPECIES DIFFERENCES

A variety of indicator media have been studied for lead, but there is still a question as to which correlate most strongly with functional effects. Even when the response measured is encephalopathy, the range of blood levels (PbB) observed is

amazingly large. Some of the variability is probably due to
different exposure histories. Since little is known about the
effects of long versus short exposures versus intermittent exposure,
etc., as these variables influence tissue levels, it is impossible
to even begin to explain the individual differences observed in
human cases. In animal experiments in which the blood levels of
lead have been carefully documented during exposure and testing, the
variability of response is still great (Laughlin, this volume; Rice,
this volume). Are the differential effects related to real
differences in sensitivity or is PbB simply a poor measure of CNS
levels of lead? NIOSH (1978) has argued that erythrocyte
protoporphyrins (measured as FEP or ZPP) may be preferable to blood
lead levels for several reasons. For example, on theoretical
grounds, it is reasonable to measure a biological response instead
of tissue content and on practical grounds, these measures are not
so easily contaminated as are blood lead measures. Needleman (1980)
has reviewed some of the advantages and disadvantages of indicators
of lead. This is an area which needs research attention.

     Blood levels and levels in hair have proven useful (Amin-Zaki
et al., 1974) as indicators of methylmercury, but brain levels
provide more information in animal studies. Of course, none of
these measures tell us whether the metal present is in a form that
has toxic potential. For example, a recent study of cell
proliferation in developing brain (Sager et al., 1982a) found a
significant difference in mitosis between male and female subjects,
despite the fact that brain and blood levels of mercury were
virtually identical. This suggests the possibility that the mercury
might be less active in female brain, a hypothesis supported by the
fact that higher doses affected mitosis in both sexes.

     With the indicators most commonly employed, such as blood
levels of metals, there are striking species differences, especially
in retention of metals (Mottet, this volume). There are also
significant differences within species over the course of development
(Rowland et al., this volume). Such differences surely play a role
in determining the effects of metals on developing brain, but more
information is needed to develop accurate dose-response or
dose-effect data.

MECHANISMS OF ACTION

     There is no evidence to suggest that lead and mercury act by
the same mechanisms, and the differences in clinical symdromes argue
against this hypothesis. In the case of both metals, the behavioral
effects at high doses are thought to arise from gross, permanent
injury to the brain. There are many reasons to think that some or
all of the brain pathology observed is a direct effect of metal
action, but it is not possible to rule out completely indirect

sources of brain injury. That is, such known toxic effects as kidney damage could contribute to brain pathology as they are thought to do in other conditions, such as aging (Kaplan and Scheibel, 1980). However, many direct effects of metals on developing nervous system have been demonstrated, and these could account for most, if not all, the functional effects.

Some major problems in relating behavioral effects to underlying brain effects are that we have few studies in which both brain and behavior were studied in the same animals, and that many of the more mechanistic studies employ doses considerably higher than those necessary to induce functional deficits. Thus, while lead and mercury are known to injure the brain morphologically and biochemically, we have few clear demonstrations that these effects occur at doses as low or lower than the threshold for functional effects. Therefore, the changes in CNS tissue reported may not necessarily be the initiators of functional effects.

For example, we know that mercury can interfere with neuron migration in developing brain (Choi, this volume) but three 5 mg/kg injections of methylmercuric chloride on days 3, 4, and 5 in mice did not alter migration patterns, although some effects were detected in differentiation of Purkinje cells at this dose (Choi et al., 1981). Migration failures are likely to be a sufficient cause for behavoral effects, but we do not know whether they are a necessary cause of mercury-induced functional disturbance. In the same vein, mercury effects on mitosis (Sager et al., 1982a) may be sufficient to cause functional abnormality, but we do not know whether these effects occur at doses below a single gavage treatment of 4 mg Hg/kg, resulting in brain levels of about 1.5 µg Hg/g in mice. A single dose of 5 mg/kg can alter subsequent rodent behavior (Eccles and Annau, 1982). Studies of structure and function at lower doses are needed to answer the question of whether interference with mitosis is causally related to functional effects. A third mechanism by which mercury may act on developing CNS is inhibition of protein synthesis as demonstrated in post-weaning animals by Syversen (1977). As with the other mechanisms, the relationship between this injury and function is not known. One of the first mechanisms suspected as a cause of methylmercury neurotoxicity was injury to the vascular system and blood/brain barrier. As Chang (1977) has pointed out, many of the early reports involved huge doses delivered into the carotid artery of adult animals. Whether effects observed under such conditions have any meaning for lower levels of exposure is not clear. Lower doses in developing animals have been reported to cause vascular changes at the EM level when the animals were examined after weaning (Chang and Hartman, 1972). These studies are also difficult to interpret, since the treatment occurred at the primitive streak stage of embryogenesis -- i.e., before the brain, vascular system or placenta are present. Perhaps such early treatment of the dam results in retention of enough methylmercury to enter the embryo at later stages, but we know virtually nothing about how such an injury might occur, or why the vascular system might be affected. Several mechanisms demonstrated in vitro could be important in developing CNS, but remain to be studied in vivo. For example, Shamoo et al., (1976) have demonstrated inhibition of several calcium-dependent processes in skeletal muscle by both mercuric chloride and methymercury. The same authors found methylmercury, but not inorganic mercury, to inhibit ACh binding to isolated ACh receptors. Such an action, if it occurs in the developing organism, could be of great importance in understanding the teratogenic effects of methylmercury on the nervous system.

Studies of lead mechanisms are plentiful, but the discrepancy between doses used to demonstrate mechanisms and those used to induce behavioral effects is often great. Some changes in neurotransmitter activity surely occur in the range of doses typical of behavioral studies (Jason and Kellogg, 1981), but many reports of "subtle" effects on CNS morphology are from studies with doses sufficient to cause gross encephalopathy and paralysis, if not death, of many subjects, and all are from studies with doses high enough to produce some behavioral effects. Thus, while changes in cell number (Krigman et al., 1978) and synaptogenesis (Averill and Needleman, 1980) are effects of lead exposure, we do not know whether they underlie behavioral deficits or occur only at very high doses of lead. Similarly, the dosing regimens used to demonstrate demyelinization (Myers et al., 1980) and hippocampal abnormalities (Alfano and Petit, 1982) were the same or greater than those used by Pentschew and Garro (1966) to induce encephalopathy.

SAFETY LEVELS

There is no question that PbB's of around 80 - 100 µg/100 ml are sufficient to produce encephalopathy in some children (Chisholm et al., 1975; Rummo, 1974); the issue is how low blood levels have to be before a "no effect" level is reached. Most retrospective human studies have found positive effects with PbB levels around 40 µg/100 ml. While most animal studies have used regimens producing peak blood levels much higher than 40 µg/100 ml, at least a few (Winneke et al., 1977; Rice, this volume) have yielded effects of lead at doses below 40 µg/100 ml. Despite some difficulty in estimating blood lead levels in the children sampled by Needleman (1980), these results may suggest differences below the 40 µg/100 ml level. One recent study found effects on event-related slow-wave potential voltage over the whole range of PbB levels from 6 - 59 µg/100 ml (Otto, 1981). It is impossible, at this time, to assess whether prenatal or postnatal exposure is more hazardous, because most studies involve only postnatal exposure (e.g., most human studies) or both pre- and post-natal exposure (many animal studies).

Because of the availability of data from shorter-term exposures in Japan and Iraq, we have at least suggestive data on some of these questions for methylmercury. We can be certain that gross neurological impairment can result from prenatal exposure at doses below those which produce symptoms in the mother (Snyder, 1971). The lower range of blood levels producing symptoms in adults is about 300 ppb. Since infants exposed in utero tend to have higher blood levels than their mothers the lowest level of methylmercury detected in symptomatic infants in 546 ppb. By extrapolating from hair levels to blood levels, it has been estimated that fetal blood levels as low as 230 ppb can produce significant developmental delays (Marsh et al., 1980). Such delays have been associated with lasting behavioral abnormalities in both human and infant animals (reviewed by Rodier, 1982). The evaluation of fetal versus maternal levels has been substantiated in animal studies. In rats, brain levels of fetuses are more than twice as high as brain levels of dams after brief exposure to mercury (Null et al., 1973). Infants exposed postnatally via mother's milk, showing blood levels over 200 ppb, produced no symptoms detectable by the investigators. Whether infants in the postnatal period are less susceptible to methylmercury poisoning than in utero is questionable, since human brain development does not end at birth, and animal studies show effects on developing postnatal brain at very low levels of mercury.

CONCLUSIONS

Discussions of what is known and what is needed were a major feature of the Rochester Conference. In addition to the speakers on the central nervous system effects, several visitors joined in these discussions and made valuable contributions. This summary includes ideas from all members of the group, but is necessarily brief and selective, and surely reflects the ideas of the author to a greater degree than is desirable. Some ideas from the larger conference group have been incorporated, as well.

Beyond the conclusion that lead compounds and methylmercury are potent neurotoxic agents in adults and developing animals, firm conclusions are few. Both lead and methylmercury affect many different behavioral measures in animals as well as humans. Both cause obvious neuropathology at high doses.

In the case of methylmercury, there is a range of maternal exposures which produce clinical effects on CNS structure and function in offspring without producing comparable effects in the mother. While the differential effect may result from the action of mercury on biological processes exclusive to developing CNS, it may result, instead, from differential brain and blood levels in mother and fetus, or from a combination of these factors. In the case of lead, while many investigators suspect that developing nervous system is more affected by lead than mature nervous system, the data do not offer a test of this hypothesis. Blood levels of lead in fetuses do not appear to be elevated over the level of the mother. Lead has some mechanisms of action (e.g., alteration of neurotransmitter activity) that could cause permanent injury to developing neurons and transient disturbance of mature neurons, but experimental comparisons of age at exposure have not addressed questions of this sort. Indeed, experimental research has rarely addressed the problem of whether lead effects are permanent, since the most common paradigms involve exposures that continue through the test period.

RECOMMENDATIONS

While the different investigators present have different views regarding the value of different models and different measures, they were in agreement on some of the experimental approaches that would provide needed information. For example, most felt that studies correlating structure, biochemistry, and behavior would be helpful, although few research groups could attempt such studies. On a more practical level, it was asked: Why are there so few studies in which animals exposed to acute dosing are examined at more than one time point on the same measure? Without such studies we know nothing about the possibility of repair of early toxic effects and little about what is happening at the time of exposure. Of course, we need to know what happens that is lasting, but more information about the progress of an injury over time is needed. In contrast, many chronic studies involve continued treatment while testing proceeds. This is an important paradigm, but it does not answer questions about whether the effects are permanent or transient. Those investigators working with long-term dosing schedules felt that sudden exposure versus gradually increasing exposure could be an important factor in response to metals. Another area of investigation neglected by most researchers is the influence of early experience on expression of functional deficits. The morphologists were anxious to see more quantitative studies in which control and treated tissues are compared "blind." Descriptive studies, especially at the EM level, are difficult to replicate. Careful selection of tissue samples is crucial for meaningful comparisons, as is the use of tissue preparations appropriate to the hypothesis (e.g., it is not reasonable to do cell counts in EM, or to describe fine structure from thick paraffin sections).

Both the investigators involved in behavioral studies and those involved in morphology or biochemistry were anxious to see more studies with low doses of metal compounds. We need to know whether the mechanisms of injury observed with high doses operate at low doses, or whether we need to search for other mechanisms. Similarly, we need to take some of the functional measures which have proven sensitive to metal effects and test successively lower doses, before we experiment with more and more new measures.

In many studies the reporting of blood and brain levels would add immeasurably to the value of the work. In fact, some simple parametric studies of doses versus brain levels would be of benefit to many investigators.

Clinical studies provide most of the hypotheses for animal work, and all investigators are anxious to see the results of prospective studies. The development of objective, culture-free tests, such as electrophysiological measures, would benefit epidemiologic studies, and might provide tests that could be transfered directly to animals.

In almost every area of investigation, the lack of direct comparisons on almost any factor was apparent. All agreed that age at treatment, species, different compounds, etc., deserved study under conditions in which all other variables are held constant. Systematic studies of such variables should not be difficult to perform and they would provide the background needed by all investigators of metal toxicity.

REFERENCES

Albert, R.E., Shore, R.E., Sayers, A.J., Strehlow, C., Kneip, T.J., Pasternak, B.S., Friedhoff, A.J., Coran, F., and Cimino, J.A., 1974, Follow-up of children overexposed to lead, Environ. Hlth. Perspect. 7:33-39.
Alfono, D.P., and Petit, T.L., 1982, Neonatal lead exposure alters the dendritic development of hippocampal dentate granule cells, Exp. Neurol. 75:275-288.
Amin-Zaki, L., Elhassani, S., Majeed, M.A., Clarkson, T.W., Doherty, R.A., and Greenwood, M., 1974, Intrauterine methylmercury poisoning in Iraq, Pediatrics 54:587-594.
Averill, D.R., and Needleman, H.L., 1980, Neonatal lead exposure retards cortical synaptogenesis in the rat, in: "Low Level Lead Exposure: The Clinical Implications of Current Research", pp. 201-210, H.L. Needleman, ed., Raven, New York.
Barthalmus, G.T., Leander, J.D., McMillan, D.E., Mushak, P., and Krigman, M.R., 1977, Chronic effects of lead on schedule-controlled pigeon behavior, Toxicol. Appl. Pharmacol. 42:271-284.
Bornschein, R., Pearson, D., and Reiter, L., 1980, Behavioral effects of moderate lead exposure in children and animal models: Part 1 - Clinical studies and Part 2 - Animal studies, CRC Crit. Rev. Toxicol. 8:43-152.
Carroll, P.T., Silbergeld, E.K., and Goldberg, A.M., 1977, Alternation of central cholingergic function by chronic lead acetate exposure, Biochem. Pharmacol. 26:397-402.

Chang, L.W., Wade, P.R., and Pound, J.G. and Reuhl, K.R., 1980,
    Prenatal and neonatal toxicology and pathology of heavy metals,
    Advances in Pharmacol. Chemother. 17:195-231.
Chang, L.W., 1977, Neurotoxic effects of mercury - A review,
    Environ. Res. 14:329-373.
Chang, L.W., and Hartman, H.A., 1972, Ultrastructural studies of the
    nervous system after mercury intoxication. I. Pathological
    changes in the nerve cell bodies, Acta Neuropath. (Berl.)
    20:122-138.
Chisholm, J.J., and Thomas, D.J., 1983, Developmental toxicity of
    metals: implications for public health (this volume).
Chisholm, J.J., Jr., Barrett, M.B., and Bellits, E.D., 1975,
    Dose-effect and dose-response relationships for lead in
    children, J. Peds. 87:1152-1160.
Choi, B.H., 1981, Effects of prenatal methylmercury poisoning upon
    growth and development of fetal central nervous system (this
    volume).
Choi, B.H., Kudo, M., and Lapham, L.W., 1981, A golgi and electron
    microscopic study of cerebellum in methylmercury-poisoned
    neonatal mice, Acta Neuropath. (Berlin) 54:233-237.
Choi, B.H., Lapham, L.W., Amin-Zaki, L., and Saleem, T., 1978,
    Abnormal neuronal migration, deranged cerebro cortical
    organization and diffuse white matter astrocytosis of human
    fetal brain: A major effect of methylmercury poisoning in
    utero, J. Neuropath. Exper. Neurol. 37:719-733.
Clarkson, T.W., 1983, Methylmercury toxicity to the mature and
    developing nervous system: possible mechanisms, in:
    "Biological Aspects of Metals in Metal-related Diseases", B.
    Sarker, ed., Raven, New York, in press.
Cory-Slechta, D., 1982, The behavioral toxicity of lead: Problems
    and perspectives, in: "Advances in Behavioral Pharmacology",
    Vol. IV, T. Thompson, and P.B. Dews, eds., Academic Press, New
    York, in press.
David, O.J., Clark, J., and Voeller, K., 1972, Lead and
    hyperactivity, Lancet 2:900-903.
de la Burde, B., and Choate, M.L., 1975, Early asumptomatic lead
    exposure and development at school age, J. Peds. 87:638-642.
Deitz, D.D., McMillan, D.E., and Mushak, P., 1979, Effect of chronic
    lead administration on acquisition and performance of serial
    position sequences by pigeons, Toxicol. Appl. Pharma.
    47:377-384.
Eccles, C.U., and Annau, Z., 1982a, Prenatal methylmercury
    exposure: I. Alterations in neonatal activity, Neurobehav.
    Tox. and Terat. 4:371-376.
Eccles, C.U., and Annau, Z., 1982b, II. Alterations in learning and
    psychotropic drug sensitivity in adult offspring, Neurobehav.
    Tox. and Terat. 4:377-382.
Ferm, V.A., and Hanlon, D.P., 1982, Metal-induced congenital
    malformations (this volume).

Garman, R.H., Weiss, B., and Evans, H.L., 1975, Alkylmercurial
    encephalopathy in the monkey (Saimiri Sciureus and Macaca
    Arctoides): A histophatologic and autoradiographic study, Acta
    Neuropath. (Berlin) 32:61-74.
Govoni, S., Memo, M., Lucci, L., Spano, P.F., and Trabucchi, M.,
    1980, Brain neurotransmitter systems and chronic lead
    intoxication, Pharmacol. Res. Comm. 12:447-460.
Govoni, S., Montefusco, O., Spano, P.F., Trabucchi, M., 1978, Effect
    of chronic lead treatment on brain dopamine synthesis and serum
    prolactin release in the rat, Toxicol. Lett. 2:333-337.
Harada, Y., 1968, Congenital (or fetal) Minamata Disease, in:
    "Minamata Disease Study Group of Minamata Disease", pp. 93-117,
    Humamoto University, Japan.
Harris-Flanagan, A.E., 1969, Differentiation and degeneration in the
    motor horn of the foetal mouse, J. Morphol. 129:281-305.
Hoffman, G.E., Felten, D.L., and Sladek, J.R., 1976, Monoamine
    distribution in primate brain. III. Catecholamine-containing
    varicosities in the hypothalamus of Macaca mullatta. Am. J.
    Anat. 147:501-514.
Hrdina, P.O., Hanin, I., and Dabas, T.C., 1980, Neurochemical
    correlates of lead toxicity, in: "Lead Toxicity", P.L. Singhal
    and J.A. Thomas, eds., pp. 273-300, Urban and Schwartzenberg,
    Baltimore, MD.
Hunter, P., and Russell, D.S., 1954, Focal cerebral and cerebellar
    atrophy in a human subject due to organic mercury compounds, J.
    Neurol. Neurosurg. Psychiat. 17:235-241.
Jacobs, J.M., Carmichael, N., and Cavanagh, J.B., 1977,
    Ultrastructural changes in the nervous system of rabbits
    poisoned with methylmercury, Toxicol. Appl. Pharmacol.
    39(2):249-261.
Jacobson, M., 1978, in: "Developmental Neurobiology", Plenum Press,
    New York.
Jason, K.M., and Kellogg, C.K., 1980, Behavioral neurotoxicity of
    lead, in: "Lead Toxicity", pp. 241-272, P.L. Singhal and J.A.
    Thomas, eds., Urban and Schwarzenberg, Baltimore, MD.
Jason, K.M., and Kellogg, C.K., 1981, Neonatal lead exposure:
    Effects on development of behavior and striatal dopamine
    neurons. Pharmacol. Biochem. Behav. 15:641-649.
Kaplan, A.S., and Scheibel, A.B., 1980, Giant spine-poor pyramidal
    cells in auditory cortex of young and aged cats, Soc. Neurosci.
    Abstr. 6:567.
Krigman, M.R., Bertram, E., Bagnell, R., and Benduch, E.G., 1978,
    Perturbation of caudate nucleus ontogenesis by low-level lead
    burdens, Fed. Proc. 37:843.
Landrigan, P.J. et al., 1976, Increased lead absorption with anemia
    and slowed nerve conduction in children near a lead smelter, J.
    Peds. 89:904-910.
Laughlin, N.K., Bowman, R.E., and Levin, E.D., 1982, Cognitive
    deficits resulting from early lead exposure in Rhesus monkeys
    (this volume).

Lucchi, L., Memo, M., and Airaghi, M.L., 1981, Chronic lead treatment induces in rat a specific and differential effect on dopamine receptors in different brain areas, Brain Res. 213:397-404.

Magos, L., and Butler, W.H., 1976, The kinetics of methylmercury administered repeatedly to rats, Arch. Toxicol. 35:25-39.

Marsh, D.O., Myers, G.J., Clarkson, T.W., Amin-Zaki, L., Libriti, S. and Majeed, M.A., 1980, Fetal methylmercury poisoning: clinical and toxicological data on 29 cases, Annals of Neurol. 7:348-353.

Miller, M.W., and Clarkson, T.W., 1973, in: "Mercury, mercurials and mercaptans", Thomas, Springfield, Illinois.

Modak, A.T., Weintraub, S.T., and Stavinoka, W.B., 1975, Effect of chronic ingestion of lead on the central cholingergic system in rat brain regions, Toxicol. Appl. Pharmacol. 34:340-347.

Mottet, N.K., Fowler, B.A., and Ferm, V.H. The congenital teratogenicity and perinatal toxicity of metals (this volume).

Myers, R.R., Powell, H.C., Shapiro, H.M., Costello, M.L., and Lambert, P.W., 1980, Changes in endoneurial fluid pressure, permeability, and peripheral nerve ultrastructure in experimental lead neuropathy, Ann. Neurol. 8:392.

Needleman, H.L., 1980, Human lead exposure difficulties and strategies in the assessment of neuropsychological impact, in: "Lead Toxicity", pp. 1-18, P.L. Singhal and J.A. Thomas, eds., Urgan and Schwarzenberg, Baltimore, MD.

NIOSH, Criteria for a recommended standard... Occupational exposure to inorganic lead. Revised criteria - 1978, USHEW, DHEW (NIOSH Pub. No. 78-158).

Null, D.H., Gartside, P.S., and Wei, E., 1973, Methylmercury accumulation in brains of pregnant, non-pregnant and fetal rats, Life Sci. 12:65-72.

Otto, D.A., 1981, Electrophysicological assessment of neurotoxicity in children, in: "Proceedings of the First International Lead Conference", R.L. Bornschein, ed., pp. 75-95, Department of Environmental Health, University of Cincinnati, Cincinnati, Ohio.

Padich, R., and Zenick, H., 1976, The effects of developmental and/or direct lead exposure on FR behavior in the rat, Pharmacol. Biochem. and Behav. 6:371-375.

Pentschew, A., and Garro, F., 1966, Lead encephalomyelopathy of suckling rats and its implications on the porphyrinopathic nervous diseases, Acta Neuropathol. 6:266-278.

Repko, J.D., Corum, C.R., Jones, P.D., and Carcia, L.S. Jr., 1978, The effects of inorganic lead on behavioral and neurologic function. Cincinnati, OH: U.S. Dept. of Health, Education, and Welfare, National Institute for Occupational Safety and Health: DEW (NIOSH) Publication No. 78-128.

Rice, D.C., 1982, Central nervous effects of perinatal exposure to lead or methylmercury in the monkey (this volume).

Rodier, P.M., 1983, Exogenous sources of malformations in development: DNS malformations and developmental repair processes, in: "Malformations of Development: Biological and Psychological Sources and Consequences", E.S. Gollin, ed., Academic Press, New York, in press.

Rodier, P.M., 1982, Critical processes in CNS development and the pathogenesis of early injuries (this volume).

Roels, H.A., Buchet, J.P., Lauwerys, R.R., Bruanx P., Claeys-Thorian, F., Lafontaine, A., and Verduyn, G., 1980, Exposure to lead by the oral and the pulmonary routes of children living in the vicinity of a primary lead smelter. Environ. Res. 22:81-94.

Rowland, I.R., Robinson, R.D., Doherty, R.A., and Landry, T.D., 1982, Are developmental changes in methylmercury metabolism and excretion mediated by the intestinal microflora (this volume)

Rummo, J.H., 1974, Intellectual and behavioral effects of lead poisoning in children, University of North Carolina, Ph.D. Thesis.

Rutter, M., 1980, Raised lead levels and impaired cognitive/behavioral functioning: A review of the evidence. Develop. Med. and Child Neurol. 221:1-26.

Sabotka, T.J., Cook, M.P., and Brodie, R.E., 1974, Effects of perinatal exposure to methylmercury on functional brain development and neurochemistry, Psychiatry 8:307-319.

Sager, P.R., Doherty, R.A., and Rodier, P.M., 1982a, Developing cerebellum is altered by low-dose methylmercury, Teratology, 74A.

Sager, P.R., Doherty, R.A., and Rodier, P.M., 1982b, Effects of methylmercury on developing mouse cerebellar cortex, Exper. Neurol. 77:179-193.

Seppalainen, A.M., and Hernberg, S., 1972, Sensitive technique for detecting subclinical lead neuropathy, Br. J. Ind. Med. 29:443-449.

Shamoo, A.E., Maclennon, D.H., and Eldefrawi, M.E., 1976, Differential effects of mercurial compounds on excitable tissues. Chem.-Biol. Interactions 12:41-52.

Shih, T.-M., and Hanin, I., 1978, Effects of chronic lead exposure on levels of acetylcholine and choline and on acetylcholine turnover rate in rate brain areas in vivo, Psychopharmacology 58:263-269.

Silbergeld, E.K., and Hruska, R.E., 1980, Neurochemical investigations of low level lead exposure, in: "Low Level Lead Exposure: The Clinical Implications of Current Research", pp. 135-157, H.L. Needleman, ed., Raven Press, New York.

Silbergeld, E.K., Hruska, R.E., Miller, L.P., and Eng, N., 1975, Effects of lead in vivo and in vitro, on GABAergic neurochemistry, J. Neurochem. 34:1712-1718.

Snyder, R.D., 1971, Congenital mercury poisoning, New Engl. J. Med. 284:1014-1016.

Syversen, T.L.M., 1977, Effects of methylmercury on in vivo protein
    synthesis in isolated cerebral and cerebellar neurons,
    Neuropath. Appl. Neurobiol. 3:225-236.
Syversen, T.L.M., 1981, Changes in protein and RNA synthesis in rat
    brain neurons after a single dose of methylmercury, Toxicol.
    Lett. 10:31-34.
Takeuchi, T., and Eto, K., 1977, Pathology and pathogenesis of
    Minamata diseas, in: "Minamata Disease", pp. 103-141, K.
    Tsubaki and K. Irukayama, eds., Elsevier/North Holland,
    Amsterdam.
Taylor, L.L., and DiStefano, V., 1976, Effects of methylmercury on
    biogenic amines in the developing rat pup. Tox. Appl.
    Pharmacol. 38:489-497.
Winneke, G., Brockhaus, A., and Baltissen, R., 1977, Neurobehavioral
    and systemic effects of long-term blood lead-elevation in rats,
    Arch. Toxicol. 37:247-263.

PRENATAL METABOLISM: METALS AND METALLOTHIONEIN

Richard K. Miller and Zahir Shaikh

Working Group: George H. Cherian, Bengt R.G. Danielsson, Lennert Dencker, Bruce Kelman, Curtis Klaassen, Arthur A. Levin, Richard K.Miller, Wendy Ng, Zahir Shaikh Tsuguyoshi Suzuki, Michael Webb, Patrick Weir

Review Article Contents:

PRENATAL METABOLISM: METALS AND METALLOTHIONEIN

Richard K. Miller[1] and Zahir A. Shaikh[2]

[1]Departments of Obstetrics and Gynecology and of
 Pharmacology, University of Rochester, Rochester, New York
[2]Department of Pharmacology and Toxicology,
 University of Rhode Island, Kingston, Rhode Island

INTRODUCTION

Many of the preceding chapters have been concerned with the
effects of metals on the developing organism. Such similarities or
differences in the effects of the various metals can be mediated
through direct action on the embryo/fetus, on the placenta and its
extraembryonic membranes or on the mother. To establish such
interactions, it is imperative that the clinician and medical
scientist understand the metabolism of these metals in question.

Metabolism is defined as the absorption, distribution,
biotransformation, disposition, and excretion of a compound. The
study of prenatal metabolism is further confounded by the unique
compartmentalization and altered biotransformational capabilities
of the pregnant female compared with the non-pregnant female or
male. All of these alterations in the pregnant female can be both
qualitatively and quantitatively different depending upon the stage
of gestation. Even greater metabolic differences can be attributed
to the stage of development of the embryo/fetus. These alterations
are all present within a given species; however, these comparisons
of effects are compromised even further when comparisons between
and among species are conducted without knowledge of the metabolism
involved.

Thus, any evaluation of metal metabolism must establish a primer which includes the species, day of conception, implantation/ gestational period, contribution of average uterine content to maternal weight gain and non-pregnant metabolism of the metal.

This chapter will be divided into five major sections: I. Metabolism During Pregnancy - a. maternal, b. placental, c. embryo/fetus, II. Metabolism of Specific Metals - a. mercury, b. cadmium, c. lead, d. other metals, III. Metallothionein, IV. Conclusions; and V. Recommendations.

I.   METABOLISM DURING PREGNANCY

The clinician, biologist and toxicologist are all confronted with a similar problem when considering xenobiotic exposure in the gravid female. At no other time do such diverse alterations in physiology, biochemistry, endocrinology and immunology appear so rapidly as during gestation.

From conception until delivery, the conceptus is modifying maternal processes. The actual recognition of pregnancy by the mother is the result of many sensitive physiological interactions between mother and the embryo-placental unit. The placenta, even at the blastocyst stage, releases its signals (protein and steroid hormones) to convert and adapt the maternal physiology to the immediate needs of the conceptus for intrauterine survival (see Miller et al., 1983).

A.   Maternal Factors

During the course of pregnancy, the plasma proteins in both mother and fetus are selectively increased. For example, thyroid binding globulins are increased in the mother by estrogen production from the placenta, and alpha-fetoprotein is increased in both fetus and mother. In addition, the maternal blood volume increases approximately 10-20 percent, and renal blood flow and plasma clearance are also increased. Due to the influences of pregnancy on the mother, the sensitivity of a target site and elimination of a metal may be modified. These maternal factors are summarized in Figure 1. However, these maternal factors cannot be studied independently of the placenta or embryo/fetus. Throughout pregnancy, maternal nutritional deprivation, altered hepatic metabolism, uteroplacental ischemia and uterotropic action, both by central, e.g., prolactin, and direct action, e.g., prostaglandins, can modify the metabolism of compounds as well as the survival of the embryo and fetus (Page et al., 1981; Miller, 1983).

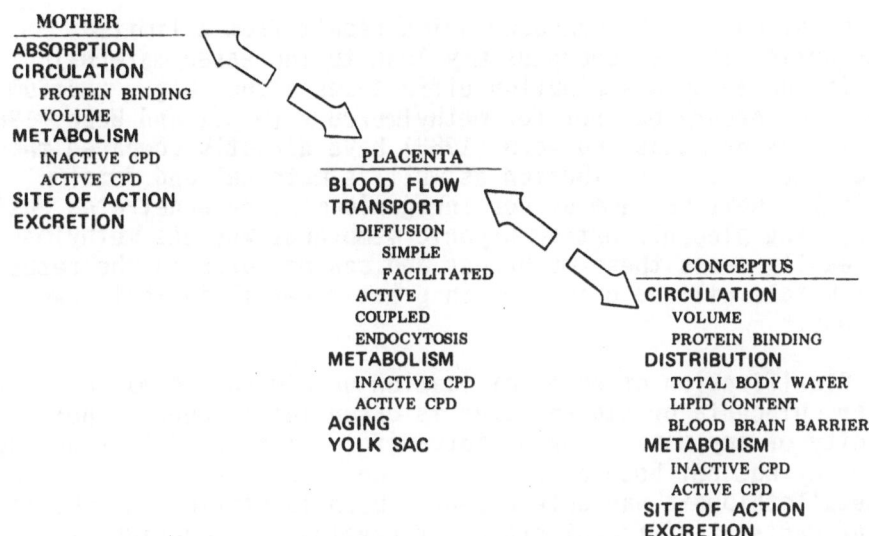

MOTHER
ABSORPTION
CIRCULATION
   PROTEIN BINDING
   VOLUME
METABOLISM
   INACTIVE CPD
   ACTIVE CPD
SITE OF ACTION
EXCRETION

PLACENTA
BLOOD FLOW
TRANSPORT
   DIFFUSION
     SIMPLE
     FACILITATED
   ACTIVE
   COUPLED
   ENDOCYTOSIS
METABOLISM
   INACTIVE CPD
   ACTIVE CPD
AGING
YOLK SAC

CONCEPTUS
CIRCULATION
   VOLUME
   PROTEIN BINDING
DISTRIBUTION
   TOTAL BODY WATER
   LIPID CONTENT
   BLOOD BRAIN BARRIER
METABOLISM
   INACTIVE CPD
   ACTIVE CPD
SITE OF ACTION
EXCRETION

Figure 1   Prenatal environmental exposures: factors related to
           mother, placenta and conceptus, Miller, 1983.

Dosing

In most animal studies, substances are normally administered
on the basis of an adult body weight; however, both maternal and
fetal toxicity can be substantially altered based upon the ratio of
uterine weight to maternal weight and the permeability of the
extraembryonic membranes to the metal. What weight of the mother
is the most accurate as a basis for a chemical exposure is open to
debate. Prepregnancy weight has been suggested as the weight at
day 7 of gestation. Most of the problems arise when the increase
in uterine contents is a large component of the total maternal
weight. This is especially true for rodents. These animals
usually have large litters and the fetuses are good size at birth.
Surface area measurements instead of weight have been used as a
denominator, but do not substantially compensate for these changes
during pregnancy. Thus, exposure during the fetal period to metals
can result in substantially different maternal toxicity when
compared to the nonpregnant adult, as demonstrated for cadmium by
Parizek (1964b), Magos and Webb (1983) and Levin et al. (1983).

If an agent does not easily penetrate the placenta/
extraembryonic membranes and does not reach the fetus in
substantive concentrations, then higher maternal tissue

concentrations of the compound which result from a limited
distribution in the conceptus may lead to increased maternal
toxicity based on distribution differences alone, e.g., cadmium and
inorganic mercury but not for methylmercury (Magos and Webb, 1983).
The studies by Magos and Webb (1983) have directly compared these
three metals for distribution as well as maternal and fetal
toxicity. Neither cadmium nor inorganic mercury penetrates easily
through the placenta/extraembryonic membranes whereas methylmercury
does easily cross these membranes and concentrates in the fetus.
These metals will be discussed in greater detail in their own
sections.

Clarification of detoxicification or biotransformation by the
mother, placenta or embryo/fetus is essential to understanding the
toxicity of any metal. Such biotransformation for metals during
pregnancy has not been documented in many species. Even the role
of metallothionein has only recently been identified in subcellular
compartments at different stages of development (Cherian et al.,
1983; this volume).

B.   Placental Factors

The placenta and the extraembryonic membranes are the critical
interfaces between maternal organism - conceptus. In addition to
synthesizing and releasing both steroid and protein hormones
(Klopper, 1982,1983), the placenta regulates the movement and
biotransformation of numerous nutrients and xenobiotics. Under
experimental conditions, the trophoblast (placenta) can be
compromised by certain metals, e.g., cadmium (Parizek, 1964a; Levin
et al., 1983). Thus, it is essential to understand the physiology
and biochemistry of the trophoblast to understand metal metabolism
during pregnancy.

The placenta is the only organ which is served by two
completely independent blood supplies. The potential for multiple
interactions is enormous. If one considers only the movement of
nutrients, oxygen, and the waste product, carbon dioxide, one may
invoke both a double-Bohr effect as well as a double-Haldane
effect. Differences in fetal plasma concentrations of various
xenobiotics may be related to the relative affinity of a metal for
the plasma proteins or the fetal hemoglobin or differences in
plasma concentrations of these proteins, e.g., methylmercury and
calcium. In addition, the placenta has the capability of producing
certain plasma protein carriers, e.g., transcobalamin II for
Vitamin B_{12} (Ng et al., 1981; Ng and Miller, 1983).

The models necessary to study the pharmacokinetics of a metal
are therefore complicated by this cellular interface, which

separates two different blood supplies. Under certain conditions,
the placenta retards the movements of certain metals, e.g., cadmium
and inorganic mercury, while allowing organic mercurials to pass
more rapidly from mother into the embryo/fetus.

Distribution of drugs and other substances within the feto-
placental unit has been investigated using a number of different
models. The discussion of pharmacokinetic models for specific
metals are discussed in Section II: Metabolism of Specific
Metals. Excellent reviews of pharmacokinetic models for acute
exposures in the feto-placental unit are presented by Levy and
Hayton (1973), Anderson et al. (1980), Waddell and Marlowe
(1981a,b), and Levy (1981). Unfortunately, neither for metals nor
other xenobiotics have chronic exposure paradigms been
systematically evaluated for the pregnant female.

Perhaps the most difficult aspect of studying placental
function, especially transport, is the tremendous species variation
in morphology and functionality of the chorioallantoic placenta
versus the other membranes, e.g., the visceral yolk sac. Even
though rodents are the most common laboratory animal for the
investigation of metal toxicity, their developmental patterns are
substantially different from the human (Miller et al., 1976;
Miller, 1983). In the rodent, the visceral yolk sac is functional
throughout gestation and has important roles both early in
gestation as well as at term. In the human after the first
trimester, little function has been attributed to this tissue.
Actually, even during early gestation in the human, little
transport function has been attributed to the yolk sac, since the
trophoblast plays the critical role even before nidation. In the
rodent, the ovary/ corpus luteum is important for the maintenance
of the pregnancy, while in the human by 6-8 weeks, an ovarectomy
can be performed without compromising the pregnancy.

In the rodent, until days 10-14, depending upon the species,
the visceral yolk sac does perform an essential nutritive role.
This earlier phase has been named histiotrophic nutrition, while
the later phase has been called hemotrophic nutrition based on the
circulatory role of the umbilical and uterine blood flows in the
chorioallantoic placenta necessary to maintain the ever enlarging
fetus (Beck, 1982).

Many of the embryo toxic effects of certain metals have been
attributed to the fact that early in gestation (before day 11) the
metals appear in the embryonic tissue. These metals also appear in
the yolk sac. If the metals are administered after days 9.5-11,
then much higher doses of the metals may be necessary to document
the appearance of the metal in the fetus. Selectivity of function/
transport for the yolk sac versus the trophoblast may be an

important species difference; the teratogenicity of certain metals
may be due strictly to the relative placental permeability of the
metal or other substances. Cadmium and inorganic mercury are
examples of this selectivity (see Section II: Metabolism of
Specific Metals).

     Besides being the critical interface between mother and
conceptus, the placenta may be an index of environmental exposures
of humans to metals (Table 1). The placenta is perhaps the most
abundant human tissue routinely available. In addition, the tissue
content of metals may represent a reasonably short-term exposure
period, 9 months. Painters, ceramic workers, and smoking women all
appear to have higher levels of specific metals. If the amount of
smoking is taken into consideration, then different regions of the
world could be studied to determine other environmental factors,
such as power plants, smelters, and increased use of fossil fuels
(see individual metals, Section II: Metabolism of Specific Metals).

C.   Embryo/Fetal Factors

     The sensitivity of the embryo/fetus to metals is not only
dependent upon the permeability of the extraembryonic membranes,
but also upon the actual development of the conceptus. The
distribution of metals is quite often dependent upon the lipid
content in the animal. As noted in Figure 1, the fetus is not a
miniature adult; rather there is substantially more water content
in the fetus when compared with the adult. Further, the amount of
lipid is also increased in proportion to the total mass of the
fetus. The blood-brain barrier is poorly developed, and more of
the cardiac output goes directly to the brain of the fetus when
compared with the adult. Also due to the ductus arteriosus,
substances entering through the placenta and the umbilical
circulation are preferentially shunted to the central nervous
tissue rather than to the lung or visceral organs (Stave, 1978).

     In addition to the circulatory differences for the central
nervous system, the liver also receives proportionally more blood
from the umbilical circulation. The liver also represents a larger
percentage of the fetal body weight and has functional differences,
e.g., production of fetal erythrocytes, when compared with the
adult liver. Perhaps this is necessary due to the relative
immaturity of the fetal liver to metabolize xenobiotic agents.
However, the ability of the fetal liver to bind zinc, copper and
cadmium is substantially greater than that seen for the normal
adult. Sasser et al. (1980) demonstrated that direct injections of
cadmium into the fetus did not increase the amount of binding of
metallothionein in this fetal tissue. From the studies of Cherian
et al. (1983), it has become apparent that the elevated fetal and

neonatal levels of metallothionein, and thus consequently cadmium, are directly related to subcellular distribution of metallothionein. In the fetus and neonate most of the metallothionein is in the nucleus, whereas in the non-induced adult most of the metallothionein is in the cytosol. For additional information, see Section III: Metallothionein. The fetal skeleton concentrates numerous metals, e.g., arsenic, chromium, lead, nickel and strontium. This is important for chromate and arsenite, which alter cartilage formation (see Section II: Metabolism of Specific Metals).

The excretion of most waste products and xenobiotics by the fetus is dependent upon the placenta because the renal and gastrointestinal tract functions are immature and can result in recirculation. In many instances it is a benefit to the fetus to have immature hepatic, renal and gastrointestinal functions since the placenta, in conjunction with the mother, performs these functions more efficiently. If many conjugates were formed by the fetus, then placental permeability would be reduced and these products would also concentrate in the amniotic fluid. All of these factors would tend to compromise the continued development of the conceptus. For reviews of the physiological processes involved, see Stave (1978).

II. THE METABOLISM OF SPECIFIC METALS

The metabolism of a metal is dependent upon its physical characteristics and especially its abilities to interact with organic compounds, whether DNA, protein, glutathione or methylation. Yet the current limitations in quantifying metals makes monitoring metal levels in any population, but especially the human population, particularly difficult.

Monitoring

Questions are constantly raised concerning the comparability of data from different laboratories and different geographical regions. Many times, the specimens are processed differently and analyzed with different levels of quality assurance. Such variability within and between studies often makes comparison between studies exceedingly difficult.

The recent Global Environmental Monitoring System study, which evaluated human exposure to the selected metals, lead and cadmium, demonstrated some of the difficulties in achieving and maintaining quality assurance standards in ten different countries (Vahter, 1982). Many of the problems which arose with quality assurance

were: 1) inadequate technic for low concentrations of metals; a
need for Delves cup technic or electrothermal atomization (furnace)
atomic absorption; 2) poor alignment between light from cathode
lamp and deuterium lamp; 3) impurities (lead) in acetylene gas;
4) improper acid washing of glassware; 5) contamination of
laboratories, personnel (e.g., smokers not wearing gloves) and
water; 6) instrument breakdown; and 7) low accuracy of analytical
balances. As any given study begins to measure more than one trace
metal, the problems associated with accurate measurements increase
exponentially.

Among the recommendations for accurate measurements of trace
metals in biological specimens are: 1) to have the standards
prepared in similar biological material which has low metal
content; and 2) to routinely have multiple internal quality control
specimens to assure reproductibility, sensitivity and accuracy.
Without such quality assurances, the surveillance of populations
around the world is in question.

Metabolism studies in animals are often less prone to these
problems for at least two reasons: a) a radioactive metal is used;
and b) the studies involve exposures which are in excess of the
background levels. Thus, in the discussions of individual metals,
three principal methods of analysis have been utilized, atomic
absorption spectroscopy, gamma scintillation spectrometry, and to a
lesser extent, neutron activation.

Metabolism

This section will review individual metals in relationship to
metabolism in the pregnant woman and animal models. Unfortunately,
little kinetic data are available due to the inaccessibility of the
embryo/fetus. Human tissues most accessible are the placenta and
the cord blood. In addition, amniotic fluid has been analyzed
(Suzuki et al., 1977; Fochtman et al., 1982). With the availability
of amniocentesis, amniotic fluid may be the only biological
specimen routinely available for multiple sampling throughout
gestation. Yet, how representative this fluid is of embryonic/
fetal tissue distribution of the metal in question is not
apparent. Hair samples from newborns have also been compared with
maternal hair for metal content (Huel et al., 1981). Procedures
are now available to measure particular segments of a single strand
of hair. Autopsy specimens are often available, but also reflect
only a single time point for the evaluation of metal metabolism.

The actual methods for evaluating the placental transfer of
metals in animal models have been discussed in a previous chapter
(Miller et al., 1976,1983). Therefore, experimental results will
be a primary focus of this review.

A.   MERCURY

The metabolism of mercury is dependent upon its form. As noted previously, the inorganic form has a different pattern of distribution when compared with the organic form, e.g., methylmercury. This distribution can account partially for the differences in embryo toxicity and lethality of the different forms.

Human Studies

As described previously organic mercurial exposure during pregnancy has resulted in human developmental disorders (Harada, 1978; Amin-Zaki et al., 1974). The actual exposure levels and distribution of methylmercury in the gravid woman were not documented at the time of exposure; however, in Iraq, detailed evaluation of infant-mother units was undertaken approximately 2-3 months following the exposure to the methylmercury fungicide in home made bread. The lowest blood level of mercury in the mothers associated with maternal symptoms was 300 ng/ml. Eight mothers had blood levels of 5-253 ng/ml with no symptoms. Infants who have blood levels of mercury in excess of 1,053 ng/ml did have symptoms. Seven infants had no symptoms with blood levels of 416 ng/ml, while an infant had no symptoms with blood levels of 636 ng/ml (Amin-Zaki et al., 1974). In Minimata Bay, Japan, umbilical cord values for methylmercury were more than 1,000 ng/ml in many cases (Harada, 1978).

When infant blood was compared with maternal blood (Clarkson et al., 1981), the levels of mercury were greater for the infant's blood. This greater ratio is also seen for cord blood (Table 1). Since methylmercury binds to red blood cells and the fetus has a higher hematocrit than the mother, this may partially account for higher cord levels of mercury. Greenwood et al. (1978) noted that the blood devised half-life in lactating women (42 days) was significantly shorter than in non-lactating women (79 days). Blood levels in prenatally exposed suckling infants tended to remain higher than the maternal levels of mercury 12 months following birth (Amin-Zaki et al., 1974). Blood levels in infants exposed to methylmercury in maternal milk eventually exceeded maternal blood levels after six months of exposure (Amin-Zaki et al., 1974). In both the prenatal and postnatal exposed groups, maternal exposure had ceased before any blood samples were collected.

Studies from many regions of the world have determined the mercury content in human placentae as well as maternal and fetal blood (Table 1).

It is known from animal studies (see Mercury Animal Models) that the different forms of mercury are distributed differently. Usually the cord blood levels of total mercury in uncomplicated pregnancies are approximately 25 percent greater than maternal blood levels (Table 1). The distribution of the mercury is dependent upon its form. Inorganic mercurials bind to both plasma proteins and hemoglobin, while organic mercurials bind primarily to red blood cells (Friberg and Vostal, 1971). Suzuki et al. (1971) postulated this distribution of mercury in maternal and cord blood based on the distribution in red blood cells. However only recently, has Kuhnert et al. (1981) measured the chemical form of mercury by gas chromatographic technic developed by Cappon and Smith (1977). Even though total mercury in the human placenta was among the lowest reported, 30 percent more methylmercury was found in the fetal erythrocytes compared with maternal erythrocytes. The placenta had the highest concentration of inorganic mercury (Table 1) compared with the bloods, which is consistent with the animal studies. Under some conditions, methylmercury was detectable in the fetal red blood cells but not in the maternal red blood cells. Further, there is a strong correlation between levels of inorganic mercury in cord and maternal bloods which suggests that some inorganic mercury does pass through the placenta. Such higher levels of methylmercury bound to fetal hemoglobin have not been adequately explained either by increased hematocrit or total binding capacity (Kuhnert et al., 1981).

The forms of mercury most commonly considered are metallic mercury, mercuric ion, phenylmercury and methylmercury. Metallic mercury and organic mercurials diffuse more rapidly across all membranes and concentrate in the brain (Berlin et al., 1969). However, metallic mercury is not readily absorbed by the gastrointestinal tract, but is by the lungs. With mercuric compounds approximately 10 percent of the total ingested is absorbed by the gastrointestinal tract. In contrast, organic mercurials are rapidly absorbed by the gastrointestinal tract (as reviewed by Koos and Longo, 1976). Phenylmercury is rapidly metabolized to inorganic mercury and excreted as such (Takeda et al., 1968). Inorganic mercury is excreted by both feces and urine with a half-life of 30 to 60 days (Friberg and Vostal, 1971), while methylmercury is excreted primarily in the feces.

Detailed studies in pregnant women involving all forms of mercury, even the methylmercury exposure data, leave numerous voids in our knowledge. Animal experimentation has provided additional information concerning the kinetics of mercurial compounds and environmental interaction in the fetus, e.g., ethanol - catalase and mercury vapor.

Table 1 The Placenta and Bloods as Indices for Mercury Exposure in Humans

	Exposure[1]	N	Maternal Blood ng/ml			Placental ng/ml	Cord Blood ng/ml			References
			Blood	RBC	Plasma		Blood	RBC	Plasma	
Tokyo, Japan	EN	9	1.68*	2.29 ± 1.19	1.24 ± 0.73	7.15 ± 2.74	2.00*	3.08 ± 2.16	1.12 ± 0.72	Suzuki et al., 1971
Nashville, TN	SU	1061	0.87			2.15 ± 2.68	1.15			Baglan et al., 1971
Iowa City, IA	SU	38	0.10			0.23 ± 0.18	0.12			Pitkin et al., 1975
Belgium-Urban Total	EN	474	1.26 ± 0.69			1.53 ± 1.41	1.42 ± 0.85*			Roels et al., 1978
Non-smokers	SU	333	1.12 ± 0.65			1.62 ± 1.50	1.36 ± 0.74*			Lauwerys et al., 1978
Smokers	SU	109	1.31 ± 0.70			1.22 ± 0.98	1.42 ± 0.80*			Buchet et al., 1978
Belgium-Rural	SU	70	1.45			0.97	1.59			Hubermont et al., 1978
Charlotte, NC	SU					1.90 ± 0.30				Karp & Robertson, 1977
Birmingham, AL	SU					1.50 ± 0.30				Karp & Robertson, 1977
Augusta, GA	SU					0.80 ± 0.10				Karp & Robertson, 1977
Cleveland, OH Total	SU	29	0.76	0.55	0.21	0.67	0.83	0.53	0.30	Kuhnert et al., 1981
Methyl Hg			0.34	0.30 ± 0.2	0.04 ± 0.02	0.14 ± 0.11	0.43	0.39 ± 30	0.04 ± 0.03	Kuhnert et al., 1981
Inorganic Hg			0.42	0.25 ± 0.18	0.17 ± 0.14	0.53 ± 0.32	0.40	0.14 ± 12	0.26 ± 0.19	Kuhnert et al., 1981

1 Suspected principal route of exposure to the metal:
  EN   Environmental
  DW   Drinking water
  OCC Occupational
  SU   Screening study or unknown route

* Significantly different from control population.

Animal Studies

METALLIC MERCURY

Metallic mercury administered as mercury vapor has been investigated in both rats and mice (Clarkson et al., 1972; Greenwood et al., 1972; Khayat and Dencker, 1982). Twenty-four hours following exposure to mercury vapor, the fetal tissue levels were 0.22 percent of the administered dose. Approximately equivalent amounts or concentrations of mercury were found in the fetus and in the placenta. During early gestation, it appears that only traces of metallic mercury are apparent in the embryonic tissues, while later in gestation substantially more mercury is present following the mercury vapor exposure (Khayat and Dencker, 1982). These observations were made using autoradiographic technics and compared with mercuric chloride. Previous studies by Clarkson et al. (1961) and Nielsen-Kudsk (1969) have suggested that even though mercury vapor is administered by inhalation, once in the body it is oxidized to mercuric ion by tissue catalase. Metabolism of mercury vapor has been proposed as the basis for increased fetal accumulation of mercury vapor as gestation progresses, since catalase activity also increases.

Additional studies utilizing ethanol to inhibit catalase have demonstrated a redistribution of mercury in the fetus as well as in the mother (Dencker et al., 1983). Thus, it appears that mercury vapor is oxidized in fetal tissues, and not transferred to the fetus in the form of mercuric ions after oxidation in the mother. Even though these autoradiographic data are not measuring the exact form of the ion, the four-fold increase in total accumulation of mercury in the fetal carcass when ethanol is present, while there was a substantial decrease in levels of mercury in the maternal carcass raises additional questions concerning environmental interactions and the potential for increased toxicity of these metals in the fetus.

MERCURIC ION

Mercuric ion has substantially different distribution compared to metallic mercury in rats, mice and guinea pigs (Berlin and Ullberg, 1963b; Clarkson et al., 1972; Suzuki et al., 1967; Kelman, 1977). Mercuric ion does not appear to penetrate well into the fetus. After 24 hours, only 0.01 percent of an injected dose of mercuric chloride was present in the rat fetus; however, 0.52 percent of injected mercuric ion could be found in the placenta (Clarkson et al., 1972). Autoradiographic data in the mouse confirmed these observations. Kelman (1977) utilized an in situ-perfused guinea pig placenta preparation during late gestation to demonstrate the

relative impermeability of mercuric ion into the fetal circulation.
In comparison studies with methylmercury, mercuric ion administered
to pregnant rats and mice had 5 to 17 times less radio-labeled
mercury in the newborns (Suzuki et al., 1967; Mansour et al., 1973;
Sasser et al., 1977). When low doses of mercuric ion are
administered to the pregnant rat on day 18 of gestation, by day 21,
only a total of 0.36 percent of the dose is present in the fetus,
following an intravenous injection of 0.7 micrograms. Suzuki et al.
(1967) demonstrated that when mice were injected subcutaneously with
40 micrograms of mercuric ion on day 14 of gestation, by day 19,
only 0.14 percent of the dose was retained by the fetus. When
pregnant rats were injected on day 12 of gestation with 1.9
micrograms of mercuric ion, by day 21 of gestation each fetus
absorbed 0.07 percent of the administered dose (Mansour et al.,
1973). From these data, it is apparent that mercuric ion, whether
measured 24 hours or 8 days later, still does not rapidly penetrate
into the conceptus, but is highly concentrated by the placenta.

These observations in the rat and mouse were confirmed and
extended by Berg and Smith (1982). Elimination and organ
distribution was followed up to 37 days after exposure in pregnant
mice administered single oral doses of mercuric oxide. Elimination
fit a three compartment model with half lives of 9 hours, 2 days and
15 days. Feces and urine in a 9:1 ratio contained 100 percent of
the dose administered. The highest organ concentrations were in
maternal liver, kidneys and placentae. Besides having the lowest
tissue concentrations, the maternal brain, fetuses and neonates also
had the slowest rates of loss for mercuric ion.

Thus, the low prenatal toxicity of mercuric ion in various
species is apparently related to the pharmacokinetics of mercuric
ion and its poor permeability into the conceptus.

ORGANO MERCURY

The metabolism of all organo mercurials is not the same. This
is especially true for phenylmercury and methylmercury. The
distribution of phenylmercury is similar to mercuric ion (Berlin and
Ullberg, 1963c, d; Suzuki et al., 1967; Garrett et al., 1972). When
levels of mercury in placental and extraembryonic membranes are
substantially higher than in the fetus, only 0.074 percent of the
maternal dose (2.5 mg/kg) was found in the fetus even four days
after injection (Suzuki et al., 1967).

These results for phenylmercury are certainly in contrast to
the disposition of methylmercury (Suzuki et al., 1967). A similar
maternal dose of methylmercury resulted in approximately 1.4 percent
of the injected dose appearing in the mouse fetus. Garrett et al.
(1972) observed similar dispositions in 14-day old fetuses. If one

compares these methylmercury values in the fetus to those in the
mother, only 11 percent of the injected dose was still present in
the mother. In contrast to direct injections of methylmercury,
Reuhl and Pounds (1981) studied the metabolism of methylmercury in
the pregnant hamster following a single oral administration of
tracer amounts of ^{203}Hg methylmercury on day 9 of gestation.
Twelve hours post intubation, the pregnant hamster absorbed slightly
more (96 versus 92 percent) of the administered dose, when compared
with the non-pregnant hamster. After twelve hours, the retention
and elimination curves were similar. In contrast to the studies of
Magos and Webb (1983), the cerebellum, pons-medulla, and spleens of
the pregnant females had more mercury present than for the
non-pregnant hamster. It should be noted that Magos and Webb (1983)
did not investigate regional differences in brain levels, but rather
whole brain levels. As has been noted for the human, monkey, mouse
and rat, the fetal brain (head) has greater concentrations of
mercury than the rest of the body (Bakir et al., 1973; Nordberg et
al., 1973; Childs, 1973; Mansour et al., 1974; Matsumoto et al.,
1967).

     The distribution of methylmercury is substantially different
dependent upon whether it represents a chronic or acute exposure.
Chronic exposure to methylmercury in utero resulted in brain levels
being higher than those of liver and kidney (Nordberg et al.,
1973). However, following a single intravenous administration of
^{203}Hg methylmercury, both the placenta and fetal brain retarded
the movement of the mercury. This decrease in movement has been
partially attributed to the extensive red blood cell binding for
methylmercury. During the seven hours of evaluation, the
concentrations of methylmercury were maternal red blood cells>fetal
red blood cells>maternal plasma>fetal plasma and fetal amniotic
fluid. Some fetal tissues concentrated methylmercury to higher
levels than in blood cells: Placenta>liver>spleen>sciatic nerve>
kidneys>ovary>muscles>skin>cerebellum>cerebrum>umbilical cord
blood. This relationship was similar whether methylmercury was
administered to mother or directly to the fetus, with the exception
of the placenta, which was about 10-fold lower when methylmercury
was administered to the fetus.

     The regional differences in methylmercury distribution in the
brain have been partially attributed to the more extensive
localization of methylmercury in gray matter (Berlin et al., 1973).
In addition to these tissue differences, it appears that even though
the placenta affords the primate fetus some protection from acute
exposure, the observation that methylmercury moves more readily into
the fetal circulation than out may also account for the fetal hazard
following chronic exposure.

     The importance of the blood brain barrier in the fetus may
relate to near term responses of the fetus, since earlier studies

during gestation were not performed. Thus, studies during early
gestation would be necessary to establish these kinetic
characteristics. However, it is apparent that whether methylmercury
is fed orally to mice in tuna fish (Childs, 1973) or intravenously
to primates, the fetal tissue distribution and relative placental
permeability to the forms of mercury compounds account for the
relative prenatal toxicity observed.

B.   LEAD

Of the metals discussed in this chapter, lead has been the most
thoroughly studied in man and animal models. Tissues that have the
highest concentration of lead in the fetus are skeleton, blood, skin,
and placenta (Barry, 1981; Dencker et al., 1983; Khera et al., 1980;
Wibberley et al., 1977; Table 2). In particular, the hemoglobin has
a high affinity for lead. This is especially true for fetal
hemoglobin (Ong and Lee, 1980). This higher affinity for fetal
hemoglobin may partially account for the concentration of lead in
the fetal blood. Yet as seen in Table 2, the fetal/neonatal blood
does not concentrate lead to higher levels than documented for the
maternal blood.

Human Studies

Various subgroups of the human population have been investigated
to determine any correlation between lead and metals in the placenta,
and/or cord bloods with higher levels of metal exposure, or
complications during pregnancy.

Substantial variation is apparent between laboratories as well
as within laboratories with alternative analytical technics
(Wibberley et al., 1977; Khera et al., 1980). Fahim and colleagues
reported a two- to four-fold higher concentration of lead in the
blood of women with premature delivery or premature rupture of the
membranes (PROM) than in women without these complications (Fahim et
al., 1976). A more recent study by Angell and Lavery (1982) did not
find substantial differences in fetal blood levels of lead for these
complications in pregnancy (Table 2). Although 154 sets of cord and
maternal blood measurements were compared and were highly correlated
as noted in Table 2, there is no significant difference between the
maternal and cord blood levels of lead. As gestation progresses,
Barry (1981) noted an increasing level of lead in blood.

Environmental exposures to lead have been associated with
higher levels of lead in the embryo/fetus. When humans are exposed
to lead in drinking water in concentrations in excess of 50
micrograms per liter, there is a significantly higher level of lead
in maternal and cord blood as well as in the placenta when compared

Table 2 The Placenta and Bloods as Indices for Lead Exposure in Humans

Location	Exposure[1]	#	Maternal Blood ng/ml	Placenta ng/gm	Cord Blood ng/ml	Reference
Germany						
rural	SU	12	–	100 ± 3	–	Thieme et al., 1974
urban	SU	55	–	350 ± 30	–	Thieme et al., 1974
Dortmund	SU	53	–	374 ± 174	–	Thurauf et al., 1975
Erlangen	SU	34	–	306 ± 88	–	Thurauf et al., 1975
Roding	SU	61	–	387 ± 147	–	Engelhardt et al., 1976
Belgium						
TOTAL		474	102 ± 37	84 ± 57	84 ± 35	Roels et al., 1978
non-smokers	EN	333	100 ± 40	83 ± 57	81 ± 35	Bucket et al., 1978
smokers	EN	109	105 ± 32	85 ± 44	89 ± 33	Lauwerys et al., 1978
TOTAL		70	120	111	101	Hubermont et al., 1978
water 50 g/L	DW	41	106	97	88	
water 50 g/L	DW	29	138*	133*	121*	
Tennessee						
Nashville	SU	234	–	305 ± 427	–	Baglan et al., 1971
Missouri						
Columbia	SU	249	–	70 ± 16	–	Fahim et al., 1976
Rolla	SU	253	–	80 ± 9.5	–	Fahim et al., 1976

1 Suspected principal route of exposure to the metal:
   EN Environmental
   DW Drinking water
   OCC Occupational
   SU Screening study or unknown route

* Significantly different from control population.

Data significantly different from Khera et al., 1980; suggested technical difficulties as an explanation for Webberley et al., 1977.

Location	Exposure[1]	#	Maternal Blood ng/ml	Placenta ng/gm	Cord Blood ng/ml	Reference
North Carolina Charlotte	SU		-	312 + 50	-	Karp and Robertson, 1977
Alabama Birmingham	SU		-	296 + 34	-	Karp and Robertson, 1977
Georgia Augusta	SU		-	275 + 50	-	Robertson, 1977
United Kingdom						
Birmingham						
Normal births	SU	24	-	930 + 640	-	Webberley et al., 1977
Malformed Stillbirths	SU	13	-	1480 + 690*	-	Webberley et al., 1977
Non-malformed Stillbirths	SU	8	-	1450 + 500*	-	Webberley et al., 1977
Premature Births	SU	24	-	960 + 280*	-	Webberley et al., 1977
Birmingham				120		Khera et al., 1980
Stoke on Trent						Khera et al., 1980

(continued)

Table 2   The Placenta and Bloods as Indices for Lead Exposure in Humans (continued)

Location	Exposure[1]	#	Maternal Blood ng/ml	Placenta ng/gm	Cord Blood ng/ml	Reference
Pottery Industry						
Transferrer	OCC	8	120	$340 + 140$	-	Barry et al., 1981
Lithographer	OCC	16	190 ± 90	340 ± 160	-	
Painter	OCC	7	240 ± 90	700 ± 150	-	
Northwest Area						
Normal Births	SU	15	-	-	123 ± 64	
Stillbirths	SU	13	-	-	106 ± 52	
1-5 Years	SU	8	-	-	188 ± 115	
11-16 Years	SU	5	-	-	164 ± 82	
Kentucky						Angel and Lowrey, 1982
Louisville						
Normal	SU	635	-	-	94 ± 41	
PROM	SU	56	-	-	98 ± 36	
Premature						
Delivery	SU	74	-	-	101 ± 45	
Pre eclambosia	SU	32	-	-	87 ± 36	
Meconium						
Staining	SU		98 ± 44	-	91 ± 39	
Normals	SU	123	-	-	97 ± 41	
Massachusetts						
Boston	EN	11837	-	-	65 ± 32	Rabinowitz and Needleman, 1982

Location	Exposure[1]	#	Maternal Blood ng/ml	Placenta ng/gm	Cord Blood ng/ml	Reference
United Kingdom						
Rural						
Ashington						
Pregnant	EN	165	122 ± 31	-	114 ± 41	(Neonate, 6 days) Alexander and Delves, 1981
non-preg.	EN	19	132 ± 29	-		
City						
Newcastle						
Upon Tyne						
Pregnant	EN	19	157 ± 27	-	-	Alexander and Delves, 1981
Non-Preg.	EN	20	170 ± 31			
Zambia						
Lead Mine Gr.	OCC	122	412 ± 144	-	370 ± 153	Clark, 1977
Control Gr.		31	147 ± 75	-	118 ± 56	

with similar tissues from women who routinely drink water with less lead (Hubermont et al., 1978). This is in contrast to the smoker, where there does not appear to be any significant differences in blood or placental levels of lead (Roels et al., 1978; Buchet et al., 1978; Lauwerys et al., 1978). In England, an investigation in the pottery industry did demonstrate that even though the numbers of exposed individuals are small, it is apparent that depending upon the occupation in the factory, whether painter or transferrer, there can be substantial differences in the amount of lead in the placenta (Khera et al., 1980). Also the length of employment in this industry was correlated with higher blood levels. Employment of less than one year's duration gave average values of approximately 300 nanograms per gram, whereas greater than six years of occupational exposure resulted in placental levels of an average of 460 nanograms per gram (Khera et al., 1980).

It should be noted that standardization of analysis is essential. Previous studies by the Khera group (Wibberley et al., 1977) in Birmingham had observed the highest levels of lead reported in placentae. Even though relative differences between normal and abnormal births (malformations) may be suggestive, the absolute values were not reproduced by the later Khera study (1980).

Correlations were reported between placental levels of lead and other environmental conditions (rural vs city vs occupational exposure) (Table 2; Thieme et al., 1974; Khera et al., 1980; Alexander and Delves, 1981). Maternal and newborn hair have also been analysed (Huel et al., 1981), but no strong correlations were established.

Neonatal/cord blood levels of lead were consistently lower than maternal values (Roels et al., 1978; Alexander and Delves, 1981; Angell and Lavery, 1982). Even though fetal hemoglobin has a higher affinity for lead, perhaps the reason for the lower neonatal/cord levels of lead may be related to a rapid distribution of the lead to other fetal organs, especially bone. Thus, besides the relative impermeability of the extraembryonic membranes to lead, redistribution within the fetus may be equally important as suggested by Alexander and Delves (1981).

The observations recorded here for human exposures to lead have been of either normal background levels or chronic exposures to lead, from drinking water or occupational sources. There are no reports of acute exposures to lead during pregnancy, which are the primary data reported for animal models.

As compared to a number of animal studies, there does remain some question whether the human placenta does concentrate lead to substantially high levels than in the maternal blood (Table 2). Yet whether for the placenta, cord blood or hair, the use of these specimens have been a means for documenting human exposure.

Animal Studies

Lead penetrates into the extraembryonic membranes and enters into the conceptus in numerous species besides man (Carpenter et al., 1973; Green and Gruener, 1974; McClain and Becker, 1975; Kimmel et al., 1980). The distribution of lead within the conceptus is dependent upon the permeability of the placenta as well as the relative affinity of the embryonic/fetal tissue among other factors.

Lead is highly concentrated by the yolk sac of the hamster following administration of lead on day 7 or 8 of gestation (Carpenter et al., 1973). Autoradiographic studies demonstrated the persistence of lead in the visceral yolk sac even five days later. At this stage of development, the yolk sac is the primary source for nutrients as well as the site for red blood cell synthesis. The developing chorioallantoic placenta, myometrium and decidua have only moderate levels of lead. Lead was present at high levels in the embryos, which had malformations or were resorbing.

Preliminary studies by Green and Gruener (1974) indicated that if lead was injected into the pregnant mouse later in gestation, more lead would appear in the newborn. Such higher levels of lead in the newborn could be attributed to 1) increasing uterine weight near term and therefore increasing maternal doses of lead; 2) less available time for excretion of lead by fetus and mother; 3) increased placental permeability of lead; and, 4) localization of lead in fetal tissues, which have differing amounts or affinities for lead, e.g., bone.

McClain and Becker (1975) resolved some of these questions by utilizing both intravenous single injections and infusions of lead into rats. When 50 mg/kg of lead acetate was injected on day 17 of gestation, the half-time of lead in the maternal plasma was approximately 5 hours. At 24 hours, the maternal plasma levels of lead were about 100 µg/ml. Fetal levels of lead rose from 0.8 µg/gm at 1 hour to 12 µg/gm at 24 hours. This teratogenic dose of lead was also largely concentrated in maternal liver, kidney and spleen. By 24 hours, the placental and fetal levels of lead were not in equilibrium. With infusion studies increasing maternal plasma levels of lead (to greater than 400 µg/ml after 60 minutes), the whole fetal levels of lead were 2.4 µg/gm. Detectable levels of lead were noted in the fetus even after two minutes of infusion. Unfortunately, no fetal blood or plasma levels of lead or tissues levels were reported.

Thus, it appears that the placenta may supply the fetus with lead even when maternal plasma levels of lead have fallen below the placental concentrations of lead. Similar maternal observations in pregnant mice were noted by Dencker et al. (1983) following intravenous administration of lead acetate. Consistently, there were higher tissue concentrations of lead in older fetuses (13-18 days of gestation). These increasing tissue levels of lead with advancing gestational age are partially attributed to the individual tissues (skeleton, liver, blood). After 24 hours, the fetal blood levels of lead are only slightly lower than the lead concentrations in the maternal blood (Dencker et al., 1983). The slowly rising fetal levels of lead have been partially attributed to reduced permeability and high placental concentrations of lead but especially in rodents were due to the fact that red blood cells are initially synthesized in the yolk sac.

Kimmel et al. (1980) in chronic low exposure lead studies (0.5-250 ppm in the drinking water) have demonstrated a dose related increase in the 21-day old fetal carcass of the rat from a control value of 0.08 to 0.75 ppm at an exposure dose of 50 ppm. The fetal brain levels of lead (0.05 ppm) did not differ significantly with dose. However, the maternal blood levels of lead increased from 4 µg percent to 3.5 (control vs 50 ppm). Thus, low level lead exposure did not produce malformations or increase perinatal mortality. Unfortunately, no other tissue levels of lead were reported, which would have been most helpful, e.g., for fetal blood and placenta.

C.   CADMIUM

There is increasing use of cadmium by the industrialized nations. Various industries utilize cadmium in paints, plastics, electroplating of steel, alloys, and batteries and for fertilizer, especially as sewage sludge (as reviewed by Friberg et al., 1974; Carmichael et al., 1982). With the increasing use of fossil fuels, more cadmium may be released into the environment. With this increasing risk of exposure to cadmium, studies have been undertaken in both pregnant humans and animal models to assess both the effects of and the metabolism of cadmium. In Japan, the association between the Itai-Itai syndrome and cadmium has not resulted in any clarification concerning the perinatal toxicity of cadmium, since the syndrome appears primarily in women over the age of 40 years (Friberg et al., 1974). In animal studies, cadmium can certainly be toxic to the developing organism. This toxicity is dependent upon the period of gestation in which the cadmium is administered (see reviews - Ferm and Hanlon, 1983; Mottet et al., 1983).

Human Studies

Even though there are no documented cases of major malformations due to cadmium exposure in the human, increasing associations with perinatal toxicity have been raised for smoking/cadmium/pregnancy, and hypertension/cadmium/pregnancy (Table 3; Huel et al., 1981). As noted for mercury and lead, cadmium is also present in the placenta. The human placenta concentrates

Table 3 The Placenta and Bloods as Indices for Cadmium Exposure in Humans

Location	Exposure[1]	#	Maternal Blood ng/ml	Placenta ng/gm	Cord Blood ng/ml	Reference
Sweden	SU	44	-	10	-	Friberg et al., 1974
Germany						
rural	SU	29	-	18 ± 1	-	Thieme et al., 1974
urban	EN	45	-	21 ± 4	-	Thieme et al., 1974
Dortmund	SU	53	-	176 ± 51	-	Thurauf et al., 1975
Erlangen						
Nurnberg	SU	34	-	129 ± 37	-	Thurauf et al., 1975
Roding	SU	61	-	152 ± 52	-	Engelhardt et al., 1976
Belgium						
rural		70	1.4	11.4	0.6	Hubermont et al., 1978
TOTAL		474	1.5 ± 1.3	13.2 ± 8.7	1.0 ± 1.2	Lauwerys et al., 1978
non-smoker		333	1.2 ± 1.2	12.5 ± 8.6	1.0 ± 1.3	Bucket et al., 1978
smoker	EN	109	2.0 ± 1.2*	15.7 ± 9.2*	0.7 ± 0.9	Roels et al., 1978
Netherlands						
Amsterdam						
non-smoker	EN	31	-	8.2 ± 3.2*	-	Van Hattum et al., 1981
smoker		30	-	10.6 ± 5.2*	-	Van Hattum et al., 1981

1 Suspected principal route of exposure to the metal:
EN   Environmental
DW   Drinking water
OCC Occupational
SU   Screening study or unknown route

* Significantly different from control population.

(continued)

Table 3 The Placenta and Bloods as Indices for Cadmium Exposure in Humans (continued)

Location	Exposure[1]	#	Maternal Blood ng/ml	Placenta ng/gm	Cord Blood ng/ml	Reference
New York						
Rochester						
non-smoker		18	-	4.3 ± 2.8	-	Miller and Gardner, 1981
smoker	EN	24	-	19.2 ± 4.6*	-	
Ohio						
Cleveland						
non-smoker		31	2.2 ± 0.8	13.7 ± 6.4	1.9 ± 0.6	Kuhnert et al., 1982
smoker	EN	41	3.5 ± 1.7*	18.1 ± 7.3*	2.2 ± 0.9	Kuhnert et al., 1982

cadmium to substantially higher levels than seen in either the maternal or fetal blood (Table 3). If one uses the placenta as an index for cadmium exposure, there are greater levels of cadmium in placentae from smoking mothers than from non-smoking mothers. Such increased levels of cadmium, along with the other components of cigarette smoke, e.g., benzo(α)pyrene, carbon monoxide, cyanide, nicotine, have been associated with decreased birth weights, small placentae, and most recently, alterations in the endothelial cells of the fetal capillaries. In preliminary reports, Assmussen (1979) described thickening of the fetal endothelium in placenta from smoking mothers. Copius Peereboom-Stegeman and associates (1982) have extended these observations in both human placentae from smokers and in rats injected with cadmium at a dose of 0.2 mg/kg until day 19 of gestation.

Further studies utilizing in vitro perfused human placentae demonstrated that in perfusions up to 7 hours, cadmium is highly concentrated by the placenta with only minor levels in the fetal perfusate (Wier et al., 1983). These gradients are produced whether trace or 10 nm/ml levels of cadmium are originally present in the maternal perfusate.

In normal human fetuses, cadmium can be detected in liver 80 percent of the time with an average content of 113 ng/gm (Chaube et al., 1973). The average renal and brain contents of cadmium were 50 ng/gm and 140 µg/gm, respectively. These values are obtained from terminated pregnancies from regions in Japan that did not have excessive levels of cadmium in the environment. Bryce-Smith et al. (1977) in England, found higher levels of cadmium than zinc in stillbirths. Even though the levels of cadmium are higher, there is currently no reason to implicate cadmium as the causative agent for the pregnancy loss.

Hair has also been an index medium for documenting exposure to metals. Detectable levels of cadmium are present in the newborn hair (0.54 µg/gm) at levels comparable to maternal values (0.43 µg/gm) (Huel et al., 1981). Interestingly, the newborn hair from mothers with hypertension was three times greater than the maternal levels of cadmium and was significantly greater than newborn hair from normotensive mothers (Huel et al., 1981). These provocative observations lead to many speculations of increased placental permeability, or altered maternal and fetal distribution of cadmium in the hypertensive pregnancy; however, analysis of other tissue compartments must be performed in both normotensive and hypertensive populations.

Cadmium is thus, normally present in the fetus due to environmental exposures; however, levels of cadmium, which are toxic in animals models have not been reported in humans.

Animal Studies

The movement between mother and conceptus is dependent upon the stage of gestation. In the mouse and hamster, cadmium does reach the embryo during early organogenesis (Ferm et al., 1969; Dencker, 1975; Dencker et al., 1983). The distribution of cadmium in the early embryo is primarily in the primitive gut wall and vitelline duct; the highest concentrations of cadmium are in the visceral yolk sac (Dencker, 1975). Once the vitelline duct is closed about day 9 in the hamster and day 9.5 in the mouse, the movement of cadmium into the embryo decreased. This period of movement of cadmium into the embryo corresponds to the maximum time for teratogenicity for cadmium in these species.

Once the chorioallantoic placenta is functional there appears to be a decreasing transfer of cadmium to the embryo/fetus (Berlin and Ullberg, 1963a; Sonawane et al., 1975). On day 20 of gestation in the rat, an intravenous injection of cadmium resulted in only 0.015 percent/gm fetus of the feto-toxic dose accumulating in the fetus (Sonawane et al., 1975a; Ahokas and Dilts, 1979; Levin et al., 1983). The one exception to this decreased permeability of cadmium by the chorioallantoic placenta was noted by Kelman and Walter (1977) using an in situ perfused guinea pig placenta. In these studies, cadmium rapidly appeared in the fetal perfusates. Perhaps this represents a species difference for the guinea pig.

Feto-toxic doses of cadmium also produce placental necrosis (Parizek, 1964a,b; Sonawane et al., 1975b; Levin and Miller, 1980). With the exception of the maternal liver, the chorioallantoic placenta accumulated the most cadmium of all tissues (Samawickrama and Webb, 1981; Levin et al., 1983). The maternal blood levels of cadmium following a subcutaneous injection of 40 μmol/kg resulted in an exponential decay with a rapid rise in placental organ concentrations followed by a linear increase (Levin et al., 1983). Thus, the placental necrosis associated with fetal toxicity may be directly related to the rapid and high levels of cadmium concentrated in this organ.

Cadmium that does reach the fetus is highly concentrated in the fetal liver. Direct injections of cadmium into the fetus results in levels of cadmium in excess of those concentrated by the maternal liver (Levin and Miller, 1980; Sasser et al., 1980; see Section III: Metallothionein; Cherian et al., 1983; Webb, 1983). Intravenous injections of metallothionein-109 cadmium results in little cadmium appearing in the fetus or placenta (Plautz et al., 1980; Levin et al., 1981).

Thus, in both animal and human studies, the placenta highly concentrates cadmium; however, its movement into the conceptus is low in most species studied and dependent upon the stage of gestation.

D.   OTHER METALS

AMERICIUM

Among the other heavy metals are the actinodes which are also radiation hazards. Weiss et al. (1980) investigated the disposition of americium in pregnant mice. The lowest dose administered would be equivalent to 32 μci for a 150 lb. man, which is in excess of the known human ingestions (approximately 0.1 μci). At the lower ranges of the dose levels examined, the percent of americium incorporated after 48 hours exposure beginning on day 16 of gestation by the fetus, placenta and maternal femur decreased from fetus - 0.038 percent/gm, placenta - 0.9 percent/gm, femur - 8 percent/gm at 0.4 μci to 0.023, 0.75, and 5 percent/gm at 3.4 μci per mouse. The maternal level increased from 10 to 17 percent/mg as did carcass. Obviously, there is a dose-exposure effect for americium as well as plutonium. From these studies it was determined that atom for atom, 10-25 times smaller amounts of americium was incorporated into fetal tissue when compared to plutonium.

ARSENIC

Arsenic exists in many forms. The three most widely examined in relationship to developmental metabolism are pentavalent (arsenate), trivalent (arsenite) and dimethylarsenic. Arsenite has been identified as more toxic than arsenate even though both are teratogenic in rodents (Ferm and Hanlon, 1983; Dencker et al., 1983). Dencker et al. (1983) have postulated that the differences in teratogenicity for arsenate and arsenite are related to the differences in direct embryonic cellular toxicity rather than arsenic metabolism in the pregnant animal.

The earliest human reports of arsenic levels during pregnancy are by Underhill and Armatrude (1923) and Eastman (1931). It appears that organic arsenicals used in the treatment of syphillis did not readily cross the placenta, but were concentrated by the placenta. However, one case report (Luego et al., 1969) indicated that a dose of arsenic taken during the third trimester of pregnancy resulted in very high arsenic levels in the liver, brain and kidney of an 1100 gm neonate who died 11 hours after birth.

With these limited human studies, investigations have been undertaken in animal models. In the adult hamster and mouse, arsenite has a three times longer half-life than arsenate. Arsenite is accumulated by the liver and excreted in the bile, whereas arsenate is predominantly excreted in the urine (Dencker et al., 1983). If arsenite is given daily in the diet to pregnant rats (0-6 days of gestation), the arsenite is persistent in skin (0.36

percent), thyroid (1.1 percent), liver (0.6 percent), uterus (0.34 percent), ovaries (0.23 percent), brain (0.1 percent), bone (0.14 percent) and lung (0.29 percent) on a gm weight basis for the dam (Gerber et al., 1982). The absorption of arsenite was approximately 20 percent. If arsenite was intraperitoneally injected on day 12 of gestation, there were two metabolic components: 95 percent of the arsenite was excreted with a half-life of six hours, while the remaining 5 percent had a half-life of 2.4 days. The placental and embryonic levels of arsenic on day 13 of gestation decreased from 0.1 percent/gm at 12 days to less than 0.01 percent/gm on day 13. These values are about 10-fold lower than maternal uterine or ovarian levels of arsenic. Individual fetal or embryonic tissue levels were not reported.

By using autoradiographic technics, the relative placental permeability of the different forms of arsenic were determined in hamster, mouse and primate (Dencker et al., 1983). Both arsenate and arsenite do readily penetrate through the rodent placenta throughout gestation. On day 10 of gestation, there was a greater accumulation of arsenate in the neuroepithelium than when arsenate is administered between days 12-14 of gestation, which demonstrated no concentration of the metal. During the fetal period, substantial arsenate is noted in the fetal skeleton which is not present for arsenite. Further large concentrations of arsenic were noted in the fetal skin, eye and upper gastrointestinal tract. Even though the adult thyroid concentrated arsenic, the fetal thyroid did not, such is consistent with the ability of the early fetal thyroid to concentrate iodine. Dencker et al. (1983) suggest that this high localization of arsenic in the skin and gastrointestinal tract may be related to the keratin deposition in these tissues and the high affinity of arsenic for keratin.

Arsenite has a fetal distribution similar to that of the mother eight hours following a single maternal injection in the near term marmoset monkey (Dencker et al., 1983). In the fetus, there was a blood brain barrier for arsenite.

Organic arsenicals in the form of dimethylarsenic are concentrated in the fetal lens but are not specifically concentrated by the fetal skin or skeleton as noted for arsenate or arsenite (Dencker et al., 1983).

Thus, the metabolism of arsenicals by the pregnant female is quite dependent upon its form, route of biotransformation, and relative tissue affinities, especially for bone, eye and skin.

CHROMIUM

In the work environment, there are two forms of chromium

commonly present: trivalent (chromium chloride III) and sextavalent (sodium chromate VI). The metabolism of these forms of chromium are different and represent an explanation for their differences in developmental toxicity (Ferm and Hanlon, 1983; Danielsson et al., 1983; Dencker et al., 1983).

In the blood, sodium chromate VI is preferentially bound to red blood cells, while chromium chloride III is bound to plasma proteins. Wallenburg et al. (1978) have demonstrated in the rhesus monkey that if red blood cells are labelled with chromium and injected into the mother even after five days, the total circulating chromium in the fetus is only 0.03 percent. These observations are in contrast with the intravenous injection of chromium itself (Danielsson et al., 1982; Dencker et al., 1983).

In the 13-day pregnant mouse, chromate VI is more rapidly transferred to the embryo and is more highly concentrated in the embryo than is chromium chloride III (0.3 µg/gm vs 0.03 µg/gm one hr after injection). During early organogenesis, no chromium chloride III could be detected by autoradiographic technics in embryonic tissues. If chromium is administered on day 13 of gestation, only a small amount of chromium is present in embryonic tissues. In the late fetal period, chromium is present in the fetus, particularily localized in calcified areas of the skeleton (Dencker et al., 1983). During these periods, chromium is highly concentrated in the visceral yolk sac.

Chromate VI readily appears in the embryo/fetus throughout gestation, even though maternal blood levels were lower than that from chromium chloride. As with chromium, chromate also concentrated in the calcified regions of the skeleton. Both chromate and chromium concentrate in the visceral yolk sac. Since chromium does appear in both the embryo and the fetus, this distribution for chromium has many similarities to cadmium and inorganic mercury.

GALLIUM

Gallium has not been studied in the pregnant woman. The only study reviewed was in the mouse (Otten et al., 1973). By using autoradiographic technics, 24 hours after intravenous injection of 67-gallium, the 6-day embryo had scattered labelling of its tissues. In the 8-13 day pregnant mouse, gallium was localized in decidua, the fetal membranes and the embryonic limb buds. By day 14, most of the gallium was localized in the skeleton. No kinetic evaluation was performed.

NICKEL

Nickel crosses the extraembryonic membranes into the conceptus (Sunderman et al., 1978). Recent studies have demonstrated in the 16 day pregnant mouse that nickel is concentrated in the visceral yolk sac, lung, gastrointestinal tract and kidney even 72 hours after injection (Olsen and Jonson, 1979). Even the 5 and 6 day embryo accumulates nickel but with a general pattern of distribution. In addition, a high concentration is noted in the pituitary gland of both mother and fetus (Clary, 1975; Sunderman et al., 1978, 1983). Maximal concentrations of nickel in both blood and placentae are noted 2 hours after an intravenous injection. Nickel is excreted by the pregnant mouse within 42 hours based upon calculated biological half-times of 33 hours and 8.9 hours (Lu et al., 1981). It also appears that the fetal kidney can filter and excrete nickel on day 16 of gestation in the mouse; however, the kinetics of these processes have not been investigated (Sunderman et al., 1978).

Nickel can be embryotoxic in animals (see Mottet et al., 1983; see Sunderman et al., 1983). If an embryotoxic dose is administered to a pregnant mouse on day 8 of gestation, 800 times higher concentrations of nickel are found 4 hours after administration in the embryonic tissues of affected embryos than in non-affected embryos (Lu et al., 1981).

NIOBIUM

Niobium has not been detected in human tissues; however, if injected into pregnant rats, niobium can be detected in the fetus (Schroeder et al., 1965). Unfortunately, this is the only report available studying the disposition of niobium.

SELENIUM

Selenium can be found in a number of different forms; however, one, bis(methylmercuric) selenide, represents a combination with mercury. Selenium does rapidly enter the conceptus. Yet selenium does not modify the movement of methylmercury; however, methylmercury does enhance the fetal accumulation of selenium (Suzuki, 1983). Selenium concentrates in the placenta and has also been reported to induce placental damage (Yonemoto et al., 1982). Perhaps this is a similar response as noted for cadmium (Parizek, 1964a,b; Levin et al., 1983a,b).

Even though selenium does penetrate into the placenta and does concentrate in the fetus, bis(methylmercuric) selenide does not easily penetrate into the fetus (Suzuki, 1983). Thus, depending upon the form of selenium, the distribution of the metal can be partially accounting for the embryo and fetal toxicity expressed.

TELLURIUM

Tellurium has been detected in the human fetus (Schroeder et al., 1963). Single injections of telluric acid have resulted in the appearance of tellurium in the embryo/fetus depending upon the stage of gestation (Agnew et al., 1968; Duckett and Ellem, 1971; Agnew, 1972). Agnew and Chang (1971) reported that tellurium is highly bound to both red blood cells and plasma proteins. In maternal tissues 4 hours following an intravenous injection of telluric acid, the highest to lowest concentrations were kidney, liver, blood, muscle, central nervous system, cerebral spinal fluid. In the same experiments, the fetal tissues ranked: blood>liver>kidney>whole brain (Agnew et al., 1968). As gestation progressed, less tellurium crossed into the fetus, even though the choriod plexus continued to contain high concentrations of tellurium (Agnew, 1972). Among the greatest concentrations of tellurium in any fetal or embryonic tissues are found in the visceral yolk sac and chorioallantoic placenta. Thus, the placenta appears to retard the movement of tellurium to the fetus late in gestation. However, the preferential concentration of tellurium by the developing choriod plexus is consistent with a direct action of tellurium in the production of hydrocephalus.

There are no data available concerning the chronic low dose exposure to tellurium during pregnancy. The half-life of tellurium in the pregnant female has not been determined. There are many forms of tellurium. To date only telluric acid has been investigated.

TIN

Tin has not been detected in fetuses and newborns (Schroeder et al., 1964); however, this is the only report available.

TITANIUM

Few investigations have been pursued in pregnant females to study the metabolism of titanium. Schroeder et al. (1963) detected titanium in some but not all fetuses. The actual kinetics of the metabolic process are not currently known.

VANADIUM

Vanadium has not been detected in human fetuses (Schroeder et al., 1963). However, no other data are available to confirm this observation.

III. ROLE OF METALLOTHIONEIN IN PRE AND POSTNATAL DEVELOPMENT

Due to its affinity for divalent cations, metallothionein may have a significant role in metal metabolism. The presence of metallothionein in liver, kidney and other tissues of adult animals and humans has been known for some time. A metallothionein-like protein has also been reported in rat placenta. It is only recently that the presence of metallothionein in fetal and neonatal animals as well as humans has been studied in more detail. The concentration of metallothionein is highest in fetal liver during late gestation and early neonatal life. It is also present in low concentrations in neonatal intestine, kidney and testes.

The function of metallothionein in fetal and neonatal liver appears to be the storage of zinc and copper. Exposure to toxic cations like cadmium and mercury, results in displacement of zinc and/or copper from the fetal and neonatal hepatic metallothionein. In certain species, additional metallothionein synthesis as a result of cadmium exposure has also been reported. The binding of cadmium and mercury to metallothionein appears to have detoxifying effects. However, the displacement of zinc and copper from hepatic metallothionein and subsequent loss of these cations from the liver may be responsible for growth retardation observed after cadmium exposure.

A.   Fetal and Neonatal Metallothionein

Hepatic Metallothionein

The amino acid composition of hepatic metallothionein in rat fetal and newborn liver is similar to the adult rat hepatic metallothionein (Wong and Klaassen, 1979a,b). In rats, it appears to function as a storage protein for zinc in the cytosol (Oh and Whanger, 1979; Charles-Shannon et al., 1981), and for copper in the subcellular particles (Webb, 1983). The dominant cation bound to cytosolic metallothionein in various species is either zinc or copper (Table 4).

Zinc-metallothionein accumulates in fetal rat liver only after 14 days of gestation (Webb, 1983; Kern et al., 1981). The highest concentration is reached between two and five days after birth, declining thereafter to the adult hepatic level by day 14 (Webb, 1983; Cherian et al., 1983). This event coincides with the maturation of the intestine. Thus, Webb (1983) postulates that the hepatic metallothionein in the neonate may participate in zinc homeostasis.

The copper content of the rat hepatic metallothionein is low at birth, but increases gradually during the next 14-15 days (Webb,

1983). The delayed accumulation of copper in hepatic metallothionein as compared with zinc suggests that during the early stages of life, copper retention is regulated by some extrahepatic mechanism; the insoluble intestinal copper complex has been suggested as a possible candidate (Webb, 1983).

Immunohistochemical studies show that metallothionein is concentrated in nuclei of the fetal and newborn rat hepatocytes. This is followed by a shift to cytoplasmic staining for metallothionein after 14 days. It has been suggested that the presence of metallothionein in the nucleus may indicate active synthesis of the protein (Cherian et al., 1983).

Intestinal Metallothionein

The neonatal rat intestine contains copper and zinc-metallothionein (Johnson and Evans, 1980). A significant proportion of the intestinal copper is also associated with larger molecular weight proteins (Mason et al., 1981). In early neonatal life, metallothionein does not appear to play a significant part in binding zinc. The binding of copper to intestinal metallothionein is also minimal in 21-day old rat pups (Mason et al., 1981). Thus, intestinal metallothionein does not appear to have a significant role in sequestration of either zinc or copper in the neonates.

Renal Metallothionein

By immunohistochemical methods, Kojima and Hamashima (1980) demonstrated the presence of metallothionein in the human fetal kidney. In neonatal rats, the renal metallothionein is a zinc-binding protein and its concentration does not change during development (Wong and Klaassen, 1979b; Webb, 1983). This is in contrast to adult rats and humans where the predominant cations renal metallothionein is copper. What role does bound to metallothionein play in copper and zinc metabolism in the kidney is not known.

Testicular Metallothionein

Testicular metallothionein in neonatal rats is a zinc metallothionein. Its concentration appears to increase steadily for the first 35 days of neonatal life. As opposed to the adult testes, which contains two isoforms of the protein, the neonatal metallothionein consists of only one isoform (Brady and Webb, 1981). Also the content of metallothionein in testes at 35 days of age has been reported by Brady and Webb (1981) to be greater than that in liver and kidney combined. In adult rat testes,

metallothionein is detected by immunochemical staining in Sertoli
and interstitial cells but not in spermatogonia (Danielsson et al.,
1982). Whether metallothionein in the testes is a store for
endogenous zinc remains to be investigated.

Table 4 Mammalian Hepatic Metallothionein in the Fetus and Neonate

Species	Predominant Cation	Reference
Rat	Zinc	Ohatke et al., 1978 Wong and Klaassen, 1979a Oh and Whanger, 1979 Bell, 1979 Waalkes and Bell, 1980b, 1981 Mason et al., 1980 Kern et al., 1982 Cherian et al., 1983
Rabbit	Zinc	Waalkes and Bell, 1980a, 1982 Bakka and Webb, 1981
Chinese Hamster	Zinc	Bakka and Webb, 1981
Syrian Hamster	Copper	Bakka and Webb, 1981
Goat	Copper	Tanabe, 1980
Sheep	Copper	Bremner et al., 1981
Cow	Copper	Porter, 1974 Hartman and Weser, 1977
Human (soluble)	Zinc	Riordan and Richards, 1980 Bakka and Webb, 1981
(insoluble)	Copper	Ryden and Deutsch, 1978 Riordan and Richards, 1980

Mammary Gland Metallothionein

While Lucis et al. (1972) were unable to detect metallothionein in mammary glands of rats injected with tracer doses of cadmium, an inducible metallothionein-like protein was reported in a human breast tumor cell by Bazzell et al. (1979). Species differences in the presence of this protein in mammary tissue and its positive identity as metallothionein remains to be investigated. Also, the function of this low molecular weight metal-binding protein in tissue is unclear.

B.   Effect of Cadmium Exposure on Metallothionein

Placental Metallothionein

Tracer doses of injected cadmium have been shown to bind to a metallothionein-like protein in rat and hamster placentae (Lucis et al., 1972; Lafont et al., 1976; Arizono et al., 1981; Hanlon et al., 1982). The identity of this protein as an authentic metallothionein has not been demonstrated. There is some suggestion that this protein may be a metallothionein dimer (Wolkowski, 1974; Hanlon et al., 1982). Its role in zinc transport to the fetus and in protecting the fetus from the toxic effects of cadmium and mercury needs to be studied.

Fetal Metallothionein

In pregnant rats and rabbits, cadmium crosses the placenta and appears in fetal liver and kidney (Lucis et al., 1972; Kelman, 1979; Kelman et al., 1979; Waalkes and Bell, 1980b; Waalkes et al., 1982; Sowa et al., 1982). A part of the cadmium in fetal liver is associated with metallothionein. Maternal exposure to cadmium in rats results in a dose-dependent decrease in both total cytosolic zinc as well as metallothionein-bound zinc in the fetal liver (Waalkes and Bell, 1980b; Sowa et al., 1982). About two-thirds of the cytosolic zinc in fetal liver is normally bound to metallothionein (Waalkes and Bell, 1980b; Waalkes et al., 1982). A decrease in metallothionein- bound zinc is possibly the cause of intrauterine growth retardation observed after cadmium exposure (Webb, 1983).

Neonatal Metallothionein

Injected cadmium appears in the liver where it binds to metallothionein possibly by displacement of zinc (Wong and Klaassen, 1980; Bell, 1981). At high doses (6 mg/kg) cadmium also stimulates the synthesis of additional metallothionein (Bell, 1980). However, this does not protect the animals from the toxic effects of cadmium, and Bell (1981) reports that 30 percent of the animals die within 48 hours.

C.   Effect of Mercury Exposure on Metallothionein

Placental Metallothionein

Exposure of pregnant rats to mercury results in an increased placental concentration of metallothionein (Webb, 1983). Whether metallothionein regulates the transfer of mercury to fetus is unknown.

Neonatal Metallothionein

In neonatal liver, mercury binds to metallothionein and by displacement of zinc (Webb and Holt, 1982). Mercury also binds to renal metallothionein as in adults. The role of metallothionein in reducing the toxicity of mercury in the neonates remains to be investigated.

IV.   CONCLUSIONS

A.   Pregnancy infers a continuum of change in the biology of the female. As such, both the effects and dispositions of metals can be altered, when compared with the non-pregnant female.

Acute exposure to metals at specific times during gestation can result in substantial differences in metabolism and expressed toxicity due to:

1. Maternal factors: hormonal changes, circulation, volume increases, relative uterine/maternal weight changes, metabolism, availability of nutrients, individual organ functions.

2. Extraembryonic membrane factors: permeability, affinity, variable functional responses of the yolk sac and placenta during gestation, age of tissue, uteroplacental blood flow changes.

3. Embryonic/fetal factors: stage of development, functional maturation of organ systems, gestational stage dependent metabolism.

B.   Unfortunately, few chronic metal exposure studies during or before pregnancy have been undertaken to evaluate the risk to

pregnant animals. This chronic exposure may be a more comparable
situation to what may occur under human exposure conditions.

     C. It is not currently possible to select a species, which
may be best to examine and extrapolate to the human concerning both
metabolism and toxicity due to differences in length of gestation,
the maternal adaptations to pregnancy by these species and the
paucity of clearly defined pharmacokinetic studies.

         1. Maternal toxicity/metabolism
         2. Placental toxicity/metabolism
         3. Embryonic/fetal toxicity metabolism

     D. It is further recognized that considerable species
variation in staging of development can result in a merging of fetal
and neonatal organ functions for one species, which would be more
equivalent to in utero development for the human. Therefore,
caution must be exercised in defining birth as the most critical
factor for metal metabolism and specific organ function in the
developing organism.

     E. Nutritional status is known to modify the distribution of
metals among tissues from mother, placenta/extraembryonic membranes,
and embryo/fetus. Essential elements, vitamins and macronutrients
have all been implicated.

     F. Other factors affecting the metabolism of metals:

         1. Environmental/pharmacological interactions have been
documented for a number of metals: mercury-ethanol and glutathione.

         2. Chelation therapy: Few investigations are available
in pregnant women or animals for any metals. An assessment of
essential nutrient/trace metal balances must be simultaneously
investigated when considering such chelation therapy. A number of
chelators are known to alter the development of the embryo/fetus.

         3. Genetic and host factors: Only a limited number of
studies have attempted to examine strain differences or unique
disease processes in relationship to metabolism or toxicity.

     G. Data on species differences which lead to changes in
pharmacokinetics of metals are insufficient and sparse. No
systematic pharmacokinetic approach to the metabolism of metals in
one or more species has been undertaken in the pregnant animal.

     H. Human exposure to metals during pregnancy has been
investigated in reasonable detail in only a few instances.
Evaluation of human tissues has been one form of monitoring. To
date, cord and maternal blood, neonatal and maternal hair samples,

amniotic fluids, and placental tissues have been studied with rare autopsy samples when available. The only correlations to human exposures have been for acute exposure to methylmercury in Japan and Iraq, chronic exposure to lead in pottery workers in England, and numerous reports of increased placental/amniotic fluid levels of cadmium in women who smoke cigarettes. The implications for the health of the mother and fetus are obvious; however, more thorough dose effect relationships must be determined.

I.   Metallothionein: The concentration of metallothionein in the liver is highest in fetal (late gestation) and neonatal stages of the life cycle, although it is also present in intestine, kidney, and testis of the newborn animal. The precise functions of metallothionein are not established. However, it appears that in fetal and neonatal liver, metallothionein may serve as a storage protein for zinc and/or copper. Thus, metallothionein may be involved in the homeostatic regulation of these essential trace metals.

Both cadmium and mercury have strong affinity for metallothionein. By sequestering cadmium and mercury, the metallothionein appears to serve a detoxifying function. On the other hand, displacement of zinc from the metallothionein may be associated with the growth retardation.

V.   RECOMMENDATIONS

A.   The most critical of these recommendations is the standardizations of analytical technics for assessing the metal and its state. Without such standardization, no geographical or interlaboratory comparisons can be established. It is further recommended that the development of non-invasine analytical methods be continued, e.g., NMR, tomochemistry, PIXIE.

B.   It is essential that thorough metabolic examination of metals in the pregnant female be performed with special attention to:

1.   Unique maternal distribution and biotransformation
2.   More than one dose exposure
3.   Multiple time points for evaluation of peak time for concentrations, half time and state of the metal in the pregnant female at varying stages of gestation.

C.   Since most current animal studies are designed to evaluate acute toxicity, we recommend that the above criteria be applied to future studies which explore chronic exposure to metals terminated before pregnancy or continued throughout gestation. These studies could then establish whether maternal tissue concentrations of these metals can be mobilized to induce toxicity/metabolism in the mother, placenta, and embryo/fetus.

D.   With the increasing use of metals, by the industrial nations, we feel that the relationship between chelation therapy to the disposition of metals during pregnancy should be thoroughly assessed in animals.

E.   When possible, human exposure to metals during pregnancy should be evaluated with regard to metabolism. Monitoring of human tissues and fluids should be part of this evaluation. The in vitro evaluation of products of conception is equally essential to the assessment of metal metabolism and risk assessment.

F.   Metallothionein:

1.   Since most of the studies reported to date have been conducted under acute exposure conditions, the effects of chronic exposure to cadmium and mercury on the maternal, fetal and neonatal metallothionein require investigation.

2.   Metallothionein has been reported to be concentrated in the hepatocyte nuclei in the newborn and fetus. The significance of this phenomenon in development and differentiation must be investigated.

3.   Species differences in permeability of the placenta to cadmium have been reported, whether there are differences in the placental binding of cadmium to the metallothionein-like protein should be further studied as a partial explanation for these differences.

4.   The identity of the low molecular weight metallothionein-like protein in the placenta must be established. It is not known whether the placenta synthesizes this protein and whether this protein acts as a detoxifying molecule for cadmium and mercury. If so, do these interactions interfere with zinc and copper metabolism in the fetus? Also can the higher levels of cadmium noted in the placenta from smoking mothers reflect binding to this protein?

5.   The relationship for species differences and relative concentrations of intestinal copper and zinc binding proteins with absorption of metals is not clear.

6.   The identity and role of metal binding proteins in mammary gland and in the transport of zinc and copper is open to investigation.

REFERENCES

Agnew, W.F. and Chang, G.A.T., 1971, Protein binding of
    tellurium-127 in the maternal and fetal tissues of the rat,
    Toxicol. Appl. Pharmacol. 20:346-356.
Agnew, W.F., Fauvre, F.M. and Pudenz, P.H., 1968, Tellurium
    hydrocephalus: Distribution of tellurium-127 between maternal,
    fetal and neonatal tissues of the rat, Exper. Neurol.
    21:120-132.
Agnew, W.F., 1972, Transplacental uptake of 127-m tellurium studied
    by whole body autoradiography, Teratology 6:331-337.
Ahokas, R.A. and Dilts, P.V. Jr., 1979, Cadmium uptake by the rat
    embryo as a function of gestational age, Am. J. Obstet.
    Gynecol. 135:219-224.
Alexander, F.W. and Delves, H.T., 1981, Blood levels during
    pregnancy, Int. Arch. Occup. Environ. Health, 48:35-39.
Amin-Zaki, L., Elhassani, S., Majeed, M.A., Clarkson, T.W., Doherty,
    R.A. and Greenwood, M.A., 1974, Intrauterine methylmercury
    poisoning in Iraq, Pediatrics 54:587-595.
Anderson, D.F., Phernetton, and Rankin, J.H.G., 1980, Prediction of
    fetal drug concentrations, Am. J. Obstet. Gynecol. 137:735-738.
Angell, N.F. and Lavery, J.P., 1982, The relationship of blood
    levels to obstetric outcome, Am. J. Obstet. Gynecol. 142:40.
Arizono, K., Ota, S. and Ariyoshi, T., 1981, Purification of
    metallothionein-like protein in rat placenta, Bull. Environ.
    Contam. Toxicol. 27:671-677.
Asmussen, I., 1979, Effects of maternal smoking on the fetal
    cardiovascular system, Cardiovasc. Med. 4:777-790.
Baglan, R.J., Brill, A.B., Schubert, A., Wilson, D., Larsen, K.,
    Dyer, N., Mansour, M., Schaffner, W., Hoffman, L. and Davies,
    J., 1974, Utility of placental tissue as an indicator of trace
    element exposure to adult and fetus, Environ. Res. 8:6470.
Bakir, F., Demuluji, S.F., Amin-Zaki, L., Murtadha, M., Khalidi, A.,
    Al-Rawi, N., Tikriti, S., Dhahir, H., Clarkson, T., Smith, J.
    and Doherty, R., 1973, Methylmercury poisoning in Iraq, Science
    181:230-241.
Bakka, A. and Webb, M., 1981, Metabolism of zinc and copper in the
    neonate: Changes in the concentrations and contents of
    thionein-bound Zn and Cu with age in the livers of various
    mammalian species, Biochem. Pharmacol. 30:721-725.
Barry, P.S.I., 1981, Concentrations of lead in the tissues of
    children, Br. J. Indust. Med. 38:61-71.
Bazzell, K.L., Coleman, R.L. and Nordquist, R.E., 1979, Induction of
    metallothionein-like protein in human breast tumor cells,
    Toxicol. Appl. Pharmacol. 50:199-205.
Beck, F., 1982, Models in teratology research, in: "Developmental
    Toxicology," K. Snell, ed., pp. 11-32, Praeger Publishers, New
    York.
Bell, J.U., 1979, A metallothionein-like protein in the hepatic
    cytosol of the term rat fetus, Toxicol. Appl. Pharmacol.
    48:139-144.

Bell, J.U., 1980, Induction of hepatic metallothionein in the immature rat following administration of cadmium, Toxic Appl. Pharmacol. 54:148-155.

Bell, J.U., 1981, Native metallothionein levels in rat hepatic cystosol during perinatal development, Toxicol. Appl. Pharmacol. 50:101-107.

Berg, G.G. and Smith, B.S., 1982, Toxicity of mercuric oxide to pregnant mice and the mechanism of resistance of prenatally exposed litters, Teratology 26:46A.

Berlin, M. and Ullberg, S., 1963a, The fate of cadmium-109 in the mouse: An autoradiographic study after a single intravenous injection of cadmium-109 C12, Arch. Environ. Hlth. 7:686-693.

Berlin, M. and Ullberg, S., 1963b, Accumulation and retention of mercury in the mouse. I. An autoradiographic study after a single intravenous injection of mercuric chloride, Arch. Environ. Hlth. 6:589-601.

Berlin, M. and Ullberg, S., 1963c, Accumulation and retention of mercury in the mouse. II. An autoradiographic comparison of phenylmercuric acetate with inorganic mercury, Arch. Environ. Hlth. 6:602-609.

Berlin, M. and Ullberg, S., 1963d, Accumulation and retention of mercury in the mouse. III. An autoradiographic comparison of phenylmercuric acetate with inorganic mercury, Arch. Environ. Hlth. 6:610-616.

Berlin, M., Fazackerley, J. and Nordberg, G., 1969, The uptake of mercury in the brain of mammals exposed to mercury vapor and to mercuric salts, Arch. Environmental Hlth. 18:719-726.

Berlin, M., Nordberg, G. and Hellberg, J., 1973, The uptake and distribution of methyl-mercury in the brain of Saimiri Sciureus in relation to behavioral and morphological changes, in: "Mercury, Mercurials and Mercaptans," M.W. Miller and T.W. Clarkson, eds., pp. 187-208, C.C. Thomas, Springfield.

Brady, F.O. and Webb. M., 1981, Metabolism of zinc and copper in the neonate, J. Biol. Chem. 256:3931-3935.

Bremner, I., Williams, R.B. and Young, B.W., 1981, Distribution of copper and zinc in the livers of developing sheep foetus, Brit. J. Nutr. 38:87-92.

Bryce-Smith, D., Deshpande, R.R., Hughes, J. and Waldron, H.A., 1977, Lead and cadmium levels in stillbirths, Lancet 1:1159.

Buchet, J.P., Rolls, H., Hubermont, G. and Lauwerys, R., 1978, Placental transfer of lead, mercury, cadmium, carbon monoxide in women, II, Environ. Res. 15:494-503.

Cappon, C.J. and Smith, J.C., 1977, Gas-chromotographic determination of inorganic mercury and organomercurials in biological materials, Anal. Chem. 49:365-370.

Carmichael, N.G., Backhouse, B.L., Winder, C. and Lewis, P.D., 1982, Teratogenicity, toxicity and perinatal effects of cadmium, Human Toxicol. 1:159-186.

Carpenter, S.J., Ferm, V.H. and Gale, T.F., 1973, Placental permeability of inorganic lead in the golden hamster: Radioautographic evidence, Experientia 29:311-313.

Charles-Shannon, V.L., Sasser, L.B., Burbank, D.K. and Kelman, B.J., 1981, The influence of zinc on the ontogeny of hepatic metallothionein in the fetal rat, Proc. Soc. Expt. Biol. Med. 168:56-61.

Chaube, S., Nishimura, H. and Swinyard, C.A., 1973, Zinc and cadmium in normal human-embryos and fetuses, Arch. Environ. Hlth. 26:237-240.

Cherian, M.G., Panemangalore, M. and Banerjee, D., 1983, The cellular accumulation and subcellular localization of metallothionein in rat and liver during postnatal development, in: "Reproductive and Developmental Toxicity of Metals," T.W. Clarkson, G. Nordberg and P. Sager, eds., Plenum Press, New York. This volume.

Childs, E., 1973, Kinetics of transplacental movement of mercury fed in a tuna matrix to mice, Arch. Environ. Hlth. 27:50-52.

Clark, A.R.L., 1977, Placental transfer of lead and its effect on the newborn, Postgraduate Medical Journal 53:673-678.

Clarkson, T., Magos, L. and Greenwood, M., 1972, The transport of elemental mercury into fetal tissues, Biol. Neonate 21:239.

Clarkson, T.W., Cox, C., Marsh, D.O., Myers, G.J., Al-Tikriti, S., Amin-Zaki, L., Dabbagh, A.R., 1981, Dose-response relationships for adult and prenatal exposures to methylmercury, in: "Measurement of Risk", G.G. Berg, H.D. Maillie and M.W. Miller, eds., Plenum Publishing Co., New York.

Clarkson, T.W., Gatzy, J. and Dalton, C., 1961, Studies on the equilibration of mercury vapor with blood, University of Rochester AEP Report No. 582.

Clarkson, T.W., Nordberg, G. and Sager, P., eds., 1983, "Reproductive and Developmental Toxicity of Metals", Plenum Press, New York, this volume.

Clary, J.J., 1975, Nickel chloride-induced metabolic changes in the rat and guinea pig, Toxicol. Appl. Pharmacol. 31:55-65.

Creason, J.P., Svendsgaard, D., Bumgarner, J., Pinkerton, C. and Hinners, T., 1975, Maternal-fetal tissue levels of 16 trace elements in 8 selected continental United States communities, Clin. Chem. 21:603-612.

Danielson, K.G., Ohi, S. and Huang, P.C., 1982, Immunochemical detection of metallothionein in specific epithelial cells of rat organs, Proc. Natl. Acad. Sci., USA 79:2301-2304.

Danielsson, B., Hassoun, E. and Dencker, L., 1982, Placental transport of chromium and its effects on cartilage formation, Teratology 26:47A.

Dawson, E.B., Croft, H.A., Clar, R.R. and McGanity, W.J., 1968, Study of seasonal variations in nine cations of normal term placentas, Am. J. Obstet. Gynecol. 102(3):354-357.

Dencker, L., 1975, Possible mechanisms of cadmium fetotoxicity in golden hamsters and mice: Uptake of the embryo, placenta, and ovary, J. Reproduct. Fertil. 44:461-471.

Dencker, L., Danielsson, B., Khayat, A. and Lindgren, A., 1983, Disposition of metals in the embryo and fetus, in: "Reproductive and Developmental Toxicity of Metals", T.W. Clarkson, G. Nordberg and P. Sager, eds., Plenum Press, New York. This volume.

Dibman, B., Tutt, M.L. and Vaughn, J.M., 1951, The retention of radioactive strontium and yttrium in pregnant and lactating rabbits and their offspring, J. Pathol. Bacteriol. 63:253.

Duckett, S. and Ellem, K.A.O., 1971, Localization of tellurium in fetal tissue, particularly brain, Experi. Neurol. 32:49-57.

Eastman, N.J., 1931, The arsenic content of the human placenta following arsphenamine therapy, Am. J. Obstet. Gynecol. 21:60-64.

Fahim, M.S., Fahim, Z. and Hall, D.G., 1976, Effects of subtoxic lead levels on pregnant women in the state of Missouri, Res. Comm. Chem. Pathol. Pharm. 13:309-331.

Ferm, V.H., 1976, Teratogenic effects and placental permeability of heavy metals, Current Topics in Pathology 62:145-150.

Ferm, V.H. and Hanlon, D.P., 1983, Metal-induced congential malformations, in: "Reproductive and Developmental Toxicity of Metals", T.W. Clarkson, G. Nordberg and P. Sager, eds., Plenum Press, New York. This volume.

Ferm, V.H., Hanlon, D.P. and Urban, J., 1969, The permeability of the hamster placenta to radioactive cadmium, J. Embryol. Exp. Morph. 22(1):107-113.

Fochtman, F.W., Kritko, C.F. and Winek, C.L., 1982, Cadmium concentrations in amniotic fluids, The Toxicologist 2(1):5.

Friberg, L., Piscator, M., Nordberg, G. and Kjellstrom, T., 1974, "Cadmium in the Environment", CRC Press, Cleveland.

Friberg, L. and Vostal, J., eds., 1971, "Mercury in the Environment. A Toxicological and Epidemiological Appraisal", PB-205 000, Nat'l. Tech. Information Svc., U.S. Dept. Commerce, U.S. Govt.

Garrett, N.E., Burrises, J., Garrett, B. and Archdeacon, J.W., 1972, Placental transmission of mercury to the fetal rat, Tox. Appl. Pharmacol. 22:649-654.

Gerber, G.B., Maes, J. and Eykens, B., 1982, Transfer of antimony and arsenic to the developing organism, Arch. Toxicol. 49:159-168.

Gibson, J.E. and Becker, B.A., 1970, Placental transfer, embryo-toxicity and teratogenicity of thallium sulfate in normal and potassium-deficient rats, Toxicol. Appl. Pharmacol. 16:120.

Green, M. and Gruener, N., 1974, Transfer of lead via placenta and milk, Comm. Chem. Pathol. Pharmacol. 8:735-738.

Greenwood, M.A., Clarkson, T.W., Doherty, R.A., Gates, A.H., Amin-Zaki, L., Elhassani, S. and Majeed, M.A., 1978, Blood clearance half-times in lactating and nonlactating members of a population exposed to methyl-mercury, Environ. Res. 16:48-54.

Greenwood, M., Clarkson, T. and Magos, L., 1972, Transfer of metallic mercury into the foetus, Experientia 28:1415.

Hadjimarkos, D.M., Bonhorst, C.W. and Mattice, J.J., 1959, A selenium concentration in the placental tissue of fetal cord blood, J. Pediat. 54:296.

Hanlon, D.P., Specht, C. and Ferm, V.H., 1982, The chemical status of cadmium ion in the placenta, Environ. Res. 27:89-94.

Hanlon, D.P. and Ferm, V.H., 1977, Placental permeability of arsenate during early embryogenesis in the hamster, Experientia 33:1121-1122.

Harada, M., 1978, Congenital minamata disease, Teratology 18:285-288.

Hubermont, G., Bucket, J.P., Roels, H., Lauwerys, R., 1978, Placental transfer of lead, mercury and cadmium in women living in a rural area, Int. Arch. Occup. Environ. Health 41:117-124.

Hartman, H.J. and Weser, U., 1979, Copper-thionein from fetal bovin liner, Biochem. Biophys. Acta 491:221-222.

Huel, G., Boudene, C. and Ibrahim, M.A., 1981, Cadmium and lead content of maternal and newborn hair: relationship to parity, birthweight, and hypertension, Arch. Environ. Hlth. 36:221-227.

Johnson, W. and Evans, G.W., 1980, Isolation of a (copper-zinc)-thionein from the small intestine of neonatal rats, Biochem. Biophys. Res. Comm. 96:10-17.

Karlog, O. and Moller, K.O., 1958, Three cases of acute lead poisoning during pregnancy, Acta Pharmacology et Toxicology 5:8-11.

Karp, W.B. and Robertson, A.F., 1977, Correlation of human placental enzymatic activity with trace metal concentration in placenta from three geographical locations, Environ. Res. 13:470-477.

Kelman, B.J., 1977, Inorganic mercury movements across the perfused guinea pig placenta in late gestation, Tox. Appl. Pharm. 41:659-665.

Kelman, B.J., 1979, Effects of toxic agents on movements of material across the placenta, Fed. Proc. 38:2246-2250.

Kelman, B.J., Ozga, J.A., Walter, B.K. and Sasser, L.B., 1979, Cadmium-binding in the pregnant and fetal rat, Toxicology Letters 4:135-141.

Kelman, B.J. and Sikov, M.R., 1981, Plutoneum movements across the hemochorioplacenta of the guinea pig, Placenta Suppl. 3:319-326.

Kelman, B.J., Steinmetz, S.E., Walter, B.K. and Sasser, L.B., 1980, Absorption of methylmercury by the fetal guinea pig during mid to late gestation, Teratology 21:161-165.

Kelman, B.J. and Walter, B.K., 1977, Passage of cadmium across the perfused guinea pig placenta, Proc. Soc. Exp. Biol. Med. 156:68-71.

Kern, S.R., Smith, H.A., Fontaine, D. and Bryan, S.E., 1982, Partition of zinc and copper in fetal liver subfractions -- appearance of metallothionein-like protein during development, Toxicol. Appl. Pharmacol. 59:346-355.

Khayat, A. and Dencker, L., 1982, Fetal uptake and distribution of metallic mercury vapor in the mouse: Influence of ethanol and aminotriogole, Biol. Res. in Pregn. 3:38-42.

Khera, A.K., Wibberley, D.G. and Dathan, J.G., 1980, Placental and stillbirth tissue lead concentrations in occupationally exposed women, Br. J. Ind. Med. 37:394-396.

Kimmel, C.A., Grant, L.D., Sloan, C.S. and Gladen, B.C., 1980, Chronic low-level toxicity in the rat, Tox. Appl. Pharmacol. 56:28-41.

Kjellstrom, T. and Nordberg, G.F., 1978, A kinetic model of cadmium metabolism in the human being, Environ. Res. 16:248-269.

Klopper, A., 1982, "Immunology of Human Placental Proteins", Praeger, New York.

Klopper, A., 1983, Steroid and protein metabolism by the trophoblast, in: "Fetal Nutrition, Metabolism and Immunology: Role of the Placenta," R.K. Miller and H.A. Thiede, eds., Plenum Press, New York, in press.

Kojima, Y. and Hamashina, Y., 1980, Immunohistological studies of metallothionein. 2. Its detection in the human fetal kidney, Acta Histochem. Cytochem. 13:277-286.

Koos, B.J. and Longo, L.D., 1976, Mercury toxicity in the pregnant women, fetus, and newborn infant, Am. J. Obstet. Gynecol. 126:390-409.

Kuhnert, P., Kuhnert, B. and Erhard, P., 1981, Comparison of mercury levels in maternal blood, fetal cord blood, and placental tissues, Am. J. Obstet. Gynecol. 139:209-213.

Kuhnert, P.M., Kuhnert, B.R., Bottoms, S.F. and Erhard, P., 1982, Cadmium levels in maternal blood, fetal cord blood, and placental tissues of pregnant women who smoke, Am. J. Obstet. Gynecol. 142:1021-1025.

Lafont, J., Rouanet, J.M., Besancon, P. and Moretti, J., 1976, Existence d'une metallothioneine dans le placenta, C.R. Acad. Sci. (Paris) 283:417-420.

Lauwerys, R., 1979, Cadmium in man, in: "The Chemistry, Biochemistry, and Biology of Cadmium", M. Webb, ed., pp. 433-455, Elsevier/North Holland, Amsterdam.

Lauwerys, R., Bucket, J.P., Roels, H. and Hubermont, G., 1978, Placental transfer of lead mercury, cadmium and carbon monoxide, I. Environ. Res. 15:278-289.

Levin, A.A., Miller, R.K. and di Sant'Agnese, P.A., 1983a, Heavy metal alterations of placental functions: A mechanism for the induction of fetal toxicity by cadmium, in: "Reproductive and Developmental Toxicity of Metals", T. Clarkson G. Nordberg, and P. Sager, eds., Plenum Press, New York. This volume.

Levin, A.A., Kilpper, R. and Miller, R.K., 1983b, Organ specific kinetics of a fetal toxic injection of $CdCl_2$ in the pregnant rat, Tox. Appl. Pharmacol., in press.

Levin, A.A. and Miller, R.K., 1980, Fetal toxicity of cadmium: Maternal vs. fetal injections, Teratology 22:1-5.

Levin, A.A. and Miller, R.K., 1981, Fetal toxicity of cadmium in the rat: decreased uteroplacental blood flow, Tox. Appl. Pharm. 58:297-306.

Levin, A.A., Plautz, J.R., de Sant'Agnese, P.A. and Miller, R.K., 1981, Cadmium: Placental mechanisms of fetal toxicity, Placenta Suppl. 3:303-318.

Levy, G., 1981, Pharmacokinetics of fetal and neonatal exposure to drugs, Obs. Gyn. 58:9S-16S.

Levy, G. and Hayton, W.L., 1973, Pharmacokinetics aspects of placental drug transfer, in: "Fetal Pharmacology," L. Boreus, ed., pp. 29-40, Raven Press, New York.

Lu, C.C., Matsumoto, H. and Iijima, S., 1979, Teratogenic effects of nickel chloride on embryonic mice and its transfer to embryonic mice, Teratology 19:137-142.

Lu, C.C., Matsumoto, N. and Iijima, S., 1981, Placental transfer and body distribution of nickel chloride in pregnant mice, Toxicol. Appl. Pharmacol. 59:409-413.

Lucis, O.J., Lucks, R. and Shaikh, Z.A., 1972, Cadmium and zinc in pregnancy and lactation, Arch. Environ. Hlth. 25:14-22.

Luego, G., Cassidy, G. and Palmisano, P., 1969, Acute maternal arsenic intoxiciation with neonatal death, Am. J. Dis. Child. 117:328-330.

Magos, L. and Webb, M., 1983, The influence of weight and other physiological changes during pregnancy and lactation on the toxicities of mercury and cadmium, in: "Reproductive and Developmental Toxicity of Metals", T. Clarkson G. Nordberg, and P. Sager, eds., Plenum Press, New York. This volume.

Mansour, M., Dyer, N., Hoffman, L., Schulert, A. and Brill, A., 1973, Maternal-fetal transfer of organic and inorganic mercury via placenta and milk, Environ. Res. 6:479.

Mansour, M., Dyer, N., Hoffman, L., Davies, J. and Brill, A., 1974, Placental transfer of mercuric nitrate and methyl mercury in the rat, Am. J. Obstet. Gynecol. 119:557-561.

Mason, R., Bakka, A., Samarawickrama, G.T. and Webb, M., 1980, Metabolism of zinc and copper in the neonate: Acumulation and function of (Zn,Cu)-metallothionein in the liver of the newborn rat. Brit. J. Nutr. 45:375-391.

Mason, R., Brady, F.O. and Webb, M., 1981, Metabolism of zinc and copper in the neonate: Accumulation of copper in the gastrointestinal tract of the newborn rat. Brit. J. Nutr. 45:391-401.

Matsumoto, H., Suzuki, A. and Morita, C., 1967, Preventative effect of penicillamine on the brain defect of fetal rat poisoned transplacentally with methyl mercury, Life Sci. 6:2321-2326.

McClain, R.M. and Becker, B.A., 1975, Teratogenicity, fetal toxicity, placental transfer of lead nitrate in rats, Tox. Appl. Pharmacol. 31:72-82.

Miller, R.K., 1983, Perinatal toxicology: Its recognition and fundamentals, Am. J. Indust. Med., in press.

Miller, R.K., Koszalka, T.R. and Brent, R.L., 1976, Transport mechanisms for molecules across placental membranes, in: "Cell Surface in Animal Development I. Cell Surface Reviews", G. Poste and G.L. Nicolson, eds., pp. 145-223, Elsevier/North Holland, Amsterdam.

Miller, R.K., Ng, W.W. and Levin, A.A., 1983, The placenta:
    Relevance to toxicology, in: "Reproductive and Developmental
    Toxicity of Metals", T. Clarkson G. Nordberg, and P. Sager,
    eds., Plenum Press, New York. This volume.
Miller, R.K. and Gardner, K.A., 1981, Cadmium in the human
    placenta: Relationship to smoking, Teratology 23:51a.
Moore, M.R., Goldberg, A., Fyfe, W.M. and Richards, W.M., 1981,
    Maternal lead levels after alterations to water supply, Lancet
    1:203-204.
Mottet, K., Fowler, B.A. and Ferm, V.H., 1983, The congenital
    teratogenicity and perinatal toxicity of metals, in:
    "Reproductive and Developmental Toxicity of Metals", T.
    Clarkson, G. Nordberg, and P. Sager, eds., Plenum Press, New
    York. This volume.
Ng, W.W., Catus, R. and Miller, R.K., 1981, Macromolecule transfer
    in the human trophoblast: Transcobalamin-Vitamin B_{12},
    Placenta Suppl. 3:145-160.
Ng, W.W. and Miller, R.K., 1983, Transport of nutrients in the early
    human placenta: Amino acid, creatine, vitamin B_{12}, in:
    "Fetal Nutrition, Metabolism and Immunology: Role of the
    Placenta", R.K. Miller and H.A. Thiede, eds., Plenum Press, New
    York, in press.
Nielsen-Kudsk, F., 1969, Uptake of mercury vapour in blood in vivo
    and in vitro from Hg- containing air, Acta Pharmacol. Toxicol.
    27:149-154.
Nordberg, G.F., Nordberg, M. and Piscator, M., 1973, Separation of
    two forms of rabbit metallothionein by isoelectric focusing,
    Biochem. J. 126:491-498.
Oh, S.H. and Whanger, P.D., 1979, Biological function of
    metallothionein. VII. Effect of age on its metabolism in
    rats, Am. J. Physiol. 237:E18-E22.
Ohtake, H., Hasegawa, K. and Koga, M., 1978, Zinc-binding protein in
    livers of neonatal, normal and partially hepatectomized rats,
    Biochem. J. 174:999-1005.
Olsen, I. and Jonsoen, J., 1979, Whole-body autoradiography of
    ^{63}Ni in mice throughout gestation, Toxicology 12:165-172.
Ong, C.N. and Lee, W.R., 1980, High affinity of lead for fetal
    haemoglobin, Br. J. Ind. Med. 37:292-298.
Otten, J.A., Tyndall, R.L., Estes, P.C., Gude, W.D. and
    Swartzendruber, D.C., 1973, Localization of gallium-67 during
    embryogenesis, Proc. Soc. Exp. Biol. Med. 142:92-95.
Page, E., Villee, C. and Villee, D., 1981, "Human Reproduction:
    Essentials of Reproductive and Perinatal Medicine", W.B.
    Saunders Co., Philadelphia.
Parizek, J., 1964a, Vascular changes at sites of estrogen
    biosynthesis produced by injection of cadmium: A destruction
    of the placenta by cadmium, J. Reproduct. Fertil. 7:263-264.
Parizek, J., 1964b, The peculiar toxicity of cadmium during
    pregnancy: An experimental toxemia of pregnancy induced by
    cadmium, J. Reproduct. Fertil. 9:111-112.

Parizek, J, Babicky, A., Ostadalova, I., Kalouskova, J. and Pavilik, L., 1969, The effect of selenium compounds on the cross-placental passage of ^{203}Hg, in: "Radiation Biology of the Fetal and Juvenile Mammal", M.R. Sikov and D.D. Mahlum, eds., pp. 137-143, U.S. Atomic Energy Commission, Washington.

Parzyck, D.C., Shaw, S.M., Kessler, W.V., Vetter, R.J., Van Sickle, D.C. and Mayes, R.A., 1978, Fetal effects of cadmium in pregnant rats on normal and zinc deficient diets, Bull. Environ. Contam. Toxicol. 19:206-214.

Peereboom, J.W. Copius, de Voogt, P., van Hattum, B., van de Velde, W. and Peereboom-Stegeman, J.H.J., 1979, The use of the human placenta as a biological indicator for cadmium exposure, Int. Conf.: Management and Control of Heavy Metals in the Environment.

Peereboom, J.W. Copius, and Peereboom, J.H.J. Copius, 1981, Exposure and health effects of cadmium. Part 2. Toxic effects of cadmium to animals and man. Tox. Environ. Chem. Rev. 4:67-178.

Peereboom-Stegeman, J.H.J., Jonsgtra-Spaapen, E., Letschert, J. and Dessing, H., 1981, Effects of cadmium exposure on female reproductive organs, Int. Conf.: Heavy Metals in the Environment.

Peereboom-Stegeman, J.H.J. Copius and Jongstra-Spaapen, E.J., 1979, The effect of a single sublethal administration of cadmium chloride on the microcirculation in the uterus of the rat, Toxicology 13:199-213.

Peereboom-Stegeman, J.H.J. Copius, van der Velde, W.J. and Dessing, J.W.M., 1982, Influence of cadmium on placental structure, Ecotox. Environ. Safety, in press.

Pitkin, R.M., Bahns, J.A., Filer, Jr., L.J. and Reynolds, W.A., 1975, Mercury in human maternal and cord blood, placenta and milk, Proc. Soc. Exp. Biol. Med. 157:565-570.

Plautz, J.R., Levin, A.A. and Miller, R.K., 1980, Fetal and maternal toxicity of cadmium, metallothionein and its distribution in the pregnant Wistar rat, Teratology 26:61a.

Plautz, J.R., Levin, A.A. and Miller, R.K., 1981, Fetal placental distributions of cadmium, metallothionein and cadmium chloride in the Wistar rat, Teratology 23:56a.

Porter, H., 1974, The particulate half-cystine-rich copper protein of newborn liver. Relationship to metallothionein and subcellular localization in non-mitochondrial particles possibly representing heavy lysosomes, Biochem. Biophys. Res. Comm. 56:661-668.

Prigge, E., 1978, Inhalative cadmium effects in pregnant and fetal rats, Toxicology 10:297-309.

Rabinowitz, M.B. and Needleman, H.L., 1982, Temporal trends in the lead concentrations of umbilical cord blood, Science 216:1429-1431.

Reuhl, K.R. and Pounds, J.R., 1981, Absorption and disposition of Hg in the pregnant and non-pregnant hamster following oral administration of ^{203}Hg methylmercuric chloride, Environ. Res. 24:131-139.

Reuhl, K.R., Chang, L.W. and Townsend, J.W., 1981, Pathological
    effects of in utero methylmercury exposure on the cerebellum of
    the golden hamster, Environ. Res. 26:281-306.
Reynolds, W.A. and Pitkin, R.M., 1975, Transplacental passage of
    methylmercury and its uptake by primate fetal tissues, Proc.
    Soc. Exp. Biol. Med. 148:523.
Riordan, J.R. and Richards, V., 1980, Human fetal liver contains
    both zinc- and copper-rich forms of metallothionein, J. Biol.
    Chem. 255:5380-5383.
Roels, H., Hubermont, G., Buchet, J.P. and Lauwerys, R., 1978,
    Placental transfer of lead, mercury, cadmium, and carbon
    monoxide in women III. Factors influencing the accumulation of
    heavy metals in the placenta and the relationship between metal
    concentration in the placenta and in maternal and cord blood,
    Environ. Res. 16:236-247.
Ryden, L. and Deutsch, H.F., 1978, Preparation and properties of the
    major copper-binding component in human fetal liver, J. Biol.
    Chem. 253:519-524.
Samarawickrama, G.P., 1979, Biological effects of cadmium in
    mammals, in: "The Chemistry, Biochemistry, and Biology of
    Cadmium", M. Webb, ed., pp. 341-421, Elsevier/North Holland,
    Amsterdam.
Samarawickrama, G.P. and Webb, M., 1979, Acute effects of cadmium
    during pregnancy and embryo fetal development in the rat,
    Environ. Hlth. Perspect. 28:345-349.
Samarawickrama, G.P. and Webb, M., 1981, The acute toxicity and
    teratogenicity of cadmium in the pregnant rat, J. Appl.
    Toxicol. 1:264-269.
Sasser, L.B., Jarboe, G.E. and Laprade, J., 1977, The influence of
    selenium on the distribution of methyl mercury and mercury
    chloride in the pregnant rat, in: "Biological Implications of
    Metals in the Environment", H. Drucker and R. Wildung, eds.,
    pp. 478-487, NTIS. CONF.-750929, Springfield.
Sasser, L.B., Levin, A.A., Miller, R.K. and Kelman, B.J., 1980, The
    effect of fetal cadmium injection on metallothionein and fetal
    and maternal rat liver, Annual Meeting of the Society of
    Toxicology.
Satoh, H. and Suzuki, T., 1979, Effects of sodium selenite on
    methylmercury distribution in mice of late gestational period,
    Arch. Tox. 42:275-279.
Scanlon, J., 1972, Human fetal hazards from environmental pollution
    with certain non-essential trace elements, Clinical Pediatrics
    11(3):135-140.
Schroeder, H.A., Balassa, J.J. and Tipton, I.H., 1963, Abnormal
    trace elements in man: Titanium, J. Chronic Dis. 16:55-61.
Schroeder, H.A., Balassa, J.J. and Tipton, I.H., 1962, Abnormal
    trace elements in man: Nickel, J. Chronic Dis. 15:51-55.
Schroeder, H.A., Balassa, J.J. and Tipton, I.H., 1964, Abnormal
    trace elements in man: Tin, J. Chronic Dis. 17:483-486.
Schroeder, H.A., Balassa, J.J. and Tipton, I.H., 1963, Abnormal
    trace elements in man: Vanadium, J. Chronic Dis. 16:1047-1050.

Schroeder, H.A., Balassa, J.J. and Tipton, I.H., 1965, Abnormal
     trace elements in man: Niobium, J. Chronic Dis. 18:229-232.
Schroeder, H.A., Balassa, J.J. and Tipton, I.H., 1965, Abnormal
     trace elements in man: Arsenic, J. Chronic Dis. 19:85-89.
Schroeder, H.A. and Balassa, J.J., 1961, Abnormal trace elements in
     man: Cadmium, J. Chronic Dis. 14:236-241.
Schroeder, H.W., Buchman, J. and Balassa, J.J., 1967, Abnormal trace
     elements in man: Tellurium, J. Chronic Dis. 20:147-152.
Shearer, T.R., Johnson, B.E., Ridlington, J.W. and Whanger, P.D.,
     1982, Chemical location of cadmium in developing rat molars, J.
     Dent. Res. 61:510-511.
Sonawane, B.R., Nordberg, M., Nordberg, G. and Lucier, G., 1975a,
     Placental transfer of cadmium in rats: Influence of dose and
     gestational age, Environ. Hlth. Perspect. 28:248-249.
Sonawane, B.R., Nordberg, M., Nordberg, G.F. and Lucier, G.W.,
     1975b, Placental transfer of cadmium in rats: Influence of
     dose and gestational age, Environ. Hlth. Perspect. 12:97-102.
Sowa, B., Steibert, E., Gralewska, K. and Piekarski, M., 1982,
     Effect of oral cadmium administration to female rats before
     and/or during pregnancy on the metallothionein level in the
     fetal liver, Toxicol. Let. 11:233-236.
Stave, U., 1978, "Perinatal Physiology", Plenum Press, New York.
Sunderman, F.W., Shen, S.K., Mitchell, J.M., Allpass, P.R. and
     Damjanov, I., 1978, Embryotoxicity and fetal toxicity of nickel
     in rats, Toxicol. Appl. Pharmacol. 43:387-390.
Sunderman, F.W., Reid, M.C., Shen, S.K. and Kevorkian, C.B., 1983,
     Embryotoxicity and teratogenicity of nickel compounds, in:
     "Reproductive and Developmental Toxicity of Metals", T.
     Clarkson, G. Nordberg, and P. Sager, eds., Plenum Press, New
     York. This volume.
Suzuki, T., 1983, Methylmercury metabolism in pregnant mice--its
     modification by selenium with particular reference to prenatal
     toxicity of these compounds, in: "Reproductive and
     Developmental Toxicity of Metals", T. Clarkson G. Nordberg, and
     P. Sager, eds., Plenum Press, New York. This volume.
Suzuki, T., Matsumoto, N., Miyama, T. and Katsunuma, H., 1967,
     Placental transfer of mercuric chloride, phenyl mercuric
     acetate, and methylmercury acetate in mice, Industr. Hlth.
     53:219-226.
Suzuki, T., Miyama, T., Katsunuma, H., 1971, Comparison of mercury
     contents in maternal blood, umbilical cord blood and placental
     tissues, Bull. Environ. Contam. Toxicol. 5: 502-506.
Suzuki, T., Takemoto, T., Shishido, S. and Kani, K., 1977, Mercury
     in human amniotic fluid, Scand. J. Environ. Hlth. 3:32-35.
Takeda, Y., Kunugi, T., Hoshino, O. and Ukita, T., 1968, Distribution
     of inorganic aryl and alkyl mercury compounds in rats, Toxicol.
     Appl. Pharmacol. 13:156-159.
Tanabe, S., 1980, Effect of zinc injection on zinc-binding in
     cytosols of several tissues of kids, Brit. J. Nutr. 44:355-360.

Thieme, R., Schramel, P., Klose, G.J., Waidl, E., 1974, The
    influence of regional environmental factors on the trace
    element composition of the placenta, Geburtsch u. Frauenheilk
    14:36-41.
Thurauf, J., Schaller, K.H., Engehardt, E. and Gossler, K., 1975,
    Der cadmiumgehalt der mensheishleu placenta, Arch. Occup.
    Environ. Hlth. 36:1927.
Underhill, F.P. and Amatrude, F.G., 1923, Transmission of arsenic
    from mother to fetus, J. Am. Med. Assoc. 81:2009-2015.
Vahter, M., 1982, Assessment of human exposure to lead and cadmium
    through biological monitoring, Natl Swedish Inst. of Environ.
    Med. Karolinska Inst. (D.E.H.), Stockholm.
Van Hattum, B., de Voogt, P., 1981, An analytical procedure for the
    determination of cadmium in human placentae, Intern. J.
    Environ. Anal. Chem. 10:121-133.
Waalkes, M.P. and Bell, J.U., 1980a, Isolation and partial
    characterization of native metallothionein in fetal rabbit
    liver, Life Sci. 27:585-593.
Waalkes, M.P. and Bell, J.U., 1980b, Depression of metallothionein
    in fetal rat liver following maternal cadmium exposure,
    Toxicology 18:103-110.
Waalkes, M.P., Thomas, J.A. and Bell, J.Y., 1982, Induction of
    hepatic metallothionein in the rabbit fetus following maternal
    cadmium exposure, Toxicol. Appl. Pharmacol. 62:211-218.
Waddell, W.J. and Marlowe, C., 1981a, Biochemical regulation of the
    accessibility of teratogens to the developing embryo, in: "The
    Biochemical Basis of Chemical Teratogenesis", M.R. Juchau, ed.,
    p. 162, Elsevier/North Holland, Amsterdam.
Waddell, W.J. and Marlow, C., 1981b, Transfer of drugs across the
    placenta, Pharm. Therap. 14:375-390.
Wallenburg, H.C.S., Van Kessel, T.H. and Brand, A., 1978, Transfer
    of 51 chromium ointments and 51 chromium ions across the term
    rhesus monkey placenta, Acta Obstet. Gynecol. Scand. 57:105-109.
Wannag, A. and Aaseth, J., 1980, The effect of immediate and delayed
    treatment with 2,3-dimercaptopropane-1-sulphate on the
    distribution and toxicity of inorganic mercury in mice and in
    foetal and adult rats, Acta Pharmacol. Toxicol. 46:81-88.
Webb, M., 1983, Endogenous metal-binding proteins in the control of
    Zn, Cu, Cd and Hg metabolism during prenatal and postnatal
    development, in: "Reproductive and Developmental Toxicity of
    Metals", T. Clarkson, G. Nordberg, and P. Sager, eds., Plenum
    Press, New York. This volume.
Webb, M. and Holt, D., 1982, Endogenous metal-binding proteins in
    relation to the differences in absorption and distribution of
    mercury in newborn and adult rats, Arch. Toxicol. 49:237-245.
Webb, M., 1979, The metallothioneins, in: "The Chemistry,
    Biochemistry, and Biology of Cadmium", M. Webb, ed., pp.
    196-266, Elsevier/North Holland, Amsterdam.
Webb, M. and Samarawickrama, G.P., 1981, Placental transport and
    embryonic utilization of essential metabolites in the rat at
    teratogenic doses of cadmium, J. Appl. Toxicol. 1:270-274.

Weischer, C.H., Kordel, W. and Hochrainer, D., 1980, Effects of
    NiCl$_2$ and NiO in Wistar rats after oral uptake and inhalation
    exposure respectively, Zbl. Bakt. Hyg., I. Abt. Orig. B.
    171:336-351.
Weiss, J.F. and Walburg, H.E. Jr., 1978, Influence of the mass of
    administered plutonium on its cross-placental transfer in mice,
    Health Phys. 35:773-777.
Weiss, J.F., Walburg, H.E. and McDowell, W.J., 1980, Placental
    transfer of americium and plutonium in mice, Health Phys.
    39:903-911.
Welch, R.M. and House, W.A., Cadmium and zinc bioavailability to
    rats from lettuce leaves and sulfate salts, U.S. Plant, Soil
    and Nutrition Lab, USDA, ARS, Ithaca, New York, U.S.A. p. 140.
Wibberley, D.G., Khera, A.K., Edwards, J.H. and Rushton, D.I., 1977,
    Lead levels in human placentae from normal and malformed
    births, J. Med. Gen. 14:339-345.
Wier, P., Miller, R.K. and Maulik, D., 1983, Cadmium: Transfer and
    accumulation by the perfused human placental labule,
    Teratology, in press.
Wolkowski, R.M, 1974, Differential cadmium-induced embryotoxicity in
    two inbred mouse strains: Analysis of inheritance of the
    response to cadmium and of the presence of cadmium in fetal and
    placental tissues, Teratology 10:243-262.
Wong, K.L. and Klaassen, C.D., 1979a, Tissue distribution and
    retention of cadmium in rats during postnatal development:
    Minimal role of hepatic metallothionein, Toxicol. Appl.
    Pharmacol. 53:343-353.
Wong, K.L. and Klaassen, C.D., 1979b, Isolation and characterization
    of metallothionein, which is highly concentrated in newborn rat
    liver, J. Biol. Chem. 254:12399-12403.
Wong, K.L. and Klaassen, C.D., 1980, Tissue distribution and
    retention of cadmium in rat during postnatal development:
    Minimal role of hepatic metallothionein. Toxicol. Appl.
    Pharmacol. 53:343-353.
Yonemoto, J., Naganuma, A., Suzuki, T., and Imura, N., 1982, Effects
    of vitamin E, glutathione and methylmercury on distribution and
    placental transfer of selenium in mice, Chemosphere, in press.
Zylber-Haran, E.A., Gershamn, H., Rosemann, E. and Spitz, I.M.,
    1982, Gonadotrophin, testosterone and prolactin
    interrelationships in cadmium-treated rats, J. Endocr.
    92:123-130.

EFFECTS AND METABOLISM OF TOXIC TRACE METALS IN THE NEONATAL PERIOD

Harold H. Sandstead, Richard A. Doherty and Kathryn Mahaffey

Working Group: Harold H. Sandstead, Richard A. Doherty,
    Kathryn A. Mahaffey, Bo Lonnerdal, Nazzareno Ballatori,
    Masyka Bhattacharyya, Ian Rowland, Jerry Stara,
    Elzbieta Komsta-Szumska, Roy Robinson, Philip J. Bushnell,
    Elsa Cernichiari

Review Article Contents:

EFFECTS AND METABOLISM OF TOXIC TRACE METALS IN THE NEONATAL PERIOD

Harold H. Sandstead,[1] Richard A. Doherty[2] and
Kathryn A. Mahaffey[3]

[1]Grand Forks Human Nutrition Research Center
 Grand Forks, North Dakota
[2]Environmental Health Sciences Center, University of
 Rochester, Rochester, New York
[3]DHHS, Food and Drug Administration
 Cincinnati, Ohio

INTRODUCTION

Exposure of the neonate to toxic metals occurs because of their presence in foods and the human biosphere. Nursing infants may ingest these metals in mother's milk. After weaning, their presence in formula, cow's milk and weanling foods is of major importance. Additional environmental metal contaminant sources become important when the infants begin to creep on the floor and have access to objects which they can chew or mouth. Infants are at particular hazard when their environment is contaminated by vapors, by metal-containing dust and particulate fallout or entrainment on articles brought into the home, or by building materials, such as plaster or lead-containing paints.

After toxic metals are ingested their bioavailiability for intestinal absorption is a major factor in affecting toxicity. Bioavailability is influenced by the composition of foods and by the maturity of homeostatic mechanisms that either exclude toxic metals from absorption or increase their excretion. Apparently exclusion mechanisms are less effective in infants than in adults. After absorption, toxic metals may have both acute and chronic effects. The clinical manifestations of injury depend on dose, chronicity of exposure and tissue retention. Long-term sequelae can significantly impair function and well being of persons later in life.

In this review we summarize experimental and clinical findings that support the above statements. Our conclusions and recommendations are based in part on discussions that occurred during this Symposium.

Maternal lactation, diet composition and intestinal absorption are the major factors that influence both the nutrition of infants and their exposure to toxic metals. Relationships between nutritional factors and susceptibility to toxic metals have been revealed through studies on experimental animals. While translation of research findings from experiments with animals directly to humans is not appropriate because of differences in physiology and rates of maturation, data from such studies should alert caretakers of infants of potential hazards and provide a guide for research on humans and prevention of injury.

Studies in rats reviewed by Kostial (this volume) suggest that the neonate has greater susceptibility to dietary lead, cadmium, mercuric mercury and manganese than older animals. When radionuclides of these elements were given orally, uptake and retention were substantially greater during the first week of life than at three or more weeks. A finding that might be particularly important for humans was the observation that all four elements were retained in infant brain to a greater extent than in older animals. High bioavailability and greater intestinal absorption (compared to adults) of lead, cadmium and mercury from milk were responsible for the high uptake of these elements by the sucklings. Apparent absorption of lead (60-80 percent), manganese (40-70 percent) and mercuric mercury (50-70 percent) were greater than apparent absorption of cadmium (20-40 percent). The high absorption of lead and manganese was primarily related to a carcass retention of 80-90 percent of the absorbed metal. In contrast, only 20-40 percent of absorbed cadmium and mercury was in the carcass. The remainder was retained by the intestinal mucosal cells. Presumably the metal retained in the intestinal mucosal cells did not traverse the mucosal cells but was returned to the intestinal lumen as cells were lost into the lumen as a consequence of cell turnover.

In contrast to metallic mercury, methyl mercury readily traverses the mucosa (Zepp et al., 1974). According to work of Kostial (this volume) and Keller and Doherty (1980a,b), it appears that the absorption of toxic metals by the neonatal rodent occurs in part through endocytosis. This phenomenon stops as the gut mucosa matures. Research in humans suggests that endocytic absorption occurs in premature and newborn infants. Permeability to protein macromolecules from milk and soy appears to diminish in humans after three months of life (Walker, 1978). Whether this phenomenon facilitates absorption of toxic metals in human infants in unknown.

Studies on rodents suggest that a feature of milk that might contribute to a greater absorption of lead (Barltrop and Khoo, 1976) is its fat content. The low contents of the elements of iron, zinc, and copper may not be factors in suckling animals because addition of iron to milk did not suppress lead absorption in suckling rats, and all of these elements did not suppress the intestinal absorption of cadmium, mercuric mercury and manganese from milk (Kostial, this volume). On the other hand, it seems possible that calcium and phophorus in milk tend to suppress lead absorption (Barltrop and Khoo, 1976; Mahaffey, 1981). Studies presented at the Symposium illustrated the complexities of these relationships in rhesus monkeys (Gilbert et al., 1982). The monkeys displayed a substantially greater absorption of lead when fed a diet based on milk, compared to a commercial monkey diet. This occurred even though the animals were not infants and had been maintained on a commercial monkey diet for a substantial interval of time prior to the feeding of the milk diet. In this experiment, the calcium and phosphorus contents of the milk diet were inadequate to suppress a facilitating effect fat may have had on lead absorption; this interpretation is consistent with findings in rodents (Kostial, et al., 1971).

Lead consumed by nursing mice appears in their milk. Thus, studies using a radioactive tracer of lead showed that suckling mice litters received a substantial portion (25 percent) of the blood lead of their intravenously dosed mothers (Keller and Doherty, 1980c), and that as much as 3 percent of total body lead acquired by rat mothers prior to lactation was passed on to the pups by suckling (Keller and Doherty, 1980b).

In contrast to lead, relatively little cadmium fed to nursing mice appears in milk. This is probably related to the retention of cadmium by the maternal intestinal mucosa, breast, and other tissues (Kostial, this volume; Chang et al., 1980). Similar phenomena occur in cattle; high dietary intakes of cadmium have little influence on milk cadmium (Miller et al., 1967).

Organ distribution of toxic metals in neonatal animals may have implications for human infants. For example, lead accumulation in brains of rats during early life has been associated with poor subsequent behavioral function (Jason and Kellogg, 1981; Zenick and Goldsmith, 1981), and lead accumulated in kidneys has been associated with increased blood pressure (Perry et al., 1979) and abnormal renin-angiotensin responsiveness to sodium deprivation in rats (Victery et al., 1982a,b).

Though not done in sucklings, cadmium accumulation in kidneys was presumably responsible for the increase in blood pressure that occurred in rats exposed to 0.01-0.5 ppm in drinking water subsequent to weaning (Perry et al., 1979; Kopp et al., 1982). (0.5 ppm cadmium was equivalent to a dose of about 10 μg/kg body weight or about 12 times the level present in infant diets noted subsequently in this review.) Chronic exposure to 1 ppm cadmium in drinking water impaired cardiac function of the rats; inorganic orthophosphate levels in heart muscle were increased and ATP was decreased (Kopp et al., 1982). These findings are consistent with in vitro effects of cadmium on oxydative phosphorylation and ATPase (Jacobson and Turner, 1980). Possible relevance of these studies for infants is suggested by observations on rats exposed to 0.06 ppm cadmium, a level believed to simulate the environment (Sabbioni et al., 1978). When exposed for 745 days, growth and development were unimpaired even though the level of intake was similar to levels associated with increased blood pressure in the studies noted previously. Of interest was a rapid early increase in tissue cadmium with a later continued gradual accumulation in kidney, lung, testicle and brain. Levels in liver did not increase after 100 days of exposure. Another effect of cadmium observed in neonatal rats that might be of some significance to humans was the effect of feeding 0.1 to 1.0 µg of cadmium daily on glucose metabolism. After 45 days, hyperglycemia and suppressed in vitro release of insulin from islet cells occurred (Merali and Singhal, 1980). Research on animals suggests that diet composition has an influence on the toxicity of dietary lead, cadmium and mercury. Interactions of some diet constituents with the toxic metals can influence their absorption. For example, intestinal absorption and toxicity of lead is influenced by the level of dietary calcium, iron, zinc, copper, protein, vitamin D and fat (Mahaffey and Michaelson, 1980; Mahaffey, 1981). When dietary calcium, iron or zinc are low, absorption and toxicity of lead is enhanced. It seems possible that plant substances, such as hemicellulose and phytate, which form insoluble complexes with some essential trace elements, might also complex with dietary lead and inhibit its absorption. Substances that enhance lead absorption include fat (Barltrop and Khoo, 1976) and vitamin D (Mahaffey and Michaelson, 1980).

The lead-vitamin D interaction is complex, lead exposure is associated with reduced serum 1,25-dihydroxy vitamin D concentrations in children (Mahaffey et al., 1982b). This vitamin D metabolite has been demonstrated to be active in stimulating lead absorption in rats (Mahaffey et al., 1979).

Cadmium toxicity is influenced by the levels of dietary zinc, iron, copper, selenium, calcium, ascorbic acid, vitamin D and protein (Fox, 1974). Low dietary zinc, iron, copper, calcium, vitamin D and protein enhance cadmium absorption and/or toxicity, while increased levels of dietary zinc, ferrous iron, copper, selenium, ascorbic acid and protein have the opposite effect. Because hemicellulose and phytate suppress zinc absorption (Sandstead, 1981), and because cadmium has chemical properties similar to zinc and competes with zinc for binding ligands (Fox, 1974), it seems likely that these plant substances will also suppress the absorption of cadmium.

The influence of dietary substances on mercury absorption is not as well characterized as for lead and cadmium. The bioavailability of methylmercury for absorption is extremely high (>90 percent) (Suzuki, 1977). Factors that inhibit the intestinal absorption of organomercury compounds are incompletely understood. Landry et al. (1979) have observed large differences in whole body methylmercury elimination rates related to quality of diet. Mice fed a high protein liquid diet excreted mercury more rapidly than mice fed a standard pellet diet. Mice fed the standard pellet diet excreted mercury more rapidly than mice fed a diet of milk. As described in this Symposium (Rowland et al., this volume), studies in mice indicate that demethylation by intestinal flora is an important mechanism contributing to methylmercury excretion in adults, but is apparently not operative until after weaning when gut flora has changed. Marked qualitative and quantitative changes in intestinal flora occur at this time. These microbial changes are correlated with a large increase in the rate of demethylation of methylmercury in the gut contents and an increase in the fecal excretion of mercury. Body burden subsequent to the methylmercury exposure is thus decreased.

Another factor in the elimination of methylmercury from the body is its secretion in bile complexed with glutathione. The rat liver develops this capacity between 2 and 4 weeks after birth (Ballatori and Clarkson, 1982). After re-entering the gut, some of the methylmercury is reabsorbed. The majority is demethylated and excreted in the feces, presumably by the microflora as noted above.

The effects of toxic metals on human infants are less well defined than in animals. This is in part related to the fortunate circumstance that severe exposure of infants to toxic elements is unusual. Some potential adverse effects of exposures to relatively low levels of toxic metals are suggested by findings in animals noted previously.

Lead

Of the toxic elements to which infants are exposed, lead is the most intensively studied. Lead is widely distributed in the infant's environment. High levels in dirt and dust represent a hazard because infants may eat dirt, may mouth lead-containing dust from their hands and toys, and thus ingest substantial amounts of lead. Similarly, lead-containing paint, plastic, newsprint and other materials that infants ingest contribute substantially to their lead intake. Parents who work in lead related industries may entrain lead on their clothing into the home and thus expose their infants to significant hazard. As indicated by data reviewed by Lin-Fu (1973) and Mahaffey (1983), environmental sources of lead are usually a greater hazard for infants than food. The most important sources appear to be lead-contaminated dirt, household dust and paint. Mahaffey (this volume) reported that children living in an urban setting had about 2,400 ppm lead on their hands when outdoor dirt contained 1,200 ppm lead, and indoor dust contained 11,000 ppm. It was estimated that young children exposed to urban street dust had an average daily intake from these sources of 50 µg of lead (range, 20-200 µg). In contrast, surveys of the U.S. Food and Drug Administration indicate that food lead intake of infants and toddlers in the U.S. has averaged 25.2 and 28.8 µg daily. On a body weight basis, the lead intake from food by U.S. infants is nearly three times greater than adult intakes. Thus, lead intake from environmental sources and food is substantially greater relative to body size in infants than in older children and adults.

In addition to the hazards engendered by their relatively higher exposures to lead, infants are also at greater risk because they absorb a greater percentage of lead via the gastrointestinal tract than do adults. According to Alexander (1974), infants may absorb more than 50 percent and retain more than 15 percent of dietary lead. These findings are supported by Ziegler et al. (1978) who found that infants with daily intakes of more than 5 µg per kilogram absorbed about 40 percent and retained about 30 percent of ingested lead. In contrast, adults are reported to absorb 5-10 percent of dietary lead (Kehoe, 1961). This difference in absorption might be related to the about one-third slower intestinal peristalsis of infants compared to adults (Barbero et al., 1958). Another speculative explanation for the greater absorption is immaturity of an unidentified heavy metal exclusion mechanism.

A third possible explanation for greater lead absorption by infants is the composition of infant diets. Observations on nonhuman primates reported at this Symposium revealed that substantially greater amounts of lead were absorbed when monkeys previously fed a commercial monkey food were given a milk formula (Gilbert et al., 1982). For most contemporary U.S. infants and toddlers, human milk, commercial formula prepared from heat treated cow milk, and cow milk are major dietary constituents during the first two years of life, providing about 46 percent and 33 percent of the food intake at six months and two years, respectively (Mahaffey, 1983). The findings in monkeys noted above may indicate that the high milk consumption of infants and toddlers is a contributory factor to their higher absorption of lead. An alternate explanation for these findings in monkeys is that binding substances, such as phyate and hemicellulose in the control food, inhibited lead absorption, and that their absence allowed high lead absorption to occur. The interpretation that milk facilitated lead absorption in the monkeys seems at variance with findings in human infants that showed an inverse retention of lead when dietary calcium was increased (Ziegler et al., 1978), and findings in rodents that show that increased dietary calcium suppresses intestinal absorption of lead (Mahaffey, 1981).

Other components of a diet in which the primary energy source is milk that might contribute to an increased susceptibility to lead is its relatively low content of zinc and iron. When weaned rats were fed low intakes of these elements, susceptibility to lead intoxication was increased (Mahaffey and Michaelson, 1980). Because rapidly growing infants and toddlers have a relatively high requirement for these elements, whose levels in milk are low, it seems conceivable that such a condition would favor increased intestinal absorption of lead. It should be noted that dietary inadequacies of iron, zinc, and calcium are apparently more common among children from lower socio-economic strata (Lin-Fu, 1973; Sandstead, 1981) than from higher strata. On the other hand, as cited previously, Kostial (this volume) did not find that the addition of iron to milk decreased the intestinal absorption of lead by suckling rats. After the first several months of life human infants and toddlers ususally consume a mixed diet consisting of foods in addition to milk or infant formula. Also human infants are much more mature than suckling rats. It seems possible, therefore, that their responses to low intakes of iron and zinc or to additions of these elements to a diet would be more like those of weaned rats than of suckling rats.

The well known consequences of severe lead poisoning have been reviewed by Goyer (1981). Less well understood are effects of lead exposure at levels that were, until recently, not considered hazardous. While central nervous system injury in infants from eating lead-containing paint has been known for at least 40 years (Byers and Lord, 1943) it is now recognized that lead exposures substantially below those associated with clinical lead poisoning can have adverse effects on the central nervous system of young children (Needleman et al., 1979; Landrigan et al., 1975; Perino and Ernhart, 1974; Thatcher et al., 1982). Studies in experimental animals have shown that uptake of lead by brains of neonates is substantially greater than in adult animals. Similar increased uptake in infants and toddlers may account for their greater susceptibility to neurobehavioral effects compared to adults. As reviewed elsewhere in this volume, the sensitivity of the brain to injury by toxic substances is much greater during early life when it is undergoing rapid growth and maturation.

Because lead is readily transferred across the placenta, blood lead concentrations of neonates are quite similar to those of their mothers. Usually blood levels of the newborn infant are within 1 to 2 µg/dl of the mother's blood lead concentration; specific studies demonstrating this association are reviewed in this volume (Mahaffey, this volume). If women are employed in lead trades or have substantial exposure to lead during pregnancy, the neonate's blood lead concentration will be comparably evaluated with that of the mother (Ryu et al., 1978,1983). The World Health Organization recommended in 1980 (WHO, 1980) that blood lead levels for female workers of child-bearing age remain under 30 µg pb/dl whole blood. At that time the 30 µg/dl level was considered to be not associated with impairment of central nervous system development and behavioral effects in young children (CDC, 1978). Current research suggests that this level may be revised downward based on greater understanding of the range of health effects produced by lead. Data from the general population of the United States, ages 6 months through 74 years, indicated that blood lead concentrations among women of child-bearing age are generally the lowest of any age and sex group (Mahaffey et al., 1982a). Between the years 1976 and 1980, women between the ages of 18 and 45 years had average blood lead concentrations between 10 and 13 μg/dl.

Body burden of lead is only estimated by blood lead concentration. Studies with experimental animals have demonstrated that the very young have higher tissue lead concentrations than mature animals having the same blood lead concentration (Mahaffey, 1983; Kostial, 1983). Depending on the balance between body burden of lead at birth, environmental lead exposure and growth rate, tissue concentrations of lead (expressed per unit body weight) may decrease but total body burden of lead increases.

Erythrocyte protoporphyrin levels reflect interference with heme synthesis as does activity of aminoevulinic acid dehydratase. These effects of lead, and others, on heme containing enzymes and cytochromes have been reviewed (Goyer, 1981; Piomelli et al., 1982). Indeed, these indices are profoundly affected by increased body level burdens in infants and children, and, because of their sensitivity, they are useful markers of lead burden and provide a means of identifying infants and children who are at risk of lead-induced central nervous system injury.

Refinements of tests of nervous system function have indicated that concentrations of blood lead observed in the upper range of those present in the general population are assocated with a significant risk of neurobehavioral deficits in young children (CDC, 1978; Needleman et al., 1979; Perino and Ernhart, 1974; Needleman, 1982).

Increased levels of lead in unconventional tissues, such as teeth, have been found associated with impaired neurobehavioral function (Needleman, 1982). Increased levels of lead in this tissue probably reflects increased lead in bone. Accumulation of bone lead stores begins during gestation (Barltrop, 1968). Animal experiments have shown that a greater percent of an ingested lead dose is retained in the femur of young animals than mature animals (Mahaffey, 1983). Human bone lead concentrations double between infancy and the late teen years (Barry, 1975). During this period skeletal mass increases about 40-fold indicating the total amount of skeletal lead increases by 80-fold. Skeletal stores of lead are a significant endogenous source of this toxic metal for critical organs under physiological conditions in vivo. Recycling rates of bone mineral are much higher in children because of the constant physiological

processes of bone remodeling during growth. The contribution of
bone lead to blood and soft tissue lead is likely to be considerable
as recycling rates for bone are 8 to 10 times higher in children
than adults (Rosen, 1983). Levels in blood are in part a reflection
of the movement of lead from bone to soft tissue. Thus, the finding
of a blood level >30µg/dl not only may reflect current intake, but
may reflect redistribution of lead previously accumulated in bone.

A recently reported national survey has shown that many
thousands of children in the United States from low socio-economic
groups, and particularly those who live in cities, have levels of
blood lead that exceed 30 µg/dl (Mahaffey et al., 1982a). The
research of Needleman et al. (1979), Landrigan et al. (1975), and
Perino and Ernhart (1974) suggest that some of these children
probably have impairments in neuropsychological function. Thatcher
et al's. (1982) findings also suggest the problem is not limited to
inner city populations or to a particular socio-economic group, but
also can occur among children in rural settings who live "down wind"
from cities and thus are exposed to fallout that contains lead.

Cadmium

In contrast to lead there is limited clinical evidence
suggesting that cadmium poisoning is a problem among infants of the
United States. Environmental sources of cadmium include dust, paint,
newsprint, cigarette smoke and objects that infants may mouth. Under
usual circumstances, diet appears to be the most important source of
cadmium for infants. Even small concentrations in food are
potentially important because of the large amounts of food consumed
by infants relative to their body size. Food and Drug Administration
surveys indicate that dietary cadmium of U.S. infants is about 4-6
µg/day. By two years of age the level is increased to about 9-10
µg/day (Mahaffey, 1983). According to Alexander et al. (1974),
infants absorb up to 55 percent of ingested cadmium as compared to
adults who absorb less than 10 percent. Of the cadmium absorbed
most is accumulated in the kidneys and liver with as much as a 200
percent increase in concentration during the first three years of
life (Henke et al., 1970). In contrast to other tissues, cadmium
accumulation in the brain is small.

Amounts of cadmium in milk are very low (0.005 ppm average in
dairy products) (Mahaffey et al., 1975). Introduction of other
foods such as cereals (0.028 ppm cadmium) and fruits (0.042 ppm
cadmium) as is common practice at 3-6 months of life substantially
increases the infants dietary cadmium relative to amounts that would
be consumed if the infant were fed only human milk or a milk based
formula. Other potentially important food sources of cadmium are
leafy vegetables (0.051 ppm), potatoes (0.046 ppm), oils and fat
(0.27 ppm), root vegetables (0.021 ppm) and garden fruits (0.019 ppm).

Observations in experimental animals cited previously in studies of biochemical effects of cadmium on activity of certain enzymes, its binding to certain amino acids such as histidine, and to DNA, and its adverse effects on oxidative phosphorylation cytochrome P450 protein synthesis and cell replication suggest that even small amounts of cadmium accumulation are undesirable (Jacobson and Turner, 1980).

Mercury

Significant exposure of the human infant to mercury compounds other than methylmercury is often presumed to be rare, but there have been important exceptions.

Acrodynia (painful extremities), also known as pink disease (red hands and feet), is now a very rare disorder, although thousands of infants were afflicted during earlier decades of this century, apparently from exposure to mercurous chloride "teething powders", mercuric oxide ointments for impetigo or mercurials administered as vermifuges (Cheek, 1972). Though hundreds of thousands of infants were repeatedly exposed, only a small fraction developed the disease. Following the nearly complete cessation of use of these medications during the last two decades, acrodynia has become an increasingly rare clinical observation.

Recently in Argentina, several thousand infants were exposed to phenylmercury-contaminated diapers (EHSC, 1982). The diaper contamination was a consequence of use of a phenylmercury fungicide in a large urban diaper washing facility. A few cases of acrodynia were observed, but clinical effects seemed to be surprisingly mild given the mercury urine levels found in exposed infants. The question of long-term adverse effects is being studied. Further exposure has been prevented by banning the use of mercury fungicides.

Significant exposure of infants to mercury vapor is always a potential hazard if liquid mercury is released in households, especially if it is trapped in rugs or carpeting or is taken up and aerosolized and vaporized through vacuum cleaners. Poisoning of a family following exposure in the home to mercury vapor generated by heating liquid mercury has also been reported (EHSC, 1978). Such exposures, except possibly for some dental offices is presumably rare.

Exposure of neonates in closed (nursery) incubators to mercury vapor generated from broken liquid mercury thermometers and hemostats has been of recent concern (Waffarn and Hodgman, 1979).

Methylmercury is exceptional among mercury compounds in that it is a normal constituent of foods, especially fish and fish products

(WHO, 1976). Methylmercury body burden is the result of degree and duration of exposure, rate and extent of absorption, and rate of elimination. It has been well documented that ingested methylmercury is nearly completely absorbed at all ages.

Using a mouse model, Doherty et al. (1973) observed that compared to adults, suckling mice excrete minimal amounts of their body burdens of methylmercury until weaned. If these findings can be applied to human infants, risks from methylmercury accumulated in utero, or by suckling or other routes postnatally, may be greater than expected from the assumption that early postnatal excretion rates are comparable to those of adults.

As noted previously, experimental studies in animals indicate that elimination of methylmercury from the body is sharply accelerated after weaning. The mechanism may involve changes in biliary excretion and markedly increased demethylation by intestinal bacteria.

The rapidly developing infant is protected to some extent by "growth dilution" i.e. distribution of body content of methylmercury into a rapidly increasing total body mass due to growth. Nevertheless, since cumulative methylmercury body burden is directly related to elimination half-times at different life cycle stages, developmental changes in mercury excretion must be considered in estimating hazards to human health from dietary intake of methylmercury.

In 1971-72 in Iraq, a large outbreak of methylmercury poisoning occurred from ingestion of bread made from seed wheat contaminated with a methylmercury fungicide. Early in the outbreak it was found that amounts of mercury in mothers' milk correlated closely with amounts of mercury in blood (Bakir et al., 1973). It was later shown that infants not exposed prenatally could accumulate a significant amount of mercury in blood (some as high as 1000 ng/ml) when suckled by mothers who consumed methylmercury-contaminated bread after delivery (Amin-Zaki et al., 1974). These infant blood mercury levels were well above the minimum toxic blood levels for adults. As shown in Figure 1, the suckled infant's blood mercury concentration remained higher than the pair mother's blood level during a number of months of breast feeding, reflecting continued methylmercury intake by suckling and perhaps reduced mercury excretion in the infant compared to the mother. In Iraq, maternal milk averaged 8.6 percent of the simultaneous mothers' blood mercury levels, but the relationship was non-linear at blood mercury levels below 50 ng/ml (Amin-Zaki et al., 1976).

Certain subpopulations with very high dietary methylmercury intake may be at special risk. Wheatley (1979) reported elevated blood mercury levels in Eskimo populations in Northern Quebec who

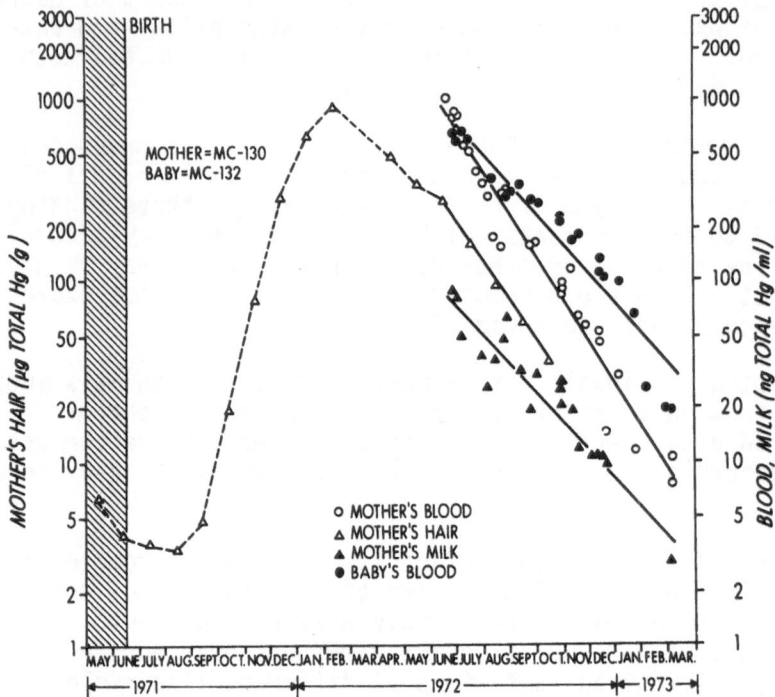

Figure 1   Concentration of total mercury in 1-cm segments of sample
           of mother's hair, whole blood and milk, and baby's blood
           (postnatal exposure). Concentrations in milk and blood
           are plotted according to dates of collection.

have large dietary intakes of seal liver. In one village of 150
families, 50 individuals were found to have blood mercury
concentrations greater than 100 ng/ml (normal range, 5-15 ng/ml).
Eleven females of child-bearing age had blood mercury levels between
100 and 200 ng/ml. A recent Canadian report describes probable
neurobehavioral effects in children born and suckled by Indian
mothers with high fresh water fish intake (McGill Report, 1980).
The fish were taken from lakes with no known industrial mercury
contamination. Hair mercury levels of 10-30 ng/ml (equivalent to
blood levels of 30-100 ng/ml) were reported to be associated with
probable adverse effects on offspring.

    The Iraqi experience documents that infants exposed only by
suckling milk of mothers heavily exposed to methylmercury through
dietary intake can ingest and absorb enough mercury to produce

significant adverse neurobehavioral effects (Amin-Zaki et al., 1980). This degree of maternal exposure is unusual and would not be expected to result from dietary intake of fish from non-industrially-contaminated lakes or oceans.

It has been established that the developing fetal and neonatal central nervous system is the critical human organ system for methylmercury toxicity. Prenatal exposure of the developing fetus to methylmercury from dietary fish intake remains the most significant potential hazard relevant to populations who consume very large quantities of fish. Safe levels of dietary methylmercury intake for pregnant women contiue to be evaluated and definitive recommendations are not yet determined. It has become evident from human and animal studies that for a small segment of certain populations exposed to methylmercury through heavy dietary fish intake, there is a potential hazard for adverse neurobehavioral effects on the developing fetus and infant mainly through transplacental exposure but possible augmented by postnatal intake from nursing.

CONCLUSIONS - POSTNATAL METABOLISM AND EFFECTS OF TOXIC ELEMENTS

1. Most of the information on early postnatal metabolism and toxic effects of metals comes from studies of experimental animals. Information from such studies must be extrapolated to humans with caution because of differences in metabolism and rates of maturation between species.

2. The long-term functional effects of "low dose" exposures to toxic elements during infancy are not well understood in either experimental animals or humans. Emerging data on humans suggests that previously unsuspected, cryptic effects can occur that have undesirable implications for health and performance.

3. The intake of toxic elements on a per kilogram basis in infants is greater than in adults. The relatively greater requirements of infants for energy, water and oxygen contribute to their greater exposure to toxic elements.

4. The absorption, distribution and excretion of toxic elements are developmentally dependent processes. In infants intestinal absorption of toxic elements is generally greater than in adults; uptake of toxic elements into soft tissues is generally greater; and excretion of toxic elements is generally less.

5. Rapidly developing organ systems appear to be particularly vulnerable to toxic elements. Thus injury to the brain during its critical postnatal period of growth and maturation can result in poorly reversable functional sequelae.

6.   From studies of rodents, a variety of dietary factors, and
      nutritional states appear to influence the absorption of metals
      and susceptibility of animals to metal toxicity. While these
      relationships are not so well defined in humans, observations
      on interactions that influence essential trace element nutriture
      in man suggest that the findings in animals on toxic element
      bioavailability are probably applicable to humans.

7.   In rodents, maternal absorption of certain toxic elements is
      increased during lactation. These elements are subsequently
      transferred in milk to pups. The amount of transfer differs
      among the elements. It is presumed that similar phenomena
      occur in humans.

8.   Exposure of human infants to toxic elements occurs not only
      from air, food and water, but from dirt, dust and fomites that
      are contaminated with these elements largely as a result of
      human activity.

RECOMMENDATIONS

1.   Pharmacokinetic data are needed to accurately define the
      relation between dose and effect in infants.

2.   Dose cannot be quantitatively extrapolated between species.
      Therefore data are needed on humans.

3.   Research should focus on functional endpoints that reflect
      damage to organ systems.

4.   Multigenerational studies at "low levels" of exposure are needed
      to ascertain if functional deficits occur.

5.   Interactions of toxic elements with nutrients and non nutrients
      that influence absorption, excretion and the effects of toxic
      elements on homeostasis, need further definition.

REFERENCES

Alexander, F.W., 1974, The uptake of lead by chidren in differing
      environments, Environ. Health Perspect. May:155-159.
Alexander, F.W., Clayton, B.E. and Delves, H.T., 1974, Mineral and
      trace-metal balances in children receiving normal and synthetic
      diets, Quarterly J. Med. New Series XLIII, 169:89-111.
Amin-Zaki, L., Elhassani, S., Majeed, M.A., Clarkson, T.W., Doherty,
      R.A. and Greenwood, M.R., 1974, Studies of infants postnatally
      exposed to methylmercury, J. of Ped. 85:81-84.

Amin-Zaki, L., Elhassani, S., Majeed, M.A., Clarkson, T.W., Doherty, R.A., Greenwood, M.R. and Giovanoli-Jakubczak, T., 1976, Perinatal methylmercury poisoning in Iraq, Amer. J. Dis. Child. 130:1070-1076.

Amin-Zaki, L., Elhassani, S., Majeed, M.A., Clarkson, T.W., Doherty, R.A. and Greenwood, M.R., 1980, Methylmercury poisoning in mothers and their suckling infants, in: "Mechanisms of Toxicity and Hazard Evaluation", B. Holmstedt, R. Lauwerys, M. Mercier and M. Roberfroid, eds, pp. 75-78, Elsevier/ North-Holland Biomedical Press.

Bakir, F., Damluji, S.F., Amin-Zaki, L., Murtadha, M., Khalidi, A., Al-Rawi, N., Tikriti, S., Dhahir, H., Clarkson, T.W., Smith, J.C. and Doherty, R.A., 1973, Methylmercury poisoning in Iraq, Science 181:230-241.

Ballatori, N. and Clarkson, T.W., 1982, Developmental changes in the biliary excretion of methylmercury and glutathione, Science 215:61-63.

Barbero, G.C., Kim, I.C. and Davis, J., 1958, Duodenal motility patterns in infants and children, Pediatr. 22:1054-1064.

Barltrop, D., 1968, Transfer of lead to the human fetus, in: "Mineral Metabolism in Paediatrics", D. Barltrop and W. Burland, eds., Vol. 56, pp. 221-225, Blackwell Scientific Publications, Oxford.

Barltrop, D. and Khoo, H.E., 1976, The influence of dietary minerals and fat in the absorption of lead, Science Total Environ. 6:265-273.

Barry, P.S.I., 1975, A comparison of concentrations of lead in human tissues, Brit. J. Ind. Med. 32:119-139.

Byers, R.K. and Lord, E.E., 1943, Late effects of lead poisoning on mental development, Amer. J. Dis. Child 66:471-494.

Center for Disease Control, 1978, Preventing lead poisoning in young children, J. Pediatr. 93:709-720.

Chang, L.W., Wade, P., Pounds, J. and Ruehl, K., 1980, Prenatal and neonatal toxicology and pathology of heavy metals, Adv. Pharmacol. Chemother. 17:195-231.

Cheek, D.B., 1972, Acrodynia, in: "Brennemann's Practice of Pediatrics", Vol. I, V.C. Kelly, ed., Chapt. 17D, pp. 1-14, Harper and Row Publishers, Inc.

Doherty, R.A. and Gates, A.H., 1973, Epidemic methylmercury poisoning: Application of a mouse model, Pediat. Res. 7:319.

EHSC, 1978, Heavy metals as environmental hazards to man, Environmental Health Sciences Center, Program Project Proposal, T.W. CLarkson, ed., pp. 447-490, Section 4, University of Rochester Medical Center, Rochester, New York.

EHSC, 1982, Exposure of infants to phenylmercury compounds, Environmental Health Sciences Center, Annual Report, T.W. Clarkson, ed., pp. 7-21, University of Rochester Medical Center, Rochester, New York.

Fox, M.R.S., 1974, Effect of essential minerals on cadmium toxicity, J. Food Sci. 39:321-324.

Gilbert, S.G., Truelove, J.F. and Rice, D.C., 1982, Effects of diet on blood lead levels in the monkey, Teratology 26:47A.

Goyer, R.A., 1981, Lead, in: "Disorders of Mineral Metabolism I", F. Bronner and J.W. Coburn, eds., pp. 159-199, Academic Press, New York.

Henke, G., Sachs, H. and Bohm, G., 1970, Cadmium-Bestimmvagen in leder und niereu von kindern und jugendlichen durch neutronenabtivierungsanalyse, Arch. Toxik. 26:8-16.

Jacobson, K.B. and Turner, J.E., 1980, The interaction of cadmium and certain other metal ions with proteins and nucleic acids, Toxicology 16:1-37.

Jason, K.M. and Kellogg, C.K., 1981, Neonatal lead exposure: effect on development of behavior and striatal dopamine neurons, Pharm. Biochem. Behav. 15:641-649.

Kehoe, R.A., 1961, The metabolism of lead in man in health and disease, II. The metabolism of lead under abnormal conditions, J. Roy. Inst. Publ. Health Hyg. 24:101-135.

Keller, C.A. and Doherty, R.A., 1980a, Bone lead mobilization in lactating mice and lead transfer to suckling offspring, Toxicol. Appl. Pharm. 55:220-228.

Keller, C.A. and Doherty, R.A., 1980b, Correlation between lead retention and intestinal pinocytosis in the suckling mouse, Am. J. Physiol. 239:G114-G122.

Keller, C.A. and Doherty, R.A., 1980c, Lead and calcium distributions in blood, plasma, and milk of lactating mouse, J. Lab. Clin. Med. 95:81-89.

Kopp, S.J., Glonek, T., Perry, H., Erlanger, M. and Perry, E., 1982, Cardiovascular actions of cadmium at environmental exposure levels, Science 217:837-839.

Kostial, K., 1983, The absorption of heavy metals by the growing organism: Experimental experience with animals, in: "Health Evaluation of Heavy Metal Exposure from Infant Formula and Junior Foods", E.H.F. Schmidt and A. Hildebrand, eds., Springer-Verlag, in press.

Kostial, K., Simonovic, I. and Pisonic, M., 1971, Reduction of lead absorption from the intestines in new born rats, Environ. Res. 4:360-363.

Landrigan, P.J., Whitworth, R.H., Baloh, R.W., Staehling, N.W., Barthel, W.F. and Rosenblum, B.T., 1975, Neuropsycholotgical dysfunction in children with chronic low level lead absorption, Lancet 1:708-712.

Landry, T.D., Doherty, R.A. and Gates, A.H., 1979, Effects of three diets on mercury excretion after methylmercury administration, Bull. Environ. Contamin. Toxicol. 22:151-158.

Lin-Fu, J.S., 1973, Vulnerability of children to lead exposure and toxicity, N. Eng. J. Med. 289:1229-1233, 1289-1293.

Mahaffey, K.R., 1981, Nutritional factors in lead poisoning, Nutr. Res. 39:353-362.

Mahaffey, K.R., 1983, Absorption of lead by infants ad young
    children, in: "Health Evaluation of Heavy Metal Exposure from
    Infant Formula and Junior Foods", E.H.F. Schmidt and A.
    Hildebrand, eds., Springer-Verlag, in press.
Mahaffey, K.R. and Michaelson, I.A., 1980, The interaction between
    lead and nutrition, in: "Low Level Lead Exposure: The
    Clinical Implication of Current Research", H.L. Needleman, ed.,
    pp. 159-200, Raven Press, New York.
Mahaffey, K.R., Corneliussen, P.E., Jelinek, C.F. and Fiorino, J.A.,
    1975, Heavy metal exposure from foods, Environ. Health
    Perspect. 12:63-69.
Mahaffey, K.R., Smith, C., Tanaka, Y. and Deluca, H.F., 1979,
    Stimulation of gastrointestinal lead absorption of
    1,25-dihydroxy vitamin D_3, Fed. Proc. 38:384 (Abstract).
Mahaffey, K.R., Annest, J.L., Roberts, J. and Murphy, R.S., 1982a,
    National estimates of blood lead levels: United States,
    1976-1980. Association with selected demographic and
    socioeconomic factors, New Engl. J. Med. 307:573-579.
Mahaffey, K.R., Rosen, J.F., Chesney, R.W., Peeler, J.T., Smith,
    C.M. and DeLuca, H.G., 1982b, Association between age, blood
    lead concentration and serum 1,25dihydroxycholecalciferol
    levels in children, Am. J. Clin. Nutr. 35:1327-1331.
McGill Report, 1980, "Methylmercury", University of McGill,
    Montreal, Canada.
Merali, Z. and Singhal, R.L., 1980, Diabetogenic effects of chronic
    oral cadmium administration to neonatal rats, Br. J. Pharm.
    69:151-157.
Miller, W.J., Lampp, B., Powell, G.W., Salotti, C.A. and Blackmon,
    D.M., 1967, Influence of a high level of dietary cadmium on
    cadmium content in milk excretion and cow performance, J. Diary
    Sci. 50:1404-1408.
Needleman, H.L., 1982, The neuropsychiatric implications of low
    level exposure to lead, Psychological Medicine 12:461-463.
Needleman, H.D., Gunnoe, C., Leviton, A., Reed, R., Peresie, H.,
    Maher, C. and Barrett, B.S., 1979, Deficits in psychologic and
    classroom performance of children with elevated dentine lead
    levels, N. Engl. J. Med. 300:689-695.
Perino, J. and Ernhart, C.B., 1974, The relation of subclinical lead
    level to cognitive and sensory motor impairment in black
    pre-schoolers, J. Learning Disabilities 7:26-30.
Perry, H.M., Erlanger, M. and Perry, E.F., 1979, Increase in the
    cystolic pressure of rats chronically fed cadmium, Environ.
    Health Perspect. 28:251-260.
Piomelli, S., Seaman, C., Zullow, D., Curran, A. and Davidow, B.,
    1982, Threshold of lead damage to heme synthesis in urban
    children, Proc. Natl. Acad. Sci. USA 79:3335-3339.
Rosen, J.F., 1983, Metabolic and cellular effects of lead: A guide
    to low level lead toxicity in children, in: "Health
    Implications of Current Levels of Lead Exposure", K.R.
    Mahaffey, ed., Elsevier/Biomedical Press, in press.

Ryu, J.E., Ziegler, E.E. and Fomon, S.J., 1978, Maternal lead exposure and blood lead concentration in infancy, J. Pediatr. 93:476-478.

Ryu, J.E., Ziegler, E.E., Nelson, S.E. and Fomon, S.J., 1983, Dietary and environmental lead exposure during the first year of life, in: "Health Implications of Current Levels of Lead Exposure", K.R. Mahaffey, ed., Elsevier/Biomedical Press, in press.

Sabbioni, E., Marafonte, E., Amantini, L., Ubertalli, L. and Pietra, R., 1978, Cadmium toxicity studies under long-term low-level exposure conditions, Sci. Total Environ. 10:131-161.

Sandstead, H.H., 1981, Zinc in human nutrition, in: "Disorders of Mineral Metabolism I", F. Bronner and J.W. Coburn, eds., pp. 93-157, Academic Press, New York.

Suzuki, T., 1977, Metabolism of mercurial compounds, in: "Advances in Modern Toxicology II, Toxicology of Trace Elements", R.A. Goyer and M.A. Mehlman, eds., pp. 1-39, Hemisphere Publishers, John Wiley and Sons, New York.

Thatcher, R.W., Lester, M.L., McMaster, R. and Horst, R., 1982, Effects of low levels of cadmium and lead on cognitive functioning in children, Arch. Environ. Health 37:159-166.

Victery, W., Vander, A.J., Shulak, J., Schoeps, P. and Julius, S., 1982a, Lead, hypertension, and reninangiotensin system in rats, J. Lab. Clin. Med. 99:354-362.

Victery, W., Vander, A.J., Markel, H., Katyman, L., Shulak, J. and Germain, C., 1982b, Lead exposure begun in utero, decreases in renin and angiotensin II in adult rats, Proc. Soc. Exptl. Biol. Med. 170:37-63.

Waffarn, F. and Hodgman, J.E., 1979, Mercury vapor contamination of infant incubators: A potential hazard, Pediatrics 64:640-642.

Walker, W.A., 1978, Antigen handling by the gut, Arch. Dis. Child. 53:527-531.

Wheatley, B., 1979, "Methylmercury in Canada," Medical Services Branch, Department of Health and Welfare, Tunney's Pasture, Ottawa, Canada.

World Health Organization, 1976, Recommended Health-Based Limits in Occupational Exposure to Heavy Metals, Technical Report Series No.647, World Health Organization, Geneva.

World Health Organization, 1980, Recommended Health-Based Limits in Occupational Exposure to Heavy Metals, Technical Report Series No.647, World Health Organization, Geneva.

Zenick, H. and Goldsmith, M., 1981, Drug discrimination learning in lead-exposed rats, Science 212:569-571.

Zepp, E.A., Thomas, J.A. and Knotts, G.R., 1974, The toxic effects of mercury, Clin. Pediat. 13:783-787.

Ziegler, E.E., Edwards, B., Jensen, R., Mahaffey, K.R. and Fomon, S.J., 1978, Absorption and retention of lead by infants, Pediat. Res. 12:29-34.

INVITED PAPERS

SESSION 1. EFFECTS OF METALS ON THE MALE REPRODUCTIVE SYSTEM

Chairpersons: *Maths Berlin and Lonnie D. Russell*

NORMAL TESTICULAR STRUCTURE AND METHODS OF EVALUATION UNDER

EXPERIMENTAL AND DISRUPTIVE CONDITIONS

Lonnie D. Russell

Department of Physiology
Southern Illinois University School of Medicine
Carbondale, Illinois

ABSTRACT

    Although there are many environmental/toxic agents which lead to
male infertility, there are few descriptions of testicular pathology
which provide meaningful mechanistic interpretations. Several
methodological guidelines are suggested. In using experimental
animals, it is necessary to obtain properly-fixed tissue; perfusion
fixation by one of several methods affords excellent tissue
preservation. Light microscopic resolution is greatly improved with
plastic embedment such that many subcellular organelles may be
distinguished with relative ease. The investigator should be
thoroughly familiar with the normal spermatogenesis and techniques
to quantitate spermatogenesis. Short periods in the transformation
of an abnormal degenerating cell may be pinpointed and the phase of
its development correlated with its known functional activity.
Through comparisons of this type, clues to the mechanisms of action
of agents may be sought. The dogma persists that a germinal cell
develops at a prescribed rate throughout spermatogenesis, and that
various agents can not speed up or slow down its progress. If it
degenerates, it is easily identifiable in early phases of
degeneration and it can be determined precisely when its development
was arrested. Treatments with short-term sacrifice provide insight
into mechanisms since damage is restricted to primary effects. Long-
term studies answer the following questions: is there testicular
damage due to a particular agent and, if so, how severely is it
capable of affecting the seminiferous epithelium? It is convenient
to describe a morphological pattern of response by assuming that the
number of pathways necessary for normal spermatogenesis is limited,
but the number of agents affecting these pathways is much greater.

INTRODUCTION

The testes of humans and other mammals are highly susceptible to damage produced by genetic disorders, environmental or occupational exposure to chemicals or other means. Specific causes of testicular damage have been catalogued by several workers (Jackson and Ericsson, 1970; Jackson, 1973; Patanelli et al., 1975; Gomes, 1977; Johnson, 1977; Lucier et al., 1977), although these listings are by no means complete. The susceptibility of the testis to one or more of the agents (the general term which will be used to refer to a cause of testicular damage irregardless of how it was provoked) is due to the complexity and long duration of the spermatogenic process. It stands to reason that the more complex the structural and biochemical pathways stimulating and leading to the production of sperm, the greater the probability that one or more pathways will be interrupted by any particular agent.

The prime means to determine whether an agent has an effect on the testis, and the mechanism by which it exerts this effect is through morphological examination of the testis. However, the very complexity which made the testis susceptible to damage also makes its evaluation difficult, especially to the investigator who is not thoroughly familiar with the spermatogenesis process. What follows are methodologies developed over the course of several years, which we and others have found most useful in evaluating the effects of various agents on spermatogenesis and testis structure. As a prelude to this, a section on understanding normal testis structure and spermatogenesis is included to provide the inexperienced investigator with a basic introduction to spermatogenesis. Selected references are also provided with which he/she may become more familiar with this complex process.

NORMAL TESTIS MICROSTRUCTURE

The mammalian testis has two basic compartments, the interstitial (intertubular) compartment and the seminiferous tubules. The interstitial compartment is highly vascularized, with cells of Leydig clustered near or around the vessels (Figures 1 and 2). Leydig cells are responsive to luteinizing hormone (LH) and secrete testosterone which is important for maintenance of spermatogenesis (Steinberger, 1975) and for development of male glands and characteristics. Leydig cells are irregularly shaped and ultrastructurally show an abundance of smooth endoplasmic reticulum and mitochondria with tubular cristae (Figure 2 inset), both of which participate in the steroid synthetic process. In most species, lipid droplets are present within these cells and serve as a reservoir of steroid precursors. Often macrophages lie adjacent to Leydig cell clumps. The lymphatics of the testis reside within the intertubular compartment (Figures 1 and 2) and the precise way

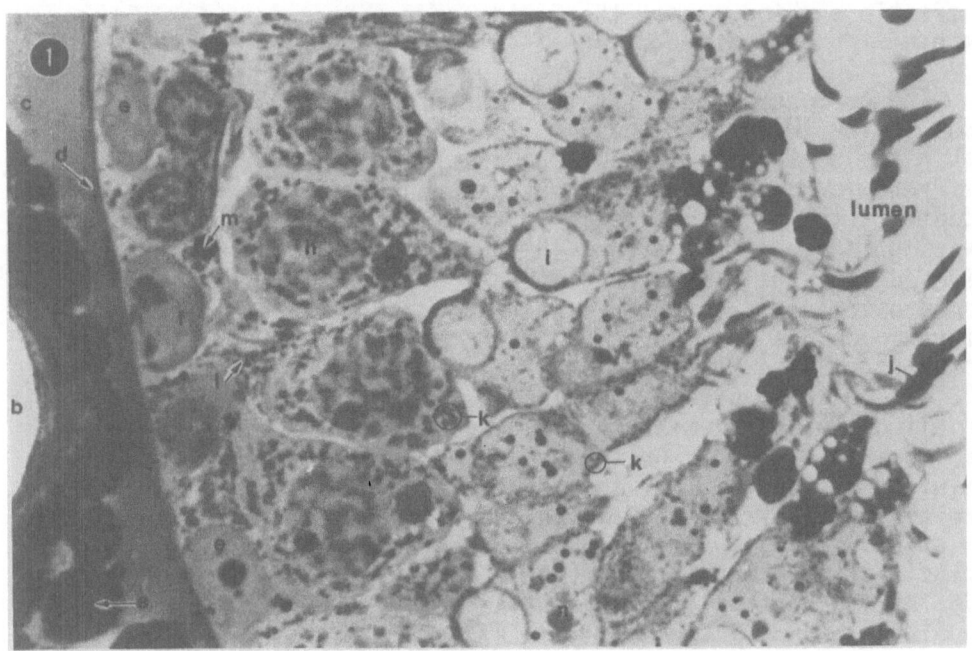

Figure 1   This light micrograph of a perfused, epoxy-embedded
           section of a rat seminiferous tubule shows the detail
           resolvable. Leydig cells (a) are seen in the interstitial
           compartment and surround a small vessel (b). The
           lymphatics (c) bathe the wall of the seminiferous tubule
           (d). Sertoli cell nuclei (e) are easy to identify, but
           the cell boundaries of the Sertoli cell are elusive.
           Indicated are spermatogonia (f); spermatocytes: leptotene
           (g) and pachytene (h); and spermatids: round (i) and
           elongate (j). Mitochondria (k), lysosome (l), lipid (m),
           Golgi (n) and other fine structures are identifiable.
           This tubule depicts cell association VIII (as indicated in
           Figure 4) in which the late spermatids are about to be
           released.

the lymphatics are organized is somewhat variable from species to
species (Fawcett et al., 1973).

     The seminiferous tubules form convoluted loops. Each end of
the loop joins the excurrent duct system within the substance of the
testis. The walls of the seminiferous tubules are comprised of
muscle-like or myoid cells, and a basal lamina with a variable
amount of collagen intervening (Figure 3). The myoid cells are
contractile and are thought to be responsible for peristaltic

contractions which propel the fluids and spermatozoa within the lumen of the seminiferous tubule (Clermont, 1958).

The peripheral cells of the seminiferous tubule rest on its basal lamina (Figures 2 and 3). Two cell populations are present within the seminiferous tubule. One of these, the germ cells, is a self-renewing population which has an embryonic origin from yolk sac endoderm. These cells undergo a process of mitotic and meiotic divisions and transformations in spermatogenesis (Figure 5). When released into the seminiferous tubule lumen, they are properly termed spermatozoa although it is recognized that epididymal maturation and a period residence in the female reproductive system are prerequisites for full fertilizing capacity (Young, 1931; Chang, 1951; Blandau and Rumery, 1964). The other population of cells, the Sertoli cells, has a mesenchymal origin and at sexual maturation, they cease dividing. For the remainder of their lifespan in the seminiferous tubule, they are closely and intimately related to the germ cells. Their configuration position, movements (Fawcett, 1975; Dym et al., 1977; Russell, 1980b), responsiveness to follicle-stimulating hormone (FSH) and testosterone (Means et al., 1976; Elkington et al., 1975) and secretory products (see Ewing et al., 1980) have led to much speculation as to their function.

The fundamental organization and integrity of the seminiferous tubules are provided by the Sertoli cells. These tall, irregularly-columnar cells (Russell and Wong, 1981) span the distance from the base of the tubule to the tubular lumen and have attachments to the basal lamina (Connell, 1974; Russell, 1977a), other Sertoli cells (Dym and Fawcett, 1970) and germ cells (Russell, 1980b). Adjacent Sertoli cells form contacts with each other at their lateral surfaces and near their base to effectively compartmentalize and separate the two populations of germ cells (Ross, 1970; Figure 3). Those germ cells near the base of the tubule (spermatogonia and young spermatocytes) are directly percolating substances from the lymph and blood (basal compartment), and those near the lumen (most spermatocytes and spermatids) are isolated from these substances (adluminal compartment) by the

Figure 2 This electron micrograph shows the intertubular and tubular compartments. A small vessel (a) is surrounded by Leydig cells and Leydig cell processes (b) and an occasional macrophage (c). The lymphatic space (d) is filled with proteinaceous material and makes contact with the tubular wall. The myoid cells (e) and basal lamina (f) are readily identifiable as are Sertoli (g) and germinal cells (h) at the periphery of the tubule. The inset shows a magnified view of Leydig cell cytoplasm which is characterized by smooth endoplasmic reticulum and numerous mitochondria.

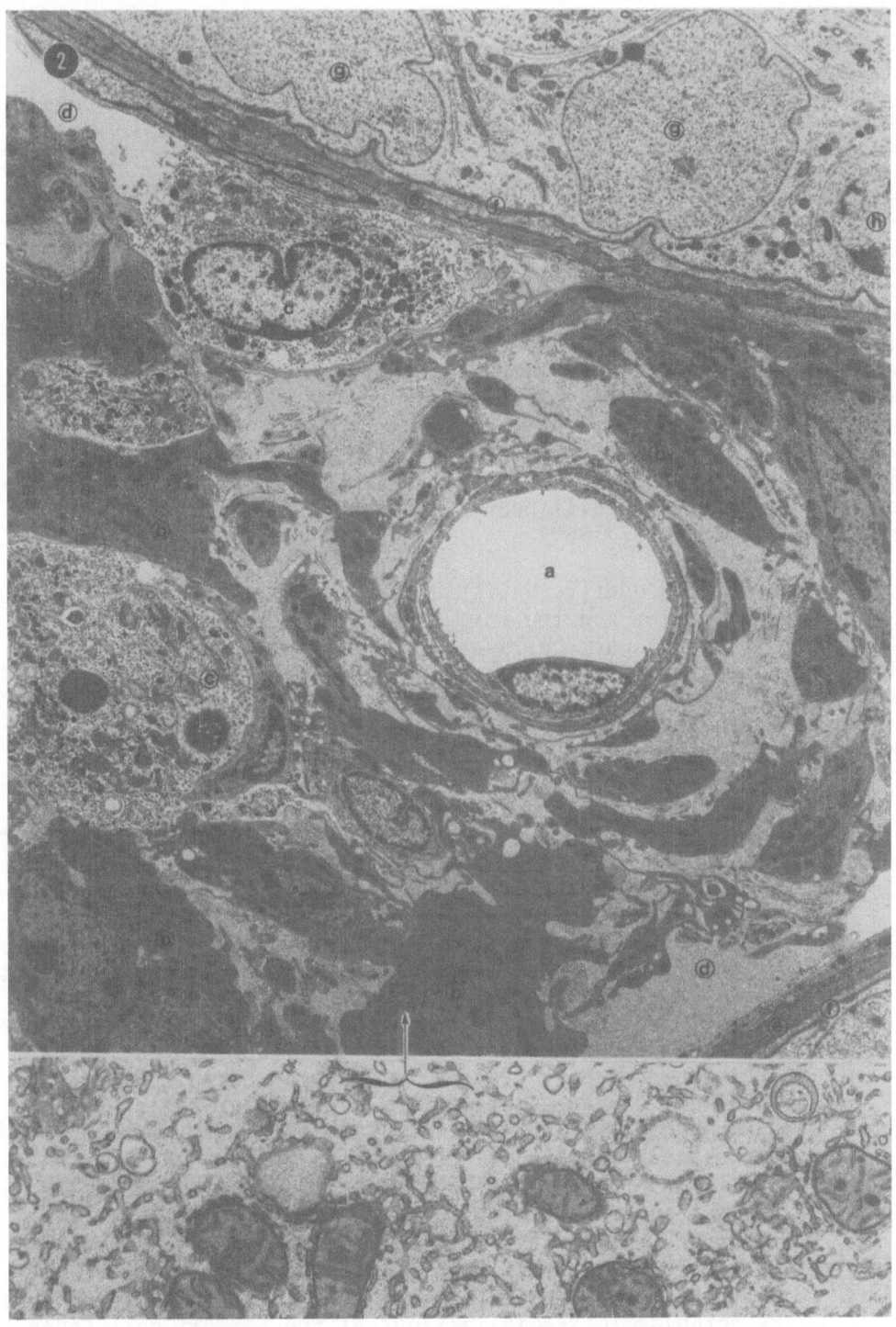

occluding junctions which form between adjacent Sertoli cells
(Gilula et al., 1976). Some germ cells are in transit through the
area of Sertoli-Sertoli contact and for a short time exist in a
separate compartment (intermediate compartment) so as not to break
the continuity of the blood-testis barrier in their transit
(Russell, 1977a). For a review of the morphological and functional
components of the blood-testis barrier, see Setchell and Waites
(1975).

The relationship of Sertoli cells with most germ cell types is
sufficiently elaborate that only rarely do germ cells face each
other without an intervening Sertoli cell process (Figure 3). The
elongate germ cells have a special relationship to the Sertoli
cell. They are positioned deep within crypts of the Sertoli cell
with their heads and proximal flagella buried within these crypts.
The distal flagella of these spermatids projects into the lumen
(Figure 3). A special mantle (ectoplasmic specialization; Russell,
1977b) at the surface of the Sertoli cell holds the head of the germ
cell in this position until near the time of sperm release
(spermiation, Russell, 1983).

In general, the undifferentiated germ cells or spermatogonia lie
near the basal lamina and the more mature germ cells are "layered"
with the most mature germ cells near the tubular lumen (Figure 3).
Since the elongate cells are embedded in the Sertoli recesses, they
often appear, with the light microscope, to lie between round germ
cells which are less differentiated. Each "layer of cells" is
precisely at the same state of differentiation. In a cross section

Figure 3   The fundamental organization of the seminiferous tubule is
           illustrated in the drawing. The cells at the base of the
           seminiferous tubule rest on the basal lamina which is
           overlaid with contractile myoid cells. The Sertoli cells
           extend from the base of the tubule to the lumen. Adjacent
           Sertoli cells compartmentalize the epithelium by forming
           contacts which ring the seminiferous tubule (paired arrows)
           such that spermatogonia (gonia) and young spermatocytes
           (not shown) are separated from mature spermatocytes and
           round and elongate spermatids. The latter cells are
           morphologically and functionally separated from blood-
           borne and lymphatic fluids which bathe the seminiferous
           tubule and the peripherally-positioned cells. Sertoli
           cells also send numerous processes between all germ cell
           types and are indented at their apical ends by elongate
           germ cells which rest within recesses of the Sertoli cell.
           The heads of elongate germ cells are held in these recesses
           by ectoplasmic specializations of the Sertoli cell (open
           arrows).

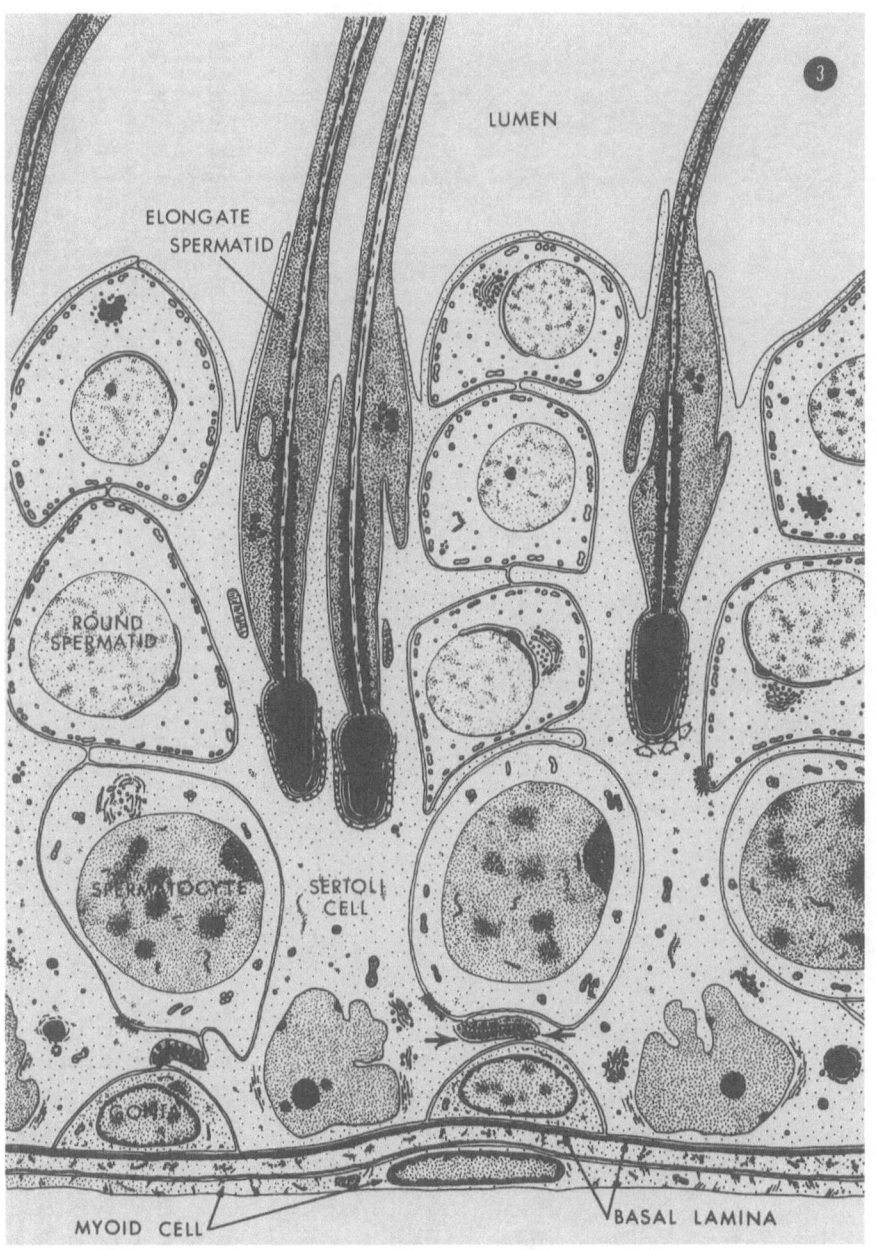

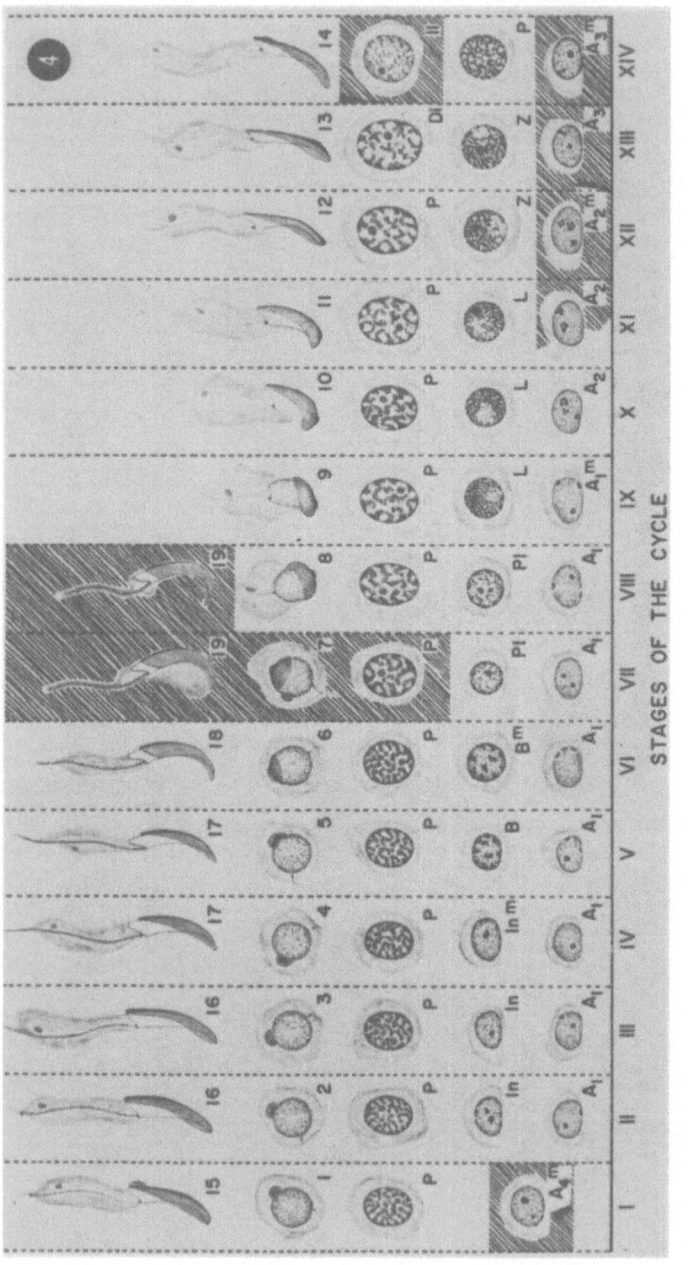

Figure 4   This drawing shows the cellular composition in the 14 stages of the spermatogenesis cycle. Vertical columns are indicated by Roman numerals and represent associations of cells seen in cross sections of seminiferous tubules (such as that shown in Figure 1). The cells are designated similar to those in Figure 5 and an M beside the designation indicates mitosis occurring as the cells progress in development to become part of the cell association in the next vertical column. Four and one-half cycles (horizontal rows) are necessary to complete spermatogenesis. The cells indicated by cross hatches are those seen degenerating in normal rats. Cross-hatched cells of Stage VII degenerate with increased frequency in response to numerous treatments which influence the LH-testosterone stimulation of the testis (Russell and Clermont, 1977; Russell et al., 1981a).

of any particular tubule, the layering and association of layers of cell types is always characteristic and has been termed a stage (Leblond and Clermont, 1952a,b). All stages or cell association are represented by vertical rows of cells as seen in Figure 4. If all appropriate cell associations are placed side-by-side in a logical order, then a map of the spermatogenic process is available for a particular species. It is obvious, from examination of such a map, that primative germ cells begin their differentiation long before the previous generation of cells has completed its development. The map, opposite page, for the rat (Figure 4) shows that the recruitment of cells occurs at periodic intervals. The time it takes cell associations to complete the developmental sequence in horizontal rows is known as a cycle; in the rat and most species there are about four and one-half cycles necessary to complete spermatogenesis. The duration of the cycle is known from thymidine incorporation studies, and the duration of any particular stage may be determined from the relative frequency of stages (Clermont et al., 1959). Hormones do not influence this strict timing (Clermont and Harvey, 1965). In most species, only one stage is evident in cross sections of seminiferous tubules; however, in some primates and in the human (Heller and Clermont, 1964), there are frequently several different cellular associations occupying parts of one tubular cross section.

Thus far consideration of spermatogenesis has been restricted to what is seen in a cross section of seminiferous tubules. Cell associations are restricted to small segments along the length of seminiferous tubules. Although some variations are common, these segments usually have a sequential ordering along the tubule. A complete series of segments is termed the "wave of the seminiferous epithelium" (Perey et al., 1961).

Unlike most cells of the body, germ cells of a clone exist connected by cytoplasmic bridges (Burgos and Fawcett, 1955). It is not until sperm release that germ cells become independent units.

Germ cells are in a continual process of differentiation and only general characteristics can be ascribed to each (Figure 5). Spermatogonia are always found at the periphery of the seminiferous tubule. Two types generally are present: 1) the stem cells which periodically undergo mitosis to give rise to 2) spermatogonia which are rapidly dividing and committed to becoming spermatozoa (Clermont and Bustos-Obregon, 1968; Huckins, 1971; Huckins and Oakberg, 1978). These divisions are normal mitosis and serve to increase the population of cells which will undergo meiosis. It is necessary that this proliferation occurs since the testes of most mammals produce millions of sperm per day which are necessary to assure fertility. After spermatogonial proliferation is initiated, each terminal stage spermatogonium (A$_4$ of Figure 5) will eventually give rise to eight spermatozoa. Once a cell differentiates from a stem cell spermatogonium, it is committed to undergo mitoses,

meioses and subsequent differentiations that culminate in the
production of spermatozoa. The only alternative is that the cell
will degenerate during this process. In the normal testis,
degenerating cells have been described (Roosen-Runge, 1973; Russell
and Clermont, 1977) and the cell loss during spermatogenesis has
been calculated (Clermont, 1962; Courot et al., 1970; Huckins, 1978).

   Two primary spermatocytes result from a single spermatogonium
and soon they enter a complicated and long meiotic prophase. After
the S phase of preleptotene cells, spermatocytes successively pass
through leptotene, zygotene, pachytene and diplotene (Figure 5)
phases of meiosis in which homologous chromosomes pair and exchange
genetic material (crossing over; Stern and Hotta, 1973) and then
separate again. Prophase meiotic cells are highly synthetic and
grow rapidly. The nucleus is also large and is characterized by the
visably condensed chromosomes. The first meiotic division separates
homologous chromosomes, reducing the chromosome number, and the
second meiotic division separates sister chromatids. The secondary
spermatocytes are formed from the first meiotic division and are
short-lived; they are present during only a portion of one stage of
the spermatogenic cycle. One secondary spermatocyte forms two
haploid spermatids. At the onset of spermiogenesis (transformation
of spermatid to a spermatozoon; Setchell, 1978), the spermatids are
relatively undifferentiated, but soon are drastically modified
(Figure 5). Early in this transformation, the Golgi apparatus

Figure 5   In this schematic representation of spermatogenesis of the
           rat, a primitive type A stem cell becomes committed to
           spermatogenesis by dividing into an A_1 spermatogonia. The
           progeny from mitoses and meioses is indicated by short dark
           arrows and the short open arrows indicate a daughter cell
           which is also not shown. Spermatogonia divide mitotically
           to form A_2, A_3, A_4, intermediate (IN) and type B
           spermatogonia. Type B spermatogonia divide mitotically
           to form spermatocytes which enter a long prophase
           (preleptotene, PL; leptotene, L; zygotene, Z; pachytene,
           P; and diplotene, not shown). These primary spermatocytes
           divide to form two secondary spermatocytes (2°); these
           quickly divide to form two round spermatids (1). The
           spermatids undergo a transformation, which lasts about ten
           days, called spermiogenesis. The number under each
           spermatid corresponds to the particular step of
           spermiogenesis assigned to it by Leblond and Clermont
           (1952) as shown in Figure 4. The spermatids develop an
           acrosome, a flagellum and an elongate condensed nucleus.
           Just prior to release as spermatozoa, some of the cytoplasm
           of the spermatid is gathered into a lobule which is
           discarded as the residual body.

packages material which initiates acrosome formation. A flagellum
forms from the centrioles and becomes associated with the nucleus.
The cell and its nucleus elongate and the nuclear chromatin becomes
condensed and lysine rich histones are exchanged for arginine rich
protamines. Late spermatids are released almost simultaneously
through the activity of the Sertoli cell (Russell, 1980b, 1983).
After release into the tubular lumen, they are called spermatozoa.
Spermatids having attained certain morphological characteristics are
assigned numbers, and these are referred to as <u>steps</u> in
spermiogenesis.

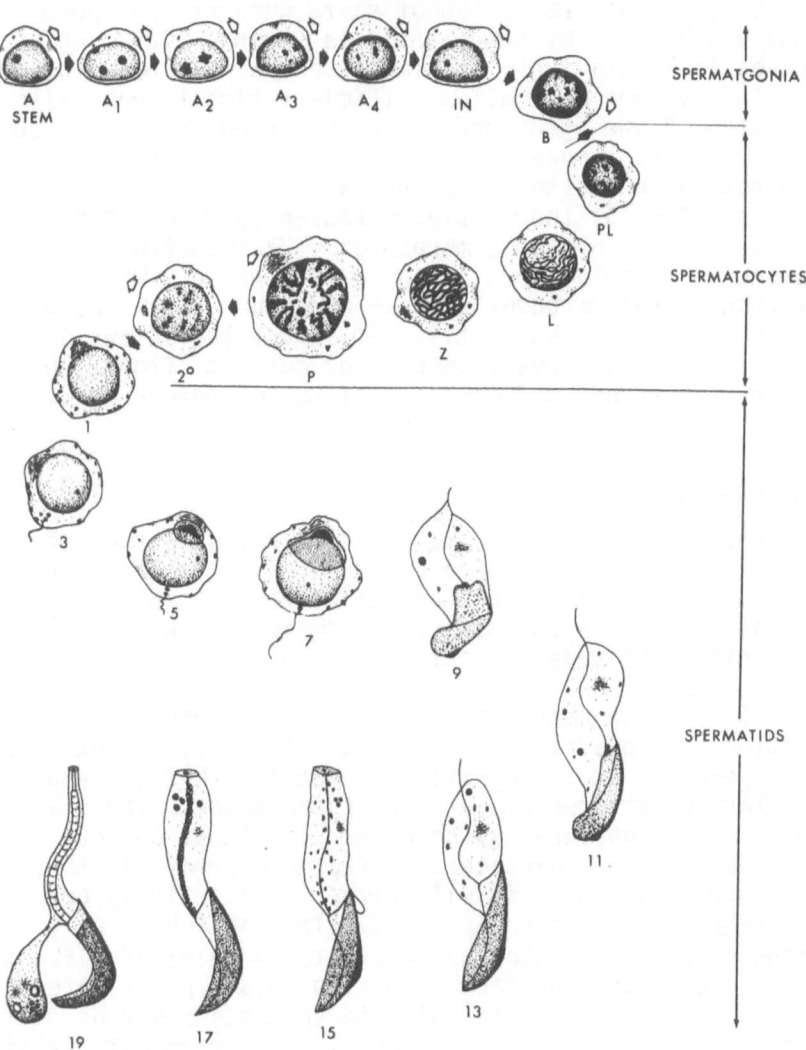

Detailed reviews of spermatogenesis and spermiogenesis are available (Roosen-Runge, 1962, 1973; Steinberger and Steinberger, 1975; Setchell, 1978; Ewing et al., 1980).

MORPHOLOGICAL EVALUATION OF THE TESTIS

Morphological analysis of the testis is the primary means for assessing damage to the testis. However, histological and cytological examination of the testis may not be the only methods to indicate testicular damage or infertility. For example, if one is simply interested in the effect of an agent on male fertility, this problem can be assessed by breeding studies (e.g., Russell and Gardner, 1974). A determination of sperm numbers and sperm morphology can be made by semen analysis (Amann, 1981), which in most species is a relatively simple procedure. In breeding or semen analysis studies, one must allow sufficient time to pass after administration of the agent under consideration for depletion of stored sperm reserves such that the results are those due to the agent and not to sperm stored in the cauda epididymis. If decreased fertility is noted, or there is a decreased sperm count or qualitative changes in sperm, morpholgical examination of the testis is indicated to pinpoint the lesion to the testis. What follows is a description of the methodologies we and others have found useful in assessing damage to the testis. It is not the intention of this section to reflect negatively on past or current efforts, but to indicate growing trends and considerations for future work.

Types of Analysis

It is relatively easy to make a determination either of a qualitative or quantitative nature in regard to spermatogenesis. On the other hand, the interpretations as to the original site or the mechanism of damage are not always as simple. Each determination requires a different type of analysis.

In the first case where it is necessary to make a simple determination of a qualitative or quantitative alteration somewhere in spermatogenesis, it is important to realize that the end products of testicular spermatogenesis are the spermatozoa. The numbers of sperm and their morphology may be examined without concern as to precisely how or when a particular defect occurred. If there is a defect in spermatogenesis, it will either qualitatively or quantitatively effect the end product. The particular cell association or stage in which sperm are to be released (like that shown in Figure 1) is important in making this type of determination. A simple subjective examination of late spermatids may be sufficient to determine if their numbers are normal or near normal, or if further study is needed. Otherwise, to be precise in one's determinations, cell quantitation must be undertaken (see below). For example, in cross sections of the same thickness and orientation through the seminiferous tubule, one can simply count the number of sperm heads captured in the section. These counts may be compared in a relative sense to counts obtained in the same manner from control animals. Another method employs squashes of whole testes which may be used to quantitate elongate spermatids in a relative or absolute way (Amann et al., 1976; Amann, 1981). This method, of course, assumes that all elongate spermatids successfully complete spermiogenesis and are released into the seminiferous tubule.

For a qualitative assessment of testicular spermatozoa, one must often rely on electron microscopic evidence. Again, the stage of release should be preferentially examined and the morphology of caput epididymal sperm as well. Defective spermatids are often not released, but phagocytosed (Russell, 1980a; Russell and Clermont, 1977; Russell et al., 1981a), so that examination of the stage following release is often useful to determine if abnormal sperm have been retained within the Sertoli cell cytoplasm.

On the other hand, if insight into mechanisms of damage is desired, it is necessary to examine the entire spermatogenic process. The very complexity of the spermatogenic process and its duration of many weeks allows one to pinpoint defects and correlate these with both biochemical and structural changes known to be taking place at particular time periods. As a general rule, germ cells which are altered in their progress or are damaged in some way will soon degenerate and be phagocytosed by nearby Sertoli cells. Except in certain types of genetic damage (Fishbein et al., 1970; Epstein et al., 1972) or in certain drug treatments (Russell et al., 1982), this dogma is generally accepted. Thus, once committed, a spermatogonium must proceed through mitosis, meiosis and complex differentiation or it will degenerate. Degenerating cells are conspicious in plastic-embedded, light microscope sections and may be recognized in the early phases of degeneration. Degenerating cells are always arrested in development and, although somewhat pyknotic, careful examination of their cytological features indicates how long they have been arrested compared to nearby germ cells which have progressed normally. By knowing the time of arrest and the processes taking place at that time, one may make an educated guess at the causal or mechanistic factors involved. For example, degenerating cells are frequently seen as meiotic divisions take place, and the degenerating cells appear to be arrested in metaphase (Russell and Clermont, 1977; Russell et al., 1981a). It is therefore thought that this cellular degeneration is due to genetic incompatibilities in the meiotic process. As Amann (1981) points out, the phrase "germ cell arrest" is often used inappropriately when applied to viable cells since, without disposal of these cells, there would, after some time, be an accumulation of immature forms.

This has never been shown to be the case since cells which are arrested soon degenerate and are phagocytosed or are sloughed into the tubular lumen.

Sometimes when a cell has been damaged, there is a short period in which the cell is viable but is morphologically abnormal prior to degeneration (Courot, 1980). For example, spermatids may be multinucleate for a short time. At a later time, they cannot undergo further differentiation in the multinucleate form, and after a certain delay, they will usually degenerate or be sloughed into the tubular lumen.

Figures 6-8 are light micrographs depicting the types of dose- and time-dependent morphological changes seen in the testis in response to an agent.

Short-Term (Mechanistic) and Long-Term Effects (End-Stage Maturation Depletion)

Different types of information are obtained with long-term and short-term exposure to (or sacrifice after administration of) an agent. Experiments should be designed to reflect the investigator's needs either to seek mechanistic answers or to determine the end

Figure 6   Short-term Response. The seminiferous epithelium is minimally altered after short-term hypophysectomy. The epithelium appears normal except for a few degenerating cells (arrows). Staging is easy since the cell associations are basically intact.

Figure 7   An intermediate type of response is produced when the numbers of degenerating cell increase and the seminiferous epithelium is severely disorganized as shown here. Secondary effects may influence the morphological response.

Figure 8   Long-term Response. After some time, a steady state is attained when the seminiferous epithelium no longer deteriorates morphologically. This figure is taken from a 96-day hypophysectomized rat seminiferous tubule. Spermatocytes are the most advanced germ cell seen and most of these will progress up to mid-pachytene before they degenerate. A few will become mid-cycle spermatids (step 7).

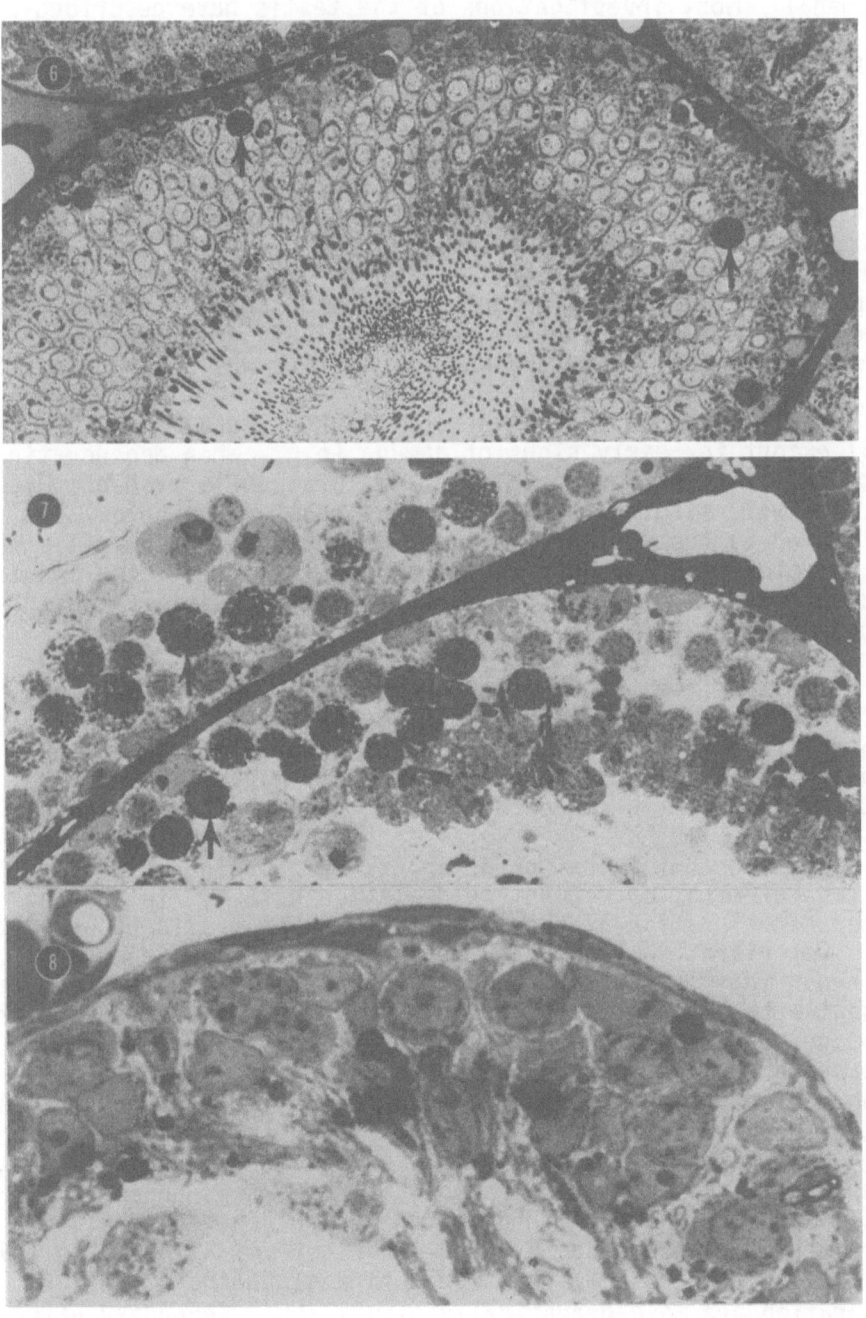

result of exposure to an agent (end-stage maturation depletion phenomena). Most investigations of the testis have described either long-term effects or intermediate effects (see below) with few demonstrating short-term effects.

In experiments which are short-term, several hours or a few days are usually necessary to produce results after single or multiple exposure to an agent. At this time, the initial morphological changes which accompany the administration of a particular agent can be noted (Russell and Clermont, 1977; Russell et al., 1981b). These alterations, which are the primary morphological indicator of a defect, provide the best clues to the mechanism of damage since they are most likely a direct consequence of the agent rather than to secondary factors which may have arisen.

Ideally, one should examine seminiferous tubules which appear normal except for early signs of damage (e.g., when degenerating cells are first seen or Sertoli cell alteration is evident; Figure 6). Moreover, staging the seminiferous tubule (see below) is facilitated by the presence of the numerous viable germ cells which are characteristic of short-term experiments. Pilot experiments might be necessary to find the correct sacrifice interval or dosage to product short-term results.

After some time, the seminiferous tubule and its contents become highly disorganized, staging is difficult, and secondary effects are often apparent (Figure 7). The morphological picture is very confusing since numerous degenerating cells may be present from stages far removed in sequence from the stage being examined.

Long-term administration of agents are herein defined as end-stage effects, or maturation depletion effects, in that no further deterioration of the morphology of the testis occurs with time. Deterioration eventually reaches a steady state after continuous administration of an agent or after a single exposure to an agent with a long-lasting effect. Experiments designed to show end-stage effects best reveal to what extent maturation of germ cells can occur under influence of an agent. For example, in hypophysectomy a few mid-pachytene spermatocytes degenerate in a short time, but rarely are cells more mature than mid-pachytene (stage VII in the rat) seen in long-term or end-stage experiments (Figure 8). This indicates that one or more steps necessary for cells to progress beyond mid-pachytene are blocked directly or indirectly by hypophysectomy. End-stage determinations show this more clearly than a short-term evaluation since the arrest and degeneration are more dramatically visualized. Secondary effects may play a role in further depleting the seminiferous epithelium and these effects will be evident in long-term but not short-term treatments.

For some agents whose effects have ended (e.g., after a single dose), there may be re-initiation of spermatogenesis. Precisely when this might occur depends on both the nature of the agent and the dose given. It is one of the difficulties which must be dealt with in making end-stage determinations.

Tissue Preparation

Testicular structure has been traditionally evaluated by light microscopy of paraffin-embedded materials which have been fixed by immersion. This type of tissue preparation is usually sufficient for a determination of major damage or a simple measurement of tubular diameters, but falls short in many respects when one's goal is to critically evaluate the testis. In the last decade, vascular perfusion techniques have replaced immersion fixation, and plastic embedment has replaced paraffin embedment. Vascular perfusion of the testis with buffered glutaraldehyde was first introduced by Christensen (1965), and the perfusion methodology for the rat was improved by Vitale et al. (1973). With experience, success with vascular perfusion is nearly 100 percent. The fixative of choice is glutaraldehyde (3-5 percent) or a glutaraldehyde: formaldehyde mixture (Forssmann et al., 1976). Generally, postfixation with osmium tetroxide is sufficient although the ferrocyanide:reduced osmium technique (Karnovski, 1971) yields improved ultrastructural images in the testis (Russell and Burguet, 1977). When appropriately fixed, the testis becomes hard and is easily sliced into one millimeter blocks and these are embedded in an epoxy plastic resin. Both light and electron microscope examination are possible with sections made at 0.5-2.0 μm in thickness on an ultramicrotome and stained with methylene or toluidine blue.

This investigator is impressed with the increasing resolution offered by the semi-thin plastic sections. Small structures including mitochondria, lipid Golgi, acrosomes, lysosomes, chromatoid body, etc., are clearly resolved (Figure 1). Hence, it is not always necessary to rely on the electron microscope to provide cytological details. In many cases, degenerating cells are identifiable as to cell type and phase of development at the time of arrest even though they are early in the process of degeneration (Russell and Clermont, 1977; Russell et al., 1981a,b). Certainly, quantitation of the seminiferous epithelial cells is best accomplished at the light microscope level since large areas may be viewed at one time.

Route of Administration and Dosage of a Particular Agent

Ideally, any agent would be administered in a manner, and by a route, which would mimic the conditions for which the agent was being tested. Environmental, occupational, contraceptive, fertility,

or other types of agents would be administered at the levels and/or
rates at which they occur naturally or are given therapeutically.
It is not always feasible, since low levels of many agents take
considerable time to accumulate or exert an effect. Other agents
are often purposefully administered in high concentrations to provoke
an effect in order to examine their mechanism of action or to
understand how agents with known effects disrupt spermatogenesic
processes (Russell, 1981b; Handel, 1979).

Agents can be administered at relatively high dosages for a
short or moderate period to determine if they show some response.
If they do, their levels and the time period they are administered
can be adjusted to provoke a minimal response. Such a response is
highly desirable, since it produces the short-term effect referred
to above.

Oral, intraperitoneal, intramuscular and subcutaneous routes of
administration are commonly used; environmental chambers and
slow-release devices are also used. Our laboratory has found
intratesticular injections valuable in the rat in several instances
where it was desirable to provoke an effect without regard to how
"naturally" the agent was to be administered. We have administered
agents at multiple sites with a 32-gauge needle; control animals
received saline by the same route. In the controls, there has never
been evidence of mechanical damage or trauma as long as we have
avoided major vessels at the time of injection (Russell et al.,
1981b). In some animals, the testicular vessels can be seen through
the skin with sufficient illumination. A small incision in the
scrotum and fascia may also be used to reveal vessels underlying the
tunica albuginea. In the rat, the agent is invariably introduced
locally into the lymphatics of the testis and from there spreads
rapidly to other regions with widespread effects.

Preliminary experiments may be necessary to arrive at an
optimum dosage regimen and an acceptable route of administration of
an agent. Similarly, single versus repeated administration of an
agent must often be tested.

Applicability of the Cycle of the Seminiferous Epithelium

Traditionally, investigators have been satisfied to describe
the general cell type damaged (i.e., spermatogonia, spermatocytes or
spermatids). This level of detail is less than satisfactory since a
spermatogonium, spermatocyte, or spermatid may be present for a week
or more and undergo numerous changes during this period. By
describing the precise phase of its development, an understanding of
the processes that previously may have been interrupted by an agent
is gained. The road maps provided for several species (human,
Clermont, 1963; dog, Ibach et al., 1976; guinea pig, Clermont, 1960;

hamster, Clermont, 1954; mouse, Oakberg, 1956; rabbit, Swierstra and Foote, 1963; rat, Leblond and Clermont, 1952a,b; monkey, Clermont and Leblond, 1959; and many others) allow precise staging of the seminiferous epithelium and also serve as a reference to which other investigators may compare their results. Although it may take several days to become familiar with a staging classification for a particular species, once familiar with the classification, it is easy to utilize this information for other species.

In regard to degenerating cells, staging is also useful in the determination of the time elapsed since the initiation of cell degeneration. For example, in the study of hypophysectomized and agent-treated animals (Russell and Clermont, 1977; Russell et al., 1981a), degenerating cells were identified even though they were often seen in stages more advanced than when they initiated degeneration. With the timing of each stage being known, it is then possible to determine precisely how long after the administration of an agent the cell in question had been arrested in development. This type of determination is most appropriate for short-term experiments.

Quantitative Determinations

The trend in histological or cytological evaluation is no longer to rely only on descriptive data, but to increasingly back this type of information with quantitative data. Methodologies for quantative analysis in the testes are numerous (Berndtson, 1977) and only a few will be cited here.

Testicular Weight. Perhaps the single most important indication of testicular damage is testicular weight. The only caution to be noted here is that a weight comparison of perfused with unfixed or immersed testis may not be valid.

Tubular Diameter. Decreased tubular diameters are good indicators of germ cell damage within the tubule. For the determinations to be valid, tubules to be measured should be cross sectioned and thus appear round in profile under the microscope. In most animals, cross-sectioned profiles can be obtained by orienting the blocks to be sectioned in such a manner that they are cut perpendicular to the long axis of the testis.

Homogenization Technique for Enumerating Elongate Germ Cells. This technique (Amann et al., 1976), mentioned above, allows enumeration of elongate germ cells which have undergone some nuclear condensation, and precludes any other morphological analysis of the same tissue.

Morphometry. Under this broad category are a variety of techniques which may be used to obtain quantitative information. The proponents of these techniques have published adequate reviews in this area and the reader is referred to them (Weibel, 1963; Weibel et al., 1966). The principles underlying morphometry assume random sampling and often employ a test system of points, lines, line intersections, grids, or bars which are used to determine relative or absolute frequency (numbers), the area or surface area, length, volume and shape of particular objects or cells. The technique may be applied to measure area or volumes of compartments of the testis (tubular vs. interstitial) or to specific cell types or to subcellular structures (employing electron micrographs). For an excellent example of the use of these techniques, see Mori and Christensen (1965). Increasingly, morphometry is being applied to study the normal and perturbed tissues.

Other Quantitation Techniques. The precise tool to be employed for cell counts depends on the specific needs of the investigator, and these needs are rarely determined until a preliminary examination of the testis has been undertaken. As indicated above, relative number of cells may be determined by morphometry. Another method employs the numbers of germ cells at a specific phase of development as determined from round profiles of seminiferous tubules. This technique is valuable, but relatively laborious, and often several hundred round germ cell types must be counted in each tubule and compared with counts from tubules at the same phase of development in control animals. Counts of this type may provide ratios of cell types obtained from controls and compared with similar ratios from tubules in experimental animals. For example, if the ratio of one germ cell type to another approaches 1 to 2 (e.g., Type B spermatogonia:pachytene spermatocytes of the same stage) in the control animal and is nearer to 1 to 1, in the agent-treated animal, there would appear to have been cell loss in the period in which one cell type developed into the next. This loss can be attributed to the agent under consideration. Cell size and shape influence counts and for this reason counts are comparable only in a relative sense.

Ratios may be very useful in another way. For example, Sertoli cells are not prone to degeneration under most adverse conditions affecting the seminiferous tubule. A ratio of Sertoli nuclei or nucleoli to a particular germ cell type can first be established in control animals and compared with those obtained from agent-treated animals. The Sertoli nuclei must be shown not to be affected by the treatment through a change in their size. Sertoli nucleoli are easily identified and provide a better reference structure to obtain ratios, since their size or shape, and thus the frequency which they are seen in sections, are not thought to be affected by most agents.

A more sensitive method for determining cell loss is by identification and quantitation of degenerating cells. The dictum provided above indicates that once cell differentiation is initiated, a cell is obligated to complete the process of spermatogenesis in a specified time and in coordination with other cells at the same phase of development, or it will degenerate. This may not be a hard and fast rule (Russell et al., 1982), but for the majority of instances it holds true.

Thus, most deleterious conditions would show some degenerating cells. These degenerating cells may be quantitated in a similar manner to viable cells. Our laboratory prefers using Sertoli nuclei or nucleoli as entities upon which ratios of degenerating cells may be based (Russell and Clermont, 1977; Russell et al., 1981a). If possible, it is best to quantitate degenerating cells in the stage following the initiation of degeneration. We have found that with most agents only a few cell types initially become necrotic, and these do so in specific stages. As a result, cell degeneration is rarely seen in all stages in short-term experiments. In longer-term experiments, degenerating cells may be present for many days and give the false impression that degenerations are initiated in each stage.

Morphological Patterns of Response

As mentioned above, there are numerous agents which affect the testis, probably due to the multiplicity of biochemical pathways necessary in the course of spermatogenesis. The number and variety of agents affecting spermatogenesis are many-fold greater than the number of pathways affected, since it is likely that more than one agent or class of agents act to disrupt any single pathway. Recent publications from our laboratory (Figure 4; Russell and Clermont, 1977; Russell et al., 1981a) illustrate this very clearly. A short-term evaluation of hypophysectomy in the rat reveals a particular morphological pattern of response whereby Leydig cells are decreased in size, and step 7 and step 19 spermatids and pachytene spermatocytes of Stage VII all degenerate in numbers significantly greater than in unoperated animals (Figure 4). A morphological pattern of response is defined as a specific set of features discernible from examination of testis structure which characterizes the effects of a particular agent under a given set of circumstances. One hypothesis is that no matter where interruption occurred along the pathway of hormonal stimulation of the testis - whether it be at synthesis or release from the pituitary, at stimulation of Leydig cells, or at binding to receptors - the same morphological pattern of response would be present. Indeed, in short-term treatment experiments, this hypothesis has been borne out (Russell et al., 1981a). Such shared morphological patterns of response are then of diagnostic value when one tests an agent which

is suspected of having, for example, an effect which would disrupt
the LH stimulation of the testis. The presence of a similar
morphological pattern of response, seen in an agent whose effects
are as yet not known, would be highly indicative of a hormonal
disruption. Shared morphological patterns of response have also
been shown with respect to agents which disrupt microtubles in the
testis (Russell et al., 1981b). Cataloging the morphological
patterns of response and the shared morphological patterns of
response for laboratory animals exposed to agents is of diagnostic
value and provides a ready reference for understanding how agents
work and of potential pathways which are interrupted.

ACKNOWLEDGEMENTS

The excellent drawings were provided by Ms. Terri Russell.

REFERENCES

Amann, R.P., 1981, A critical review of methods for evaluation of
    spermatogenesis from seminal characteristics, J. Androl.
    2:37-58.
Amann, R.P., Johnson, L., Thompson, D.L., Jr. and Pickett, B.W.,
    1976, Daily spermatozoal production of epididymal spermatozoal
    reserves and transit time of spermatozoa through the epididymis
    of the rhesus monkey, Brit. Reprod. 15:586-592.
Berndtson, W.E., 1977, Methods for qualifying mammalian
    spermatogenesis: A review, J. Anim. Sci. 44:818-833.
Blandau, R.J. and Rumery, R.E., 1964, The relationship of swimming
    movements of epididymal spermatozoa to their fertilizing
    capacity, Fertil. Steril. 15:571-579.
Burgos, M.H. and Fawcett, D.W., 1955, Studies on the fine structure
    of the mammalian testis. I. Differentiation of the spermatids
    in the cat (Felis domestica), J. Biophys. Biochem. Cytol.
    1:287-299.
Chang, M.C., 1951, Fertilizing capacity of spermatozoa deposited
    into the Fallopian tubes, Nature (London) 168:697-698.
Christensen, A.K., 1965, The fine structure of testicular
    interstitial cells in guinea pigs, J. Cell. Biol. 26:911-935.
Clermont, Y., 1954, Cycle de l'epithelium seminal et mode de
    renouvellement des spermatogonies chez le hamster, Rev. Can.
    Biol. 13:208-245.
Clermont, Y., 1958, Contractile elements in the limiting membrane
    of the seminiferous tubules of the rat, Exp. Cell Res.
    15:438-440.
Clermont, Y., 1960, Cycle of the seminiferous epithelium of the
    guinea pig, Fert. Steril. 11:563-573.

Clermont, Y., 1962, Quantitative analysis of spermatogenesis of the rat: A revised model for the renewal of the spermatogonia, <u>Am. J. Anat.</u> 111:111-129.

Clermont, Y., 1963, The cycle of the seminiferous epithelium in man, <u>Am. J. Anat.</u> 112:35-45.

Clermont, Y. and Leblond, C.P., 1959, Differentiation and renewal of spermatogonia in the monkey, <u>Macacus rhesis</u>, <u>Am. J. Anat.</u> 104:237-272.

Clermont, Y. and Harvey, S.C., 1965, Duration of the cycle of the seminiferous epithelium of normal, hypophysectomized and hypophysectiomized-hormone treated albino rats, <u>Endocrinol.</u> 76:80-89.

Clermont, Y. and Harvey, S.C., 1967, Effects of hormones on spermatogenesis in the rat, <u>Ciba Found. Colloq. Endocrinol.</u> 16:173-196.

Clermont, Y. and Bustos-Obregon, E., 1968, Re-examination of spermatogonial renewal in the rat by means of seminiferous tubules mounted "in toto," <u>Am. J. Anat.</u> 122:237-242.

Clermont, Y., Leblond, C.P., and Messier, B., 1959, Duree du cycle de l'epithelium seminal du rat, <u>Arch. Anat. Microsc. Morph. Exp.</u> 48:36-56.

Connell, C.J., 1974, The Sertoli cell of the sexually mature dog, Anat. Rec. 178:291.

Courot, M., 1980, The regulation of testicular function by pituitary gonadotrophins, <u>Proc. 9th Int. Cong. Anim. Reprod.</u> 2:155-162.

Courot, M., Hochereau-de Rivers, M.T. and Ortavant, R., 1970, Spermatogenesis, <u>in</u>: "The Testis", Vol. I, A.D. Johnson, W.R. Gomes and N.L. Van Demark, eds., pp. 339-432, Academic Press, New York.

Dym, M. and Fawcett, D.W., 1970, The blood-testis barrier in the rat and the physiological compartmentation of the seminiferous epithelium, <u>Biol. Reprod.</u> 3:308-326.

Dym, M., Madhwa Raj, H.G. and Chemes, H.E., 1977, Response of the testis to selective withdrawal of LH or FSH using antigonadotropic sera, <u>in</u>: "The Testis in Normal and Infertile Men", P. Troen and H.R. Nakin, eds., pp. 97-124, Raven Press, New York.

Elkington, J.S.H., Sanborn, B.M. and Steinberger, E., 1975, The effect of testosterone propionate on the concentration of testicular and epididymal androgen binding protein activity in the hypophysectomized rat, <u>Mol. Cell. Endocrinol.</u> 2:157-170.

Epstein, S.S., Arnold, E., Andrea, J., Bass, W. and Bishop, Y., 1972, Detection of chemical mutagens by the dominant lethal assay in the mouse, <u>Toxicol. Appl. Pharmacol.</u> 23:288-325.

Ewing, L.L., Davis, J.C. and Zirkin, B.R., 1980, Regulation of testicular function: A spatial and temporal view, <u>in</u>: "Reproductive Physiology III", R.O. Greep, ed., pp. 41-115, University Park Press, Baltimore.

Fawcett, D.W., 1975, Ultrastructure and function of the Sertoli cell, in: "Handbook of Physiology", Section 7, "Endocrinology", R.O. Greep and E.B. Astwood, eds., pp. 21-55, Williams and Wilkins Co., Baltimore.

Fawcett, D.W., Neaves, W.B. and Flores, M.N., 1973, Comparative observations on intertubular lymphatics and the organization of the interstitial tissue of the mammalian testis, Biol. Reprod. 9:500-532.

Fishbein, L., Falk, L.H. and Flamm, W.G., eds., 1970, "Chemical Mutagens", Academic Press, New York.

Forssmann, W.G., Ito, S., Weihe, E., Aoki, A., Dym, M., Fawcett, D.W., 1976, An improved fixation method for the testis, Anat. Rec. 188:307-314.

Gilula, N.B., Fawcett, D.W. and Aoki, A., 1976, The Sertoli cell occluding junctions and gap junctions in mature and developing mammalian testis, Dev. Biol. 50:142-168.

Gomes, W.R., 1977, Pharmacological agents and male fertility, in: "The Testis", Vol. IV, A.D. Johnson and W.R. Gomes, eds., pp. 605-628, Academic Press, New York.

Handel, M.A., 1979, Effects of colchicine on spermiogenesis in the mouse, J. Embryol. Exp. Morph. 51:73-83.

Heller, C.G. and Clermont, Y., 1964, Kinetics of the germinal epithelium in man, Recent Prog. Horm. Res. 20:545-575.

Huckins, C., 1971, The spermatogonial stem cell population in adult rats. 1. Their morphology, proliferation and maturation, Anat. Rec. 169:533-558.

Huckins, C., 1978, The morphology and kinetics of spermatogonial degeneration in normal adult rats: An analysis using a simplified classification of the germinal epithelium, Anat. Rec. 190:905-926.

Huckins, C. and Oakberg, E.F., 1978, Morphological and quantitation analysis of spermatogonia in mouse testes using whole mounted seminiferous tubules. I. The normal testes, Anat. Rec. 192:519-528.

Ibach, B., Weissbach, L. and Hilscher, B., 1976, Stages of the cycle of the seminiferous epithelium in the dog, Andrologia 8:297-307.

Jackson, H., 1973, Comparative effects of some antispermatogenic chemicals, in: "The Regulation of Mammalian Reproduction", S.J. Segal et al., eds., pp. 257-270, Thomas, Springfield, Illinois.

Jackson, H. and Ericsson, R.J., 1970, Bibliography on effect of chemical agents and hormones on spermatogenesis and the epididymis, Bibliogr. Reprod. 14:453-600.

Johnson, A.D., 1977, The influence of cadmium on the testis, in "The Testis", Vol. IV, A.d. Johnson and W.R. Gomes, eds., pp. 565-576, Academic Press, New York.

Karnovski, M.J., 1971, Use of ferrocyanide-reduced osmium tetroxide in electron microscopy, J. Cell Biol. Abstract 284.

Leblond, C.P. and Clermont, Y., 1952a, Definition of the stages of the cycle of the seminiferous epithelium in the rat, Ann. N.Y. Acad. Sci. 55:548-573.

Leblond, C.P. and Clermont, Y., 1952b, Spermiogenesis in rat, mouse, hamster and guinea pig as revealed by the periodic acid-fuchsin sulfurous acid technique, Am. J. Anat. 90:167-215.

Lucier, G.W., Lee, I.P. and Dixon, R.L., 1977, Effects of environmental agents on male reproduction, in: "The Testis", Vol. IV, A.D. Johnson and W.R. Gomes, eds., pp. 578-604, Academic Press, New York.

Means, A.R., Fakunding, J.L., Huckins, C., Tindall, D.J. and Vitale, R., 1976, Follicle stimulating hormone, the Sertoli cells, and spermatogenesis, Recent Prog. Horm. Res. 32:477-527.

Mori, H. and Christensen, A.K., 1980, Morphometric analysis of Leydig cells in the normal rat testis, J. Cell Biol. 84:340-354.

Oakberg, E.F., 1956, A description of spermiogenesis in the mouse and its use in analysis of the cycle of the seminiferous epithelium and germ cell renewal, Am. J. Anat. 99:391-413.

Patanelli, D.J., 1975, Suppression of fertility in the male, in "Handbook of Physiology", Section 7, "Endocrinology", R.O. Greep, ed., pp. 245-258, American Physiological Society, Washington, D.C.

Perey, B., Clermont, Y. and Leblond, C.P., 1961, The wave of the seminiferous epthelium in the rat. Am. J. Anat. 108:47-77.

Roosen-Runge, E.C., 1962, The process of spermatogenesis in mammals, Biol. Rev., 37:343-377.

Roosen-Runge, E.C., 1973, Germinal-cell loss in normal metazoan spermatogenesis, J. Reprod. Fertil. 35:339-348.

Ross, M.H., 1970, The Sertoli cells and the blood-testicular barrier: An electron microscopic study, Fortechrotte der Andrologie 1:83-86.

Russell, L.D., 1977a, Movement of spermatocytes from basal to adluminal compartment of the rat testis, Am. J. Anat. 148:313-328.

Russell, L.D., 1977b, Observations on rat Sertoli ectoplasmic ('junctional') specializations in their association with germ cells of the rat testis, Tissue and Cell 9:475-498.

Russell, L.D., 1980a, Deformities in the head region of late spermatides of hypophysectomized-hormone treated rats, Anat. Rec. 197:21-31.

Russell, L.D., 1980b, Sertoli-germ cell interrelations: A review, Gamete Research 3:179-202.

Russell, L.D., 1983, Spermiation (sperm release): Ultrastructural interpretations and unresolved problems, in: "Current Topics in Ultrastructural Research," Martinus Nijhoff Publ., Boston (in press).

Russell, L.D. and Gardner, P.J., 1974, Ultrastructure of the testes and fertility of the restricted color (H_{re}) rat, Biol. Reprod. 11:631-643.

Russell, L.D. and Burguet, S., 1977, Ultrastructure of Leydig cells as revealed by secondary tissue treatment with a ferrocyanide-osmium mixture, Tissue and Cell 9:751-766.

Russell, L.D. and Clermont, Y., 1977, Degeneration of germ cells in normal, hypophysectomized and hormone-treated hypophysectomized rats, Anat. Rec. 187:347-366.

Russell, L.D. and Wong, V., 1981, Three dimensional reconstruction of a rat Sertoli cell: Size configuration and general relationship to germ cells, J. Andrology 2:24.

Russell, L.D., Malone, J.P. and Karpas, S., 1981a, Morphological pattern elicited by agents affecting spermatogenesis by disruption of its hormonal stimulation, Tissue and Cell 18:369-380.

Russell, L.D., Malone, J.P. and MacCurdy, D., 1981b, Effects of the microtubule disrupting agents, colchicine and vinblastine, on seminiferous tubule structure in rat, Tissue and Cell 13:349-367.

Russell, L.D., Lee, I.P., Ettlin, R.A., Peterson, R.N. and Malone, J.P., 1982, Asynchronization of the spermatogenic cycle after administration of procarbazine, Anat. Rec., 178:291.

Setchell, B.P., 1978, "The Mammalian Testis", Paul Elek, London.

Setchell, B.P. and Waites, G.M.H., 1975, The blood-testis barrier, in: "Handbook of Physiology", Vol. 5, Section 7, R.O. Greep and E.B. Astwood, eds., pp. 143-172, Williams and Wilkins Co., Baltimore.

Steinberger, E., 1975, Hormonal regulation of the seminiferous tubule function, in: "Hormonal Regulation of Spermatogenesis", F.S. French, V. Hansson, E.M. Ritzen, and S.N. Nayfeh, eds., pp. 337-352, Plenum Press, New York.

Steinberger, E. and Steinberger, A., 1975, Spermatogenic function of the testis, in "Handbook of Physiology", Section 7, "Endocrinology", R.O. Greep, ed., pp. 1-19, American Physiological Society, Washington, D.C.

Stern, H. and Hotta, Y., 1973, Biochemical controls of meiosis, Ann. Rev. Genet. 7:37-66.

Swierstra, E.E. and Foote, R.H., 1963, Cytology and kinetics of spermatogenesis in the rabbit, J. Reprod. Fert. 5:309-322.

Vitale, R., Fawcett, D.W. and Dym, M., 1973, The normal development of the blood-testis barrier and the effects of clomiphene and estrogen treatment, Anat. Rec. 176:333-344.

Weibel, E.R., 1963, "Morphometry of the Human Lung", Springer Verlag, Berlin, Academic Press, New York.

Weibel, E.R., Kistler, G.S. and Scherle, W.F., 1966, Practical stereological methods for morphometric cytology, J. Cell Biol. 30:23-38.

Young, W.C., 1931, A study of the function of the epididymis. II. Functional changes undergone by spermatozoa during their passage through the epididymus and vas deferens in the guinea pig, J. Exptl. Biol. 8:151-162.

EFFECTS OF ENVIRONMENTAL METALS ON MALE REPRODUCTION

Insu P. Lee

Laboratory of Reproductive and Developmental Toxicology
National Institute of Environmental Health Sciences
Research Triangle Park, North Carolina

ABSTRACT

A review of the literature has revealed that the reproductive effects of metals such as aluminum, boron, nickel, vanadium, chromium, lead, mercury, methylmercury and cadmium on male laboratory animals are inconsistent among studies. Varying physiochemical, pharmacokinetic, and pharmacodynamic factors along with interactions between two or more metals, the nutritional status of animals, and genetic factors complicate reproductive toxicity of metals. Although attention is usually focused on the so-called "heavy metals", the general reactivity of metallic ions and their role in biological processes demand a broader review. Occupational exposure to such elements as arsenic, beryllium, boron, cadmium, chromium, lead, mercury, nickel and vanadium is a concern. In humans, only lead has been reported to have male reproductive effects while data concerning cadmium, mercury, nickel, chromium, vanadium and aluminum suggest no effect. In most of the laboratory studies, animals were treated with high parenteral doses of the metals for short periods of time. Humans, however, are usually exposed to low level doses for prolonged periods of time. Hence, discrepancies in dose, duration and route of exposure drastically complicate extrapolation of laboratory data to man. Furthermore, the entire process of gametogenesis and the hypothalmic-pituitary axis is an important target for toxicity. More sensitive approaches may evolve from more basic studies of molecular and reproductive biology, hormonal action and regulation, accessory sex organ function, and improved animal models. Only with improved laboratory techniques will we be able to reliably assess toxic chemicals and determine health risks in humans.

INTRODUCTION

Naturally occurring metals and metalloids are widely
distributed in the environment. Under normal conditions, their
distribution remains relatively constant because of natural and
biological processes, and they do not pose serious public health
problems. However, when used in industrial processes, they may
re-enter the environment and disrupt the natural balance. The
annual industrial production for arsenic, cadmium, chromium, mercury
and nickel is approximately 60,000; 16,000; 7,000,000; 10,100 and
660,000 tons, respectively (Friberg et al., 1975). The presence in
high concentrations of boron, cadmium, cobalt, copper, chromium,
mercury, nickel, lead and zinc in waste water and sewage sludge
reflects widespread environmental contamination (Diamant, 1977).

Trace elements are widely distributed in human populations.
Analysis for 24 trace elements in the dry and ash content of 29
different tissues of 150 U.S. adults who died instantly has been
previously reported (Tipton and Cook, 1963). From this report, the
percentages of both essential and non-essential macro- and
micro-trace elements in the testes and prostate glands have been
compiled and are listed in Table 1. The distribution of both macro-
and micro-trace elements in these tissues is fairly constant and the
organs appear to operate and maintain the delicate balance of other
essential elements. Furthermore, when essential trace elements are
deficient, a dysfunction may be produced; conversely, when they are
in excess, toxicity may result. Aluminum, lead, tin, and chromium
are present in human testes and prostate glands in greater than 70
percent of tissues examined. Other non-essential trace elements
such as silver, titanium, nickel, bismuth, cadium, gold, and boron
are found in testes and prostate glands in less than 34 percent of
tissue samples examined. The toxicological significance of these
non-essential elements in male reproductive tissue is unclear.
While there is considerable literature pertaining to the general
toxicology of these elements, there is a paucity of reproductive
toxicity studies involving trace elements. In this paper, an
attempt has been made to review and bring together relevant
information on the toxic effects of non-essential trace elements on
the male reproductive tissues.

ALUMINUM

There is no report of animal or human toxicity attributed to
aluminum occurring naturally in the environment. Aluminum sulfate,
aluminum oxide and aluminum hydroxide have been used as growth
stimulants for rabbits, chickens, sheep, cattle, and hogs where
these elements composed no more than 1 to 2 percent of the diet
(Sorenson et al., 1974). It seems very unlikely that grazing
animals would ever encounter such concentrations naturally. Acute

Table 1   Trace Elements in Human Testes and Prostate Glands of U.S. Adults[a]

Element	Percent Incidence in Tissues		Median μg/g Tissue	
	Testes[b]	Prostate Glands[b]	Testes	Prostate Glands
K[c]	100	100	180,000	180,000
P[c]	100	100	120,000	90,000
Mg[c]	100	100	10,000	15,000
Ca[c]	100	100	8,000	21,000
Fe[c]	100	100	2,100	2,400
Zn[c]	100	100	1,400	7,500
Cu[d]	100	100	80	100
Mn[d]	100	100	12	14
Sr	100	100	4.3	11
Ba	75	88	1.1	2.1
Mo[d]	3	4	< 4	< 4
Co[d]	8	60	< 2	< 2
Al	100	100	30	46
Pb	94	88	12	10
Cr	92	82	1.6	6.9
Sb	75	84	11	14
Ag	34	50	< 0.1	< 0.1
Ti	26	32	< 5	< 5
Ni	24	18	< 5	< 5
Bi	22	88	< 2	< 2
Cd	15	40	< 50	< 50
Au	15	20	< 10	< 10
B	1	18	< 10	< 10
V	-	2	-	< 1

[a]Data compiled from Tipton and Cook, 1963.
[b]From 65 to 72 tissue samples.
[c]Macronutrients.
[d]Essential micronutrients.

toxicity studies involving laboratory animals showed the LD_{50} for aluminum nitrate to be 0.26 g/kg (Sorenson et al., 1974). Chronic toxicity results in several phosphorous metabolism imbalances including excretion of phosphorous, decreased incorporation of phosphorous into phospholipids, and a drop in ATP levels in blood. Aluminum poisoning in humans appears to be rare. Ingestion of 150 mg of aluminum per day is without obvious effects on a normal human;

200 mg per day, however, may give rise to mild catharsis which increases with dosage (Sorenson et al., 1974).

Although aluminum occurs in all human testes in approximately the same molar concentration as the essential elements, very few studies have considered the possible reproductive effects of aluminum. One study reported that, while a single subcutaneous administration of salts of aluminum caused no discernible effects on the rat testes, repeated injections to mice for 30 days (2.6 μmole/ kg/day) produced shrinkage of testes and spermatogenic cell arrest without any damage to the Leydig cells (Kamboji and Kar, 1964). In contrast to these findings, the inclusion of aluminum chloride in the drinking water of young adult male Sprague-Dawley rats at levels as high as 500 mg/1 (equivalent to 50 mg/kg/day) for a period up to 90 days, did not affect male fertility nor cause testicular damage (Dixon and Lee, 1979).

BORON

Soviet scientists have reported infertility associated with oligospermia and decreased libido among men working in factories in which boric acid is produced and in communities where boron concentration is high in artesian well water (Khachatrian and Nazarenko, 1973; Krasovskii et al., 1976; Tarasenko et al., 1972). In contrast, in the United States, much less attention is given to the possible health hazards associated with boron compounds. To date, the mechanism of boron toxicity is not well understood. Although death due to acute ingestion of 15-20 g of boric acid in adults and 5-6 g in infants has been reported (Goldbloom and Goldbloom, 1953; Valdes-Dapena and Arey, 1962; Locksley and Farr, 1955), little information is available about the toxic effects of chronic exposure at low-dose levels in man. In animal studies, however, it has been shown that chronic exposure to boron at 1170 ppm (23-30 mg of boron ingested per day) for 90 days causes testicular atrophy in the rat (Weir and Fisher, 1972). Further studies with boron at doses of 0, 500, 1000 or 2000 ppm in the diet for 30 or 60 days, demonstrated that male rats receiving 1000 or 2000 ppm of boron displayed a significant germinal aplasia associated with a significant increase of plasma follicle stimulating hormone (FSH) and a variable increase of plasma luteinizing hormone (LH) (Lee et al., 1978). Serial mating studies demonstrated reduced fertility without change in copulatory behavior (Tables 2 and 3). The duration of reduced fertility was greater at the higher dose and the longer duration of exposure. Germinal aplasia, elevated FSH, and infertility persisted for at least 8 months following cessation of boron exposure at the higher dose. These studies suggest that the minimum boron concentrations of 6-8 μg/g testis is necessary to cause progressive germ cell depletion, and that the testicular lesion can persist long after toxic exposure to boron has occurred (Table 4).

Table 2 Effects of Borax (Boron) Treatment on Male Rat Fertility (30-day Treatment)[a]

Weeks Following Exposure	Percentage Pregnant/ Number with Vaginal Plugs				Average Litter Size			
	0 ppm	500 ppm	1000 ppm	2000 ppm	0 ppm	500 ppm	1000 ppm	2000 ppm
1	100/80	100/100	20/60[b]	0/60[b]	10.4	9.6	9.0	-
2	80/80	100/100	20/80	0/80[b]	10.8	9.6	2.0	-
3	80/100	80/100	0/80[b]	0/100[b]	11.0	10.5	-	-
4	100/100	80/100	100/80	0/100[b]	10.6	12.5	9.8	-
5	100/100	100/100	60/100	0/100[b]	8.0	10.4	11.3	-
6	100/100	100/100	100/100	0/100[b]	10.5	9.2	9.8	-
7	100/100	100/100	100/100	25/100[b]	10.4	10.6	9.8	-
8	40/100	100/100	80/100	0/100	11.0	12.4	12.0	-
9	100/100	100/100	80/100	50/100	10.8	10.6	11.2	12.5
10	100/100	100/100	80/100	50/100	13.0	12.5	10.8	6.0
Overall	88	94	66	10	10.6	10.7	10.3	9.2

[a]Lee et al., 1978. Each treatment group was composed of five males with the exception of the 2000-ppm dose which had four.
[b]Significantly different from control ($p < 0.05$).

Table 3 Effects of Borax (Boron) Treatment on Male Rat Fertility (60-day Treatment)[a]

Weeks Following Exposure	Percentage Pregnant/ Number with Vaginal Plugs				Average Litter Size			
	0 ppm	500 ppm	1000 ppm	2000 ppm	0 ppm	500 ppm	1000 ppm	2000 ppm
1	80/80	60/60	20/60	0/60[b]	11.0	12.3	4.0[c]	-
2	20/20	60/60	0/60	0/60	12.0[c]	9.0	-	-
3	100/100	100/100	0/80[b]	0/80[b]	10.2	9.2	-	-
4	100/80	80/100	20/80[b]	0/100[b]	11.8	13.0	3.0[c]	-
5	80/100	100/100	60/100	0/100[b]	12.0	10.8	13.0	-
6	100/100	100/100	80/100	0/100[b]	12.0	10.8	12.0	-
7	100/100	100/100	80/100	0/100[b]	10.2	11.4	11.2	-
8	100/100	100/100	80/100	0/100[b]	9.6	10.0	10.8	-
9	100/100	100/100	80/100	0/100[b]	11.4	9.2	11.8	-
10	100/100	100/100	80/100	0/100[b]	10.2	10.4	11.5	-
11	80/100	-	80/100	0/100[b]	10.8	-	10.2	-
12	80/100	-	60/100	0/100[b]	12.5	-	11.3	-
Overall	87	90	52	0	11.0	10.6	10.9	-

[a]Lee et al., 1978. Each treatment group was composed of five males.
[b]Significantly different from control (p < 0.05).
[c]Based on one animal.

Table 4   Boron Concentrations in Plasma and Testes of Male Rats
          Receiving Dietary Borax (500, 1000, or 2000 ppm as Boron
          Equivalent) for 30 and 60 Days[a]

Exposure	Control	500 ppm	1000 ppm	2000 ppm
30 days				
Plasma	0.2[b]	0.9	3.8	5.5
Testes	0.3	0.9	-	-
60 days				
Plasma	0.1	2.6	4.3	6.8
Testes	0.3	2.1	6.1	8.5

[a]Lee et al., 1978.
[b]All boron values (in parts per million) are the means
of two samples.

     In contrast to these findings, boron concentrations of 6 mg/l
of drinking water (0.15 mg of boron ingested per day) for 90 days
failed to cause infertility in male rats in spite of a slight
reduction in sperm numbers (Dixon et al., 1976). However, when
boron concentrations in the drinking water were increased to 150 or
300 mg/l (3 or 6 mg of boron ingested per day), testicular atrophy
and azoospermia occurred (Seal and Weeth, 1980).

     The relevance of these observations to humans depends on
whether such chronic boron exposure could occur in man. Although
there are little data on boron levels in food and water in the
United States, boron concentrations in water in some areas of the
Soviet Union have been reported to be 0.4 - 1.2 mg/l. Further
studies are necessary to determine whether such low concentrations
of boron in food and drinking water accumulate to toxic levels and
affect male reproduction.

NICKEL

     Nickel is used primarily in the metallurgical industry, chiefly
in ferro alloys. Nickel carbonyl, $Ni(CO)_4$, a volatile liquid
which is an intermediate product in nickel metallurgy, is the most
toxic nickel compound, particularly if inhaled. Acute nickel
carbonyl poisoning usually occurs as a consequence of an industrial
accident. The general population is normally not exposed to air
containing this compound.

Numerous other nickel compounds and salts have been shown to be carcinogenic in both man and animals (Haro et al., 1968; Heath and Daniel, 1964). Carcinogenicity appears to be related to the solubility of the compounds in aqueous media rather than the route of administration (Hueper, 1955; Hueper and Payne, 1962; Lou et al., 1972). Intratesticular injection of Ni_3S_2 induces testicular sarcomas (Damjanov et al., 1978). The testicular sarcoma is thought to be derived from pluripotential mesenchymal cells in the interstitial compartment, not derived from germ cells.

It has been reported that administration of soluble nickel salts to rats per os (Manthur et al., 1977a; Stoner et al., 1976), dermal (Von Waltschewa et al., 1972a), subcutaneous (Hoey, 1966; Manthur et al., 1977a,b) and intratesticular routes (Kamboji and Kar, 1964) produces testicular damage with degeneration of seminiferous tubules and/or arrest of spermatogenesis. Nickel fed in the diet of rats at 250, 500 or 1000 ppm did not have any significant effects on male reproduction. Since nickel salts are poorly absorbed, 90 percent of the intake was excreted in the feces (Phatak and Patwardhan, 1950). However, adverse effects on male reproduction were observed in rats following treatment with soluble nickel salts (nickel sulfate). The acute and chronic effects on the rat testes of nickel sulfate given subcutaneously at 0.04 mmole/kg included hyperemia of intertubular capillaries and degeneration of spermatozoa 18 hours after a single dose (Hoey, 1966). Inhibition of spermatogenesis has also been observed after oral administration of daily doses of nickel sulfate at 25 mg/kg. Male rats given this dose for 120 days were found to be completely infertile (Von Waltschawa et al., 1972b). Nickel sulfate given continuously for 3 generations at 5 ppm in the drinking water of rats caused a decrease in the average litter size of each succeeding generation (Schroeder and Mitchner, 1971). Possible mechanisms for nickel's inhibition of spermatogenesis and promotion of testicular carcinogenesis are not known, but it has been suggested that nickel penetrates the cell nucleus in vivo and may bind tightly to DNA with consequent inhibition of DNA-dependent RNA synthesis (Sunderman, 1977a,b).

Epidemiological studies conclude that several nickel compounds are carcinogenic in humans following chronic exposure by inhalation. Increased incidence of mainly respiratory cancers, but also of laryngeal, gastric and renal cancers (Sunderman, 1977a,b) have been reported among workers in nickel refineries and in a variety of other nickel-related industries. However, no changes in fertility among nickel industrial workers have yet been identified.

VANADIUM

Vanadium is considered to be both an essential and a toxic element, but is not particularly toxic to man. Not only is vanadium

poorly absorbed from the gastrointestinal tract, but it causes
minimal irritation to the lungs when inhaled. The LD_{50} for mice
given vanadium trioxide orally is 130 mg/kg and for vanadium
pentoxide and trichloride, it is 23 mg/kg (National Research
Council, 1974). Vanadium is found in fossil fuel sources such as
coal, oil shale, and crude oil (Lee and Von Lehmden, 1973). The
concentration of this trace element is known to increase in the
close physical environments of various industrial operations (Parker
et al., 1978). Further exploitation of fossil fuels for energy
purposes is likely to accelerate redistribution of this metal in the
ecosystem.

Vanadium is essential for growth in rats and chickens (Hopkins
and Mohr, 1971; Schwarz and Milne, 1971). Rats fed a diet deficient
in vanadium produced fewer offspring in the third and fourth
generations (Hopkins and Mohr, 1974). When male Wistar rats were
given vanadyl trichloride ($^{48}VOCl_3$) in doses of vanadium ranging
from 0.1 to 8 mg/kg of testicular tissue, blood to testis vanadium
concentration ratios 5 days after the treatment were found to be 4.2
to 2.9, respectively (Scharma et al., 1980). This suggests that
vanadium crosses the blood-testis barrier and accumulates in rat
testes. Furthermore, following hypophysectomy, vanadium accumulates
in rat testes. The reduced hepatic levels of coenzyme A are
influenced by both LH and FSH levels (Peabody et al., 1980). Since
vanadium is known to inhibit the activity of monoamine oxidase,
serotonin may accumulate, with a consequent increase in the
permeability of blood vessels to chemicals in the testes. The
reduced hepatic levels of coenzyme A also reflect the reduced
availabilty of cysteine, a precursor of coenzyme A. Coenzyme A
plays a key role in many biosynthetic and oxidative pathways (Bergel
et al., 1958). The reduction of coenzyme A levels is followed by
decreased levels of triglycerides, phospholipids, cholesterol, and
ascorbic acid (Azarnoff et al., 1961; Snyder and Cornatzer, 1958;
Roshchin et al., 1965). Lowered serum acid levels are followed by a
lowering of hemoglobin levels, probably because of the reduced
facilitation of iron removal from ferritin by ascorbate. It remains
to be determined whether testicular androgen biosynthesis is reduced
because of reduced levels of cholesterol, and whether this is
followed by inhibition of spermatogenesis with subsequent
alterations in male fertility.

CHROMIUM

Chromium is used mainly in chrome-plating or in alloys, and for
manufacturing ball points for pens. It is also widely used in
tanning and photography, as a mortant in dyes, and as a catalyst for
organic and inorganic reactions. Because of its high resistance to
heat, it is also used to manufacture refractors. Human exposure
occurs in chromium mining and in industrial applications utilizing

chromium when the atmosphere is contaminated with a variety of
trivalent and hexavalent chromium compounds. Hexavalent chromium,
which originates from the production of chromates and dichromates,
is about 100 times more toxic than trivalent chromium (National
Academy of Sciences, 1974; Baetjer, 1956).

Hexavalent chromium compounds have been recognized as
nephrotoxic, hepatotoxic and cardiotoxic agents (Kaufman et al.,
1970; Evan and Dail, 1974). The increased risk of lung cancer among
chromium-exposed workers has been known for more than 40 years. The
less soluble trivalent chromium compounds, on the other hand, have
been regarded as relatively biologically inert (Baetjer et al.,
1974a,b). However, chromic acetate, chromite ore roast (Hueper and
Payne, 1962) and a few other trivalent chromium salts (Morris, 1964)
have been found to be carcinogenic when inhaled, ingested or
otherwise brought into contact with tissues. Hexavalent chromium
compounds are reduced biochemically to a less toxic trivalent form
in mammalian systems.

When rabbits were treated intraperitoneally with daily
administration of a 2 mg/kg dose of either trivalent or hexavalent
chromium for 3 or 6 weeks, testicular succinic dehydrogenase,
ATPase, and acid phosphatase activities were reduced significantly,
coincident with the presence of multinucleated germ cells and the
degeneration of spermatocytes in the seminiferous tubules.
Spermatogenic cell degenerations were more severe in the animal
group treated with trivalent chromium than in that treated with
hexavalent chromium, whereas the interstitial cell compartment of
the former appeared normal. In contrast, the interstitial cell
compartment of the hexavalent-treated animals was edematous at both
3 and 6 weeks, following 3- and 6-week treatments. When male rats
were treated intraperitoneally with 1, 2 or 3 mg of trivalent
chromium/kg for 30 or 60 days, the accumulation of trivalent chromium
in the testes was found to be dependent both upon dose and duration
of treatment (Behari et al., 1978). At a daily dose of 1 mg
trivalent chromium/kg for 60 days, the concentrations of trivalent
chromium in the liver, kidney, testis, and brain were 14.1, 8.1, 3.2
and 2.8 µg/g tissue, respectively. Lower accumulations of trivalent
chromium were found in the testis and brain than in the liver or
kidney. The lower concentration of chromium in the testis and brain
is most likely due to the action of both the blood-testis barrier
and blood-brain barrier. It has been suggested that the accumulation
of chromium in the testes is related to the extent of spermatogenic
cell damage in the seminiferous tubules (Tandon et al., 1979).

Pulmonary carcinoma in humans after chronic exposure to chromium
appears to be linked to hexavalent chromium; however, the effects of
hexavalent chromium on antispermatogenic and carcinogenic action
appear to be mediated by its ability to modify DNA bases.
Furthermore, mutagenicity of chromates is not modified in DNA

repair-deficient bacteria and therefore, the hexavalent ion's interaction with DNA may be a direct modification of DNA bases (Venitt and Levy, 1974). Chromate modification of DNA may also be mediated by interaction with calcium which stabilizes DNA bases (Angjileri, 1973).

LEAD

Lead has been used extensively because of its resistance to erosion and because of its several physiochemical attributes. The principle source of lead intake by members of the general population is via diet. Lead intake by adults without undue lead exposure is usually between 100 and 300 µg/day. If blood lead levels are correlated with daily dietary lead intake as given in recent published studies (Coulston et al., 1972; Tepper and Levin, 1972; Rabinowitz et al., 1974), it is estimated that every 100 µg of long-term daily intake of dietary lead contributes about 10 µg of blood lead per 100 ml of blood. When blood lead levels are in the range of 20-30 µg/100 ml, air lead present in the ambient environment contributes relatively little to blood lead levels (ca. 0.3 - 1.75 µg lead/100 ml blood per µg lead/m^3 air). For children, these estimates are more difficult to obtain and are less well established. Dietary lead intake for children 1-3 years of age in the United States has been estimated to be about 100 µg per day (Kolbye et al., 1974), but absorption may be as high as 50 percent (Alexander, 1974). A high rate of uptake by growing bone, however, tends to hold the blood level close to adult values.

Acute or overt lead poisoning has been a major toxicological problem. Because of the cumulative nature of lead in the body, chronic intake may culminate in severe clinical disease. Furthermore, other factors, such as calcium, iron, protein, vitamin D, ascorbic and nicotinic acid deficiencies, and the presence of excess zinc or lead were found in 94 percent of testicular samples which contained a median lead concentration of 12 µg/g testis (Table 1). Histochemical studies have demonstrated that lead is found in various loci of the testis including the tail of the spermatozoa and the cells around the intratubular blood vessels (Timm and Schultz, 1966). Following the parenteral administration of lead or in chronic lead poisoning in animals, lead deposits are visible in the lumen of the seminiferous tubules and excreted in the rete-testis fluid (RTF). Furthermore, lead concentrations in the testes, epididimedes and seminal vesicles are about equally distributed (Tarabaeva, 1959).

Mutagenic, teratogenic and embroyotoxic effects of lead have recently been reviewed (Gerber et al., 1980). It has been reported that feeding male rats 0, 5, or 100 µg/Pb per day resulted in blood lead levels of 14, 19, and 30 µg/100 ml of blood. When whole blood

lead levels were greater than 30 µg/100 ml, the animals showed the
following: 1) a two-fold increase in the size of prostate glands
due to prostatic hyperplasia; 2) a male refusal to copulate with
estrus females or, in other words, impotence; 3) less mobile sperm;
and 4) a 70 percent reduction in testicular weight in 20 percent of
the males in the treatment group. Histopathology showed seminiferous
tubular damage and spermatogenic cell arrest (Hilderbrand et al.,
1973). Furthermore, in another study, transplantable interstitial
tumors were induced with lead acetate (Fahim and Khare, 1980).

In contrast, exposure to low doses of lead in drinking water at
1, 10, or 100 mg Pb/l of water for as long as 90 days did not show
any significant changes with respect to testicular morphology, plasma
gonadotrophin levels, and male fertility (Dixon and Lee, 1979). In
multigeneration studies, male rats exposed to lead orally at 0.2
mg/kg or 20 mg/kg showed fertility decreased to 65 percent of the
control level (Ivanova-Chemishanska et al., 1980). These results
suggest that potential risk may be realized eventually by human
offspring born from fathers occupationally exposed to significant
concentrations of lead. However, such specific reports are not yet
available and further study with experimental animals is needed to
gather data which can be extrapolated to humans. The possible
mechanisms for the antispermatogenic effects of lead in experimental
animals are not clear. Lead is reported to inhibit the hepatic
microsomal detoxification system; whether lead can alter androgen
biosynthesis mediated by cytochrome P-450 system of the interstitial
cells of testes needs to be ascertained. A precise mechanism for
lead-induced antispermatogenic effects and prostatic hyperplasia is
unclear and needs further investigation.

Evidence in humans for the deleterious effects of lead on the
germ cells of both sexes has been previously reviewed (Hamilton and
Hardy, 1949). The prevalence of sterile marriages, abortions, and
stillbirths is thought to be related to toxic effects of lead on the
testes of male lead workers. These findings related to occupational
exposures (presumably very high) occurred before modern industrial
hygiene standards had come into effect. Epidemiological studies
concerning male reproductive function following occupational exposure
to lead indicate that workers with blood lead concentrations between
23 and 75 µg/100 ml exhibited infertility associated with
asthenospermia, oligospermia, and teratospermia. Leydig cell
function, based on both testosterone levels and histopathology
apparently was not altered in rats (Lancranjan et al., 1975).

MERCURY

Mercury and organomercurials have been used extensively
throughout the world. Mercury is found in various chemical forms
which have different pharmacokinetic properties of absorption,

distribution, accumulation and excretion. Elemental mercury, inorganic mercury compounds, short-chain alkylmercurials, and other organomercury compounds can be distinguished by their toxicological properties. Normal human tissues contain mercury ions because of daily environmental exposure. However, increasing concern with mercury stems from repeated outbreaks of epidemics of methylmercury poisoning, worldwide contamination with methylmercury, and the conversion of elemental mercury and mercury compounds into methylmercury in the environment. The incidence of Minamata disease in Japan in 1953 has raised a worldwide concern about alkylmercury toxicosis which is mainly a neurologic disease affecting many species, including man (Takeuchi, 1970).

Food, mainly fish and fish products, is the main source of methylmercury for humans due to the avid accumulation of methylmercury in aquatic food chains after biotransformation of inorganic mercury. Methylmercury has been reported to be cytotoxic (Kim, 1971), and teratogenic (Rizzo and Furst, 1972). In eukaryotes, organomercury compounds have been shown to act directly upon genetic material as well as on chromosomal segregation. It is assumed that its effects on cell division are due to interaction with the sulfhydryl groups of the protein forming the mitotic spindle (Ramel, 1972). Ethyl- and methylmercury compounds also induce non-disjunction and sex-linked recessive lethals in Drosophila melanogaster (Ramel and Magnusson, 1969). In vitro treatment with methylmercury and other alkyl mercury compounds at concentrations ranging from 0.1 to 5 x 10^{-6}M caused C-mitosis in human leukocytes (Fiskerjo, 1970), as well as inhibition of HeLa cell growth (Umeda et al., 1969), and increased frequency of polyploidy, as well as aneuploidy in human fibroblast cells (Ochi and Tonomoura, 1975). Methylmercury-induced chromosome damage in the lymphocytes of 23 humans who had consumed fish contaminated by methylmercury has been reported (Skerfving et al., 1970). A statistically significant increase in frequency of cells with chromatid type aberrations, unstable chromosome type aberrations and aneuploidy was noted. Aneuploid cells were also found in people who were exposed occupationally to low concentrations of mercury (Vershaeve et al., 1976). In spite of strong evidence of the mutagenic qualities of methylmercury in both experimental animals and in the exposed human populations, there is no evidence to link methylmercury to carcinogenicity.

Pharmacokinetic and reproductive studies with mercury compounds are very few. In vivo uptake of mercuric chloride and methylmercury into CDF1 mouse testes showed that the initial uptake of methylmercury into the testes was approximately four times greater than that of mercuric chloride; the subsequent decay rate of methylmercury was also faster than that of mercuric chloride. The testicular half-life of methylmercury was 3.4 days, whereas that of inorganic mercury was approximately 56 days. The concentration of methylmercury in the testes rose very rapidly to a peak value within the first 12 hours after injection. The mercury level also fell very rapidly during the following 16 days. On the other hand, the peak levels of mercuric chloride in the testes were reached at 24 hours after injection, with subsequent slow elimination (Lee and Dixon, 1975). This finding is further supported by a similar study in which Swiss albino male mice were injected with methylmercury, either intraperitoneally or subcutaneously (Mehra and Kanwar, 1980). The peak activity in the testes was found at 12 hours (intraperitoneal) and at 24 hours (subcutaneous). Methylmercury activity was higher in the testes than in either the seminal vesicles or the epididymides. Other similar studies with a mouse strain (C57BL/6J) also demonstrated that, following a single subcutaneous injection of methylmercury, the highest radioactivity was found by 7 hours in all organs but testis and brain (Mehra and Choi, 1981). The peak radioactivity in testis and brain was found at one and two days posttreatment, respectively.

The differences in the uptake of both mercury and methylmercury were also reflected in their uptake into various spermatogenic cells. The radioactive profile of mercury and methylmercury indicated that methylmercury in spermatogonial cells and early spermatids was approximately 3 times higher than that of mercuric chloride in these cell types (Lee and Dixon, 1975). Both mercuric chloride and methylmercury inhibited the synthesis of DNA in spermatogonia (Table 5). These findings are in agreement with other reports in which thymidine uptake into the spermatogonial cell nuclei was significantly inhibited (Sakai and Takeuchi, 1972). The inhibition of DNA, RNA synthesis (Takeuchi, 1970) and meiotic cell arrests have also been observed (Ramal and Magnusson, 1969).

Serial mating studies indicate no evidence for dominant lethal effects (Schroeder and Balassa, 1961; Tipton and Stewart, 1969) and therefore, neither mercuric chloride nor methylmercury appears to have mutagenic effects on mammalian germ cells. However, there were dose-related reductions in mean litter size and the number of fertile matings during the interval 5 to 20 days posttreatment. In mice, however, there was only a slight reduction in the average litter size and no effect on the frequency of fertile matings. These findings are somewhat different from those of other studies in which methylmercury hydroxide affected fertility of male mice (CDF1) during the interval 21 to 49 days posttreatment corresponding to both spermatocyte and spermatogonial stage spermatogenesis (Lee and Dixon, 1975) (Table 6). On the other hand, mercuric chloride-induced infertility occurred during the interval 28 to 49 days posttreatment and the magnitude of infertility was significantly less than that induced by methylmercury. These differences in male infertility induced by mercuric chloride and methylmercury were correlated with the observed inhibition of thymidine uptake.

Table 5   Effect of Varying Concentrations of CH_3HgOH and $HgCl_2$ on the Incorporation of Thymidine into Spermatogonia[a]

M	Thymidine Uptake: Percent of Control	
	CH_3HgOH	$HgCl_2$
10^{-3}	40.6[b]	78.8[b]
10^{-4}	60.2[b]	93.8[b]
10^{-5}	64.2[b]	93.9[b]
10^{-6}	66.5	
10^{-7}	71.6	
10^{-8}	96.7	

[a]Lee and Dixon, 1975
[b]Significantly different ($p < .05$) by Student's t test

Table 6   Percent Fertility[a]. The mercury compounds at a dosage of 1 mg/kg were administered intraperitoneally once to hybrid DBA_2/Balb c mice.

Days	Control	CH_3HgOH	$HgCl_2$
-14	100	90	100
-7	100	100	90
R_x>0	90	100	100
7	100	90	90
14	90	80	90
21	100	40[a,b]	80
28	90	50[c,b]	70[d]
35	100	60[c,b]	50[c,b]
42	100	0[a,b]	60[c,b]
49	90	20[a,b]	60[b]
56	100	70[d]	80
63	100	90	90
70	90	90	100

[a]Lee and Dixon, 1975
[b]$p < .01$ vs. controls
[c]$p < .01$ vs. pretreatment values
[d]$p < .05$ vs. controls
[e]$p < .05$ vs. pretreatment values

Fertility studies have further shown that mercuric chloride affects both spermatogonia and premeiotic spermatocytes, whereas methylmercury affects spermatogonia, premeiotic spermatocytes and early spermatids. Spermatogonial cells appear to be the most sensitive of all the spermatogenic cells to both mercury ions. Additionally, greater effects obtained with methylmercury than mercuric chloride could be attributed to both its level in target cells and to its greater inhibition of spermatogonial DNA synthesis (Table 5). Whether mercury effects on premeiotic spermatocytes are due to meiotic arrest (at fertility interval 21-35 days in Table 6) similar to the meiotic nondisjunction in Drosophila induced by methylmercury treatment (Ramel and Magnusson, 1969) needs to be ascertained.

The exact mechanism by which mercury inhibits DNA, RNA and protein synthesis in spermatogenic cells is not clear. However, it has been reported that many metal ions can interact with both phosphate and base sites on the DNA molecule (Eichhorn et al., 1971). Interactions of inorganic mercury and methylmercury with DNA have been extensively studied (Gruenwadel and Davidson, 1966). One experiment dealt with the Hg^{2+}-DNA complex, assuming that each Hg^{2+} is attached to purine and pyrimidine bases on two polynucleotide chains (Eichhorn and Clark, 1963). Ultracentrifugation and spectrophotometric studies of CH_3Hg^+-DNA interaction demonstrated that CH_3Hg^+ cannot bind two complementary strands of DNA by the chelation process as the Hg^{2+} ion can, since the reaction of CH_3Hg^+ with native DNA causes denaturation (Gruenwadel and Davidson, 1967). Therefore, mercury-bound DNA could affect the unwinding and rewinding of DNA which is essential for replication and transcription. Intercalation of DNA in turn affects RNA transcription and protein synthesis. In addition, the mercuric ion may chelate sulfhydryl sites of enzyme or structural proteins to inhibit metabolism and/or both mitosis and meiosis. Further careful studies are needed to elucidate exact mechanisms of action of mercuric chloride and methylmercury on male reproductive organs.

CADMIUM

The concentration of cadmium in the biosphere varies from one geographical area to another, depending on natural deposits and on man-made pollution (Friberg et al., 1971; Schroeder and Balassa, 1961). In the United States, an estimate of human daily intake of as much as 200 to 500 µg of cadmium has been reported (Tipton and Stewart, 1969). This element accumulates progressively with age in the living organism (Schroeder, 1967). Cadmium is not generally considered an essential element.

Numerous studies of cadmium-induced toxicities have been reported in the past. One of the target organs for cadmium, when given parenterally, is the male gonads and the effects of cadium on the testes have been studied more extensively than those of any other element to date (Gunn et al., 1966; Gundland and Gould, 1970). The toxic effects of cadmium on the testes are very selective; as low a dose as 1.12 to 2.24 mg/kg of cadmium can cause testicular damage without pathological changes in other organs (Parizek and Zahor, 1956; Gunn et al., 1963a). Cadmium causes damage to the blood vessels of the testes. It accumulates in the interstitial compartment where it produces endothelial cell damage, particularly in the arterioles. Vascular permeability increases when cadmium doses of 6 µmole/kg or greater are given, resulting in hemorrhagic edema (Gunn and Gould, 1970). Electron microscropic studies of the initial changes in the rat testis confirm that damage to the tubules is due to ischemia (Gunn et al., 1963a; Setchell and Waites, 1970). The intraperitoneal or subcutaneous administration of 27 to 30 µmole/kg of cadmium chloride resulted in leakage of fluids from testicular blood vessels into the interstitial tissue compartment 1-3 hours after treatment. Following this, the passage of carbon particles into the walls of capillaries and venules indicated that there were discontinuities in the endothelium. By 3 hours after treatment, intravascular accumulation of red blood cells was evident, and at 4 hours, there was obstruction of microvascular circulation with consequent necrosis of spermatogenic cells. Thus, as numerous experimental data now indicate, the spermatogenic epithelium is not the primary, but the secondary, site of injury.

The uptake studies of cadmium into the testes of rats and mice demonstrated that, when a trace amount or a 12 µmole/kg dose of cadmium-109 was administered, testicular cadmium levels reached the highest point at day 1 (0.44 percent of the administered dose) (Gunn et al., 1968). The testes are vulnerable to as little as 0.15 µg of cadmium per gram of tissue. Autoradiographic studies with cadmium-109 failed to detect the metal in the seminiferous tubules of mice at 16 days following administration (Berlin and Ullberg, 1963). Cadmium-109 distribution studies in the rat suggest that cadmium is confined to nonspermatogenic tissue at all times (1 hour to 4 weeks) in contrast to zinc, which concentrates in both interstitial and germ cell compartments (Berlin and Ullberg, 1963). In contrast to these findings, cadmium levels in the rete-testis fluid following a single injection of a trace amount of cadium-109 were found to be 7-8 percent of the total plasma level during the first 30 minutes of infusion time (Dixon et al., 1975). Since 99.5 percent of the cadmium was bound to plasma protein, the concentration ratio of rete-testis fluid to that of plasma was based on the unbound plasma concentration. In spite of the rapid decrease of plasma cadmium, the ratio of cadmium concentration in rete-testis fluid to the unbound plasma concentration approaches 40, suggesting an accumulation of this metal in the seminiferous tubules and perhaps a

special transport process. Furthermore, when animals were treated
either with zinc and cadmium simultaneously or with zinc alone 4
hours prior to cadmium treatment, the cadmium transport into the
rete-testis fluid was dramatically inhibited (Table 7). These data
support previous reports that zinc can reverse cadmium effects on
endothelial cells (Gundland and Gould, 1970; Gunn et al., 1966; Aoki
and Foffer, 1978; Niewenhuis, 1980; Guthrie, 1964) and on elongated
spermatids (Lee and Dixon, 1973).

The mechanism of action of cadmium on testes is not well
understood. It has been postulated that the mechanism of toxicity
may be via decreased utilization of zinc by spermatogenic cells due
to a competitive action of cadmium. The spermatogenic cell types
which incorporate cadmium and zinc and the interaction of these two
metals (cadmium-109 and zinc-65) were studied (Lee and Dixon,
1973). After intraperitoneal injection of either cadmium or zinc,
peak radioactivity was present in the spermatogenic cell fraction
which sediments at 2.2 mm/hr (late elongated spermatids). The
affinity of cadmium for these cells was 2.5 to 2.9 times that of
zinc at equimolar concentrations (Table 8); the incorporation of
these two metals into the late elongated spermatids appeared to be
competitive (Table 9). Serial mating fertility studies indicated
that cadmium affected all spermatogenic cell types, with the
exception of mature spermatozoa, and significantly decreased
fertility during a 55-day period after a single cadmium injection.
Pretreatment of mice with zinc completely blocked the biochemical
and functional effect of cadmium on spermiogenic cells but not on
spermatogonial cells. Therefore, the primary action of cadmium
seems to be both an effect on zinc utilization by spermiogenic cells

Table 7   Ratio of Cadmium Concentration in Rete-testes Fluid (RTF)
          to the Cadmium Concentration in Plasma during the First
          30 Minutes of Infusion[a]

Treatment	(RTF):(plasma)
Cd only	0.066
	0.077
	0.075
Cd with ZnCl$_2$ (1 mg/kg)	0.004
	0.012
Treated with ZnCl$_2$ (1mg/kg) 4 hours before Cd administered	0.005
	0.009

[a]Dixon et al., 1975.

Table 8 The in vitro Incorporation of ^{109}Cd and ^{65}Zn by the Late Elongated Spermatids[a]

Concentration of Cd and Zn M	Cellular Incorporation 10^{-9} M/10^6 cells		Ratio Incorporated
	Cd	Zn	Cd/Zn
1×10^{-4}	4.1	1.4	2.9
2×10^{-4}	10.2	4.1	2.5
4×10^{-4}	17.0	6.6	2.6
8×10^{-4}	20.0	8.0	2.5

[a]Lee and Dixon, 1973.
[b]Varying concentrations of equimolar ^{109}Cd and ^{65}Zn were incubated simultaneously with seminiferous tubules at 32°C for 30 minutes prior to cell fractionation and radioactivity determination.

Table 9 Effects of Zinc Pretreatment on the Uptake of Cadmium by Late Elongated Spermatids[a,b]

Zinc pretreatment mg/kg body weight	Cadmium Uptake (% of control)[c]
0.125	79.4 + 8.5[c]
0.25	68.2 + 6.2
0.5	54.2 + 4.3
1.0	43.4 + 8.4

[a]Lee and Dixon, 1973.
[b]CDF1 mice were injected peritoneally with varying concentrations of $ZnCl_2$ 19 hours prior to injection of 100 μCi of ^{109}Cd per mouse (4 μCi/g). Mice were sacrificed 2 hours later, testicular cells were fractionated and radioactivity was determined. Control cells incorporated 8.3×10^{-11} M Cd/10^6 cells (2.8×10^4 dpm/10^6 cells).
[c]Mean ± S.D.

as well as an inhibition of DNA synthesis by spermatogonial cells
(Table 5). Although the dose of cadmium used (5.4 μmole/kg) was not
associated with vascular damage or intertubular edema by histological
examinations, a significant increase in testicular angiotensin-
converting enzyme activity was noted 24 hours after intraperitoneal
administration of cadmium chloride (5.4 μmole/kg) to mice. This
suggests a possible permeability change across the blood-testis
barrier (Kim et al., 1981). Cadmium-induced infertility, inhibition
of DNA, RNA and protein synthesis, and inhibition of androgen
synthesis are further supported by several recent studies (Cihak and
Inoue, 1979; Saksena and Lau, 1979; Nicholls and Rakhra, 1981).

        The exact mechanism by which cadmium inhibits DNA synthesis in
the spermatogonia is not clear. However, it has been reported that
divalent metal ions can interact with both phosphate and base sites
on DNA (Eichhorn et al., 1971). It is interesting that the
inhibition of DNA synthesis in spermatogonial cells was not reversed
by zinc (Lee and Dixon, 1973). Another study indicates that
stronger inhibition of testicular DNA synthesis was achieved by
cadmium plus zinc than by cadmium alone (Cihak and Inoue, 1979).
Furthermore, the inhibition of testicular protein synthesis induced
by cadmium was attributed to significantly decreased aminoacyl-tRNA
in ribosomes (Nicholls and Rakhra, 1981).

        Although Leydig cell tumors and sarcomas were induced by
various cadmium salts in mice and rats (Guthrie, 1964; Gunn et al.,
1963b), epidemiological studies with respect to the mutagenicity and
carcinogenicity of cadmium are still not definite. Some studies
suggest that workers occupationally exposed to cadmium showed
chromosomal aberrations in white blood cells and a possible
increased rate of prostate carcinoma (Holden, 1969; Friberg et al.,
1971), but these studies are complicated by a variety of factors
including possible exposure to other heavy metals via diet. Further
study is needed to obtain molecular mechanisms of cadmium toxicity
as well as both synergistic and antagonistic cadium interaction with
other metals in male reproductive organs.

REFERENCES

Alexander, R.F., 1974, The uptake of lead by children in differing
        environments, Environ. Health Pers. 7:155-160.
Angjileri, L.J., 1973, Calcium metabolism in tumors. Its
        relationship with chromium complex accumulation, Oncology
        27:30-44.
Aoki, A. and Foffer, A.P., 1978, Reexamination of the lesions in rat
        testis caused by cadmium, Biol. Reprod. 18:579-591.
Azarnoff, D.L. Brock, F.E. and Curran, G.L., 1961, A specific site
        of vanadium inhibition of cholesterol biosynthesis, Biochem.
        Biophys. Acta 51:397.

Baetjer, A.M., 1956, Relation of chromium to health, in: "Chromium, Vol. 1: Chemistry of Chromium and its Compounds", M.J. Voly, ed., American Chemical Soc. Monogr. No. 132:76-104.

Baetajer, A.M., Birmingham, D.J., Enterline, P.E., Mertz, W. and Pierce, J.O., 1974a, "Chromium", National Academy of Sciences, Washington, D.C., p. 42.

Baetjer, A.M., Birmingham, D.J., Enterline, P.E., Mertz, W. and Pierce, J.O., 1974b, "Chromium", National Academy of Sciences, Washington, D.C., p. 74.

Behari, J., Chandra, S.V. and Tandon, S.K., 1978, Comparative toxicity of trivalent and hexavalent chromium to rabbits, Acta Biol. Med. Ger. 37:463.

Bergel, F., Bray, R.C. and Harrap, Y.R., 1958, A model system for cysteine desulphydrase action, Nature 181:1654.

Berlin, M. and Ullberg, S., 1963, The fate of Cd-109 in the mouse, Arch. Environ. Health 7:686-693.

Cihak, A. and Inoue, H., 1979, Synthesis of DNA in the liver and testes of cadmium-treated partially hepatectomized rats, J. Biochem. 86:657-662.

Coulston, F., Goldberg, L., Groffer, T.B. and Russell, J.C., 1972, The effects of continuous exposure to airborne lead. I. Exposure of rats and monkeys to particulate lead at a level of 21.5 mg/m^3, Final report to the EPA. Publication of the Department of Environmental Health, College of Medicine, University of Cincinnati, Ohio.

Damjanov, I., Sunderman, F.W., Jr., Mitchell, J.M., Allpass, P.R., 1978, Induction of testicular sarcomas in Fisher rats by intratesticular injection of nickel sulfate, Cancer Res. 38:268-276.

Diamant, R.M.E., 1977, Chemistry of sewage purification, in: "Environmental Chemistry", J. O'mblocklis, ed., pp. 95-119, Plenum Press, New York.

Dixon, R.L. and Lee, I.P., 1979, Assessment of environmental factors affecting male fertility, Environ. Health Pers. 30:53-68.

Dixon, R.L., Okumura, K. and Lee, I.P., 1975, Studies of the blood-testis barrier in rats, Proc. Europ. Soc. Tox., Excerpta Medica ICS 345:242-247.

Dixon, R.L., Sherins, R.J. and Lee, I.P., 1976, Methods to assess reproductive effects of environmental chemicals: Studies of cadmium and boron administered orally, Environ. Health Pers. 13:59-67.

Eichhorn, G.L. and Clark, P., 1963, The reaction of mercury (II) with nucleotides, J. Amer. Chem. Soc. 85:4020-4024.

Eichhorn, G.L., Barger, N.A., Butzow, J.J., Clark, P., Rifkind, J.M., Shin, Y.A. and Tarien, E., 1971, The effect of metal ions on the structure of nucleic acids, Adv. Chem. Ser. 100:135-154.

Evan, A.P. and Dail, W.G., 1974, The effects of sodium chromate on the proximal tubules of the rat kidney, Lab. Invest. 30:704.

Fahim, M.S. and Khare, N.K., 1980, Effects of subtoxic levels of lead and cadmium on urogenital organs of male rats, Arch. Androl. 4:357-362.

Fiskerjo, G., 1970, The effect of two organic compounds on human leukocytes in vitro, Hereditas 64: 142-146.

Friberg, L., Piscator, M. and Nordberg, G.F., 1971, "Cadmium in the Environment", CRC Press, Cleveland, Ohio.

Friberg, L., Nordberg, G. and Vouk, V.B., 1975, "Handbook on the Toxicology of Metals", L. Friberg, G. Nordberg and V.B. Vouk, eds., Elsevier/North Holland, Amsterdam.

Gerber, G.B., Leonard, A. and Jacquet, P., 1980, Toxicity, mutagenicity and teratogenicity of lead, Mutation Res. 76:115-141.

Goldbloom, R.B. and Goldbloom, A., 1953, Boron acid poisoning, J. Pediat. 43:631-643.

Gruenwadel, D.W. and Davidson, N., 1966, Complexing and denaturation of DNA by methylmercuric hydroxide, J. Mol. Biol. 21:129-144.

Gruenwadel, D.W. and Davidson, N., 1967, Complexing and denaturation of DNA by methylmercuric hydroxide. II. Ultracentrifugation studies, Biopolymers 5:847-861.

Gundlund, S.A. and Gould, T.B., 1970, Specificity of the vascular system of the male reproductive tract, J. Reprod. Fert. Suppl. 10:75-95.

Gunn, S.A. and Gould, T.C., 1970, Cadmium and other mineral elements, in: "Testis", Vol. 3, A.D. Johnson, W.R. Gomes and N.L. Vandemark, eds., pp. 378-467, Academic Press, New York.

Gunn, S.A., Gould, T.C. and Anderson, W.A.D., 1963a, The selective injurious response of testicular and epididymal blood vessel to cadmium and its prevention by zinc, Amer. J. Pathol. 42:685-702.

Gunn, S., Gould, A., Clark, T. and Anderson, W.A.D., 1963b, Cadmium-induced interstitial cell tumors in rats and mice and their prevention by zinc, J. Nat. Cancer Inst. 31:745-751.

Gunn, S.A., Gould, T.C. and Anderson, W.A.D., 1966, Loss of selective injurious vascular response to cadmium in regenerated blood vessels of testis, Amer. J. Pathology 48:959-969.

Gunn, S.A., Gould, T.C. and Anderson, W.A.D., 1968, Selectivity or organ response to cadmium injury and various protective measures, J. Pathol. Bacteriol. 96:89-94.

Guthrie, J., 1964, Histological effects of intratesticular injections of cadmium chloride in domestic fowl, Br. J. Cancer 18:255-260.

Hamilton, A. and Hardy, H.L., 1949, "Industrial Toxicology", Harper, New York.

Haro, R.T., Furst, A., Payne, W.W. and Falh, H., 1968, A new nickel carcinogen, Proc. Am. Assoc. Cancer Res. 9:28.

Hart, M.M. and Adamson, R.H., 1971, Antitumor activity and toxicity of salts of inorganic group IIIa metals: Aluminum, gallium, indium, and thalium, Proc. Nat. Acad. Sci. (USA) 68:1623-1626.

Heath, J.C. and Daniel, M.R., 1964, The production of malignant tumors by nickel in the rat, Br. J. Cancer 18:261-264.

Hilderbrand, D.C., Der, R., Briffin, W.T. and Fahim, M., 1973, Effect of lead acetate on reproduction, Amer. J. Obstet. Gynecol. 115:1058-1061.

Hoey, M.J., 1966, The effects of metallic salts on the histology and
    functioning of the rat testis, J. Reprod. Fert. 12:461-471.
Holden, H., 1969, Cadmium toxicology, Lancet 2:54.
Hopkins, L.L., Jr. and Mohr, H.E., 1971, in: "Newer Trace Elements
    in Nutrition", W. Mertz and W.E. Cornatzer, eds., pp. 195-213,
    Marcel Dekker, New York.
Hopkins, L.L., Jr. and Mohr, H.E., 1974, Vanadium as an essential
    nutrient, Fed. Proc. 33:1773-1775.
Hueper, W.C., 1955, Cancer produced by parenterally introduced
    metallic Ni, J. Nat. Cancer Inst. 16:55-74.
Hueper, W.C. and Payne, W.W., 1962, Experimental studies in metal
    carcinogenesis, Arch. Environ. Health 5:445-462.
Ivanova-Chemishanska, L., Antov, G. and Hristeva, V., 1980,
    Multigeneration studies of white rats, obtained from male
    parent generation, exposed to lead acetate, Toxicol. Letters
    Spec. Issue, No. 1, p. 111.
Kamboji, V.P. and Kar, A.B., 1964, Antitesticular effects of
    metallic salt and rare earth salts, J. Reprod. Fert. 7:21-28.
Kaufman, D.B., DiNicola, W. and McIntosh, R., 1970, Acute potassium
    dichromate poisoning, Am. J. Dis. Child. 119:374.
Khachatrian, T.S. and Nazarenko, A.F., 1973, Hygienic evaluation
    of boron in drinking water, Zh. Eksp. Klin. Med. 13:29-34.
Kim, S.U., 1971, Neurotoxic effects of alkylmercury compounds on
    myelinating cultures of mouse cerebellum, Exp. Neurol.
    32:237-246.
Kim, S.J., Roberts, J.F. and Lee, I.P., 1981, Testicular angiotensin
    converting enzyme activity in cadmium-treated mice,
    Pharmacologist 23(3):116.
Kolbye, A.C., Mahaffey, K.R., Finine, J.A., Cornelius, S.N. and
    Jelinus, D.F., 1974, Food exposure to lead, Environ. Health
    Pers. 7:65-74.
Krasovskii, G.N., Varshavskaya, S.P. and Borisova, A.F., 1976, Toxic
    and gonadotrophic effects of cadmium and boron relative to
    standards for these substances in drinking water, Environ.
    Health Pers. 13:69-75.
Lancranjan, I., Popescu, H.I., Gavanescu, O., Klepsch, I. and
    Serbanescu, M., 1975, Reproductive ability of workmen
    occupationally exposed to lead, Arch. Environ. Health
    30:396-399.
Lee, I.P. and Dixon, R.L., 1973, Effect of cadmium on
    spermatogenesis studied by velocity sedimentation cell
    separation and serial mating, J. Pharmacol. Exp. Ther.
    187:641-642.
Lee, I.P. and Dixon, R.L., 1975, Effects of mercury on
    spermatogenesis studied by velocity sedimentation cell
    separation and serial mating, J. Pharmacol. Exp. Ther.
    193:171-181.
Lee, I.P., Sherins, R.J. and Dixon, R.L., 1978, Evidence for
    induction of germinal aplasia in male rats by environmental
    exposure to boron, Toxicol. Appl. Pharmacol. 45:577-590.

Lee, R.E. and Von Lehmden, D.J., 1973, Trace metal pollution in the environment, J. Air Pollut. Control Assoc. 23:853-857.

Locksley, H.G. and Farr, L.E., 1955, The tolerance of large doses of sodium borate intravenously by patients receiving neutron capture therapy. J. Pharmacol. Exp. Ther. 114:484-489.

Lou, T.J., Hackett, R.L. and Sunderman, W., 1972, The carcinogenicity of intravenous nickel carbon in rats, Cancer Res. 32:2253-2258.

Manthur, A.K., Chandra, S.V., Behari, J. and Tandon, S.K., 1977a, Biochemical and morphological changes in some organs of rats in nickel intoxication, Arch. Toxicol. 37:159-164.

Manthur, A.K., Datta, K.K., Tandon, S.K. and Dikshith, T.S.S., 1977b, Effect of nickel sulfate on male rats, Bull. Environ. Contam. Toxicol. 17:241-248.

Mehra, M. and Choi, B.H., 1981, Distribution and biotransformation of methyl mercuric chloride in different tissues of mice, Acta Pharmacol. Toxicol. 49:28-37.

Mehra, M. and Kanwar, K.C., 1980, Absorption, distribution, and excretion on methylmercury in mice, Bull. Environ. Contam. Toxicol. 24:627-633.

Morris, G.E., 1964, Toxic hazards, chrome hazards, N. Eng. J. Med. 263:364.

National Academy of Sciences, 1974, Chromium, National Academy of Sciences, Washington.

National Research Council, Committee on Biologic Effects of Atmospheric Pollutants, 1974, Vanadium: National Academy of Sciences, Washington, 117p.

Nicholls, D.M. and Rakhra, G.S., 1981, Testicular protein synthesis during the response to subtoxic levels of cadium, Hormon. Res. 14:56-69.

Niewenhuis, R.J., 1980, Effects of cadmium upon regenerated testicular vessels in the rat, Biol. Reprod. 23:171-179.

Ochi, H. and Tonomoura, A., 1975, The low-dose effect of two organic mercury compounds on cultured human fibroblastic cells, Mutation Res. 31:268.

Parizek, J. and Zahor, Z., 1956, Effect of cadmium salts on testicular tissue, Nature (London) 177:1036.

Parker, R.D., Sharma, R.P. and Miller, G.W., 1978, Accumulation and depletion of vanadium in selected tissues of rats treated with vanadyl sulfate and sodium orthovanadate. J. Environ. Pathol. Toxicol. 2:235-245.

Peabody, R.A., Wallach, S., Verch, R.L. and Lifschitz, M., 1980, Effect of LH and FSH on vanadium distribution in hypophysectomized rats (40984), Proc. Soc. Exp. Biol. Med. 165:349-353.

Phatak, S.S. and Patwardhan, V.N., 1950, Toxicity of nickel, J. Sci. Ind. Res. 9b930:70-76.

Rabinowitz, M.B., Wetherrill, G.W. and Kopple, J.D., 1974, Studies of human lead metabolism by use of stable isotope tracers, Environ. Health Pers. 7:145-154.

Ramel, C. 1972, "Genetic Effects in Mercury in the Environment", L. Friberg and J. Vostal, eds., pp. 169-181, CRC Press Cleveland, Ohio.

Ramel, C. and Magnusson, J., 1969, Genetic effects of organic mercury compounds II. Chromosome segregation on Drosophila melanogaster, Hereditas 61:231-254.

Rizzo, A.M. and Furst, A., 1972, Mercury teratogenesis in the rat, Proc. West. Pharmacol. Soc. 15:52-54.

Roshchin, I.V., Il'nitskaya, A.V., Lutsendo, L.A. and Zhidkova, L.A., 1965, Effect on organism of vanadium trioxide, Fed. Proc. Trans. Suppl. 24:611.

Sakai, K. and Takeuchi, T., 1972, Biological reaction of tissue cells to alkylmercury, in: "Environmental Mercury Contamination", Ann Arbor, Michigan, Vol. 74:280.

Saksena, S.K. and Lau, I.F., 1979, Effects of cadmium chloride on testicular steroidogenesis and fertility of male rats, Endokrinologie 74:6-12.

Scharma, R.P., Oberg, S.G. and Parker, R.D.R., 1980, Vanadium retention in rat tissues following acute exposures to different dose levels, J. Toxicol. Environ. Health 6:45-54.

Schroeder, H.A., 1967, Cadmium, chromium, and cardiovascular disease, Circulation 35:570-582.

Schroeder, H.A. and Balassa, J.J., 1961, Abnormal trace metals in man: cadmium, J. Chronic Dis. 14:236-258.

Schroeder, H.A. and Mitchner, M., 1971, Toxic effects of trace elements on the reproduction of mice and rats, Arch. Environ. Health 23:102-106.

Schwarz, K. and Milne, D.B., 1971, Growth effects of vanadium in the rat, Science 174:426.

Seal, B.S. and Weeth, H.J., 1980, Effect of boron in drinking water on the male laboratory rat, Bull. Environ. Contam. Toxicol. 25:782-789.

Setchell, B.P. and Waites, G.M.H., 1970, Changes in the permeability of the testicular capillaries and of the blood-testis barrier after injection of cadmium chloride in the rat, J. Endocrinol. 47:81-86.

Skerfving, S., Hansson, K. and Kindsten, J., 1970, Chromosome breakage in humans exposed to methylmercury through fish consumption, Arch. Environ. Health 21:133-139.

Snyder, F. and Cornatzer, W.E., 1958, Vanadium inhibition of phospholipid synthesis and sulfhydryl activity in rat liver, Nature 182:462.

Sorenson, R.J., Campbell, I.R., Tepper, L.B. and Lingg, R.D., 1974, Aluminum in the environment and human health, Environ. Health Pers. 8:3-95.

Stoner, G.D., Shimkin, M.B., Troxell, M.C., Thompson, T.L. and Terry, L.S., 1976, Test for carcinogenicity of metallic compounds by the pulmonary tumor responses in strain A mice, Cancer Res. 36:1744-1746.

Sunderman, F.W. Jr., 1977a, A review of the metabolism and toxicology of nickel, Annals Clin. Lab. Sci. 7:377-398.

Sunderman, F.W. Jr., 1977b, The metabolism and toxicology of nickel, in: "Clinical Chemistry and Chemical Toxicology of Metals", S.S. Brown, ed., pp. 231-259, Elsevier/North Holland, Amsterdam.

Takeuchi, T., 1970, Biological reactions and pathological changes of human beings and animals under the condition of organic mercury contamination, International Conference on Environmental Mercury Contamination, Ann Arbor, Michigan.

Tandon, S.K., Behari, J. and Kachru, D.N., 1979, Distribution of chromium in poisoned rats, Toxicol. 13:29-34.

Tarabaeva, G.I., 1959, Distribution of radioactive lead in the sexual organs of animals, Izv. Akad. Nauk Kaz. S.S.R., Ser. Med. I. Fiziol 2:95-101.

Tarasenko, N.Y., Kasparova, A.A. and Strongina, O.M., 1972, The effect of boric acid on the generative function of the male organism, Gig. Tr. Prof. Zabol. 16(3) 11:13-16.

Tepper, L.B. and Levin, L.S., 1972, A survey of air and population lead levels in selected American communities. Final report to the EPA. Publication of the Department of Environmental Health, College of Medicine, University of Cincinnati, OH.

Timm, F. and Schultz, G., 1966, Hoden und Schwermetalle, Histochemie 7:15-21.

Tipton, I.H. and Cook, M.J., 1963, Trace elements in human tissue. Part II. Adult subjects from the United States, Health Physics 9:103-145.

Tipton, I.H. and Stewart, P.L., 1969, Patterns of elemental excretion in long-term balance studies, II, in: "Internal Dosimetry", W.S. Snyder, ed., Health Physics Division Annual Progress Report for period ending July 31.

Umeda, M., Saito, K., Hirose, K. and Saito, M., 1969, Mercuric compounds on HeLa cells, Jap. J. Exp. Med. 39:47-58.

Valdes-Dapena, M.A. and Arey, J.B., 1962, Boric acid poisoning, J. Pediat. 61:531-546.

Venitt, S. and Levy, L.S., 1974, Mutagenicity of chromates in bacteria and its relevance to chromate carcinogenesis, Nature 250:493-493.

Verschaeve, L., Kirsch-Volders, M., Suzanne, C., Groetenbriel, C., Haustermans, R., Lecomte, A. and Roossels, D., 1976, Genetic damage induced by occupationally low mercury exposure, Environ. Res. 12:306-316.

Von Waltschewa, W., Slatewa, M. and Michailow, I.W., 1972a, Testicular changes due to long-term administration of nickel sulfate in rats, Exptl. Pathol. 6:116-120.

Von Waltschewa, W., Slatema, M. and Michailow, I.W., 1972b, Hodenveranderugen bei weissen Ratten durch chonische Verabreichung von Nickelsulfat, Exp. Path. Bd. 6:116-120.

Weir, R.J., Jr. and Fisher, R.S., 1972, Toxicologic studies of borax and boric acid, Toxicol. Appl. Pharmacol. 23:351-364.

EFFECTS OF OCCUPATIONAL EXPOSURE TO LEAD ON SPERM AND SEMEN

Karl Wildt[1], Rune Eliasson[2], and Maths Berlin[1]

[1]Institute of Environmental Health
 University of Lund, Solvegatan, Lund, Sweden
[2]Department of Physiology I,
 Karolinska Institute, Stockholm, Sweden

ABSTRACT

Semen qualities were studied in samples from workers exposed to lead in a factory for storage batteries. The study included two groups with different degrees of exposure. The mean lead-blood concentration (Pb-B) values for the men in the two groups during the six months preceding the study were 45 µg/100 ml and 22 µg/100 ml, respectively. Each man delivered at least one semen sample during a test period and most of the men participated in both test periods, which took place within a six-month interval. The size of each of the four groups, was 16 or more men. The semen qualities assessed included sperm count, sperm motility (qualitative and quantitative), sperm morphology, sperm chromatin stability when exposed to sodium dodecyl sulphate, and release of LDH-X into the seminal plasma. The secretory function of the prostate was assessed by analyses of such markers as acid phosphatase, zinc, and magnesium. Fructose was used as the marker for the secretory function of the seminal vesicles. All semen samples had values within the expected limits for that population. A subtle but significant difference was found between the two groups for sperm chromatin stability, indicating that the exposure to lead had decreased the stability of the spermatozoa. Moreover, a decreased secretory function of the accessory genital glands was noted more frequently among the men with the higher degree of exposure than among those in the other group. For all other semen variables, there were no differences between the groups.

INTRODUCTION

It is a well established fact that occupational lead exposure
can cause disturbances in female fertility and fetal development
(Rom, 1976). Less is known about the effect of occupational lead
exposure on male fertility and reproductive organs. Studies in
animals indicate that high exposure to lead may cause testicular
changes and changes in semen quality. Testicular atrophy and
impaired spermatogenesis have been observed in the mouse (Eyden et
al., 1978), in the rat (Hildebrand et al., 1973) and in the dog
(Stowe et al., 1973) after ingestion of toxic doses of lead via the
food. Hildebrand et al. (1973) observed that the sperm motility was
impaired in semen samples from rats with blood lead (Pb-B)
concentrations exceeding 39 μg/100 ml. Monkiewiez et al. (1975)
observed in bulls a negative correlation between lead content of
seminal plasma and sperm survival time at 46.5°C.

In old clinical reports, a remarkable decrease of fertility in
lead-poisoned workers is described (Oliver, 1911). However, little
information is available as to whether these observations are a
secondary sign due to lead intoxication or a direct effect of lead
on the reproductive organs. Lancranjan et al. (1975) reported an
epidemiological study on lead-exposed workers in a battery
industry. They observed increased astenospermia, oligozoospermia
and teratospermia in workers with Pb-B concentrations between 23 and
75 μg/100 ml blood. There are, however, some serious shortcomings
in their study, and their results cannot be considered conclusive.
Sandstead et al. (1970) reported increased urinary levels of
gonadotrophin in 7 out of 12 patients with lead intoxication, and
Braunstein (1978) reported decreased libido in exposed patients,
decreased levels of plasma testosterone and slightly increased
levels of plasmatic luteinizing hormone (LH), suggesting Leydig cell
damage. Human chorion gonadotrophin injections increased the
testosterone levels but not clomifene or gonadotrophin-releasing
hormone, suggesting a hypopituitarism, secondary or primary.
Altamura et al. (1978) likewise, in a study on battery plant
workers, observed a slight trend towards oligozoospermia in exposed
workers, but the sperm count reduction could not be regarded as
statistically significant.

In a study published by Ruse et al. (1977), it is claimed that
lead intoxication causes interference with spermatogenesis; however,
the data are not conclusive. Plechaty et al. (1977) confirmed the
presence of lead in seminal plasma. However, no association between
lead concentration in seminal plasma and changes in sperm quality
was observed. The available data on effects of occupational lead
exposure at moderate and subtoxic exposure levels did not permit any
definite conclusions as to adverse effects of lead exposure on male
reproductive organs. A study was therefore performed on lead-exposed
battery plant workers in whom the lead exposure was continuously

monitored by repeated determinations of concentrations of
lead-blood (Pb-B) and zinc protoporphyrine (ZPP) in blood.

MATERIAL AND METHODS

The investigation was performed on employees at a battery
factory in the south of Sweden with about 250 male workers. The
workers were exposed to respirable lead particles or lead oxide
particles with an aerodynamic particle diameter between 1 and 5 μm.
All exposed workers, had since 1968, been regularly examined for
determinations of Pb-B. Workers with Pb-B values exceeding 2.2
μmol/l (45 μg/100 ml) were examined monthly. Workers with Pb-B
values exceeding 2.9 μmol (60 μg/100 ml) were removed from further
exposure until the Pb-B values had returned to about 2 μmol/l (40
μg/100 ml). Since January 1977, all workers have been regularly
monitored by hematofluorometric determinations of ZPP in blood.

The study was made in two steps - a pilot study in September
1978, i.e., three months after the period with the lowest exposure
risk of the year, and the second, main study in April 1979, three
months after the period with the highest risk of lead exposure
during the work year. The three-month interval was selected in view
of the length of the spermatogenetic cycle (74 days) and the time
for sperm transfer through the epididymis. The study included not
only the number and quality of the sperm cells but also the
secretory function of accessory glands, prostate and vesicles. The
endocrine function of the testicles was not studied.

The Studied Groups

Thirty-one men, 18-61 years of age, whose lead exposure had
been followed as described above for at least one year before the
intended study, and whose Pb-B levels during the six months prior to
the study exceeded 2.4 μmol/l (50 μg/100 ml) at least once, were
selected. Another group of 31 men, matched to the first group with
respect to age, ethnic and social factors, whose Pb-B levels
exceeded 1.45 μmol/l (30 μg/100 ml) only occasionally and whose ZPP
blood levels never exceeded 0.1 μmol/l (50 μg/100 ml) were selected
as a reference group. For all selected persons, the available case
sheets and results of earlier health examinations were thoroughly
checked in order to reveal any past or current clinical condition
which could interfere with the reproductive function. All 62
persons in the two groups of occupationally-exposed workers were
invited to take part in the investigation on semen quality. As a
result of the check of the case sheets and earlier health
examinations, two persons were excluded from the exposed group - one
man with extremely high Pb-B values and symptoms of poisoning, which
resulted in a thorough clinical investigation and treatment, and

another man with azoospermia as a result of resection of the
prostate gland. From the reference group, one man was excluded due
to postoperative testicular atrophy and azoospermia.

Methods of Pb-B and ZPP Determinations

The Pb-B concentrations were determined by atomic absorption
analysis on venous blood collected in lead-free vacutainers. All
analyses were performed by a laboratory authorized by the Swedish
Labor Protection Board, which requires taking part in the scheduled
national and international quality controls. The determination of
ZPP in blood was performed by hematofluorometric method, using a
Aviv fluorometer. The principle for the analysis is based on front
surface optics (Blumberg et al., 1977; Eisinger et al., 1978).

Semen Analysis

Semen samples were collected in clean plastic bottles by
masturbation after three to five days of abstinence. All plastic
material had been carefully tested for possible interference and
found acceptable (Belsey et al., 1980). After liquefaction, the
sample was transferred to a graded centrifuge tube and the volume,
possible occurrence of non-liquefied material, color and viscosity
were noted (for ref. to all methods and reference values, see
Eliasson, 1981).

Sperm count, motility and morphology. The number of
spermatozoa per ml was determined, after careful mixing and
dilution, with the hematocytometer method. All counts and motility
determinations were done with phase contrast microscopy.

Sperm motility was assessed subjectively with regard to the
percentage of motile spermatozoa (with 5 percent interval) and the
mean progressive motility score (0=none, 1=poor, 2=medium, 3=good).
The assessment was made in phase contrast microscopy 1-2 hours after
ejaculation and repeated four hours after ejaculation. In the
meantime, the samples were kept at 37°C.

The percentage live spermatozoa was determined with a
supravital staining technique using 0.5 percent eosin Y in phosphate
buffer and negative phase contrast microscopy (1200x), as described
by Eliasson and Treichl (1971).

Sperm morphology was evaluated from smears stained with a
modified Papanicolaou technique (Belsey et al., 1980). The whole
spermatozoon was assessed and defects in head, midpiece and/or tail
were noted separately. With this technique, the sum of different
abnormalities will exceed the figure for "abnormal" spermatozoa

since each spermatozoon can have up to four different abnormalities
in the system we used (for details, see Belsey et al., 1980, and
Eliasson, 1981).

   Chromatin stability. The stability of the nucleus was
determined by exposing the spermatozoa to a 1 percent solution of
sodium dodecyl sulphate (SDS) in a borate buffer (0.05 M, pH 9.0).
In such a solution, the head of the mature spermatozoon will remain
intact (the cell may lose its tail) but the head of "immature"
spermatozoon will swell. After 60 minutes of exposure, the
spermatozoa were fixed with 2.5 percent glutaraldehyde and the
morphology was assessed in phase contrast microscopy (1250x). The
degree of swelling of the heads was assessed as "none" (group I),
"moderate" (group II) or "significant" (group III). The percentage
of totally intact spermatozoa (no swelling of the head + remaining
tail) was also determined. The reactivity of spermatozoa is
dependent upon zinc and the sensitivity to SDS was, therefore, also
tested on spermatozoa which had been exposed to EDTA (for details,
see Kvist, 1980; Kvist and Eliasson, 1980).

   Lactic dehydrogenase, isoenzyme X (LDH-X or LDS-C4).
Spermatozoa and spermatids contain an isoenzyme of LDH which is
specific for these cells, i.e. LDH-X or LDH-C4. Quantitative
analysis of this isoenzyme in the seminal plasma will therefore give
a measure of the leakage of this enzyme from the spermatozoa,
provided the semen does not contain immature germinal cells.

   The semen samples were incubated at 37°C for 4 hours. Seminal
plasma was obtained by centrifugation at 2.800 g and LDH was
determined by conventional spectrophotometric technique (NADH). The
isoenzymes were separated by electrophoresis on agarose gel and
localized with the tetrazolium technique. The quantitative
distribution was then assessed with a scanning procedure and the
activity of LDH-C4 expressed in nanokatal per 100 million spermatozoa
(for details, see Eliasson et al., 1967, 1980).

   Secretory function of the accessory genital glands. The
secretory function of the seminal vesicles was evaluated from the
fructose concentration in the seminal plasma. Fructose was analyzed
with a colorimetric technique (Karvonen and Malm, 1955). The
secretory function of the prostate was assessed by analyses of acid
phosphatase, zinc and magnesium in the seminal plasma as described
by Lindholmer and Eliasson (1972).

Evaluation of the Semen Analysis

   The limits presented in Table 1 are based on results from
analyses of semen samples given by men who, within a three-month
period before or after the semen analysis was performed, had made a

woman pregnant and who had not been patients for an infertility
problem.

Statistical Analyses

The results from clinical and laboratory examinations were
analysed by the Department of Statistics, University of Lund, using
the Mann-Whitney's rank sum test; the significance tests were
two-tailed. Factors which could interfere, e.g. age and time
between ejaculation and the first analysis, were checked with
covariance analysis. All relevant controls of the data entered in
the computer were run.

RESULTS

In the pilot study, 15 exposed and 24 non-exposed men gave
semen samples for examination. In the main study, 17 exposed and 17
non-exposed men participated. Of these, 14 and 15, respectively,
took part in both studies.

Table 1   Normal Limits for Variables Related to Properties of Human
          Semen Samples

Variable	Normal	Doubtful	Abnormal
Volume, ml	2 - 6	1.5 - 2.0	< 1.5
Sperm count, 10^6/ml	20 - 250	10 - 20	< 10
Sperm count, 10^6/ejaculate	> 80	20 - 80	< 20
Motile spermatozoa a)	> 50	35 - 50	< 35
Progressive motility a)	Good/very good	Medium	Poor/none
Live spermatozoa a)	> 50	35 - 50	< 35
Normal spermatozoa	> 45	30 - 45	< 30
Amorphous heads	< 40	40 - 50	> 50
Midpiece defects b)	< 20	21 - 25	> 25
Tail defects	< 20	21 - 25	> 25
Chromatin stable heads	> 70	65 - 70	< 65
LDH-C4, nanokatal/10^8sperm	< 30	30 - 40	> 40
Fructose, mmol/1 c)	6.7 - 33	4.4 - 6.6	< 4.4
Acid phosphatase mkat/1 c)	> 6.94	4.17 - 6.92	< 4.17
Zinc, mmol/1 c)	1.2 - 3.8	0.8 - 1.2	< 0.8
Magnesium, mmol/1 c)	2.9 - 10.3	2.1 - 2.8	< 2.1

aEvaluated 1-2 hours after ejaculation.
bDefect midpieces include also protoplasma droplets
 larger than half the sperm head.
cValid if volume is 2-6 ml.

The preliminary analysis revealed that one man in each group had azoospermia for reasons not related to the study. Later, one man was found to have an extremely high lead value in his blood, even after a long period of exclusion from the factory. He was therefore not included and will be discussed in a separate report.

The distribution of the remaining men, exposure criteria, and the lead and ZPP values are presented in Figure 1 and Tables 2 through 4. From these tables it is clear that the age distribution is equal and there is a highly significant difference ($p < 0.00001$) between the two groups with regard to Pb-B and ZPP.

Clinical data

During the pilot study in September 1978, 10 men in the control (non-exposed) group had subjective symptoms indicating prostatitis (or prostate-vesiculitis). The diagnosis was confirmed in three cases with cytological analysis of the expressed prostatic fluid. In four cases, no objective signs of a past or present infection could be found. Of the remaining men, one had recently had a severe infection in a tooth and two men had previously had urogenital infections but were at the moment free from symptoms. None of the men in the exposed group had symptoms or medical histories indicating urogenital infections. This difference between the two groups is not reflected in the semen qualities as they are presented in Table 5 but is hinted at in the statistical evaluations of motility and viability data (Table 6).

Sperm number and motility. From Table 5, it can be noted that in the control groups (both periods), five samples had low sperm count and four had low motility. However, these samples originated from four individuals, three of whom participated in both studies. For this reason, it cannot be concluded that there was a difference between the two groups. Mean values for motile and live spermatozoa were lower in the non-exposed group than in the exposed (< 0.05; Table 6, Figures 2 through 5).

Sperm morphology. Samples classified as abnormal with regard to the percentage of "normal spermatozoa" and "tail defects", respectively, originated from four men. One of the exposed men participated in both studies. In the pilot study, one sample from each group is included in both "<40 percent normal" and ">25 percent tail defects", since they had a combination of defects. Therefore, no difference can be noted between the exposed and non-exposed men with regard to sperm morphology.

Semen volume. The semen samples included in the two groups ">1 ml but <2 ml" and "<1 ml" originated from eight men. All of these samples were classified as normal with regard to sperm count,

Table 2 Individual Exposure Criteria for Men with Low or No Exposure

No.	Born	March 1978 – Pb-B[a]		August 1978 ZPP[a]		October 1978 – Pb-B		March 1979 ZPP		Length of service/ Exposure in months
		mean	range	mean	range	mean	range	mean	range	
01	1918	19.6	25-17	36.6	39-34	19.7	22-18	30.5	34-27	20
02	1924	11.5	12-11	38.0	40-36	12.6	14-11	31.0	36-30	291
03	1925	17.5	20-15	31.0	36-26					20
04	1930	15.3	17-14	33.3	35-31	15.0	17-14	24.2	28-20	255
05	1933	26.5	30-23	36.0	47-25	28.2	31-26	32.2	37-26	32
06	1935	23.5	24-23	43.5	47-40					60
07	1935	27.5	31-24	42.5	45-40					183
08	1937					16.5	24-09	37.0	41-36	49
09	1937	23.3	29-20	29.0	32-26	26.5	32-23	26.2	28-22	85
10	1940	13.0	13-13	20.0						23
11	1945	23.3	25-20	44.6	49-37	23.0	27-17	35.2	45-29	39
12	1946	26.0	26-26	38.0	38-38	24.0	29-20	33.2	34-30	87
13	1946	23.0	24-22	32.0	34-26	24.7	25-23	25.7	31-21	111
14	1948	18.3	19-17	24.6	32-21	24.2	26-22	19.7	27-14	21
15	1948	15.6	18-14	30.6	34-28	24.7	19-15	27.0	31-24	24
16	1949	20.5	22-19	32.5	33-32					84
17	1951					14.0	20-08	20.3	27-18	4
18	1951	23.6	28-20	26.3	28-26	27.7	37-20	20.2	24-19	19
19	1951	15.5	16-15	33.0	34-32	13.0	14-12	26.5	27-26	52
20	1952	25.6	28-23	28.6	33-25					99
21	1953	25.0	29-22	34.0	35-33					32
22	1954	20.0	22-16	32.6	35-30					31
23	1954	25.0	30-20	34.5	36-33	23.7	30-17	26.2	28-25	39
24	1955	17.6	20-16	30.0	38-24					22
25	1957	29.0	39-22	36.6	40-33	26.7	31-24	31.5	38-26	12
Mean Value		21.1		33.4		21.5		27.9		
Number		23		23		16		16		

[a]All values are presented as µg/100 ml blood.

Table 3 Individual Exposure Criteria for Men in the Exposed Group

No.	Born	March 1978 - August 1978 Pb-B[a]		ZPP[a]		October 1978 - March 1979 Pb-B		ZPP		Length of service/ Exposure in months
		mean	range	mean	range	mean	range	mean	range	
26	1925	52.5	60-44	95.4	105-90	39.7	44-36	51.0	63-44	39
27	1930	48.4	67-32	95.8	100-91	28.7	33-35	51.2	62-63	39
28	1930					50.8	56-37	120.6	144-74	23
29	1931	33.0	34-32	45.0	45-45					99
30	1933	54.8	65-47	161.4	181-95	49.8	54-40	115.2	126-103	183
31	1939	42.3	48-38	139.6	159-126	40.2	43-38	117.0	144-104	32
32	1943	42.3	42-43	95.0	109-82	34.5	44-25	67.5	81-54	27
33	1946	53.8	62-38	117.6	151-76	46.8	54-40	43.4	53-40	147
34	1947	51.4	61-42	123.2	133-75	51.2	58-44	123.6	137-99	147
35	1948	46.0	57-37	106.0	116-91	42.6	48-40	108.8	114-105	99
36	1948	44.6	53-23	66.8	83-34					12
37	1949	39.0	37-27	47.0	50-44	34.2	39-28	41.2	46-37	23
38	1950	46.7	57-38	92.0	113-63	40.5	43-39	67.7	68-67	41
39	1954	47.0	56-33	238.0	269-194	47.6	54-43	270.1	320-194	26
40	1955					47.5	54-40	54.5	80-43	18
41	1955	43.5	52-37	130.0	147-123	47.3	53-44	176.1	192-157	28
42	1957					61.8	75-46	162.1	206-127	9
43	1960					50.6	54-44	70.6	104-40	9
Mean Value		46.1		110.9		44.6		102.1		
Number		14		14		16		16		

a All values are presented as µg/100 ml blood.

Table 4 Background Information for Men Included in the Study (April 1979)

Variable	Non-Exposed Group Mean Values µg/100ml	mmol/l	Range µg/100ml	mol/l	Exposed Group Mean Values µg/100ml	mmol/l	Range µg/100ml	mmol/l
PbB 1979	20.1	9.7	9-31	(4.3-14.9)	42.3	20.4	25-54	(12.0-2)
PbB 1978	21.7	10.4	13-28	(6.2-13.5)	45.6	22.0	34-56	(16.4-2)
PbB 1977	21.6	10.4	13-29	(6.2-13.9)	43.3	20.9	13-61	(6.2-2)
PbB 1976	20.0	9.6	13-32	(6.2-15.4)	39.2	18.9	8-82	(3.8-3)
PbB 6months	19.8	9.5	13-28	(6.2-13.5)	44.4	21.4	30-62	(14.4-2)
PbB 6-12 months	20.2	9.7	12-29	(5.7-13.9)	38.1	18.3	13-55	(6.2-2)
Max PbB	30.1	14.5	17-40	(8.2-19.3)	62.9	30.3	41-78	(19.8-3)
ZPP 1979	28.3	4.5	19-38	(3.0- 6.0)	101.9	16.3	42-295	(6.7-47)
ZPP 1978	32.5	5.2	22-44	(3.5- 7.0)	108.7	17.3	46-231	(7.3-37)
ZPP 1977	34.7	5.5	24-55	(3.8- 8.8)	116.1	18.5	43-195	(6.8-31)
ZPP 6 man	27.4	4.4	17-37	(2.7- 5.9)	101.8	16.2	41-270	(6.5-43)
Max ZPP	41.9	6.7	32-67	(5.1-10.7)	174.0	27.2	57-320	(9.1-51)

Table 5   Distribution of Semen Samples in Different Groups with
           Reference to their Properties

	Pilot Study		Test Period	
	Control	Exp	Control	Exp
Normal properties in semen sample	16	5	10	5
Number <40x10^6 per ejaculate	2	0	3	0
Decreased motility[a]	2	0	2	0
Less than 40 normal spermatozoa	1	1	0	1
More than 25 tail defects	2	2	0	1
Volume >1 but <2 ml	1	4	1	3
Volume <1 ml	0	0	1	1
Decreased prostatic function	1	2	1	5
Decreased vesicular function	2	1	1	3
Number of samples examined[b]	23	14	16	16

[a]Less than 40 percent motile and/or poor progressive
motility 1-2 hour after ejaculation.
[b]The sum of the numbers in the table is not equal to
the number of samples examined since a semen sample can
have more than one abnormality and is then listed more
than once in the table.

motility and morphology, and biochemistry. One man in the control
group, and two men in the exposed group participated in both studies.

The difference between the control and exposed groups was
interesting since on a relative basis, 28 percent (4 out of 14) of
the exposed men had a low volume, compared to 4 percent (1 out of
23) in the control group. In the test period, the corresponding
figures were 25 percent (4 out of 16) vs. 12.5 percent (2 out of
16). The study was, however, too small to allow any conclusions.

Secretory functions of the prostate and seminal vesicles.
Altogether, seven men had "decreased prostatic function". One man
in each group participated in both studies. In the test period one
of the exposed men presented a semen sample with low values for both
prostatic and seminal vesicular markers. In the summary, three men
in the control group and eight men in the exposed group had
biochemical signs of decreased secretory function of the prostate
and/or the seminal vesicles. If we consider only men participating
in the test period, 43.8 percent (7 out of 16) of the exposed men
and 12.5 percent of the non-exposed men had decreased function of
the accessory genital glands. The statistical analysis showed a
significant difference only for zinc (p<0.05; Table 6).

Table 6 Statistical Evaluation of the Results from the Test Period (April 1979). Only Variables with Significant Deviations have been Included

	Non-exposed				Exposed				Significance
	Mean	Median	Range	N	Mean	Median	Range	N	P
Motile sperm, 1h	54	53	25-70	14	64	68	50-75	12	0.029
Motile sperm, 4h	44	49	10-65	15	56	57	40-70	13	0.034
Live spermatozoa, 1h	55	57	26-75	14	69	69	58-81	12	0.008
Live spermatozoa, 4h	51	51	43-59	7	71	69	64-80	2	0.040
SDS-test intact heads	92	93	82-97	16	88	88	76-97	16	0.033
SDS-test intact sperm	66	65	49-79	16	51	49	31-82	16	0.004
SDS-EDTA intact sperm	22	18	6-57	16	13	11	4-37	16	0.003
LDH act. nkat/10^8 sperm	41	35	9-83	15	29	22	13-70	16	0.033
Zinc in seminal plasma, mM	2.5	2.1	0.3-6.1	16	1.9	1.4	0.7-5.7	16	0.036

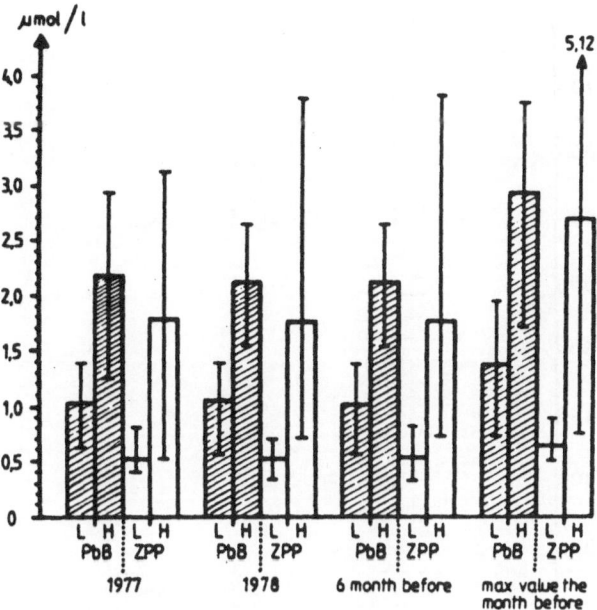

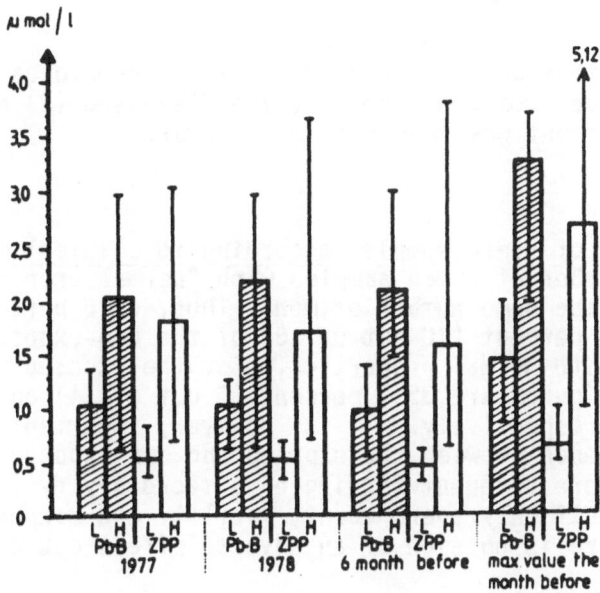

Figure 1   Mean Pb-B and ZPP values for the indicated period. L = non-exposed, H = exposed workers. Lines indicate range of individual means. Column heights are group means. Sept. 1978, above, is the pilot study. April, 1979, below, is the main study.

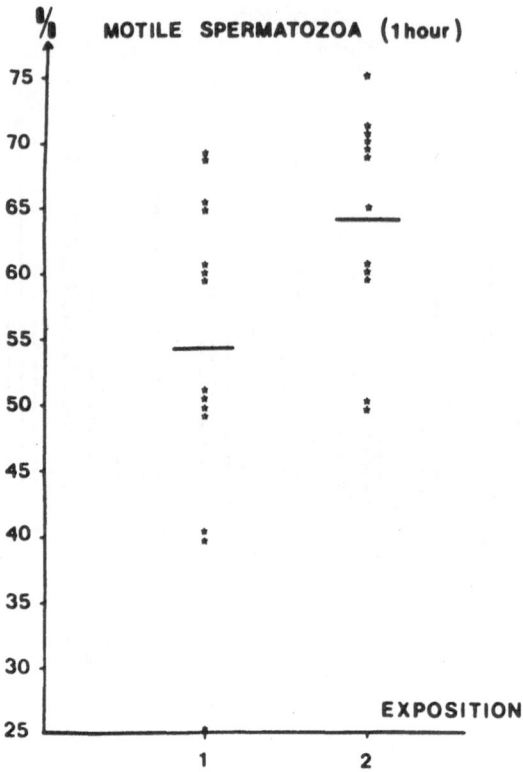

Figure 2   Distribution of percentage motile spermatozoa in semen
           samples from non-exposed (1) and exposed (2) men.
           Assessment was made within one hour.

        Evaluation of semen samples according to clinical routine.   In
Table 5, the number of semen samples with "normal properties"
corresponds to the same number of men. Thus, 69.6 percent (16 out
of 23) and 62.5 percent (10 out of 16) of the non-exposed men had
semen samples with normal properties. For the exposed men, the
corresponding figures are 35.7 percent (5 out of 14) and 31.3 percent
(5 out of 16), respectively. It is, however, important to consider
that the difference between the exposed and non-exposed groups is due
mainly to the more frequent finding of a secretory dysfunction in the
exposed group. If only sperm count, motility and morphology are
considered, there is no sign of an adverse effect caused by the lead
exposure.

        Special investigations of the spermatozoa. The stability of
the spermatozoa against SDS treatment was within the normal range
for all samples. However, in the statistical analysis, a clear
difference was noted between the two groups; spermatozoa from

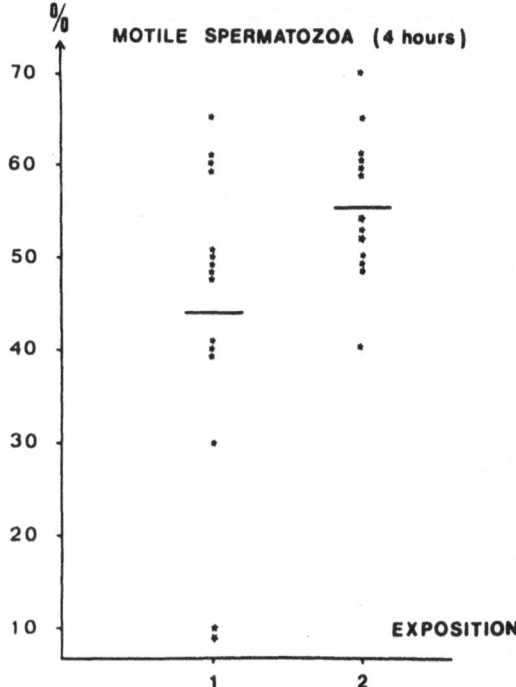

Figure 3   Distribution of percentage motile spermatozoa in semen
           samples from non-exposed (1) and exposed (2) men.
           Assessment was made four hours after ejaculation.

exposed men had a lower resistance than those from the control group
(Table 6; Figures 6 through 8). The release of the LDH-C4 was less
in semen samples from men in the exposed group than from the
controls (Table 6).

DISCUSSION

     Studies of the effects of xenobiotic factors on the human male
reproductive tract are very few (MacLeod, 1964; Eliasson, 1981).
One reason for this is the many moral and ethical obstacles that
still prevail with regard to semen collection and analysis. Another
limiting factor has been the lack of methods which could reflect
different functional properties of the organs contributing to the
semen, not only for sperm count, motility and morphology.

     Unfortunately, most research workers have presented their
projects as "studies on male fertility". This has been

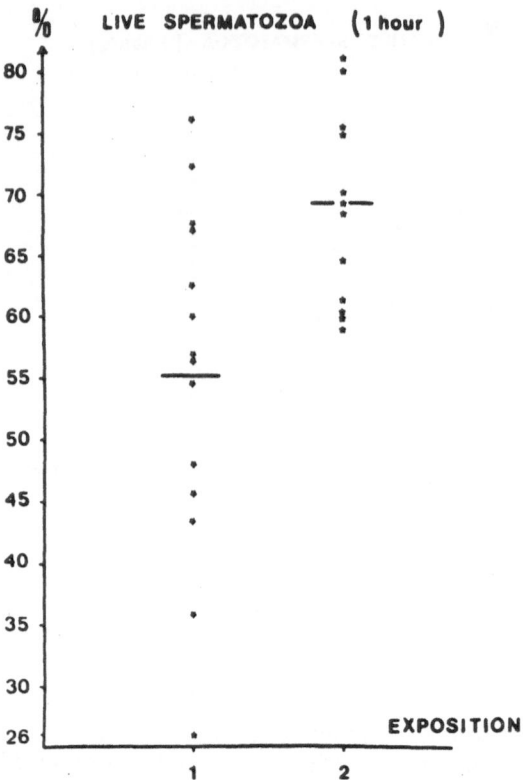

Figure 4   Distribution of percentage live spermatozoa in semen
           samples from non-exposed (1) and exposed (2) men.
           Assessment was made within one hour.

scientifically incorrect since usually only sperm count and motility
have been assessed. A decrease in sperm output and/or in sperm
motility indicates a dysfunction of the testes and/or the
epididymis, but the relation between these changes and male
fertility is obscure unless they are very drastic changes, e.g.
azoospermia or total lack of motility.

     From scientific and social points of view, it is important to
inform those who are going to participate in studies on the effects
of xenobiotic factors on the male reproductive system that such a
study can give information only about the functional status of
different organs and not about the fertility or virility of the
men. Secondly, it is important to include methods which evaluate
the secretory function of the accessory genital glands and some
functional properties of the spermatozoa. The present report has
demonstrated that such studies are possible to perform. A good

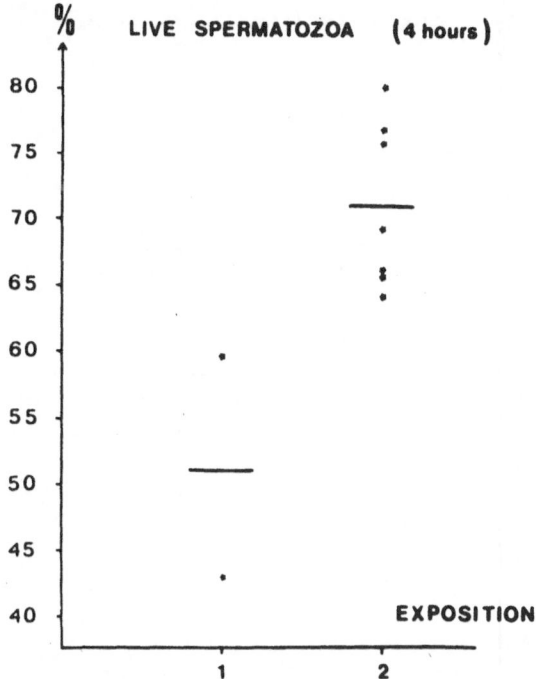

Figure 5 Distribution of percentage live spermatozoa in semen
         samples from non-exposed (1) and exposed (2) men.
         Assessment was made four hours after ejaculation.

contact with both management and union was established and all men
selected were given relevant and straightforward information about
the aim, methods, limitations of the methods and aspects related to
the study.

    Despite the efforts to obtain a control group which matched the
exposed group, there was a clear difference between them. In the
control group, ten men had symptoms of a present or past urogenital
infection, but none in the exposed group reported or showed similar
symptoms. One possible explanation for this difference could be
that for men in the exposed group, the exposure in itself was a
sufficient motivation for participating, but in the control group,
the men with acute or previous symptoms were more eager to
participate than those without any symptoms. A larger number of men
with urogenital problems in the control group could explain the
difference between the semen samples from the two groups with regard
to sperm motility and viability. It is well known that men with
prostatitis more frequently have semen with lower sperm motility and
viability.

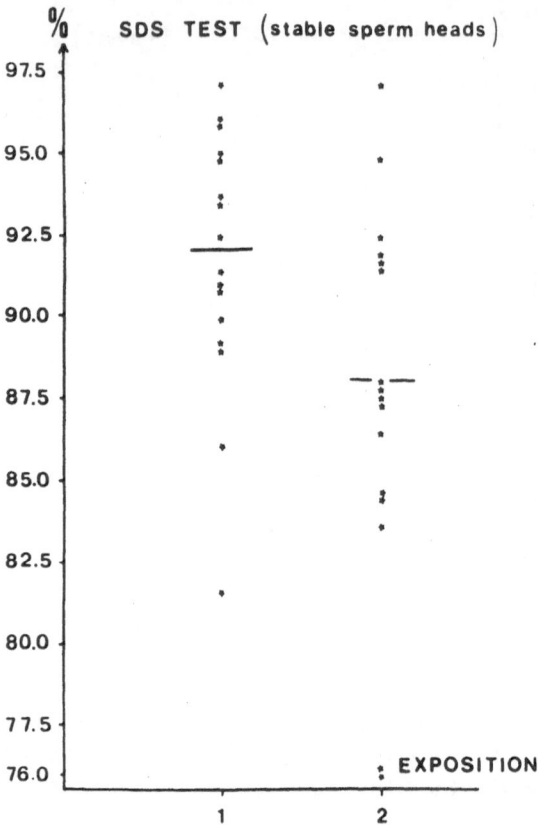

Figure 6   Distribution of percentage stable sperm heads in semen
           samples from non-exposed (1) and exposed (2) men. The
           samples were exposed to 1 percent dodecyl sulphate
           solution (SDS) for one hour.

     The resistance to SDS revealed a more interesting difference
between the two groups. According to our present opinions,
spermatozoa gain an increased resistance to SDS during their passage
through the epididymides. The resistance against SDS could thus be
seen as a test of "functional maturation". Despite the fact that
all semen samples had a percentage of stable spermatozoa within the
limits regarded as normal for a population of men whose wives were
in early pregnancy, there was a significant difference between the
two groups. This indicates that lead could interfere with the
maturation process, i.e., by interacting with zinc. Further studies
in animal models are needed to clarify this particular problem.

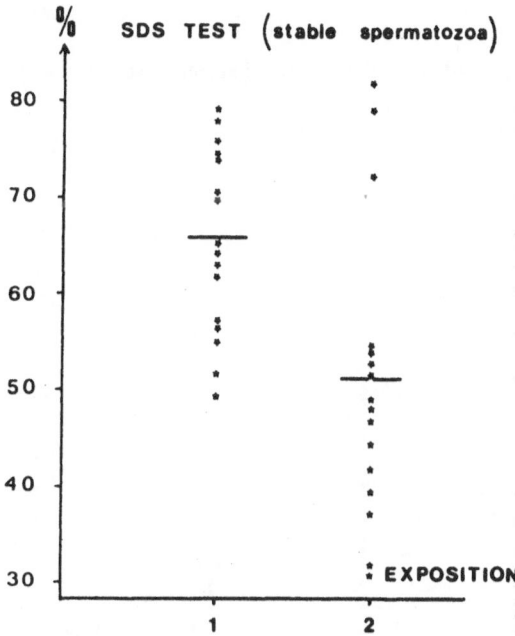

Figure 7 Distribution of percentage stable spermatozoa in semen
samples from non-exposed (1) and exposed (2) men. The
samples were exposed to 1 percent sodium dodecyl sulphate
(SDS) for one hour.

It is difficult to assess the significance of the finding that
a decreased secretory function of the accessory genital glands
occurred more frequently among the exposed men than among the
controls. However, it should be noted that Kvist and Eliasson
(1980) demonstrated a correlation between decreased prostatatic
function and the decreased resistance of spermatozoa to SDS. The
lower resistance of spermatozoa to SDS in the exposed group could
therefore be due not only to an interference on the epididymal level
but also to the secretory dysfunction of the accessory gential
glands. The results from the investigations showed that a moderate
exposure to lead, as defined according to Swedish law, does not give
changes in semen samples that are of clinical importance; the
fertility of the exposed men did not seem to be influenced. To
clarify whether the decrease in the semen volume and in the
secretory function of the prostate and seminal vesicles are the
result of the exposure to lead, one has to perform perspective
studies on men from the start to cessation of lead exposure.

In this study, we have not measured effects on sexual hormone
balance. In a recent study on battery storage plant workers,

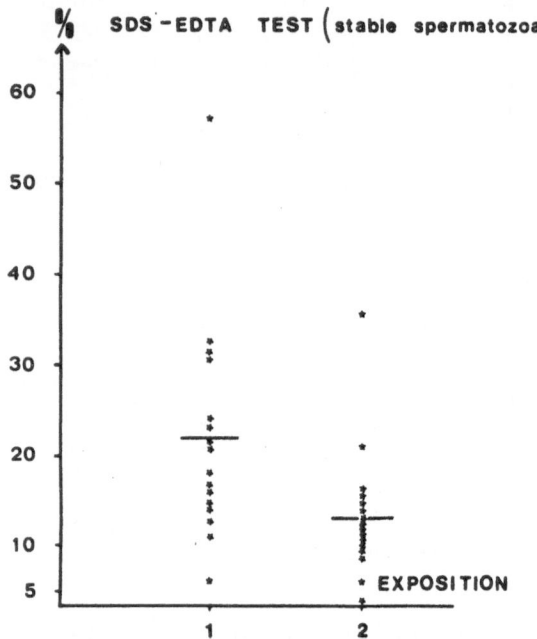

Figure 8 Distribution of percentage stable spermatozoa. The samples
were first exposed to EDTA and then to a 1 percent sodium
dodecyl sulphate (SDS) solution for 1 hour.

Molinini et al. (1981) reported testosterone, FSH, LH and prolactin
values in blood plasma of lead-exposed workers. They found no
difference for these variables in comparison with those of a
reference group.

CONCLUSION

The results show that studies of qualities of semen samples
from men exposed to xenobiotic factors can be performed if adequate
techniques for information and sampling are employed. Moderate lead
exposure close to present occupational health standards causes
subtle changes in some semen parameters, indicating direct or
indirect effects of lead on accessory genital glands function and
sperm maturation. The functional significance of the observed
changes is unknown.

REFERENCES

Altamura, B., Gagliano Candela, R. and Assennato, G., 1978, Acta of
    the conference about "Hazards and Toxicity by Lead Pollution",
    p. 229, M. Negri Institute, Milan.
Belsey, M.A., Eliasson, R., Gallegos, A.J., Moghissi, K.S., Paulsen,
    C.A. and Prasad, M.R.N., 1980, WHO Laboratory Manual for the
    Examination of Human Semen and Semen-cervical Mucus Interaction,
    Press Concern, Singapore.
Blumberg, W.E., Eisinger, J., Lamola, A.A. and Zucherman, D.M., 1977,
    The hematofluorometer, Clin. Chem. 23:270-274.
Braunstein, G., Dahlgren, J. and Loriaux, D.L., 1978, Hypogonadism
    in chronically lead-poisoned men, Infertility, 1:33-51.
Eisinger, J., Blumberg, W., Fischbein, A., Lilis, R. and Selikoff,
    I., 1978, Zinc-protoporphyrin in blood as a biological
    indicator of chronic lead intoxication, J. Environ. Pathol.
    Toxicol. 1(6):897-910.
Eliasson, R., 1981, The analysis of semen, in: "The Testis",
    (Comprehensive Endocrinology), H. Burger and D. deKretser,
    eds., pp. 381-399, Raven Press, New York.
Eliasson, R. and Treichl, L., 1971, Supravital staining of human
    spermatozoa, Fertil. Steril. 22:134-137.
Eliasson, R., Haggman, K. and Wiklund, B., 1967, Lactate
    dehydrogenase in human seminal plasma, Scand. J. Clin. Lab.
    Invest. 20:353-359.
Eliasson, R., Eliasson, L. and Virji, N., 1980, LDH-x in human
    seminal plasma as an indicator of the functional integrity of
    spermatozoa, (Abstract) J. Andrology 1:76.
Eyden, B.P., Maisin, J.R. and Mattelin, G., 1978, Long-term effects
    of dietary lead acetate on survival, body weight and seminal
    cytology in mice, Bull. Env. Contam. Toxicol. 19:266-272.
Hildebrand, D.C., Der, H., Griffin, W. and Fahim, M.S., 1973, Effect
    of lead acetate on reproduction, Am. J. Obst. Gynecol.
    115:1058-1065.
Karvonen, M.J. and Malm, M., 1955, Colorimetric determination of
    fructose with indol, Scand. J. Clin. Lab. Invest. 7:305-307.
Kvist, U., 1980, Sperm nuclear chromatin decondensation ability,
    Acta Physiol. Scand. suppl. 486:1-24.
Kvist, U. and Eliasson, R., 1980, Influence of seminal plasma on the
    chromatin stability of ejaculated human spermatozoa, Int. J.
    Andrology 3:130-142.
Lancranjan, I., Popescu, H.I., Gavenescu, O., Klepsch, I. and
    Serbanescu, M., 1975, Reproductive ability of workmen
    occupationally exposed to lead, Arch. Environ. Health
    30:396-401.
Lindholmer, C. and Eliasson, R., 1972, Zinc and magnesium in human
    spermatozoa, Int. J. Fertil. 17:153-160.
MacLeod, J., 1964, Human seminal cytology as a sensitive indicator
    of the germinal epithelium, Int. J. Fertil. 9:281.

Molinini, R., Assennato, G., Altamura, M., Gagliano Candela, R., Gagliardi, T. and Paci, C., 1981, Lead effects on male fertility in battery workers, Communication at the International Occupational Health Congress, Cairo.

Monkiewiez, J., Jaczewski, S. and Dynarowicz, I., 1975, Content of heavy metals in the semen of bulls from various environments, Med. Weter 31:681-686.

Oliver, T., 1911, Lead poisoning and the race, B. Med. J. May 13, 1096-1099.

Plechaty, M.M., Noll, B. and Sunderman Jr, F.W., 1977, Lead concentrations in semen of healthy men without occupational exposure to lead, Ann. Clin. Lab. Sci. 7:515-518.

Rom, W.N., 1976, Effects of lead on the female and reproduction: A review, Mt. Sinai J. Med. 43:542-552.

Ruse, M., Suciu, I. and Zegreanu, O., 1977, Zur Mitbeteiligung von Gonaden bei Chronischen Vergiftungen mit Schwermetallen, Zschr. Inn. Med. 32:469-470.

Sandstead, H.H., Orth, D.N., Abe, K. and Stiel, J., 1970, Lead intoxication: effect on pituitary and adrenal function in man, (Abstract) Clin. Res. 18:76.

Stowe, H.D., Goyer, R.A. and Krigman, M.M., 1973, Experimental oral lead toxicity in young dogs, Arch. Pathol. 95:106-116.

CADMIUM AND REPRODUCTION: A PERSPECTIVE AFTER 25 YEARS

Jiri Parizek

Institute of Nuclear Biology and Radiochemistry
Czechoslovak Academy of Sciences
Prague, Czechoslovakia

ABSTRACT

Research on cadmium and reproduction, which started a quarter of a century ago, is discussed from the viewpoint of the model situations produced by, and the mechanisms possibly involved in, the reproductive effects of cadmium.

The fact that a single parenteral dose of cadmium produces similar effects in the testes, in the non-ovulating ovaries of prepubertal rats and rats in persistent oestrus, and in the placentae, is of importance for any consideration of the mechanisms involved. The selective toxic syndrome observed in cadmium-treated rats towards the end of pregnancy is strictly dependent on the presence of the placenta. The interactions of cadmium with zinc and selenium are reviewed. The difference between a single dose and repeated or long-term exposure to cadmium is considered in relation to metallothionein. The use of parenteral cadmium administration as a tool for research on reproduction and development is discussed.

INTRODUCTION

Please allow me first to express my thanks for the invitation to address this meeting - in my personal capacity - on the subject of cadmium and reproduction. It is now more than 25 years since the publication of the first reports (Parizek and Zahor, 1956; Parizek, 1957) on the rapidly progressing necrosis of the testes induced by a single subcutaneous injection of cadmium salts. A certain caution is needed when a scientific problem has to be revisited after several decades. A quarter of a century is a long time in modern science and in the life of man, and the questions asked and the pathway used when approaching the problems in the past have to be understood in this historical perspective.

The main reason for the work described, at least in the first papers, was scientific curiosity. It was felt (Parizek, 1960) that cadmium could be used as a probe, a tool in research on gonadal function, in the sense of a "localized intoxication" in experimental research, a general methodological principle which was conceived by Fontana, J. Muller, and in particular by Claude Bernard in the last century. This approach should explain the mode of administration of cadmium salts and the dose used; the dose had to be high enough to get a clear-cut effect combined with a good survival of intoxicated animals, and this did not seem feasible with peroral administration. For the sake of clarity, I will restrict my presentation to the very specific effects obtained after parenteral administration of a single dose of cadmium salts.

Even with this restriction, the time and space allotted for this presentation does not allow me to mention all the results, and to pay adequate tribute to all those papers which have been published since the appearance of the first reports on cadmium and reproduction. However, I understand that the task given to me is to re-examine a few selected questions posed in the first original papers in the light of present experience referring, for a more detailed review, to some other publications (Parizek, 1960, 1969, 1972; Gunn and Gould, 1967, 1970; Friberg et al., 1974, 1975). In addition, more recent results of studies on biochemical and ultrastructural aspects of cadmium action, on teratogenic effects of cadmium, and results of animal studies with long-term exposure to metals will be presented in certain other papers at this meeting.

There is one rather personal reason why I am particularly glad to come to speak on cadmium in Rochester. The work on cadmium brought me into a long-lasting personal contact with a most noble man and a great scientist, who, for a long time was connected with scientific life at this University, and who contributed, among many other scientific achievements, to a better understanding of the reproductive effects of cadmium (Mason et al., 1964; Mason and Young, 1967). May I pay here today, a special tribute to the memory of the late Professor Karl E. Mason.

GONADAL EFFECTS OF CADMIUM SALTS

It is now well established that parenteral injection of a single dose of cadmium salts results in complete necrosis of the testes. The dose used in our experiments - usually 20 or 40 μmole per kg body weight - was quite high, however, well survived by both male and non-pregnant female rats. Most of the experiments were done on rats, but similar testicular effects of cadmium were also seen in mice, guinea-pigs, golden hamsters, and rabbits (Parizek, 1960).

Already within the first few hours following the injection, a vascular reaction occurs characterized by oedema and, later, haemorrhages. The complete destruction of tubules with spermiogenic epithelium results, of course, in permanent sterility. However, androgen-producing elements gradually regenerate, forming large masses of Leydig cells underneath the tunica albuginea, several months after cadmium injection. Details of these studies, including descriptions of the vascular reaction, necrosis of the testes, new formation of large masses of Leydig cells, and related endocrine effects, were already included in the first reports on the testicular effects of cadmium (Parizek, 1960). In some later studies, the masses of Leydig cells, observed after cadmium administration or surgical ligation of the testes vasculature, were considered to be testicular interstitial cells tumours (Gunn et al., 1963, 1965; Gunn and Gould, 1967).

In contrast to males, the parenteral administration of an equimolar dose of cadmium salts to adult female rats does not result in subsequent sterility (Parizek, 1957, 1960). However, Kar and his co-workers (1959) reported that parenteral administration of cadmium salts to prepubertal rats resulted in ovarian haemorrhages. Confirming these results on prepubertal rats, we suspected that cyclic processes connected with ovulation could modify the sensitivity of the adult ovary towards cadmium. To test this possibility, the single 20 or 40 μmole per kg body weight dose of cadmium salts was given parenterally to adult female rats in persistent oestrus, induced by a well known method of androgen administration within the first days of postnatal life. In all of these non-ovulating adult rats in persistent oestrus, cadmium administration resulted in massive ovarian haemorrhages, localized in the theca folliculi and in the ovarian interstitium (Parizek et al., 1968b). Whatever the response mechanism could be, it is clear that even the adult ovaries could be induced to react to cadmium in a similar way as do the testes.

The typical gonadal damage was also produced - both in males and in females in persistent oestrus - when cadmium was given to animals after hypophysectomy (Parizek, 1960; Parizek et al., 1968b), indicating that the cadmium effect is not mediated through, or dependent on the hypophysis, but rather is determined by a certain quality of the gonads as such.

CADMIUM SALTS ADMINISTRATION DURING PREGNANCY

In further experiments, the question was whether the same metabolic situation, the same specific characteristics of the target tissue responsible for the reaction of the gonads to cadmium, could be present in the placenta. Our experiments revealed that parenteral administration of cadmium salts to pregnant rats resulted in haemorrhages and destruction of the fetal part of the placenta with death of fetuses (Parizek, 1964). In addition, towards the end of pregnancy, cadmium administration resulted in a specific lethal syndrome affecting a high proportion of pregnant rats, characterized by convulsions, lung oedema, and bilateral haemorrhagic renal necrosis (Parizek, 1965; Parizek et al., 1968a). Similar effects were not observed in cadmium-treated, non-pregnant rats or in rats given cadmium salts after delivery (Figures 1, 2 and Table 1). In addition, no similar reaction was observed in pregnant rats, when cadmium was given after hysterectomy or after removal of the fetuses with placentae from the uteri. However, removal of fetuses only, leaving the placentae in situ, was not sufficient to abolish this peculiar reaction (Table 2), indicating that the syndrome is strictly dependent on the presence of the placenta in the pregnant rat, and resulting most probably from the placental damage produced by cadmium. However, it cannot be excluded at present that the placenta could sensitize the pregnant organism to the effects of cadmium, also by other mechanisms (Figure 3).

POSSIBLE MECHANISMS OF ACTION AND PERSPECTIVES

Table 3 summarizes the effects of parenteral administration of a single dose of cadmium which are related to reproduction. What conclusion can be drawn from these experiments performed and described a long time ago, and what can be envisaged as a perspective for research on cadmium and reproduction?

For any consideration of the mode of action of cadmium, it should be noted that parenteral administration of cadmium salts can induce selective and, for cadmium, specific damage in different organs connected with reproduction: in the testes and the spermatozoa-containing epididymis, in the non-ovulating ovaries of prepubertal rats or rats in persistent oestrus, and in the placentae. The character of the changes induced indicates that the mechanisms of action of cadmium must rely on some common denominator present in all these organs. In addition to this conclusion, several other facts have to be taken into consideration when attempting to identify the mechanisms involved. These include the development of the ability of the testes to respond to parenteral cadmium administration associated with the ontogenetic development during the second decade (days 10-20) of postnatal life of rats, (Parizek, 1960) as well as genetic determinants of resistance to testicular effects of cadmium in inbred mice (Taylor et al., 1973).

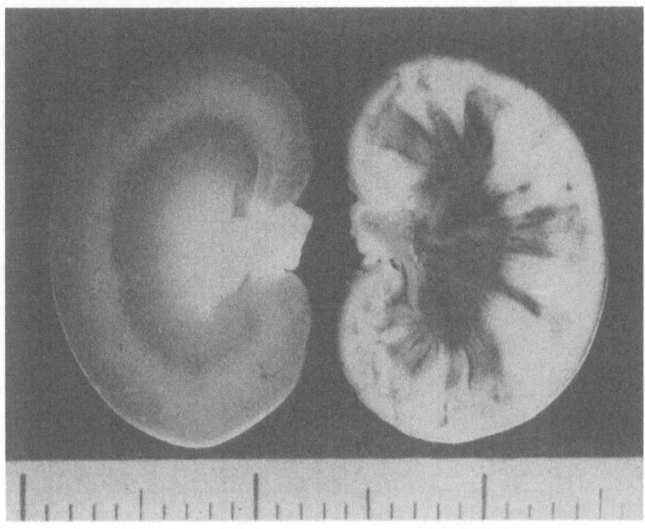

A   B

Figure 1   Toxic effects of cadmium administration during pregnancy:
           renal effects. Kidneys of rats (Wistar, Konarovice), 3
           days after subcutaneous injection of 40 μmole cadmium
           acetate/kg body weight. Left: non-pregnant rat; right:
           rat given cadmium on the 20th day of pregnancy. For a
           detailed description of the toxic syndrome including early
           death of some rats during the first day after injection
           and development of renal effects with resulting death
           about 4 days after cadmium injection, see Parizek, 1965
           and Parizek et al., 1968a.

As already stated in the first reports, vascular changes could
be observed within the first hours following cadmium injection and
they can be regarded as a triggering mechanism involved in further
damage (Parizek and Zahor, 1956; Parizek, 1957, 1960). A number of
further studies, reviewed in detail elsewhere, (Mason et al., 1964;
Mason and Young, 1967; Gunn and Gould, 1967, 1970; Friberg et al.,
1974, 1975) have underlined the role of the vascular system in
cadmium-induced testicular necrosis. However, the basic question
discussed two decades ago (Parizek, 1960) still remains: what makes
the vascular system in several different reproductive organs so
sensitive to cadmium action   In other words, is a specific
molecular target present in the vascular bed in these organs, or is
the vascular system sensitized to cadmium action by some local
factor, or is the vascular effect induced by an intermediate? It
should be noted in this connection that already two decades ago,

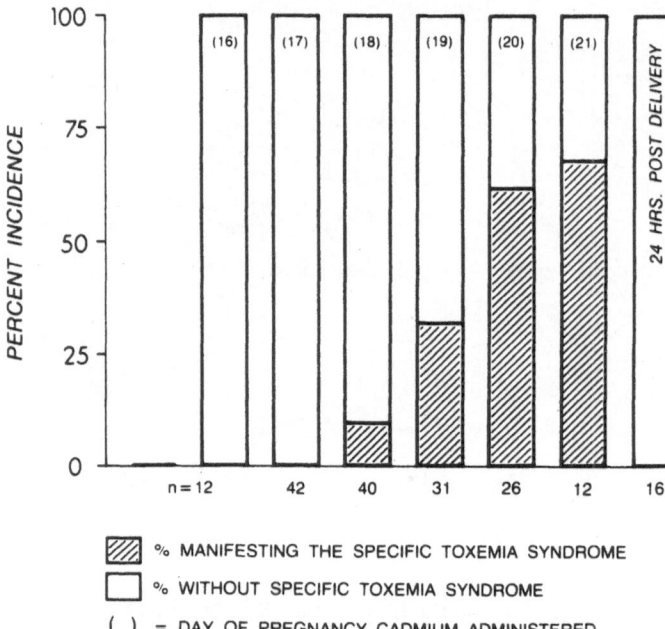

Figure 2 The specific lethal "Toxaemia" syndrome: dependence of
          the incidence of the selective toxic effect of cadmium on
          the stage of pregnancy. Animals showing specific toxic
          effects. Cadmium acetate was given subcutaneously as a
          single dose of 40 μmole/kg body weight as determined on
          the first day of pregnancy. For details, see Parizek,
          1965, 1969; Parizek et al., 1968a, 1969b.

          n = the number of animals injected on each day.

evidence was presented (Berlin and Ullberg, 1963) indicating uptake
of administered cadmium in the testicular interstitium. More
recently, it has been observed that dilatation of interendothelial
clefts in the small vessels of the testes can be detected as early
as 15 minutes after intravenous injection of cadmium salts (Gabbiani
et al., 1974).

    When discussing the mechanism of action of cadmium, it should
be noted that the effects of cadmium on the testes and other
reproductive organs can be prevented by administration of zinc salts
(Parizek, 1957, 1960) and also by administration of selenium
compounds (Kar et al., 1960; Mason et al., 1964; Mason and Young,

Table 1 The Toxic Effects of Cadmium During Pregnancy: Percentage of Rats Manifesting the Specific Lethal "Toxaemia" Syndrome

Subcutaneous Injection on the	Dose of Cadmium Acetate (μmole/kg body weight)		
	20	30	60
17th day of pregnancy	0% (3)	0% (12)	0% (9)
20th day of pregnancy	69% (35)	92% (13)	50% (4)

The numbers in brackets indicate the total number of animals in the group. In all animals, the typical placental damage and death of the fetuses were observed. For detailed description, see Parizek, 1965, 1969; Parizek et al., 1968a, 1969b.

Table 2 The Dependence of the Specific Lethal "Toxaemia" Syndrome on the Presence of the Placenta

Subcutaneous Injection of Cadmium given after	Number of Animals	% Incidence of the Specific Syndrome
Total hysterectomy	14	0
Surgical removal of placentae and fetuses	14	0
Removal of fetuses only (leaving placentae in situ)	9	78

Cadmium acetate was given as a dose of 40 μmole/kg body weight as determined on the first day of pregnancy. The subcutaneous injection was given on the 21st day of pregnancy immediately after the surgery which was performed with ether anesthesia. For further details, see Parizek, 1965, 1969; Parizek et al., 1968a, 1969b.

A.

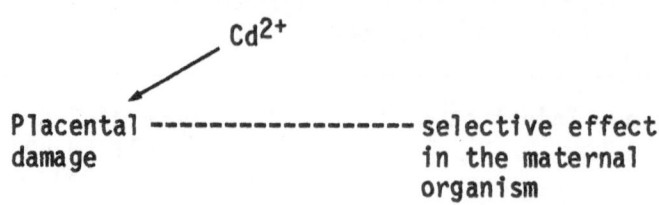

$$Cd^{2+}$$

Placental --------------------- selective effect
damage   in the maternal
                                organism

B.

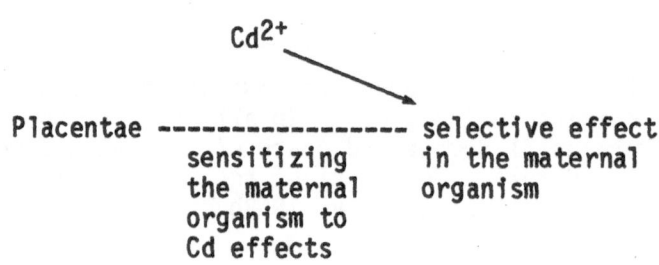

$$Cd^{2+}$$

Placentae ------------------ selective effect
          sensitizing   in the maternal
          the maternal   organism
          organism to
          Cd effects

C.   Combination of both mechanisms

Figure 3   Possible mechanisms involved in the dependency of the
           cadmium-induced selective lethal "Toxaemia" syndrome on
           the presence of the placenta.

1967). Zinc and selenium metabolism in the testes and other
reproductive organs deserve special attention (review Parizek, 1960;
NAS, 1976). However, the protective effect of zinc (Parizek et al.,
1969a) and also of selenium (Parizek et al., 1968a) is more general
in character and not confined to the reproductive organs. Moreover,
an interaction analogous to that between selenium and cadmium does
exist between selenium and inorganic salts of mercury, (Parizek and
Ostadalova, 1967; Parizek et al., 1971, 1974) and it is known, of
course, that salts of inorganic mercury do not produce the
reproductive damage typical for cadmium (Parizek, 1960, 1964;
Parizek et al., 1968b). From present knowledge, it is possible to
understand the protective action of zinc, and that of selenium, as
independent of the possible role of these trace elements in the
testes. The existence of extra-gonadal interactions discussed in
detail elsewhere, (Parizek and Ostadalova, 1967; Parizek et al.,
1969a,b, 1971, 1974; Nordberg, 1978) does not exclude, of course,
the possibility of cadmium effects being related to zinc and/or
selenium metabolism in the target tissues as well.

Table 3   Specific Reproductive Effects of Parenteral Administration
         of a Single Dose of Cadmium

Effects on gonads	Effects during pregnancy

Testes and epididymis:
    haemorrhagic necrosis
    (Parizek and Zahor,
    1956; Parizek, 1957,
    1960, 1969; Gunn and
    Gould, 1970)
	Placentae:
	    destruction of fetal parts
	    of placentae independent
	    of the presence of the fetus
	    but resulting in fetal death
	    (Parizek, 1964)

Ovaries of prepubertal rats:
    haemorrhagic necrosis
    (Kar et al., 1959)
	Selective lethal "toxaemia"
	    syndrome dependent on the
	    presence of placentae with
	    cadmium exposure from the 18th

Ovaries of rats in persistent
    oestrus:
    haemorrhagic necrosis
    (Parizek et al., 1968b)
	day of pregnancy in rats
	    (Parizek, 1965; Parizek et al.,
	    1968a, 1969b)

The first reports on the protection of the testes against
cadmium by parenteral administration of zinc (Parizek, 1957, 1960)
appeared before the discovery of metallothionein (Kagi and Vallee,
1960) and before the elucidation of the effects of exposure to
certain metals on the level of this protein, which is able to
sequester cadmium or certain other metals (review by Kagi and
Nordberg, 1979). As shown by Nordberg (1971), the injection of
cadmium-containing metallothionein does not produce the testicular
damage which results regularly from injection of inorganic cadmium
salts. However, metallothionein injection produces renal damage and
this switching of the target from the testis to the kidney,
resulting from binding of cadmium to thionein, is of pivotal
importance when interpreting the difference between a single
parenteral exposure to a high dose of cadmium and long-term exposure
through oral or respiratory pathway. The same mechanism could also
explain that not only zinc but also pretreatment with small doses of
cadmium can prevent the deleterious effects of cadmium on the testis
(Ito and Sawauchi, 1966; Nordberg, 1971; Webb, 1972).

After a quarter of a century, the effects of cadmium on
reproduction are still a challenging scientific problem. To clarify
why parenteral administration of cadmium results in specific damage
of certain reproductive organs, would help in understanding both

mechanisms, the action of cadmium in biological systems and the
specificity of the metabolic situation within the affected organs.

In addition, cadmium administration produces model situations,
useful in studies on reproductive physiology and pathophysiology.
So, for instance, the conversion of the testis into a purely
endocrine organ is a rather unique situation, useful for studying
problems of reproductive endocrinology (Parizek, 1960) or even
behavior (Madlafousek et al., 1971). The question of the
sensitivity of the ovaries to cadmium remains of interest in
relation to the mechanism of action of gonadotrophins, ovarian
receptors, and ovulation. Further studies on the toxic syndrome
produced by cadmium selectively during the last period of pregnancy,
can be of interest from point of view of the involvement of the
placenta in the pathology of pregnancy. Finally, it is not without
interest that the studies on the clear-cut acute testicular effects
of cadmium were the first to reveal the antagonism between cadmium
and zinc, (Parizek, 1957, 1960) and led to new studies on the
interaction between cadmium and selenium (Kar et al., 1960; Mason et
al., 1964; Mason and Young, 1967; Gunn and Gould, 1967).

The pathway of exposure and the high doses used in the
experiments revealing acute reproductive effects are, of course,
quite different from the prevailing conditions of human exposure to
cadmium (Friberg et al., 1974, 1975). Furthermore, the recognition
of metallothionein (Kagi and Vallee, 1960; Kagi and Nordberg, 1979)
and its involvement in differences between the effects of
single-dose and repeated or long-term exposure (Nordberg, 1971) are
highly significant for the evaluation of the health risks in this
regard. However, this does not exclude the need for further
research on the mechanism of action of cadmium responsible for the
reproductive effects, as well as the need for further studies on
animals undergoing long-term exposure. The effects of cadmium
exposure during pregnancy seem to be of particular interest in this
respect.

Parenteral administration of cadmium remains an interesting
experimental probe - and the effects a challenging problem of
nuclear biology. It is evident that certain physicochemical
qualities make the cadmium ion a useful tool in studies on
reproduction and on developmental mechanisms connected with
maturation.

A multifactorial approach is needed to understand the complex
sequence of pathogenetic processes resulting in gonadal and
epididymal necrosis, or in cadmium "toxaemia". The presence or
absence of some of these processes at certain stages of ontogenesis
will determine the outcome of cadmium exposure. Some of the problems
raised by our old results (Parizek, 1969, 1972; Parizek et al.,
1969b) underline this developmental aspect and are very much alive in
our considerations today.

What is the new quality - determining the response to cadmium which appears in the developing testes during the second decade of postnatal life (Parizek, 1960)? What is the significance of the necrotising effect in the caput epididymis and its full development with maturation and the presence of spermatozoa (Parizek, 1969)? On the contrary, why is the prepubertal ovary so sensitive to cadmium (Kar et al:, 1959; Parizek et al., 1968b)? Why only after the completion of the 17th day of gestation, do pregnant rats start to respond to cadmium in a very unusual way (Parizek, 1965, 1969; Parizek et al., 1968a, 1969b) (Figure 2)?

I am grateful that I had the chance to discuss these questions for many years with Karl E. Mason. I deeply regret that he is not with us today.

REFERENCES

Berlin, M. and Ullberg, S., 1963, The fate of [109]Cd in the mouse, Arch. Environ. Health 7:686-693.

Friberg, L., Kjellstrom, T., Nordberg, G. and Piscator, G., 1975, Cadmium in the environment III - A toxicological and epidemiological appraisal, U.S. Environmental Protection Agency, Office of Research and Development, Washington, DC.

Friberg, L., Piscator, M., Nordberg, G. and Kjellstrom, T., 1974, "Cadmium in the Environment", 2nd ed., Chemical Rubber Company Press, Cleveland, OH.

Gabbiani, G., Badonnel, M.-C., Mathewson, S.M. and Ryan, G.B., 1974, Acute cadmium intoxication - early selective lesions of endothelial clefts, Lab. Invest. 30:686-695.

Gunn, S.A. and Gould, T.C., 1967, Specificity of response in relation to cadmium, zinc and selenium, in "Selenium in Biomedicine", O.H. Muth, ed., pp: 395-413, Avi Publishing Co., Westport, CN.

Gunn, S.A. and Gould, T.C., 1970, Cadmium and other mineral elements, in "The Testis", Vol. 3, A.D. Johnson, W.R. Gomes, and N.L. VanDemark, eds., pp. 377-481, Academic Press, New York.

Gunn, S.A., Gould, T.C. and Anderson, W.A.D., 1963, Cadmium-induced interstitial cell tumors in rats and mice and their prevention by zinc, J. Nat. Cancer Inst. 31:745-759.

Gunn, S.A., Gould, T.C. and Anderson, W.A.D., 1965, Comparative study of interstitial cell tumors of rat testis induced by cadmium injection and by vascular ligation, J. Nat. Cancer Inst. 35:329-335.

Ito, K. and Sawauchi, K., 1966, Inhibitory effects on cadmium-induced testicular damage by pretreatment with smaller cadmium doses, Okajimas Folia Anat. Jap. 42:107-117.

Kagi, J.H.R. and Nordberg, M., eds., 1979, "Metallothionein," Birkhauser Verlag, Basel, Boston, Stuttgart.

Kagi, J.H.R. and Vallee, B.L., 1960, Metallothionein: a cadmium- and zinc-containing protein from equine renal cortex, J. Biol. Chem. 235:3460-3465.

Kar, A.B., Das, R.P. and Karkun, J.N., 1959, Ovarian changes in
    prepubertal rats after treatment with cadmium chloride, Acta
    Biol. Med. Germ. 3:372-399.
Kar, A.B., Das, R.P. and Mukerji, F.N.I., 1960, Prevention of
    cadmium induced changes in the gonads of rat by zinc and
    selenium - a study in antagonism between metals in the
    biological system, Proc. Nat. Inst. Sci. India, Pt.
    B26(suppl.):40.
Madlafousek, J., Hlinak, Z. and Parizek, J., 1971, Sexual behaviour
    of male rats sterilized by cadmium, J. Reprod. Fertil.
    26:189-196.
Mason, K.E., Brown, J.A., Young, J.O. and Nesbit, R.R., 1964,
    Cadmium-induced injury of the rat testis, Anat. Rec.
    149:135-148.
Mason, K.E. and Young, J.O., 1967, Effectiveness of selenium and
    zinc in protecting against cadmium-induced injury of the rat
    testis, in "Selenium in Biomedicine", O.H. Muth, ed.,
    pp. 383-394, Avi Publishing Co., Westport, CN.
National Academy of Sciences, 1976, "Selenium", Washington, DC.
Nordberg, G.F., 1971, Effects of acute and chronic cadmium exposure
    on the testicles of mice, with special reference to protective
    effects of metallothionein, Environ. Physiol. Biochem.
    1:171-187.
Nordberg, G.F., 1978, Factors influencing metabolism and toxicity of
    metals, Environ. Health Perspect. 25:3-41.
Parizek, J., 1957, The destructive effect of cadmium ion on
    testicular tissue and its prevention by zinc, J. Endocrin.
    15:56-63.
Parizek, J., 1960, Sterilization of the male by cadmium salts,
    J. Reprod. Fertil. 1:294-309.
Parizek, J., 1964, Vascular changes at sites of oestrogen
    biosynthesis produced by parenteral injection of cadmium salts:
    the destruction of placenta by cadmium salts, J. Reprod.
    Fertil. 7:263-265.
Parizek, J., 1965, The peculiar toxicity of cadmium during pregnancy
    - an experimental "toxaemia of pregnancy" induced by cadmium
    salts, J. Reprod. Fertil. 9:111-112.
Parizek, J., 1969, Influence of trace amounts of metals on the
    reproductive function, in "Yearbook of the Czechoslovak Academy
    of Sciences", pp. 111-126, Academia, Publishing House of the
    Czechoslovak Academy of Sciences, Prague.
Parizek, J., 1972, Toxicological studies involving trace elements.
    A survey paper, in "Nuclear Activation Techniques in the Life
    Sciences", pp. 177-194, International Atomic Energy Agency,
    Vienna.
Parizek, J. and Zahor, Z., 1956, Effect of cadmium salts on
    testicular tissue, Nature 177:1036-1037.
Parizek, J. and Ostadalova, I., 1967, The protective effect of small
    amounts of selenite in sublimate intoxication, Experientia
    23:142-143.

Parizek, J., Ostadalova, I., Benes, I. and Babicky, A., 1968a, Pregnancy and trace elements: the protective effect of compounds of an essential trace element - selenium - against the peculiar toxic effects of cadmium during pregnancy, J. Reprod. Fertil. 16:507-509.

Parizek, J., Ostadalova, I., Benes, I. and Pitha, J., 1968b, The effect of a subcutaneous injection of cadmium salts on the ovaries of adult rats in persistent oestrus, J. Reprod. Fertil. 17:559-562.

Parizek, J., Benes, I., Kalouskova, J., Babicky, A. and Lener, J., 1969a, Metabolic interrelations of trace elements, the effect of zinc salts on the survival of rats intoxicated by cadmium, Physiol. Bohemoslov. 18:89-93.

Parizek, J., Benes, I., Ostadalova, I., Babicky, A., Benes, J. and Pitha, J., 1969b, The effect of selenium on the toxicity and metabolism of cadmium and some other metals, in "Mineral Metabolism in Paediatrics", D. Barltrop and W.L. Burland, ed., pp. 117-134, Blackwell Scientific Publications, Oxford and Edinburgh.

Parizek, J., Ostadalova, I., Kalouskova, J., Babicky, A. and Benes, J., 1971, The detoxifying effects of selenium: interrelations between compounds of selenium and certain metals, in "Newer Trace Elements in Nutrition", W. Mertz and W.E. Cornatzer, eds., pp. 85-122, Marcel Dekker, New York.

Parizek, J., Kalouskova, J., Babicky, A., Benes, J. and Pavlik, L., 1974, Interaction of selenium with mercury, cadmium and other toxic metals, in "Trace Element Metabolism in Animals - 2", G.W. Hoekstra, J.W. Suttie, H.E. Ganther and W. Mertz, eds., pp. 119-131, University Park Press, Baltimore, Butterworths, London.

Taylor, B.A., Heiniger, H.J. and Meier, H., 1973, Genetic analysis of resistance to cadmium-induced testicular damage in mice (37380), Proc. Soc. Exp. Biol. Med. 143:629-633.

Webb, M., 1972, Protection by zinc against cadmium toxicity, Biochem. Pharmacol. 21:2767-2771.

SESSION 2. EFFECTS OF METALS ON THE FEMALE REPRODUCTIVE SYSTEM

Chairpersons: *Donald R. Mattison and Allen H. Gates*

OVARIAN TOXICITY: EFFECTS ON SEXUAL MATURATION, REPRODUCTION AND MENOPAUSE

Donald R. Mattison

Pregnancy Research Branch
National Institute of Child Health and Human Development
Bethesda, Maryland

ABSTRACT

The ability to become pregnant requires the integrated functioning of the hypothalamus, pituitary, ovary, fallopian tubes, uterus and cervix. Successful completion of reproduction with the birth of a living infant requires a more complex sequence of integrated events involving the complete maternal organism. The ovary as the repository of oocytes, as well as the source of hormones which control the functional development of the maternal organs, plays a major role in fertility and initiation of a successful gestation. In this section, I will review the development of the ovary, and mechanisms of integrated function along the hypothalamic-pituitary-ovarian-uterine axis in the sexually mature individual. Selected examples of reproductive dysfunction following prenatal and/or postnatal exposure to toxins, including metals, or experiments of nature will be discussed. The comparison of these examples of toxic and spontaneous reproductive dysfunction help in assigning the site of reproductive toxicity. Cooperation between reproductive biologists, pharmacologists, and toxicologists will be required to explore the mechanisms of reproductive toxicity. Hazards to human reproduction can only be determined by extrapolation from experiments in rodents, carefully designed studies in non-human primates, or close observation and follow up of environmentally, accidentally or occupationally exposed populations.

INTRODUCTION

The ability to become pregnant requires integrated functioning of the hypothalamus, pituitary, ovary, fallopian tubes, uterus and cervix (Figure 1). Successful completion of reproduction with the birth of a living infant requires a more complex sequence of integrated events involving the complete maternal organism. The ovary as the repository of oocytes, as well as the source of hormones which control the functional development of the maternal organs, plays a major role in fertility and initiation of a successful gestation. In this section, I will review the development of the ovary and mechanisms of integrated function along the hypothalamic-pituitary-ovarian-uterine axis in the adult. Selected examples of prenatal and postnatal ovarian toxicity produced by metals and other xenobiotics, and experiments of nature will be presented and compared to demonstrate the effects of toxins on fertility and reproductive function. Although data from experimental animals (both rodents and primates) will be reviewed in this section, my constant point of reference will always be primate reproduction. Interested readers are referred to several recent reviews of reproductive biology (Greep and Astwood, 1973; Greep and Koblinski, 1977; Yen and Jaffe, 1978), reproductive toxicology (Dixon, 1980; Messite and Bond, 1980; Mattison, 1981a, 1982), ovarian function (Jones, 1978; Zuckerman and Weir, 1977) and gonadal metabolism of xenobiotics (Heinrichs and Juchau, 1980). Growing interest and concern about xenobiotic hazards to reproduction has led to the establishment of a medical letter devoted to reproductive toxicology (Fabro and Brown, 1982).

OVARIAN DEVELOPMENT

The development of the ovary begins early in the first third of gestation with migration of primordial germ cells from an extra-embryonic location near the yolk sac into the hind gut region of the embryo (Gondos, 1978; Merchant-Larios, 1978). Differential tissue growth and continued migration of the primordial germ cells in response to an uncharacterized chemo-attractant bring the germ cells into the urogenital ridge. Cessation of germ cell migration in the urogenital ridge may result from recognition of cells in this region, or be controlled simply by the gradient of the chemo-attractant. Both during migration, and after reaching the urogenital ridge, germ cells proliferate. Embryonic or urogenital ridge controls of germ cell proliferation are not understood, however, evidence to be discussed later suggests that there may be some ability of primordial germ cell or oogonial number to respond to ovarian toxicants by continued proliferation, replacing destroyed cells (Mandl, 1964; Felton et al., 1978).

Oogonial Differentiation

After taking up residence in the urogenital ridge, primordial germ cells differentiate into oogonia, precursors of the oocytes. For some time after differentiation, oogonia will also proliferate. Oogonial proliferation, however, is somewhat different from the

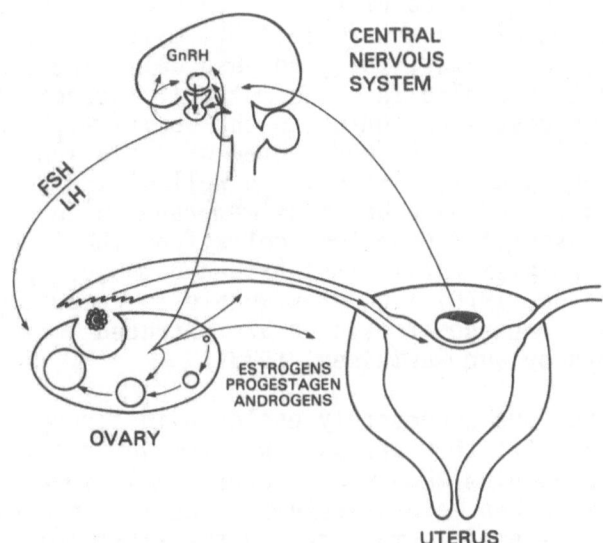

Figure 1   Schematic of the female primate reproductive system.
           Pulsatile release of GnRH by the hypothalamus appears
           to play a major role in the ovarian cycle. Estrogen
           and progesterone produced by the dominant follicle/
           corpus luteum control gonadotropin release for ovula-
           tion and endometrial proliferation in preparation for
           implantation.

proliferation of other cells in that after mitosis the daughter
cells do not separate but remain attached to each other by
cytoplasmic bridges (Gondos, 1978). This appears similar to the
proliferation of spermatogonia with interconnecting cytoplasmic
bridges observed in Sertoli cells (Burgos and Fawcett, 1955). These
interconnecting cytoplasmic bridges observed between oogonia
represent one of several kinds of specialized cell-cell contact
utilized in the reproductive system for communication and metabolic
support. These interconnecting cytoplasmic bridges also help explain
the frequent observation of nests of follicles in the ovary, and may
be responsible for the formation of follicles containing more than
one oocyte.

Folliculogenesis and Initiation of Meiosis

     At some point during oogonial proliferation, all of the
interconnected oocytes within a syncytial mass will recruit
granulosa cells from the surrounding ovarian stroma and enter
meiosis. The mechanism of this process, termed folliculogenesis or

the formation of follicle complexes, is unknown. Just as
proliferating oogonial cells were in close metabolic association
through cytoplasmic bridges, the granulosa cells and oocyte found in
a follicle complex are also in close metabolic association through
granulosa cell processes extending to the oocyte membrane (Brower
and Schultz, 1982). Some further degree of isolation of the oocyte
from the surrounding ovarian stroma, as well as the general
circulation is provided by a basement membrane which surrounds each
oocyte and its associated granulosa cells from the time of formation
of the follicle complex until it is broken down just prior to
ovulation (Bjersing, 1978). Oocytes unable to recruit granulosa
cells for support undergo atresia or are extruded from the surface
of the ovary (Byskov and Rasmussen, 1973).

    Oocytes which are successfuly enclosed in a supporting follicle
continue meiosis until they are part way through the first meiotic
division. These oocytes then become arrested in meiosis until just
prior to ovulation when meiosis resumes. Just before ovulation, the
first meiotic division is completed and the first polar body is
extruded. The second meiotic division is completed near the time of
fertilization, with subsequent formation of the second polar body.
Oocytes therefore remain arrested in meiosis for a minimum of 12 to
13 years and as long as 30 to 35 years, before ovulation and
fertilization (Schwartz and Mayaux, 1982) or atresia. Anecdotal
reports have suggested that the duration of meiotic arrest may be
longer than 50 years in some women (Wharton, 1964). During this
long period of meiotic arrest, the primary oocyte remains vulnerable
to genetic and/or epigenetic damage which may destroy the oocyte
(Gulyas and Mattison, 1979), or impair its ability to develop after
fertilization.

    Profound differences in gametogenesis between the male and
female lead to differences in response to reproductive toxins. The
testis, in the absence to reproductive toxins, retains spermatogonia
and the capability of repopulating the testis with sperm throughout
the life of the male (Russell, this volume; Lee, this volume).
Complete destruction of sperm, with preservation of spermatogonia,
will result in temporary infertility (Mandl, 1964; Mattison, 1981b).
In the ovary after completion of folliculogenesis, which occurs in
the latter portion of gestation, no oogonial cells persist. The
ovary can not replace oocytes destroyed by toxins. In fact,
throughout the life of a female, the number of oocytes remaining in
the ovary is continuously decreasing until at menopause the ovary is
essentially depleted of oocytes (Block, 1951a,b, 1952). Complete
destruction of oocytes prepubertally will result in primary
amenorrhea, with failure to pass through puberty (Styne and
Grumbach, 1978). Complete destruction of oocytes after puberty will
produce premature ovarian failure or premature menopause and
subsequent infertility (Rebar, 1982; Chapman et al., 1979a,b).

Prenatal Ovarian Toxicity

Compounds which produce prenatal ovarian toxicity in humans as well as experimental anmals have been identified and are summarized in Table 1. Our understanding of the site and mechanism of action of these compounds is limited and they are presently identified by secondary effects resulting from absence of, or a considerable decrease in the number of oocytes. Although several experimental protocols have evaluated selected reproductive effects of prenatal exposure to metals, it is not known if they alter ovarian development.

Human syndromes associated with abnormal formation of the ovary, manifest by decreased oocyte number, are listed in Table 2. These syndromes provide clear demonstration of the clinical signs and symptoms which would be observed in a population of women exposed prenatally to a toxin which blocked germ cell migration, germ cell proliferation, urogenital ridge formation, oogonial differentiation, or folliculogenesis.

Table 1   Prenatal Ovarian Toxins

Compound	Endpoint	Species	Reference
Galactose	Fertility Oocyte Number	Human Rodent	Chen et al., 1982; Kaufman et al., 1981
Benzo(a)pyrene	Fertility Oocyte Number	Rodent (?Human)	Mackenzie and Angevine, 1981; Felton et al., 1978; Dobson et al., 1978; Mattison, 1982
Ionizing Radiation	Fertility Oocyte Number	Human Rodent	Mandl, 1964; Ash, 1980
6-Mercaptopurine	Fertility	Rodent	Reimers et al., 1980; Mattison et al., 1981c

Table 2   Human Syndromes Mimicking Prenatal Ovarian Toxicity

Human Syndrome	Clinical Features	Reference
Glactosemia	Amenorrhea Infertility (+/-) Hypergonadotropic Hypogonadism	Kaufman et al., 1981
Premature Ovarian Failure	Amenorrhea Infertility (+/-) Hypergonadotropic Hypogonadism	Rebar, 1982

Depending on the exent of oocyte destruction, or block to oocyte proliferation produced, the individuals will experience prepubertal, peripubertal or postpubertal ovarian failure. Morphologically, the ovary will have a monotonous afollicular appearance. Circulating levels of the gonadotropins (follicle-stimulating hormone and luteinizing hormone) will be elevated and ovarian hormones (estrogen and progesterone) will be decreased. In the absence of oocytes, these individuals will obviously be infertile, and depending on the age of ovarian failure, may fail to reach all or some of the pubertal milestones.

SEXUAL MATURATION AND HYPOTHALAMIC, PITUITARY, OVARIAN AND UTERINE FUNCTION

Ovulation and ovarian hormone production require integrated functioning of the hypothalamus, pituitary, and ovary. Higher centers of the central nervous system may also play a role in subtle modulation of the hypothalamic-pituitary-ovarian axis by integrating exogenous and endogenous stimuli. As ovarian function impacts directly on endometrial events which are readily appparent both to the patient and the physician, these events are frequently discussed simultaneously.

Prepubertal

The hypothalamus integrates a variety of stimuli including levels of ovarian hormones and responds with the release of gonadotropin-releasing hormone (GnRH) Knobil, 1980). At the present time, it is thought that a single releasing hormone controls the release of the two gonadotropic hormones, follicle stimulating hormone (FSH) and luteinizing hormone (LH). Although the mechanism by which a single releasing hormone would control the release of the two gonadotropins remains to be elucidated, it may involve differences in the pulse frequency and amplitude of GnRH release.

Prepubertally, the hypothalamus secretes little GnRH, and as a result, there are infrequent pulses of FSH and LG (Styne and Grumbach, 1978). The pituitary, however, is capable of responding to GnRH during this period with secretion of adult levels of gonadotropins (Wildt et al., 1980). During the peripubertal period, the frequency of GnRH pulsation increases as do the gonadotropins. The ovary, like the pituitary, appears fully competent shortly after birth, and responds to this increased stimulation with increased estrogen secretion. Finally, in the sexually mature organism, the GnRH pulse frequency and amplitude is such that it permits integrated functioning of the pituitary and ovary (Carmel et al., 1976).

Shortly after birth, in rodents and primates including humans, an elevation of FSH occurs (Fuller et al., 1982; Williams, 1980). Suppression of this elevation in rodents with lead or mercury has been associated with subsequent dysfunction of the reproductive system (Table 3A,B). Other xenobiotics (including diethylstilbestrol, certain halogenated polycyclic aromatic hydrocarbons and other estrogen agonists) can produce similar hypothalamic dysfunction in rodents (Table 4). As the mechanism and role of elevated FSH may differ considerably in rodents and primates, it is not known if prepubertal exposure to these compounds would alter subsequent reproductive function in humans (Mattison, 1981a). Prenatal treatment of women with DES appears to exert its major adverse effects on the developing vagina, cervix and uterus with minimal effects on the hypothalamus and pituitary (Mattison, 1981b).

Other factors may also modify the age-dependent sensitivity of the reproductive system. The prepubertal primate gonad is thought to be more resistant to gonadotoxic antitumor agents than the adult gonad (Mattison, 1981b). Age-dependent alterations in reproductive tract sensitivity to other toxins (including metals) may also occur. The mechanisms for the increased resistance of the prepubertal gonad may reside in a decreased rate of gonadal cell proliferation (Mattison, 1981b) or alterations in the distribution of the toxin to gonadal cells (Setchell and Sharp, 1981; Janson, 1975). For some toxins, the prepubertal gonad may be more sensitive than the sexually mature gonad. As an example, the level of glutathione is lower in the immature rodent gonad than in the mature gonad (Figure 2). Xenobiotics detoxified by glutathione may be more toxic to the developing than the developed gonad. The relationship between changing ovarian glutathione and prepubertal cadmium toxicity is not understood (Kar et al., 1959).

Table 3A   Effects of Lead on the Hypothalamic–Pituitary–Ovarian–Uterine Axis

Compound	Reproductive Effect	Site	Mechanism	Reference
Lead Acetate (po)	Delayed Vaginal Opening	Hypothalamus Pituitary	Decreased FSH	Grant et al., 1976
Lead Acetate (po)	Ovarian Atrophy	Ovary Hypothalamus Pituitary	Decreased FSH Direct Toxicity	Stowe and Goyer, 1971 Vermande-Van Eck and Meigs, 1960
Lead Acetate (po)	Decreased Fertility (blocked implanta- tion)	Ovary	Decreased Progesterone Secretion	Jacquet et al., 1977
Lead Acetate (iv)	Decreased Fertility (blocked implanta- tion)	Uterus	Increased Endometrial Estrogen Receptor	Wide, 1980
Triethyl Lead (po)	Decreased Fertility (blocked implanta- tion)	Uterus/Ovary	Unknown	Oldenbro and Kihlstrom, 1977

Table 3B   Effects of Mercury on the Hypothalamic-Pituitary-Ovarian-Uterine Axis

Compound	Reproductive Effect	Site	Mechanism	Reference
Mercuric Chloride (po)	Altered Ovarian Cycle	Ovary	Direct Toxicity	Stadnicka, 1980
Mercuric Chloride (sq)	Altered Ovarian Cycle	Ovary Hypothalamus	Direct Toxicity	Lamperti and Printz, 1973 Lamperti and Niewenhuis, 1976
Mercuric Nitrate	Altered Ovarian Cycle	Ovary	Direct Toxicity	Lach and Srebro, 1972
Methyl Mercuric Chloride	Altered Ovarian Cycle	Ovary	Direct Toxicity	Busta, 1979

Table 3C Effects of Cadmium on the Hypothalamic-Pituitary-Ovarian-Uterine Axis

Compound	Reproductive Effect	Site	Mechanism	Reference
Cadmium Chloride (ip)	Follicle Necrosis	Ovary	Vascular Toxicity	Copius Peereboom-Stegeman and Jongstra-Spaapen, 1979
	Microcirculation	Uterus	Vascular Toxicity	
Cadmium Chloride (ip)	Persistant Diestrus	Ovary Hypothalamus Pituitary	Unknown	Der et al., 1977
	Decreased Weight	Pituitary Ovary Uterus	Direct Toxicity	
Cadmium	Follicular Atresia	Ovary	Direct Toxicity	Kar et al., 1959
Cadmium Chloride (sq)	Follicle Necrosis (prepubertal) (persistent estrous)	Ovary	Direct Vascular Toxicity	Parizek et al., 1968
Cadmium Chloride (sq)	Ovarian Hemorrhage	Ovary	Direct Vascular Toxicity	Watanabe et al., 1977
	Blocked Ovulation (PMSG, HCG stimulated)	Ovary	Receptor Toxicity Vascular Toxicity	
	Aneuploidy	Ovary Oocyte	Unknown	

Table 4 Xenobiotics Toxic to the Hypothalamic-Pituitary-Ovarian-Uterine Axis

Compound	Mechanism	Site	Reference
Diethylstilbestrol	Prenatal Mutagenesis Estrogen Agonist	Prenatal Developing Reproductive Tract	Barrette et al., 1981 Haney et al., 1979 Herbst et al., 1971 Korach et al., 1979 Rudiger et al., 1979
	Postnatal Mutagenesis Estrogen Agonist	Postnatal Hypothalamus, Pituitary Endometrium	
Halogenated Polycyclic Hydrocarbons	Postnatal Estrogen Agonist Microsomal Mono-oxygenases	Hypothalamus Pituitary Liver	Kupfer, 1975
	Postnatal "Critical Period" Estrogen Agonist	Hypothalamus	Gellert and Heinrichs, 1975
Polycyclic Aromatic Hydrocarbons	Prenatal Chemical Reactivity	Developing Gonad	Mackenzie and Angevine, 1981
	Postnatal Chemical Reactivity Microsomal Monooxygenases	Ovary Liver	Mattison and Nightingale, 1982a Welch et al., 1971
Alkylating Agents	Prenatal/Postnatal Chemical Reactivity	Gonad	Sieber and Adamson, 1975 Chapman et al., 1979a,b

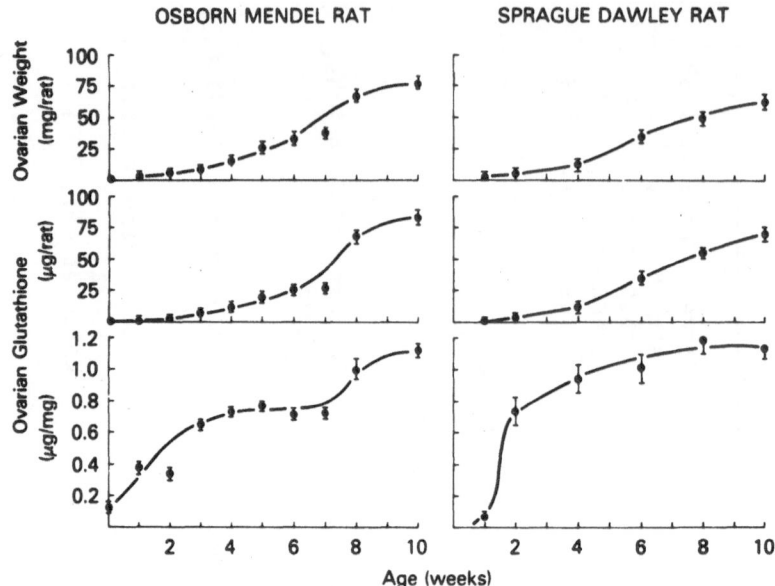

Figure 2   Ontogeny of ovarian glutathione in Osborn Mendel and
           Sprague-Dawley rats.   The animals were sacrificed at the
           indicated ages and ovarian glutathione determined by the
           method of Tietze (1969).   (D.R. Mattison, K. Shiromizu,
           J.A. Pendergrass and S.S. Thorgeirsson, personal
           communication).

The Ovarian Cycle

     Hormonal integration along the hypothalamic-pituitary-ovarian-
uterine axis is schematized in Figure 3.   As indicated, the
hypothalamus is thought to play a permissive role in the ovarian
cycle in primates.   In experimental situations with sexually
immature non-human primates, or in surgical preparations with the
hypothalamus isolated from the central nervous system, a GnRH pulse
interval of about 60 minutes will produce the appropriate pulsatile
release of gonadotropins into the circulation and support the
ovarian cycle (Knobil, 1980; Pohl and Knobil, 1982).

     If we consider day one of the cycle to be the first day of
menses and use the mid-cycle gonadotropin surge as the dividing
point of the cycle, we can conveniently explore the hormonal and
morphological alterations which occur during this period (Yen, 1978).
From the prospective of the ovary, the pre-surge interval is the
follicular phase, the post-surge interval the luteal phase.   In terms
of uterine events, the pre-surge interval is the proliferative phase,
the post-surge interval the secretory phase.

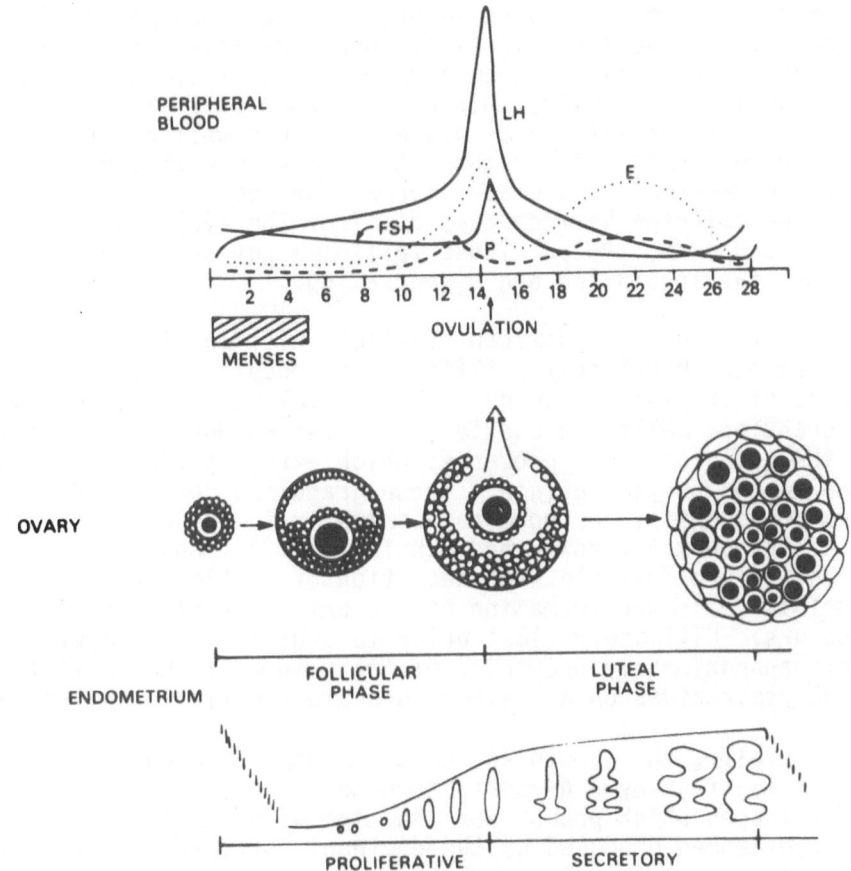

Figure 3   Schematic illustrating endocrine, ovarian and uterine
events during the primate ovarian cycle.

The Follicular or Proliferative Phase

The follicular or proliferative phase begins with menses.
Diminishing levels of progesterone and estrogen during the previous
cycle, have led to vasospasm of the spiral arterioles which support
the endometrium. Progressive vasospasm results in endometrial
necrosis, edema and eventual shedding during the first three to five
days of the cycle (Noyes et al., 1950).

Near the time of menses, a cohort of follicles begins to
develop. Follicular growth begins with enlargement of the
supporting granulosa cells, followed by granulosa cell
proliferation. Shortly after the onset of granulosa cell

proliferation, the oocyte begins to grow and the zona pellucida begins to develop. During this time, thecal cells which surround the follicle and represent the outermost component of the follicular complex begin to proliferate. Although a group of follicles begins to develop during the follicular phase, only one will develop sufficiently to respond to the gonadotropin surge with ovulation. This follicle destined to ovulate, termed the dominant follicle, is thought to be selected between days 5 - 7 of the cycle (diZerega and Hodgen, 1981; Hodgen, 1982). Those follicles not selected will undergo atresia, involuting and degenerating.

After selection, the dominant follicle will continue to grow by granulosa and thecal cell proliferation, oocyte growth and enlargement of the zona pelucida. The special interrelationship between granulosa cells and oocyte is maintained during this period through the granulosa cell processes which extend through the zona pellucida to the oocyte surface. These granulosa cell processes appear to be essential for hormonal communication to and metabolic support of the oocyte (Brower and Schultz, 1982). Continued development of the follicle with secretion of follicular fluid by the granulosa cells and formation of the antrum or fluid filled cavity occurs. Ultimately, just prior to ovulation, the cavity represents approximately one-third of the volume of the follicle, and the oocyte resides on a stalk of granulosa cells in this antrum.

Peripherally, the growth and development of the dominant follicle is manifest by a gradual, then more rapid increase in the level of estrogen which peaks near the time of ovulation. This increasing estrogen produced by the dominant follicle is responsible for endometrial proliferation and the changing levels of gonadotropins by first negative and then positive feedback on the hypothalamus and pituitary. The follicle complex, by its secretion of varying amounts of estrogen, plays the major controlling role in the menstrual cycle. As a reflection of this, the major variation in menstrual cycle length occurs during the pre-ovulatory phase (Yen, 1978). Following the mid-cycle gonadotropin surge, the time to menses is generally invariant and fixed at 14 days. Biologically, this is also reasonable as a gonadotropin surge in the absence of a ripe follicle serves no purpose. The follicle complex, containing the oocyte and secreting the hormones which control gonadotropin, release and synchronize the accessory organs of the reproductive tract, represents the cornerstone of the menstrual cycle. Abnormalities of development of the follicle complex during this period, through alteration in granulosa cell proliferation and estrogen secretion, have a profound influence on fertility during that cycle (diZerega and Hodgen, 1981a). Xenobiotics, like alkylating agents (Table 4) or heavy metals (Table 3), that are toxic to proliferating cells would be expected to alter the growth of the follicle complex, producing menstrual irregularities, aberrant luteal phase or amenorrhea.

Endometrial growth begins during the proliferative phase of the cycle. Under the influence of increasing levels of estrogen, the stroma and vascular elements as well as the glandular and epithelial components of the endometrium begin to develop. This estrogen-stimulated endometrial development progresses to the time of ovulation when the endometrium is penetrated by straight arterioles, and narrow, straight endometrial glands. The glandular cells have abundant secretions packaged in sub-nuclear vacuoles giving the appearance of an orderly arrangement of cobblestones surrounding the lumen of the gland.

Under the positive feedback of high levels of estrogen, the pituitary releases the pre-ovulatory mid-cycle surge of gonadotropins. As a result of this gonadotropin surge, the follicle gradually thins and finally breaks down on the surface of the ovary. This provides a route for release of the oocyte into the peritoneal cavity. Peri-ovarian neural and hormonal signals may act to position the fimbriated end of the fallopian tube over the dominant follicle to pick up the oocyte in its investing cumulus after ovulation. The gonadotropin surge and loss of the oocyte from the follicle produce a major change in the structure and function of the follicle. This change in the function of the follicle, manifest by decreased secretion of estrogen and increasing secretion of progesterone, produces significant changes in the accessory organs, including the endometrium.

The Luteal or Secretory Phase

Following ovulation, the basement membrane surrounding the granulosa cells breaks down and is penetrated by capillaries. The originally round compact granulosa cells differentiate into large polygonal corpus luteum cells and the luteal complex composed of thecal luteal cells and corpus luteum cells begins to secrete increasing quantities of progesterone. Under the influence of increasing quantities of progesterone, the structure of the endometrium begins to change.

During the luteal phase of the ovarian cycle, the thickness of the endometrium increases slightly. The arterial supply to the endometrium does increase, however, forming the characteristic spiral arteries by proliferation of the originally straight endometrial arteries. The length of the endometrial glands also increases, producing a convoluted tortuous gland. Glandular secretions, which were intially sub-nuclear and away from the lumen of the gland, move above the nucleus and are secreted into the lumen of the glands.

The endometrial stroma, which was edematous and relatively acellular following ovulation, becomes increasingly cellular with larger cuboidal cells. Stromal proliferation begins first in the

region of the spiral arteries, then spreads throughout the
endometrium. All of these changes produced by progesterone are
dependent on earlier modifications of the endometrium produced by
estrogen secretion during the proliferative phase, linking
endometrial development in the secretory phase to follicle complex
development during the proliferative phase. The biological rationale
for these changes in the endometrium is to prepare the uterus for
implantation and support of a fetus should fertilization occur. In
the absence of fertilization and support of the corpus luteum through
production of chorionic gonadotropin by the conceptus, luteal
function and progesterone secretion declines and the endometrium is
shed.

Toxicity to the Hypothalamic-Pituitary-Ovarian-Uterine Axis

The assessment of reproductive toxicity can be an extremely
difficult task. An instructive example of this difficulty occurs in
patients exposed prenatally to diethylstilbestrol (DES). A host of
studies have examined the male and female DES progeny, with
conflicting results (Mattison, 1981a,b). Careful analysis of the
data suggests that impaired reproductive function can occur in
exposed female offspring, and may occur in exposed male offspring.
The best data base is a group of patients who were participants in a
double-blind study in which both drug and placebo groups were
matched. Even with this study, design subtle defects which impair
fertility may be difficult to characterize. Similar well matched
groups will be difficult to obtain in settings of occupational or
environmental exposure.

Similarly, the time of evaluation of the selected end point may
influence the outcome. Xenobiotics which alter hypothalamic
patterning in rodents may not produce adverse reproductive effects
until several months after the attainment of sexual maturity
(Mattison, 1981a). Reproductive toxins may not alter functioning in
the non-stressed organisms but may produce profound alterations in
the reproductive performance of the stressed animal. For example,
the dynamic reproductive function of the non-pregnant animal may be
normal but the animal may be infertile because it cannot adapt to
the physiologic or metabolic demands of pregnancy. Just such a
mechanism may explain the increased rate of spontaneous abortion
among female metal workers over 30 years old compared to those
younger than 30 (Hemminki et al., this volume). The experiments of
Sunderman et al. (this volume), demonstrating decreased fetal weight
and hematocrit in offspring of female rats treated with nickel
subsulfate before breeding, also suggest that pre-pregnancy toxicity
can alter subsequent reproductive performance. As increasing numbers
of women are delaying their first pregnancy for schooling and/or
work, the effect of pre-pregnancy systemic toxicity on subsequent
metabolic adaptations to pregnancy becomes an increasing concern.

Because of these observations, it may be necesary to devise a variety of reproductive testing paradigms which evaluate reproductive performance in young and old, healthy and diseased, stressed and non-stressed animals.

Just as end points or sites for reproductive toxicity may be difficult to evaluate, the site or sites of toxic interaction may also be elusive. Because interactions along the hypothalamic-pituitary-ovarian-uterine axis are dynamic, impaired function may result from direct toxin interaction with one of these organs (Mattison, 1981a). For example, DES, a potent estrogen agonist can impair reproduction in the sexually mature female by inhibiting FSH and LH release at the level of the hypothalamus and pituitary (Table 4). Several halogenated hydrocarbons are also potent estrogen agonists and can alter hypothalamic function (Kupfer, 1975; Kimbrough, 1974). Impaired reproduction may also result indirectly as a result of metabolic alterations which disrupt hormonal interactions along the axis. This mechanism of action has been suggested for polycyclic aromatic and halogenated hydrocarbons (Mattison, 1981a; Welch et al., 1971) and also appears to account for the decreased effectiveness of oral contraceptives and increased clearance of replacement estrogens in patients using anticonvulsants (Aronson and Grahame-Smith, 1981).

Despite all these caveats, many xenobiotic compounds, including metals, have been implicated in reproductive dysfunction along the hypothalamic-pituitary-ovarian-uterine axis (Tables 3A,B,C and 4). The broad range of compounds listed on these tables demonstrates the vulnerability of the hypothalamic-pituitary-ovarian-uterine-endometrial axis to toxin insult. The nonmetal reproductive toxins are included with the metals for comparison of mechanism and site of action. The effects of these xenobiotics on the reproductive tract can also be evaluated by comparison to human syndromes of reproductive dysfunction (Table 5). These and other experiments of nature represent defined or partially characterized disorders of reproduction which provide a data base of clinical and endocrinological parameters essential for evaluation of reproductive toxins (Mattison and Ross, 1982).

Lead

Postnatal exposure to lead during the critical period for hypothalamic programming (Gorski, 1971) has been demonstrated to alter the development and function of the reproductive system in female rodents. The initial observation of delayed vaginal opening, a reflection of delayed ovarian estrogen secretion, suggested toxicity to the ovary, hypothalamus or pituitary (Grant et al., 1976). Subsequent investigation demonstrated decreased levels of circulating FSH during the pre-pubertal surge, and decreased pituitary content of FSH (Petrusz et al., 1979).

Table 5 Human Syndromes Mimicking Hypothalamic, Pituitary, Ovarian or Uterine Toxicity

Site	Syndrome	Clinical Features	Endocrine Parameters
Hypothalamus Pituitary	Hypogonadotropic Hypogonadism	Amenorrhea Anovulation	Decreased FHS, LH Decreased E, P
Ovary	Gonadotropin Resistant Ovary	Amenorrhea Anovulation Infertility	Increased FSH, LH Decreased E, P Follicles Present
	Oocyte Depletion: Premature Ovarian Failure Alkylating Agent Therapy Ionizing Radiation	Amenorrhea Menopausal	Increased FSH, LH Decreased E, P
	Corpus Luteum Inadequate Luteal Phase	Infertility Inadequate Endometrial Proliferation	Decreased P
	Polycystic Ovary	Anovulation	Decreased FSH, LH Increased E, T
Uterus	Endometrial Destruction Asherman's Syndrome	Amenorrhea Endometrial Cavity Scarring Infertility	Normal

Other investigators have also demonstrated that lead produces ovarian atrophy, suggesting that multiple sites of toxicity along the hypothalamic-pituitary-ovarian-endometrial axis are possible (Stowe and Goyer, 1971; Vermande-Van Eck and Meigs, 1960). Leonard et al. (this volume) and Jacquet et al. (1977) also have evidence suggesting that direct ovarian toxicity from lead, which decreases the secretion of progesterone, is responsible for endometrial alterations at the time of implantation.

Wide (this volume and 1980) has evidence suggesting that in addition to effects of progesterone secretion, lead also alters uterine estrogen receptors which may further impact on the initiation and maintenance of pregnancy. A similar impairment of implantation was observed in triethyl lead-treated mice (Odenbro and Kihlstrom 1977). The mechanism of reproductive toxicity of lead appears to result from enzyme dysfunction during treatment.

Mercury

Postnatal treatment of young female rats with mercuric chloride has been reported to disturb the estrus cycle, resulting in prolongation of diestrus. Subsequent investigators have demonstrated mercury deposition in ovarian macrophages, granulosa and luteal cells, suggesting direct ovarian toxicity (Stadnicka, 1980). Similar alterations in the estrus cycle have been observed in rodents treated with mercuric nitrate and methylmercuric chloride (Busta, 1979; Lach and Srebro, 1972). Busta (1979) has also observed an increase in follicle atresia in rats treated with methylmercuric chloride, however it is not known if this represents direct follicle toxicity or withdrawal of gonadotropin support of the follicle.

A comprehensive series of experiments by Lamperti and coworkers has demonstrated that short-term subcutaneous treatment with mercuric chloride blocks follicular growth in the hamster (Lamperti and Printz, 1973, 1974). This treatment schedule appears to alter both pituitary secretion of gonadotropins and ovarian steroid secretion (Lamperti and Niewenhuis, 1976).

Cadmium

Postnatal treatment of rats with cadmium decreased uterine, ovarian and pituitary weight and produced persistent diestrus (Der et al., 1977) without apparent morphological alterations (Gunn et al, 1961). Kar et al. (1959) have demonstrated cadmium-induced follicular atresia in prepubertal rats and Parizek et al. (1968) have demonstrated ovarian necrosis in adult rats in persistent estrus treated with cadmium. Watanabe et al. (1977) have demonstrated ovarian hemmorhage, inhibition of ovulation and aneuploidy in oocytes recovered from mice treated with cadmium chloride. Copius Peereboom-Stegeman and Jongstra-Spaapen (1979), in a careful light and electron microscopic study, have demonstrated necrosis of pre-ovulatory rat follicles and damage to the uterine microcirculation following cadmium treatment in sexually mature cycling female rats.

Where the authors have explored the mechanism of action of cadmium in producing these forms of reproductive toxicity, vascular damage, as well as the presence or absence of cytosolic binding proteins, as in the testis, appears to play a major role in modulating the toxicity.

CONCLUSION

Integrated function of the hypothalamus, pituitary, ovary and uterus can be disrupted by a variety of xenobiotic compounds, including metals. Although some xenobiotics are toxic to the reproductive system of rodents and primates, many remain to be characterized with respect to effects on experimental animals and to human hazard. With the exception of a few detailed investigations of metal-induced reproductive toxicity, there appear to be large gaps of knowledge even in experimental animal systems. Further exploration of the effects of metals on the development and function of the female reproductive system should be encouraged.

ACKNOWLEDGEMENTS

I would like to thank Dr. G.T. Ross and Mrs. Maria S. Nightingale for many helpful discussions and Dr. G.D. Hodgen for support, encouragement and stimulation. As always, Ms. L. Baldwin deserves special thanks for careful attention to the preparation of this manuscript.

REFERENCES

Aronson, J.K. and Grahame-Smith, D.G., 1981, Clinical pharmacology, adverse drug interactions, Brit. Med. J. 282:288-291.
Ash, P., 1980, The influence of radiation on fertility in man, Brit. J. Radiol. 53:271-278.
Barrette, J.C., Wong, A. and McLachlan, J.A., 1981, Diethyl-stilbestrol induces neoplastic transformation without measurable gene mutation at two loci, Science 212:1402-1404.
Bjersing, L., 1978, Maturation, morphology and endocrine function of the follicular wall in mammals, in: "The Vertebrate Ovary, Comparative Biology and Evolution", R.E. Jones, ed., pp. 181-214, Plenum Press, New York.

Block, E., 1951a, Quantitative morphological investigations of the
    follicular system in women. Methods of quantitative
    determinations, Acta Anat. Scandinav. 12:267-285.
Block, E., 1951b, Quantitative morphological investigations of the
    follicular system in women. Variations in the different phases
    of the sexual cycle, Acta Anat. Scandinav. 8:33-54.
Block, E., 1952, Quantitative morphological investigations of the
    follicular system in women. Variations at different ages, Acta
    Anat. Scandinav. 14:108-123.
Brower, P.T. and Schultz, R.M., 1982, Intercellular communication
    between granulosa cells and mouse oocytes; existence and
    possible nutritional role during oocyte growth, Dev. Biol.
    90:144-153.
Burgos, M.H. and Fawcett, D.W., 1955, Studies on the fine structure
    of the mammalian testis. I. Differentiation of the spermatids
    in the cat (Felis domestica), J. Biophys. Biochem. Cytol.
    1:287-300.
Busta, A., 1979, Doctoral Thesis, Academy of Medicine, Krakow,
    Poland, as reported by Stadnicka, 1980.
Byskov, A.G. and Rasmussen, G., 1973, Ultrastructural studies of the
    developing folicle, in: "The Development and Maturation of the
    Ovary and its Function", H. Peters, ed., pp. 55-62, Excerpta
    Medica, Amsterdam.
Carmel, P.W., Araki, S. and Ferin, M., 1976, Pituitary stalk portal
    blood collection in rhesus monkeys: evidence of pulsatile
    release of gonadotropin-releasing hormone (GnRH), Endocrinology
    99:243-248.
Chapman, R.M., Sutcliff, S.B. and Malpas, J.S., 1979a, Cytotoxic-
    induced ovarian failure in women with Hodgkins disease. I.
    Hormone function, J. Am. Med. Assoc. 242:1877-1881.
Chapman, R.M., Sutcliff, S.B. and Malpas, J.S., 1979b, Cytotoxic-
    induced ovarian failure in women with Hodgkins disease. II.
    Effects on sexual function, J. Am. Med. Assoc. 242:1882-1884.
Chen, Y.T., Mattison, D.R., Feigenbaum, L., Fukai, H. and Schulman,
    J.D., 1982, Reduction on oocyte number following prenatal
    exposure to a high galactose diet, Science 214:1145-1147.
Chiquoine, A.D., 1965, Effect of cadmium chloride on the pregnant
    albino mouse, J. Reprod. Fertil. 10:263-265.
Copius Peereboom-Stegeman, J.H. and Jongstra-Spaapen, E.J., 1979,
    The effect of a single sublethal administration of cadmium
    chloride on the microcirculation in the uterus of the rat,
    Toxicol. 13:199-213.
Der, R., Fakim, Z., Yousef, M. and Fakim, M., 1977, Effects of
    cadmium growth, sexual development, and metabolism in female
    rats, Res. Comm. Chem. Path. Pharmacol. 16:485-505.
Dixon, R.L., 1980, Toxic responses of the reproductive system, in:
    "Toxicology. The Basic Science of Poisons", J. Doull, C.D.
    Klaasen, and M.O. Admur, eds., pp. 332-354, MacMillan
    Publishing Co., New York.

diZerega, G.S. and Hodgen, G.D., 1981a, Luteal phase dysfunction infertility: a sequel to aberrant folliculogenesis, Fertil. Steril. 35:489-499.

diZerega, G.S. and Hodgen, G.D., 1981b, Folliculogenesis in the primate ovarian cycle, Endocrine Rev. 2:27-49.

Dobson, R.L. Koehler, C.G., Felton, J.S., Kwan, T.C., Wuebbles, B.J. and Jones, D.C.L., 1977, Vulnerability of female germ cells in developing mice and monkeys to tritium, gamma rays, and polycyclic aromatic hydrocarbons, in: "Developmental Toxicology of Energy-Related Pollutants", D.C. Mahlum, M.R. Sikov, P.L. Hackett and F.D. Andrew, eds., D.O.E. Symposium Series 47, Conf. 771017.

Fabro, S. and Brown, N.A., 1982, "Reproductive Toxicology. A Medical Letter on Environmental Hazards to Reproduction", Reproductive Toxicology Center, 2425 L Street, N.W., Washington, DC.

Felton, J.S., Kwan, T.C., Wuebbles, B.J. and Dobson, R.L., 1978, Genetic differences in polycyclic-aromatic-hydrocarbon metabolism and their effects on oocyte killing in developing mice, in: "Developmental Toxicology of Energy-Related Pollutants", D.C. Mahlum, M.R. Sikov, P.L. Hackett and F.D. Andrew, eds., D.O.E. Symposium Series 47, Conf. 771017.

Fuller, G.B., Faiman, C., Winter, J.S.D., Reyes, F.I. and Hobson, W.C., 1982, Sex-dependent gonadotropin concentrations in infant chimpanzees and rhesus monkeys, Proc. Soc. Exp. Biol. Med. 169:494-500.

Gellert, R.J. and Heinrichs, W.L., 1975, Effects of DDT homologs administered to female rats during the perinatal period, Biol. Neonate 26:283-290.

Gondos, B., 1978, Oogonia and oocytes in mammals, in: "The Vertebrate Ovary. Comparative Biology and Evolution", R.E. Jones, ed., pp. 120-183, Plenum Press, New York.

Gorski, R.A., 1971, Gonadal hormones and the perinatal development of neuroendocrine function, in: "Frontiers in Neuroendocrinology", C. Martini and W.F. Ganong, eds., pp. 237-290, Oxford University Press, New York.

Grant, L.D., Kimmel, C.A., Martinez-Vargas, C.M. and West, G.L., 1976, Assessment of developmental toxicity associated with chronic lead exposure, Environ. Health Perspect. 17:290.

Greep, R.O. and Astwood, E.B., 1973, "Endocrinology, Volume II, Female Reproductive System", Parts 1 and 2, Handbook of Physiology, American Physiology Society, Washington, DC.

Greep, R.O. and Koblinsky, M.A., 1977, "Frontiers in Reproduction and Fertility Control. A Review of the Reproductive Sciences and Contraceptive Development", The MIT Press, Cambridge, Massachusetts.

Gulyas, B.J. and Mattison, D.R., 1979, Degeneration of mouse oocytes in response to polycyclic aromatic hydocarbons, Anat. Res. 193:863-882.

Gunn, S., Gould, T. and Anderson, W., 1961, Zinc protection against cadmium injury to rat testis, Arch. Pathol. 71:52-57.

Haney, A.F., Hammond, C.B., Soudes, M.R. and Creasman, W.T., 1979, Diethylstilbestrol induced upper genital tract abnormalities, Fertil. Steril. 31:142-146.

Heinrichs, W.L. and Juchau, M.R., 1980, Extrahepatic drug metabolism: the gonads, in: "Extrahepatic Metabolism of Drugs and Other Foreign Compounds", T.E. Gram, ed., pp. 319-332, SP Medical and Scientific Books, New York.

Herbst, A.L., Ulfelder, H. and Poskanzer, D.C., 1971, Adenocarcinoma of the vagina, association of maternal stilbestrol therapy with tumor appearance in young women, N. Engl. J. Med. 284:878-881.

Hodgen, G.D., 1982, The dominant ovarian follicle, Fertil. Steril. 38:281-301.

Jacquet, P., Gerber, G.B., Leonard, A. and Maes, J., 1977, Plasma hormone levels in normal and lead-treated pregnant mice, Experiencia 33:1375-1377.

Janson, P.O., 1975, Effects of luteinizing hormone on blood flow in the follicular rabbit ovary, as measured by radioactive microspheres, Acta Endocrinologica 79:122-133.

Jones, R.E., 1978, "The Vertebrate Ovary: Comparative Biology and Evolution", Plenum Press, New York.

Kar, A., Das, A. and Karkun, J., 1959, Ovarian changes in prepubertal rats after treatment with cadmium chloride, Acta Biol. Med. Germ. 3:372-399.

Kaufman, F.R., Kogut, G.N., Donnell, A. and Goebelsmann, C., 1981, Hypergonadotropic hypogonadism in female patients with galactosemia, N. Engl. J. Med. 304:994-998.

Kimbrough, R.D., 1974, The toxicity of polychlorinated polycyclic compounds and related chemicals, Crit. Rev. Toxicol. 2:445-489.

Knobil, E., 1980, The neuroendocrine control of gonadotropin secretion in the rhesus monkey, Recent Prog. Horm. Res. 36:53-88.

Korach, K.S., Metzer, M. and McLachlan, J.A., 1979, Diethylstilbestrol metabolites and analogs, new probes for the study of hormone action, J. Biol. Chem. 254:8963-8968.

Kupfer, D., 1975, Effects of pesticides and related compounds on steroid metabolism and function, Crit. Rev. Toxicol. 4:83-124.

Lach, H. and Srebro, Z., 1972, The oestrus cycle of mice during lead and mercury poisoning, Acta Biol. Crac. Ser. Zool. 15:121-191.

Lamperti, A.A. and Printz, R.H., 1973, Effects of mercuric chloride on the reproductive cycle of the female hamster, Biol. Reprod. 8:373-387.

Lamperti, A.A. and Printz, R.H., 1974, Localization, accumulation and toxic effects of mercuric chloride on the reproductive axis of the female hamster, Biol. Reprod. 11:180-186.

Lamperti, A.A. and Niewenhuis, R., 1976, The effects of mercury on the structure and function of the hypothalamo-pituitary axis in the hamster, Cell Tiss. Res. 170:315-324.

Mackenzie, K.M. and Angevine, D.M., 1981, Infertility in mice exposed in utero to benzo(a)pyrene, Biol. Reprod. 24:183-191.

Mandl, A.M., 1964, The radiosensitivity of germ cells, Biol. Rev. 39:288-371.

Mattison, D.R., 1981a, Effects of biologically foreign compounds on
    reproduction, in: "Drugs During Pregnancy, Clinical
    Perspectives", R.W. Abdul-Karim, ed., pp. 101-125, George F.
    Stickley, Philadelphia.
Mattison, D.R., 1981b, Drugs, xenobiotics and the adolescent:
    implications for reprduction, in: "Drug Metabolism in the
    Immature Human", L.F. Soyka and G.P. Redmond, eds., pp.
    129-143, Raven Press, New York.
Mattison, D.R., 1982, The effects of smoking on fertility from
    gametogenesis to implantation, Environ. Res. 28:410-433.
Mattison, D.R. and Nightingale, M.S., 1982, Oocyte destruction by
    polycyclic aromatic hydrocarbons is not linked to the
    inductability of ovarian aryl hydrocarbon (benzo(a)pyrene)
    hydrozylase activity in (DBA/2N x C57BL/6N) F_1 x DBA/2N
    backcross mice, Ped. Pharmacol. 2:11-211.
Mattison, D.R. and Ross, G.T., 1982, Oogenesis and ovulation, in:
    "Laboratory Methods for Evaluating and Predicting Specific
    Reproductive Dysfunctions", V. Voulk, ed., John Wiley
    Interscience (in press).
Mattison, D.R., Chang, L., Thorgeirsson, S.S. and Shiromizu, K.,
    1981, The effects of cyclophosphamide, azathioprine and
    6-mercaptopurine on oocyte and follicle number in C57BL/6N
    mice, Res. Comm. Chem. Path. Pharmacol. 31:155-161.
Merchant-Larios, H., 1978, Ovarian differentiation, in: "The
    Vertebrate Ovary. Comparative Biology and Evolution", R.E.
    Jones, ed., pp. 47-81, Plenum Press, New York.
Messite, J. and Bond, M.B., 1980, Reproductive toxicology and
    occupational exposure, in: "Developments in Occupational
    Medicine", C. Zenz, ed., pp. 59-129, Year Book Medical
    Publishers, Chicago.
Noyes, R.W., Hertig, A.T. and Rock, J., 1950, Dating the endometrial
    biopsy, Fertil. Steril. 1:3-25.
Odenbro, A. and Kihlstrom, J.E., 1977, Frequency of pregnancy and
    ova implantation in triethyl lead-treated mice, Toxicol. Appl.
    Pharmacol. 39:359-363.
Parizek, J., Ostadalova, I., Benes, I. and Pitha, J., 1968, The
    effect of subcutaneous injection of cadmium salts on the
    ovaries of adult rats in persistent oestrus, J. Reprod. Fertil.
    17:559-562.
Petrusz, P., Weaver, C.M., Grant, L.D., Mushak, P. and Krigman,
    M.R., 1979, Lead poisoning and reproduction: effects on
    pituitary and serum gonadotropins in neonatal rats, Environ.
    Res. 19:383-391.
Pohl, C.R. and Knobil, E., 1982, The role of the central nervous
    system in the control of ovarian function in higher primates,
    Ann. Rev. Physiol. 44:583-593.
Rebar, R.W., 1982, Hypergonadotropic amenorrhea and premature
    ovarian failure: A review, J. Reprod. Med. 27:179-186.
Reimers, T.S., Sluss, P.M., Goodwin, J. and Seidel, G.E., 1980,
    Bigenerational effects of 6-mercaptopurine on reproduction in
    mice, Biol. Reprod. 22:367-375.

Rudiger, H.W., Haenisch, F., Metzler, M., Oesch, F. and Glatt, H.R.,
    1979, Metabolites of diethylstilbestrol induce sister chromatid
    exchange in cultured human fibroblasts, Nature 281:392-394.
Schwartz, D. and Mayaux, M.J., 1982, Female fecundity as a function
    of age, N. Engl. J. Med. 307:404-406.
Setchell, B.P. and Sharp, R.M., 1981, Effect of injected human
    chorionic gonadotropin on capillary permeability, extracellular
    fluid volume and the flow of lymph and blood in the testis of
    rats, J. Endocr. 91:245-254.
Sieber, S.M. and Adamson, R.H., 1975, Toxicity of antineoplastic
    agents in man: chromosomal aberrations, antifertility effects,
    congenital malformations and carcinogenic potential, Adv.
    Cancer Res. 22:57-155.
Stadnicka, A., 1980, Localization of mercury in the rat ovary after
    oral administration of mercury chloride, Acta Histochem.
    67:223-227.
Stowe, D. and Goyer, R.A., 1971, The reproductive ability and
    progeny of F_1 lead-toxic rats, Fertil. Steril. 22:755-760.
Styne, D.M. and Grumbach, M.M., 1978, Puberty in the male and
    female: its physiology and disorders, in: "Reproductive
    Endocrinology, Physiology, Pathophysiology and Clinical
    Management", S.S.C. Yen and R.B. Jaffe, eds., pp. 189-240, W.B.
    Saunders, Philadelphia.
Tietze, F., 1969, Enzymatic method for quantitative determination of
    nanogram amounts of total and oxidized glutathione: applications
    to mammalian blood and other tissues, Anal. Biochem. 27:507-522.
Vermande-Van Eck, G.J. and Meigs, J.W., 1960, Changes in the ovary
    of the rhesus monkey after chronic lead intoxication, Fertil.
    Steril. 11:223-234.
Watanabe, T., Shimada, T. and Endo, A., 1977, Mutagenic effects of
    cadmium on the oocyte chromosomes of mice, Japanese J. Hygiene
    32:472-481.
Welch, R.M., Levin, W., Kuntzman, R., Jacobson, M. and Conney, A.H.,
    1971, Effect of halogenated hydrocarbon insecticides on the
    metabolism and uterotropic acton of estrogens in rats and mice,
    Toxicol. Appl. Pharmacol. 19:234-246.
Wharton, L.J., 1964, Normal pregnancy with living children in women
    past the age of fifty, Am. J. Obstet. Gynec. 90:672-681.
Wide, M., 1980, Interference of lead with implantation in the
    mouse: effect of exogenous estradiol and progesterone,
    Teratology 21:187-191.
Wildt, L., Marshall, G. and Knobil, E., 1980, Experimental induction
    of puberty in the infantile female rhesus monkey, Science 207:
    1371-1375.
Williams, R.F., 1980, Factors regulating pituitary gonadotropin
    secretion in male and female infant monkeys, Biol. Reprod.
    Abstract 134, 87A.
Yen, S.S.C., 1978, The human menstrual cycle, integrating function
    of the hypothalamic-pituitary-ovarian-endometrial axis, in:
    "Reproductive Endocrinology, Physiology, Pathophysiology and

Clinical Management", S.S.C. Yen and R.B. Jaffe, eds., pp.
126-151, W.B. Saunders, Philadelphia.
Yen, S.S.C. and Jaffe, R.B., 1978, eds., "Reproductive Endocrinology,
Physiology, Pathophysiology and Clinical Management", W.B.
Saunders, Philadelphia.
Zuckerman, S. and Weir, B.J., 1977, "The Ovary", Volumes I, II and
III, Second Edition, Academic Press, New York.

LEAD AND DEVELOPMENT OF THE EARLY EMBRYO

Mariann Wide

Department of Zoology
Uppsala University
Uppsala, Sweden

ABSTRACT

Lead is suspected of interfering with fetal development. Very few reports deal with the effects of lead on early embryonic stages. Spermatogenesis, cleavage of the fertilized ovum and implantation have been shown to be disturbed in experimental animals exposed to lead. The mechanism of action of lead in causing implantation failure in the mouse has been studied.

Trophoblast invasion was more susceptible to lead than attachment and early postimplantation development. Blastocysts isolated from lead-treated mice were capable of "implanting" in vitro and in pregnant foster mothers, where they could also develop into late fetal stages. Ultrastructural investigation revealed: 1) the presence of intracellular lead in electron dense phagolysosomes; and 2) that endometrial surfaces in lead-treated mice around implantation were not normal for the stage of development. Oestradiol and progesterone given at implantation could completely counteract the effect of lead. No significant differences from control levels were found of oestradiol and progesterone in serum from lead-treated mice. Uterine cytosol receptors for oestradiol-17-β had significantly higher maximum binding capacity in lead-treated mice than in controls. It was assumed that lead had caused inhibition of implantation by interfering with ovarian steroid hormone stimulation of the endometrium. Since it has been shown that an early developmental stage like implantation can be disturbed by lead, it seems important to pay more attention to possible negative effects of lead on the fertility of lead-exposed women.

INTRODUCTION

It has been recognized for at least a 100 years that lead may interfere with the development of the human fetus, causing miscarriages, stillbirths, and a high neonatal loss (see review by Rom, 1976). Structural malformations of the fetus, as a result of exposure to lead, have been reported only in experimental animals. Inorganic lead was given in high doses during the organogenic period and the malformations observed were restricted to the posterior parts of the body, ranging from missing tail vertebrae to the complete absence of hind limbs (Ferm and Ferm, 1971; McClain and Becker, 1975). These reports are all concerned with lead effects mainly during the latter half of pregnancy. However, there is another important field in metal toxicology in reproduction that has hitherto not been much studied, and that is the interference with the very early stages of development, from gametogenesis and fertilization to cleavage of the zygote, blastulation and implantation. A disturbance during this period can be difficult to detect in the human, as all these different stages take place before the existence of a pregnancy can be confirmed, and an interference with any of these stages would simply result in a reduced number of offspring in a population. There are, in fact, some reports in the literature pointing to a decrease in fertility in men and women occupationally exposed to lead (Rom, 1976) as well as in experimental animals exposed to lead in the drinking water, (Schroeder and Mitchener, 1971) or in the diet (Varma et al., 1974). What is known about the effects of lead specifically on some of the earliest events of embryonic development?

Spermatogenesis has been reported to be disturbed in lead workers with blood lead levels of 50-75 µg/100 ml. The findings included a significant increase in hypospermia, astenospermia and teratospermia in these workers (Lancranjan et al., 1975). An increase in abnormal sperm following lead exposure has been reported also in the rat (Eyden et al., 1978).

Cleavages of fertilized mouse ova were delayed or inhibited by the addition of lead to the diet of pregnant animals (Jacquet et al., 1976).

Blastocyst formation, the first stage of differentiation of a mammalian embryo, results in the development of two different populations of cells - the trophectoderm and the inner cell mass. In the mouse, this developmental stage was found not to be affected by lead given during late cleavage stages (Jacquet, 1977) or during the morula stage (Wide and Nilsson, 1977). But when the lead treatment was extended further, implantation of the blastocysts failed to occur (Jacquet, 1977; Wide and Nilsson, 1977). However, nothing was known about the mechanisms of action of lead in disturbing these processes.

We have been studying the effect of lead upon the implantation process. The mouse was chosen as an experimental animal, as implantation in this species has great similarities with that in the human. During implantation in these species the blastocyst, hatched from the zona pellucida, establishes a close contact with the uterine wall. This is termed the attachment phase of implantation and lasts for several hours before the trophoblast cells start to invade the endometrium, breaking up the capillary walls, until direct contact is reached with the maternal blood. During invasion and immediately after its completion, the inner cell mass of the blastocyst differentiates into the three germ layers: the ectoderm, endoderm and (by primitive streak formation) mesoderm. The initiation and subsequent progress of implantation is governed by ovarian steroid hormones. Implantation constitutes a critical step in development, since it involves close cellular interactions of two different individuals and is known to be susceptible (at least in the mouse) to a number of exogenous factors such as stress, odours, noise and some drugs.

EXPERIMENTS

Pregnant mice were injected in the tail vein on the day before implantation (= day 4 of pregnancy) with 1 mg of lead chloride in aquaeous solution. This dose, giving blood lead levels of about 14 μmoles/l, did not cause any sign of discomfort in the animals, but implantation was completely inhibited.

Was there any difference in susceptibility for any particular stage during the period of implantation? To test this, groups of pregnant mice were given 1 mg of lead chloride; 1) before attachment of the blastocyst to the endometrial surface; 2) before invasion of the endometrium by the trophoblast; or 3) in early postimplantation before the period of primitive streak formation. We found that all these stages were affected by the lead treatment and that the group of mice injected before trophoblast invasion had significantly fewer normal embryos, as judged by light microscopy, than mice treated at the two other stages of development (Wide and Nilsson, 1977). Lead is known to interfere with the activity of a great number of enzymes, which affects protein synthesis and cellular oxidative processes (Vallee and Ulmer, 1972); the fact that invasion also involves many different enzymatic activities (Sherman and Wudl, 1976) could explain why this period was more seriously affected.

The question we asked was, had the treatment of the mothers with lead rendered the blastocysts unable to interact with the endometrium and to invade? We tested this by transferring blastocysts from uteri of lead-treated mice to: 1) an in vitro culture system, where close observation of trophoblast attachment and out-growth is possible; 2) pregnant foster mothers for implantation and possibly further development. It was then found that blastocysts from lead-treated mice had the same ability to "implant" in vitro as blastocysts from non-treated mice (Wide, 1978). Nor was there any lack of ability to implant in a pregnant foster mother. When development was allowed to go further (until 2 days before parturition), blastocysts transferred from lead-treated mice were found to have developed equally well compared to blastocysts transferred from non-treated mice as regards stage of development, fetal weight and external morphology (unpublished observations). These results perhaps suggest that a mouse embryo, whose mother has been exposed to lead before implantation, is completely unaffected by this treatment. We know from preliminary measurements of oxygen consumption of single blastocysts, using a microspectrophotometric method, that significantly less oxygen is taken up by lead-blastocysts than by normal ones (unpublished observations). However, this disorder does not seem to interfere with the ability to implant, once the blastocysts have become transferred to a lead-free environment. We have not been able so far to measure any uptake of lead in blastocysts from the uterine secretions, but work is in progress using a proton microbeam technique. Lead levels in uterine tissue, however, were measured on the day of implantation (24 hours after the lead injection) and found to be about 4 µg/g wet weight (Wide, 1978).

Careful examination of the endometrial cells was then performed in order to: 1) localize lead at the subcellular level; 2) look for intracellular changes that might help explain the mechanism of impairment of implantation by lead; and 3) closely examine the surfaces of blastocysts and uterine epithelial cells in implantation sites. Different modes of electron microscopy were used in these studies.

By the use of X-ray microanalysis in the transmission electron microscope, it was possible to detect lead in one type of organelle only where it was present in very high concentrations, namely in phagolysosomes with a granular, highly electron dense appearance (Wide and Ljung, 1981). Work is in progress trying to trace lead also in other parts of the cell.

Probably due to the short time of lead exposure, no intracellular changes were found like those reported by other investigators to be characteristic of lead effects in different tissues, such as abnormal mitochondria and intranuclear inclusion bodies (Goyer and Krall, 1969; Goyer et al., 1970).

However, the study of sections of uteri containing blastocysts revealed surface ultrastructures that were not normal for the stage of development (see Plate 1): no attachment had taken place between trophoblast and uterine epithelium and the surfaces of both were covered by abundant microvilli instead of being smooth and undulating; some blastocysts were still encased in their zonae pellucidae and the uterine lumen between blastocysts was open instead of being closed with interlocking microvilli (Wide and Nilsson, 1979). The condition seen was similar to that before the attachment stage of normal implantation or before the oestrogen-induced attachment reaction occurs in progesterone-treated, ovariectomized mice (experimental delay of implantation). The findings suggested that the implantation failure might be due to a subnormal stimulation of the endometrium by ovarian steroid hormones.

This hypothesis was tested by giving pregnant mice 1 mg of progesterone and 0.1 μg of oestrogen on the day of lead treatment and 24 hours later (= day of implantation). This treatment caused a complete counteraction of the lead effect (see Table 1) in that the group of lead plus hormone-treated mice had successful implantations in the same frequency as the non-treated group (Wide, 1980).

To find out if the lead-treated mice had lower serum levels of ovarian steroid hormones, which might explain the implantation failure, radioimmunoassays of oestrogen and progesterone were performed. It was then found that the levels of oestrogen were almost identical in the lead-treated group and in the control group, the mean values being 53.25 ± 3.56 pmol/l in the lead group and 54.85 ± 4.28 pmol/l in the control group. Progesterone levels, however, showed a great interindividual variation in both groups. The mean values obtained were 54.75 ± 12.55 nmol/l in the lead group and 67.14 ± 10.8 nmol/l in the control group but this difference was not statistically significant. The latter results do not exclude the possibility of a lead-induced damage to the hypothalamus-pituitary complex or ovaries. However, the uterus has to be considered as the possible site of interference by lead. Evidence had been presented that the binding of ^{3}H-labelled oestradiol to receptors in uterine cytosol was decreased if heavy metals (and among those, lead) were added during the incubation (Young et al.,

Table 1 Effect of Exogenous Oestradiol-17-β and Progesterone on Implantation in Lead-Treated Mice

	Controls	PbCl$_2$ on day 4	PbCl$_2$ on day 4 plus ovarian steroids
Number of mice with implantations	15/20 (75%)	4/20[*] (20%)	18/24 (75%)

*Differences from controls, p<0.002 (Fischer's exact test).

1977). Therefore, an estimation of oestradiol receptor activity in uteri of lead-treated mice was made.

In four different experiments, cytosol was prepared from uteri of lead-treated and non-treated mice of day 5 of pregnancy and incubated with labelled estradiol-17-β. In all four experiments the cytosol from lead-treated mice was found to bind significantly larger amounts of the labelled hormone than the cytosol from the non-treated mice, whether measured per uterus, per g uterine wet weight or per protein content of the cytosol. Additional experiments, in which the results were plotted according to Scatchard (1949), showed that this was due to a higher maximum binding capacity (larger number of receptors) rather than to an increase in affinity between the hormone and its receptor, Figure 1, (Wide and Wide, 1980).

How is the number of uterine steroid receptors regulated in the animal, and how can lead be thought to be implicated? It is known for the steroid hormones that the number of receptors is regulated by the action of the hormones themselves, in that oestrogen causes the synthesis of receptors for oestrogen and also for progesterone. Progesterone has the opposite effect, namely inhibition of synthesis of receptors for both oestrogen and progesterone (see review by Janne et al., 1978). In the lead-treated mice, the mean value for progesterone in serum was about 80 percent of that of the controls, although this difference was not statistically significant. However, it cannot be excluded that a possible decrease in progesterone levels (such a decrease is suggested by Dr. Leonard in a following paper) has contributed to a decreased inhibition of oestrogen receptor synthesis with an ensuing higher binding capacity of the cytosol from the lead-treated mice. A decrease in progesterone might also be thought to be connected with the interference with implantation, due to an insufficient stimulation of the endometrium. Another explanation for the implantation failure may also be proposed. It has been shown that if rats in experimental delay are given high doses of oestrogen (10 μg), implantation is inhibited (Sartor et al., 1978). Since the observed increase in oestrogen binding in the present study may have caused an increased oestrogen stimulation, it may be suggested that such a stimulation, being greater than normal due to an increased number of receptors, has caused the implantation failure.

CONCLUSION

The results from our studies, together with those from other investigators working in the field of metal toxicology in early pregnancy stages, have shown that these stages are indeed susceptible to the effects of maternal and possibly paternal, lead exposure. This emphasizes the need for further attention to

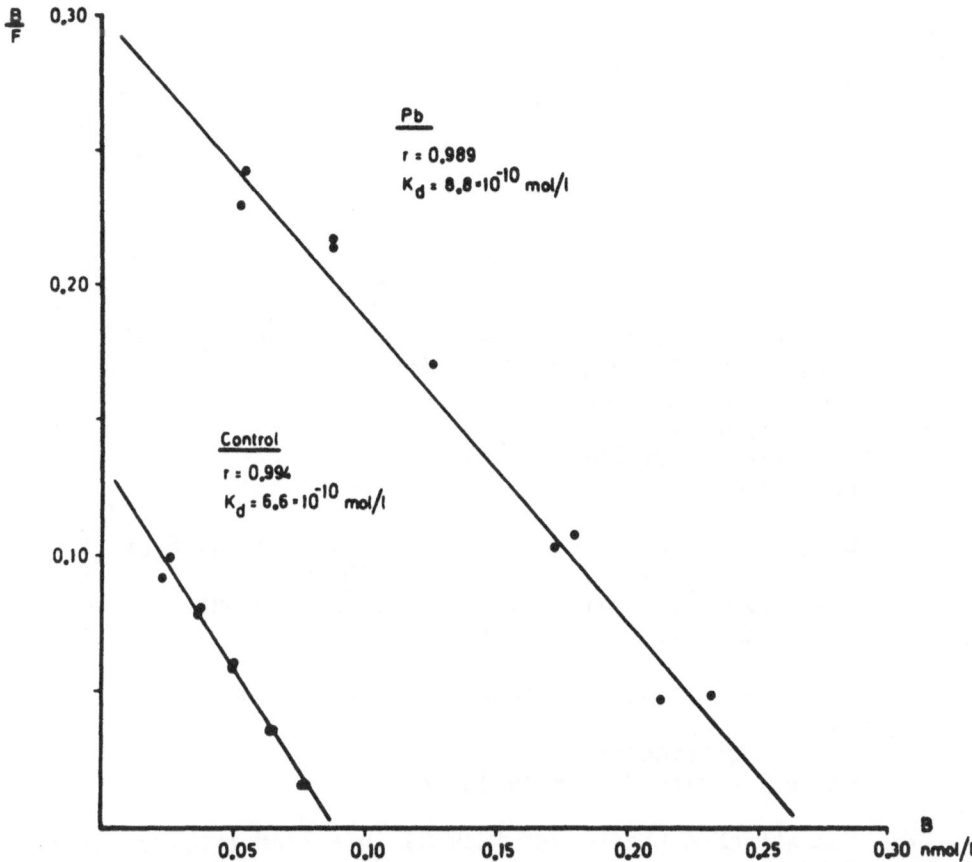

Figure 1   Scatchard plot showing the difference in binding of
            17β-estradiol to uterine cytosol from one group of control
            mice and one group of lead-treated mice, r, correlation
            coefficient; K_d, dissociation constant. (Wide, M. and
            Wide, L., 1980, courtesy of Fertility and Sterility)

possible negative effects of lead on the fertility of lead-exposed
individuals. In view of the fact that a great increase is expected
in industrial use as well as in environmental levels of a large
number of metals other than lead, it seems of great importance to
study also their possible effects on early pregnancy. Here again we
do have some information about effects on later embryonic stages,
from animal experiments, whereas virtually nothing is known about
the effects on preimplantation and implantation stages.

Plate 1

1. Blastocyst attached to the endometrium on day 5 of
    pregnancy. Control animal. 500 x
    icm - inner cell mass
    T - trophoblast cell
    Ue - uterine epithelial cells
    bc - blood capillary

2. Blastocyst flushed out from the uterus on day 5 of
    pregnancy. Lead-treated animal. 500 x
    T - microvillous trophoblast cell bulging out
        photo: T. Sensenbaugh

3. Blastocyst attachment (day 5) in control animal.
    2000 x
    bl.cl - blastocoel
    (arrow) - closed uterine lumen

4. Non attached blastocyst (day 5) in a lead-treated animal.
    2000 x
    zp - zona pellucida

5. Control blastocyst invading the endometrium late on day 5.
    Smooth cell contact (arrow). 24,000 x

6. No contact between trophoblast and uterine epithelium late
    on day 5 in a lead-treated animal. 24,000 x
    m - microvillous linings of the cells

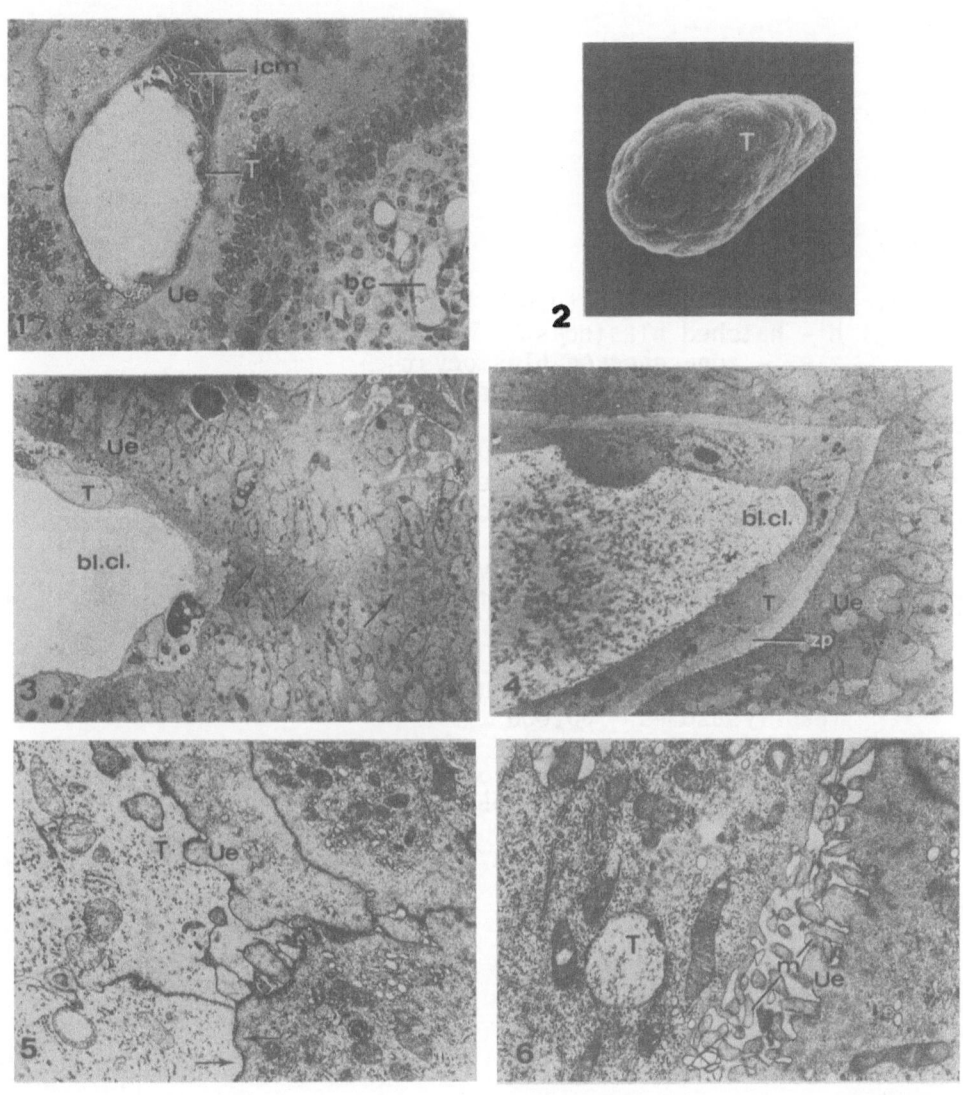

Plate 2

7. Blastocysts in culture. 150 x
    h - hatched blastocyst
    z.e. - zona encased blastocyst
    zp - free zonae pellucidae

8. Blastocyst outgrown in culture. 150 x
    gT - giant trophoblast cell
    eb - embryoblast (inner cell mass)

9. Corpus luteum cells of ovary. 9000 x
    e.l.i. - electron dense inclusions of lead
    lip - lipid granules

10. Corpus luteum cell, granular electron-dense
    lead-lysosomes. 30,000 x

11. Spectrum from X-ray microanalysis of a lead-lysosome,
    showing lead peaks at 10550 KeV (Lα shell)
                         12600 KeV (Lβ shell)
                         14700 KeV (Lγ shell)

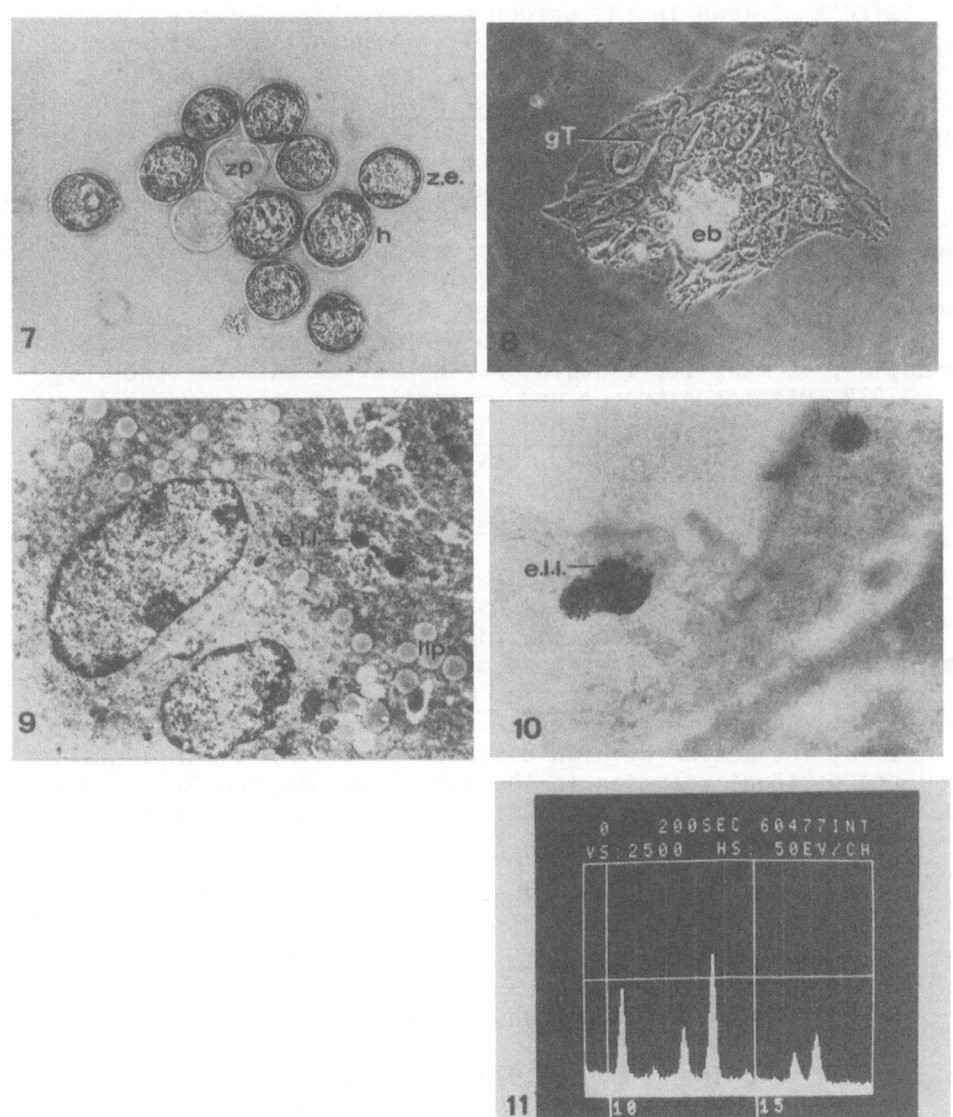

REFERENCES

Eyden, B.P., Maisin, J.R. and Mattelin, G., 1978, Long term effects
    of dietary lead acetate on survival, body weight and seminal
    cytology in mice, Bull. Environ. Contam. Toxicol. 19:266-272.
Ferm, V.H. and Ferm, D.W., 1971, The specificity of the teratogenic
    effect of lead in the golden hamster, Life Sciences 10:35-39.
Goyer, R.A. and Krall, R., 1969, Ultrastructural transformation
    in mitochondria isolated from kidneys of normal and
    lead-intoxicated rats, J. Cell Biol. 41:393-400.
Goyer, R.A., Leonard, D.L., Moore, J.F., Rhyne, B. and Krigman,
    M.R., 1970, Lead dosage and the role of the intranuclear
    inclusion body. An experimental study, Arch. Environ. Health
    20:705-711.
Jacquet, P., 1977, Early embryonic development in lead-intoxicated
    mice, Arch. Pathol. Lab. Med. 101:1641-1643.
Jacquet, P., Leonard, A. and Gerber, G.B., 1976, Action of lead
    on early divisions of the mouse embryo, Toxicology 6:129-132.
Janne, O., Isomaa, V., Isotalo, H., Kokko, E. and Vierikko, P.,
    1978, Uterine estrogen and progestin receptors and their
    regulation, Uppsala J. Med. Sci. Suppl. 22:62-70.
Lancranjan, I., Popescu, H.I., Gavanescu, D., Klepsch, I. and
    Serbanescu, M., 1975, Reproductive ability of workmen
    occupationally exposed to lead, Arch. Environ. Health
    30:396-401.
McClain, R.M. and Becker, B.A., 1975, Teratogenicity, fetal
    toxicity, and placental transfer of lead nitrate in rats,
    Toxicol. Appl. Pharmacol. 31:72-82.
Rom, W.N., 1976, Effects of lead on the female and reproduction:
    A review, The Mount Sinai J. Med. 43:542-552.
Sartor, P., Dupont, H., Dupont, M.A., Duluc, A.J. and Mayer, G.,
    1978, The action of high doses of eostradiol on implantation
    and decidual reaction in the rat, Anim. Reprod. Sci. 1:93-96.
Scatchard, G., 1949, The attraction of proteins for small
    molecules and ions, Ann. N.Y. Acad. Sci. 51:660-672.
Schroeder, H.A. and Mitchener, M., 1971, Toxic effects of trace
    elements on the reproduction of mice and rats, Arch. Environ.
    Health 23:102-106.
Sherman, M.I. and Wudl, L.R., 1976, The implanting mouse
    blastocyst, in: "The Cell Surface in Animal Development",
    G. Poste and G.L. Nicholson, eds., pp. 1-74, North Holland,
    Amsterdam.
Vallee, B.L. and Ulmer, D.D., 1972, Biochemical effects of
    mercury, cadmium and lead, Ann. Rev. Biochem. 41:91-128.
Varma, M.M., Joshi, S.R. and Adeyemi, A.O., 1974, Mutagenicity
    and infertility following administration of lead sub-acetate to
    Swiss male mice, Experientia 30:486-487.
Wide, M., 1978, Effect of inorganic lead on the mouse blastocyst
    in vitro, Teratology 17:165-170.

Wide, M., 1980, Interference of lead with implantation in the
    mouse: Effect of exogenous oestradiol and progesterone,
    Teratology 21:187-191.
Wide, M. and Nilsson, O., 1977, Differential susceptibility of
    the embryo to inorganic lead during periimplantation in the
    mouse, Teratology 16:273-276.
Wide, M. and Nilsson, B.O., 1979, Interference of lead with
    implantation in the mouse: A study of the surface
    ultrastructure of blastocysts and endometrium, Teratology
    20:101-114.
Wide, M. and Wide, L., 1980, Estradiol receptor activity in
    uteri of pregnant mice given lead before implantation, Fertil.
    Steril. 34:503-508.
Wide, M. and Ljung, L., 1981, Detection of intracellular lead
    with analytical electron microscopy of mouse uteri and ovaries,
    J. Ultrastr. Res., Abstr., 76:344.
Young, P.C.M., Cleary, R.E. and Ragan, W.P., 1977, Effect of
    metal ions on the binding of 17β-estradiol to human endometrial
    cytosol, Fertil. Steril. 28:459-463.

EFFECT OF LEAD ON REPRODUCTIVE CAPACITY AND DEVELOPMENT OF MAMMALS

A. Leonard, G.B. Gerber and P. Jacquet

Department of Radiobiology
Centre d'etude de l'energie Nucleaire
Mol, Belgium

ABSTRACT

The hazards of lead to reproduction are reviewed on the basis of the concentrations found in the environment. It appears evident that lead has no direct action on male reproductive capacity. Most likely, indeed, alterations in sperm morphology reported by several authors reflect the general cytotoxicity of the metal and not any mutagenic action since recent reviews concluded that lead is neither mutagenic nor clastogenic. This is also confirmed by the outcome of the dominant lethality and fertility tests which gave negative results. Lead crosses the placental barrier, a fact demonstrated in man as well as in experimental animals, but the human placenta presents a partial barrier to the transfer of lead. Given to pregnant mice, lead delays embryonic development and also has an indirect effect by modifying hormonal production needed for the implantation process. The toxic action on the fetus at late stages of pregnancy is caused mainly by an interference with heme synthesis but also by a lowered blood flow through the placenta.

INTRODUCTION

Great amounts of lead are utilized in industrialized societies, mainly for the manufacture of batteries, alloys, pigments and, as alkyl derivatives, for antiknock additives to gasoline. Environmental atmospheric pollution emanates from vehicle exhaust fumes, to a lesser extent from burning coal and, at certain sites, from smelting and similar operations. Air concentrations of lead in rural areas are below 500 ng/m³, but near roads with heavy traffic or near smelting plants may reach 14,000 ng/m³ (WHO, 1977).

However, the general population receives lead mainly via the diet, about 200-300 µg/day. Ingestion of excessive amounts of lead may occur near smelters or by children who ingest lead paints in old houses. Lead content in water usually does not exceed 50 µg/l, except in certain areas where soft water is conducted through leaden pipes, and levels of several mg/l have been observed.

The concentrations mentioned above are those we have to consider in our review of the hazards of lead to reproduction. A much smaller number of persons is subject to lead poisoning in industry today and lead as a suicidal, abortifacient or poisonous agent is not anymore in fashion. Most information on the effect of lead originates, however, from animal experiments with much larger doses; the problem of extrapolation to lower doses and from animal to man must be kept in mind when evaluating such information. Moreover, the birth of a normal child has as prerequisites many factors, starting from the fertilization of healthy oocyte by a healthy sperm cell in a female body suitably prepared by hormones for implantation and followed by an exactly-timed development of fetal tissues which are subject to many maternal influences. Sophisticated techniques, such as in vitro fertilization and culture or transplantation of embryos into foster mothers are required to sort out all the possible mechanisms by which an agent may affect fertility. In the case of lead, only a fragmentary beginning has been made to use such techniques, therefore it seems still best to describe the observations under the headings of effects or lead on male reproductive capacity and on embryonic development.

EFFECT OF LEAD ON MALE REPRODUCTIVE CAPACITY

A recent review by Bell and Thomas (1980) concludes that lead can affect the male reproductive organs. Indeed, lead readily enters testicular tissues but, in contrast to cadmium, does not produce specific degeneration of the testes. The changes observed in rats by Golubovits et al. (1968) have not been confirmed by Hildenbrand et al. (1973) or Der et al. (1977). Lead can, however, affect sperm morphology of mice after intraperitoneal injection (Heddle and Bruce, 1977; Eyden et al., 1978; Wyrobek and Bruce, 1978), but the dose which doubles the normally occurring frequency of abnormalities is rather high, i.e. in the order of 80 mg/kg. Alterations in sperm morphology have also been reported for workers in a plant manufacturing batteries (Lancranjan et al., 1975). Most likely, however, these changes reflect the general cytotoxicity of lead and not any mutagenic action, since recent reviews by Gerber et al. (1980) and Leonard et al. (1982) concluded that lead is neither mutagenic nor clastogenic. This is also confirmed by the outcome of the dominant lethality test by Kennedy and Arnold (1971) and Kennedy et al. (1971) who mated untreated females with male mice that had received lead acetate or tetraethyl lead and no dominant lethals in meiotic or postmeiotic male germ cells were observed, even after administration of maximal tolerable doses. Our own observations (Leonard et al., 1972) also did not demonstrate any effect of lead on fertility. In these experiments, groups of 20 couples of BALB/c mice received in their drinking water doses ranging from 0.18 mg/l to 1.8 g/l of lead acetate (0.1 mg/l to 1 g/l of lead) for 9 months. Control groups received either tap water (pH 7) or water adjusted with acetic acid to the pH of the lead acetate solutions (pH 3.3). Drinking solutions were renewed weekly. From the amount of liquid consumed, the total amount of lead ingested could be calculated to be about 31 g/kg for the highest dose given (1 g/l) (Table 1). This corresponds, for a 70 kg man, to the ingestion of 2.2 kg of lead in nine months. The fertility of the animals (number of litters, litter size at birth and at weaning) in all groups given lead did not differ from that of animals given acidified drinking water (Table 2). But, due to an increased interval between pregnancies, the number of offspring produced by the animals on acidified water was statistically lower than that of the animals drinking tap water. This difference probably has physiological causes related to water metabolism since the mice on acid water consumed only 60 percent of the amount of water of those on tap water. Similar negative findings are reported by Azar et al. (1972) with rats ingesting diets containing 0, 10, 50, 100, 1000 or 2000 ppm of lead as lead acetate for two years. Varma et al. (1974), in a dominant lethality test on Swiss mice concluded that in animals given a 2 percent aqueous solution of lead subacetate in drinking water for 28 days, the overall incidence of pregnancies was reduced by 50 percent but that the preimplantation as well as the postimplantation loss was not modified. The results of Kennedy and coworkers (1971) as well as our own observations demonstrate that the reduction of male fertility reported by Varma et al. (1974) is probably to be attributed to the acidity resulting from addition of lead acetate to the drinking water.

EFFECT OF LEAD ON FEMALE GERM CELLS AND ON INTRAUTERINE DEVELOPMENT

Lead has probably exerted its deleterious influence on human development since antiquity - indeed the decadence of the Roman empire has been ascribed to lead intoxication (Gilfillan, 1965), yet it was only a century ago that Paul (1860) recognized this toxic action of lead; during some time lead was used as a fashionable and easily accessible, but not always harmless, abortifacient (Hall, 1905; Taussig, 1936). The effects of lead on development as well as its teratogenic action have been studied experimentally only since 1970. In view of the fact that Dr. Ferm, who has made the principal observations on the teratogenic action of lead, also presents a paper here, we shall restrict our review to the general toxic action of lead on mammalian development.

Table 1 Mean Quantities of Liquid and Lead Ingested Per Pair of
         Mice

Treatment	Mean quantity (ml) of liquid ingested per pair		Mean quantity (mg) of lead ingested per kg body weight	
	During 9 months	Per day	During 9 months	Per day
water	3,252	11.61	-	-
water + HAc	1,924	6.87	-	-
0.0001 gPb/1	1,996	7.13	3.3	0.01
0.001 gPb/1	2,047	7.31	33.3	0.11
0.01 gPb/1	1,950	6.91	325.0	1.16
1.1 gPb/1	2,170	7.75	3617.0	12.90
1.0 gPb/1	1,901	6.79	31683.0	113.00

Lead crosses the placental barrier, a fact demonstrated in man as well as in experimental animals such as rat and mouse (McClain and Becker, 1972) and goat (McLellan et al., 1974), but the human placenta presents a partial barrier to the transfer of lead (Harris and Holley, 1972; Scanlon, 1971). As pointed out by Barltrop (1969), distribution and entry of lead at specific stages of pregnancy, particularly during organogenesis, is certainly more important than the amount found at term. We (Gerber et al., 1982) studied the transfer of radioactive lead given to female mice by being added to the food prior to implantation or during the entire pregnancy or by being injected intraperitoneally at critical stages of organogenesis on day 12. Only small amounts of lead reach the preimplantation embryo when feeding is started at fertilization but transfer is rapid and efficient when lead is injected during organogenesis. Moreover, transfer of lead from the diet to the fetus is about 2-3 times greater when the animals are maintained on a calcium-deficient diet. These experiments were carried out to complement the observations on the effects of lead in the fetus and embryo outlined below. In conclusion, lead can certainly reach the human embryo during critical phases of development although a quantitative extrapolation of data obtained on lower mammals to man is uncertain due to the differences in the structure of the placenta and in metabolism of lead.

Lead can effect embryonic development and provoke prenatal loss if a sufficient concentration enters the pregnant female. This has been demonstrated in sheep (James et al., 1966), dogs

Table 2 Fertility of the Mice

Treatment	Mean number of litters produced per pair ($\pm$ S.E.)	Mean number of offspring at birth ($\pm$ S.E.)		Mean number of offspring at weaning ($\pm$ S.E.)	
		Produced per pair during 9 months	Produced per litter	Produced per pair during 9 months	Produced per litter
Water	8.13 $\pm$ 0.36	47.80 $\pm$ 2.16	5.88 $\pm$ 0.14	41.40 $\pm$ 2.44	5.09 $\pm$ 0.16
Water + HAc	6.50 $\pm$ 0.63	35.83 $\pm$ 1.64	5.51 $\pm$ 0.34	29.25 $\pm$ 4.02	4.50 $\pm$ 0.44
0.0001 gPb/1	6.50 $\pm$ 0.29	32.50 $\pm$ 2.40	5.00 $\pm$ 0.28	28.83 $\pm$ 2.66	4.43 $\pm$ 0.33
0.001 gPb/1	7.07 $\pm$ 0.29	40.43 $\pm$ 1.92	5.72 $\pm$ 0.33	35.28 $\pm$ 2.05	4.99 $\pm$ 0.30
0.01 gPb/1	6.21 $\pm$ 0.34	33.00 $\pm$ 2.32	5.31 $\pm$ 0.23	28.31 $\pm$ 2.07	4.56 $\pm$ 0.22
0.1 gPb/1	6.67 $\pm$ 0.29	39.39 $\pm$ 3.54	5.91 $\pm$ 0.41	34.00 $\pm$ 2.60	5.10 $\pm$ 0.40
1 gPb/1	6.05 $\pm$ 0.47	30.94 $\pm$ 4.79	5.11 $\pm$ 0.35	24.94 $\pm$ 2.90	4.11 $\pm$ 0.33

(Azar et al., 1972), guinea-pigs (Weller, 1915), hamsters (Ferm
and Carpenter, 1967), rats (Stowe and Goyer, 1971; Kimmel et al.,
1976; Zegarska et al., 1974; McClain and Becker, 1972) and mice
(Schroeder and Mitchener, 1971; Jacquet et al., 1975; 1976; 1977b;
Maisin, 1978). Negative findings reported by a few authors can
probably be explained by the low doses used and/or route of
administration. This probably explains why Leonard et al. (1972)
as well as Azar et al. (1972) did not find a reduction in fertility
when lead was given in the drinking water.

The mechanisms by which lead causes prenatal death have been
investigated in a series of studies in our laboratory. Lead was
added to the diet at levels of 0, 0.125, 0.25, 0.5 and 1 percent
from the day of the vaginal plug, and the animals were sacrificed
at day 16 or 18. The number of pregnancies, i.e. the number of
females having at least one implant, diminished with increasing
doses of lead (Table 3). The number of postimplantation deaths
increased, although to a less marked degree. The number of
preimplantation losses decreased somewhat, probably as a result of
the entire elimination of the most sensitive pregnancies, (Jacquet
et al., 1975). These data thus suggest two mechanisms of action
of lead, one on implantation and the other, mainly at higher
doses, on fetal development. Implantation is a complex process
requiring not only a normal development of the embryo but also a
proper hormonal preparation of the maternal uterus. Both aspects
seem to be affected by lead. Indeed, when embryos were isolated
from pregnant females 48 hours after mating (Jacquet et al., 1976),
more embryos were found in the four-cell stage compared to the
eight-cell stage as the dose of lead increased from 0 to 0.125,
0.25 or 0.5 percent of lead in the diet. At a still higher dose
of 1 percent, the number of undivided eggs also increased while
the number of four cell embryos decreased (Table 4). Similar
toxic effects of lead were observed also in cultured embryos by
Streffer et al. (1978). Hormonal control of implantation in the
mouse proceeds in two slightly overlapping phases: on day 4, the
uterus is sensitized by estrogen which permits blastocyst
formation; and on day 5, the embryos are activated and the
deciduous response is induced by progesterone. The latter hormone
is needed also for the maintenance of pregnancy. In mice given
0.5 percent of dietary lead, the first estrogen dependent response
appears to proceed normally. Blastocysts, although of somewhat
reduced size, are formed (Jacquet, 1977), and serum estrogen
levels are comparable to those found in controls (Jacquet et al.,
1977a; Gerber et al., 1979). Later, however, the deciduous
response fails and implantation of the embryo after formation of
trophoblastic giant cells does not take place. Simultaneously,
one observes the absence of the normal increase in serum
progesterone and a poor development and early involution of the
corpora lutea. Thus, instead of an increase in serum progesterone
on day 5.5 of pregnancy to 18.36 ($\pm$ 3.46) ng/ml and on day 6 to

23.87 (+ 2.64) ng/ml as in controls, levels in lead-treated animals reached values of 11.61 (+ 3.03) and 11.74 (+ 1.69) ng/ml on days 5 and 6, respectively. Moreover, it is possible to force the implantation of the embryo by injecting large amounts of progesterone (Jacquet, 1978). Consequently, it appears that the mother, at least under the conditions employed here, is the decisive factor for the action of lead on pregnancy.

Lead also acts on the implanted embryo. Aside from the teratogenic action which is discussed by Dr. Ferm (this volume) and which to a certain extent is related to calcium metabolism (Jacquet and Gerber, 1979), non-teratogenic, general toxic effects also affect fetal growth. This growth is greatly retarded, especially from day 16 to 18. Newborns, following a dose of 0.5 percent dietary lead, have an average weight only half that of controls and some fetuses die during the period following major oganogenesis. The reduction in growth could be again a result of the toxic action of lead on the mother or on the fetus. Indeed, alterations are found in both. Blood flow through the mouse placenta, as measured by radioactive microspheres, is somewhat reduced although the uptake of an amino acid substrate seems nearly normal (Gerber et al., 1978). On the other hand, heme concentration in the fetus is slightly reduced, porphyrine levels are increased, and delta aminolevulinic acid dehydratase, a key enzyme in heme synthesis, is diminished to about one half when the

Table 3   Results of the Dissection on Day 16 or 18 of Pregnancy in Females Exposed to Dietary Lead Levels from Day 1 of Pregnancy

Lead (% in diet)	Pregnant females (%)	Corpora Lutea (mean per female)	Live fetuses (mean per female)	Postimplantation deaths (mean per female)	Preimplantation loss (mean per female)
0	52	13.54	8.31	1.23	4.00
0.125	56	13.61	8.25	1.46	3.98
0.250	22[a]	12.55	8.27	1.91	2.36[b]
0.500	16[a]	11.50	7.50	2.38[b]	1.63[a]

Comparison of treated animals to controls in the χ^2 test
[a]significant at $p < 0.01$ level
[b]significant at $p < 0.05$ level

Table 4   Distribution of the Embryos According to the Number of
         Cells Present at 48 Hours after Vaginal Plug

Lead in diet (%)	Number embryos examined	Stages reached			
		One-cell %	Two-cell %	Four-cell %	Eight-cell %
0	115	52	2	5	41
0.125	119	50	1	22	27
0.250	197	46	2	23	29
0.500	124	52	1	27	20
1.000	154	64	1	7	28

The χ^2 values for the comparison of divided embryos of controls with lead-treated embryos are 15.56, 14.8, 24.5, and 1.98 for 0.125, 0.25, 0.5 and 1 percent of lead, respectively. Comparison of divided cells with non-divided embryos yields for the 1 percent group $\chi^2 = 4.00$.

pregnant mother has received 0.5 percent of lead in the diet (Jacquet et al., 1977a). The lack of a significant reduction in heme concentration may, of course, reflect the fact that the growth of the embryo is limited by the amount of heme enzymes and hemoglobin available. Incorporation of iron into fetal heme increases markedly from day 16 to day 18 of pregnancy, and this increase is lacking or delayed when the animals have received 0.125 to 0.5 percent of lead in the diet (Gerber and Maes, 1978). In consequence, it appears that the toxic action on the fetus at later stages of pregnancy is mainly caused by an interference with heme sythesis but also by a lowered blood flow through the placenta.

CONCLUSIONS

A quantitative extrapolation to man from animal data on lead reproductive toxicity is not feasible due to the differences in metabolism; otherwise, we should expect an action only after very high oral doses. Nevertheless, it appears from the data that all the effects mentioned appear only above a certain threshold dose. In man, even assuming extreme conditions, the dose, most likely, would not be more than 1-2 orders of magnitudes lower than that which gives an effect in animals. Thus, levels of environmental contamination would probably not affect male fertility. Evaluating toxicity is more difficult with respect to the female. The long-term experiments with lead in the drinking water suggest that an effect is unlikely at environmental levels of contamination. The doses needed to alter hormonal metabolism were very large but given only for a short period of time. The event in the developing fetus most relevant to human exposure is most likely not fetal death or general growth retardation but the action of lead on the developing central nervous system.

This work represents publication No 1874 of the Radiation Protection Program of the Commission of the European Communities.

REFERENCES

Azar, A., Trochimowicz, H.J. and Maxfield, M.E., 1972, Review of lead studies in animals carried out at the Maskell laboratory: Two year feeding study and response to hemmorhagic study, in: "Proceedings of the International Symposium on the Environmental Health Aspects of Lead", Amsterdam, pp. 199-209.

Barltrop, D.A., 1969, Transfer of Lead to the human fetus, in: "Mineral Metabolism in Pediatrics", D. Barltrop and W. L. Barland, eds., pp. 135-151, Davis, Philadelphia.

Bell, J.U. and Thomas, J.A., 1980, Effects of lead on mammalian reproduction, in: "Lead Toxicity", R.L. Singhal and J.A. Thomas, eds., pp. 169-185, Urban and Schwarzenberg, Baltimore-Munich.

Der, R., Yousef, E., Fahim, Z. and Fahim, M., 1977, Effects of lead and cadmium on adrenal and thyroid functions of the rat, Res. Commun. Chem. Pathol. Pharmacol. 17:237-253.

Eyden, B.P., Maisin, J.R. and Mattelin, G., 1978, Long-term effects of dietary lead acetate on survival, body weight and seminal cytology in mice, Bull. Environ. Contami. Toxicol. 19:226-272.

Ferm, V.H. and Carpenter, S., 1967, Developmental malformations resulting from the administration of lead salts, Exp. Mol. Pathol. 7:208-213.

Gerber, G.B. and Maes, J., 1978, Heme synthesis in the lead intoxicated mouse embryo, Toxicology 9:173-179.

Gerber, G.B., Maes, J. and Deroo, J., 1978, Effects of dietary lead on placental blood flow and fetal uptake of a-aminoisobutyrate, Arch. Toxicol. 41:125-131.

Gerber, G.B., Jacquet, P., Leonard, A. and Maes, J., 1979, Evolution des taux d'oestradiol, de progesterone et de prostaglandines E et F2a durant la gestation chez la souris, C.R. Soc. Biol. 173:644-649.

Gerber, G.B., Leonard, A. and Jacquet, P., 1980, Toxicity, mutagenicity and teratogenicity of lead, Mutation Res. 76:115-141.

Gerber, G.B., Maes, J., Deroo, J. and Jacquet, P., 1982, Transfer of
    lead in utero in normal and calcium deficient mice, Toxicology
    (in press).
Gilfillan, S.C., 1965, Lead poisoning and the fall of the Roman
    Empire, J. Occup. Med. 7:53-60.
Golubovits, E.Y., Auhimenko, M.M. and Chirkova, E.M., 1968,
    Biochemical and morphological changes in the testicles of rats
    as the results of small doses of lead, Toxicol. Nov. Pro. Khin.
    Veschestv. 10:64.
Hall, A., 1905, Increasing use of lead as abortifacient, Brit. Med
    J. 48:584-587.
Harris, P. and Holley, M.R., 1972, Lead levels in cord blood,
    Pediatrics 49:606-608.
Heddle, J.A. and Bruce, W.R., 1977, Comparison of tests for
    mutagenicity and carcinogenicity using assays for sperm
    abnormalities, formation of micronuclei and mutations in
    Salmonella, in: "Origins of Human Cancer", Vol. 4, H.H. Hiatt,
    J.D. Watson and J.A. Winsten, eds., pp. 1549-1557, Cold Spring
    Harbor Laboratory Press, New York.
Hildenbrand, D.C., Olds, M., Der, R. and Hafim, M. S., 1973, Effect
    of lead acetate on reproduction, Am. J. Obstet. Gynecol.
    115:1058-1065.
Jacquet, P., 1976, Effets du plomb administre durant la gestation a
    des souris C57B1, C. R. Soc. Biol. 170:1319-1322.
Jacquet, P., 1977, Early embryonic development in lead intoxicated
    mice, Arch. Pathol. Lab. Med. 101:1641-1643.
Jacquet, P., 1978, Influence de la progesterone et de l'oestradiol
    exogenes sur les processus de l'implantation embryonnaire chez
    la souris femelle intoxiquee par le plomb, C. R. Soc. Biol.
    172:1037-1040.
Jacquet, P. and Gerber, G.B., 1979, Teratogenic effects of lead in
    the mouse, Biomedicine 30:223-229.
Jacquet, P., Leonard, A. and Gerber, G.B., 1975, Embryonic death in
    mouse due to lead exposure, Experientia 31:1312-1313.
Jacquet, P., Leonard, A. and Gerber, G.B., 1976, Action of lead on
    the early divisions of the mouse embryo, Toxicology 6:129-132.
Jacquet, P., Gerber, G.B., Leonard, A. and Maes, J., 1977a, Plasma
    hormone levels in normal and lead treated pregnant mice,
    Experientia 33:1375-1376.
Jacquet, P., Gerber, G.B. and Maes, J., 1977b, Biochemical studies
    in embryos after exposure of pregnant mice to dietary lead,
    Bull. Environ. Contam. Toxicol. 18:271-277.
James, L.F., Lazar, V.A. and Binns, W., 1966, Effects of sublethal
    doses of certain minerals on pregnant ewes and fetal
    development, Am. J. Vet. Med. 27:132-135.
Kennedy, G.L. and Arnold, D.W., 1971, Absence of mutagenic effects
    after treatment of mice with lead compounds, E.M.S. News Letter
    5:37.
Kennedy, G.L., Arnold, D.W., Keplinger, M.L. and Calandra, C.J.,
    1971, Mutagenic and teratogenic studies with lead acetate and
    tetraethyl lead, Toxicol. Appl. Pharmacol. 19:370.

Kimmel, C.A., Grant, L.D. and Sloan, C.S., 1976, Chronic lead exposure: Assessment of developmental toxicity, Teratology 13:27A-28A.

Lancranjan, T., Popescu, H., Gavenescu, O., Klepsch, J. and Serbanescu, M., 1975, Reproductive ability of workmen occupationally exposed to lead, Arch. Environ. Health 300:396-401.

Leonard, A., Linden, B., Gerber, G.B., 1972, Etude chez la souris des effets genetiques et cytogenetiques d'une contatmination par le plomb, Proceedings of the International Symposium on Environmental Health Aspects of Lead, Amsterdam, pp. 303-309.

Leonard, A., Gerber, G.B. and Jacquet, P., 1982, Carcinogenicity, teratogenicity and mutagenicity of heavy metals, Plenum Press (in press).

Maisin, J.R., 1978, Toxicite du plomb pour les embryons de la souris, C. R. Soc. Biol. 172:1041-1043.

McClain, R.M. and Becker, B.A., 1972, Teratogenicity, fetal toxicity and placental transfer of lead nitrate in rats, Toxicol. Appl. Pharmacol. 31:72-82.

McLellan, J.S., Vonsmolinski, A.W., Bederka, J.P. and Boulos, B.M., 1974, Developmental toxicity of lead in the mouse, Fed. Proc. Abstr. 33:288.

Paul, C., 1860, Edude sur l'intoxication lente par des preparations de plomb; de son influence sur le produit de la conception, Arch. Gen. Med. 15:513-533.

Scanlon, J., 1971, Umbilical and cord blood concentrations, relationships to urban or suburban residency during gestation, Am. J. Dis. Child. 121:325-326.

Schroeder, H.A. and Mitchener, M., 1971, Toxic effects of trace elements on the reproduction of mice and rats, Arch. Environ. Health 23:102-106.

Sharma, R.M. and Buck, W.B., 1976, Effects of chronic lead exposure on pregnant sheep and their progeny, Vet. Toxicol. 18:186-188.

Stowe, D.H. and Goyer, R.A., 1971, The reproductive ability and progeny of F1 lead toxic rats, Fertil. Ster. 22:755-760.

Streffer, C., van Beuningen, D., Molls, M., Schulz, A.P. and Zambogliou, N., 1978, The in vitro culture of preimplantated mouse embryos. A model for studying combined effects, in: "Late Biological Effects of Ionizing Radiation, II", STI/PUB/489, IAEA, Vienna.

Taussig, F.G., 1936, "Abortions, Spontaneous and Induced," Mosby, St. Louis.

Varma, M.M., Joshi, S.R. and Adeyemi, A.O., 1974, Mutagenicity and infertility following administration of lead subacetate to Swiss male mice, Experientia 30:486-487.

Weller, V.C., 1915, The blastophoric effects of chronic lead poisoning, J. Med. Res. 33:271-293.

World Health Organization, 1977, Lead, Environmental Health Criteria, World Health Organization, Geneva.

Wyrobek, A.J. and Bruce, W.R., 1978, The induction of sperm cell abnormalities in mice and humans, in: "Chemical Mutagens, Principles and Methods for their Detection", Vol. 5, A. Hollaender ed., pp 257-285, Plenum Press, New York.

Zegarska, Z., Kilkowska, K. and Romankiewicz-Wocniczko, G., 1974, Development defects in white rats caused by acute lead poisoning, Folia Morphol. (Warszawa) 33:23-28.

SPONTANEOUS ABORTION AS RISK INDICATOR IN METAL EXPOSURE

Kari Hemminki, Marja-Liisa Niemi, Pentti Kyyronen,
Kari Koskinen, and Harri Vainio

Institute of Occupational Health
Helsinki, Finland

ABSTRACT

We have used a nation-wide hospital discharge register to
retrieve cases of spontaneous abortion. The frequency of
hospitalized spontaneous abortions has been studied in relation to
occupational factors. Three study schemes are presented in the
application of the spontaneous abortion register in relation to
metal work and exposure to metals. Scheme 1 involved a study on the
female members of the Union of Metal Workers covering years 1973 -
1979. Eleven hundred spontaneous abortions were recorded for the
women. The age-standardized frequency of spontaneous abortions in
relation to pregnancies was slightly higher (7.8 percent) for the
pregnancies conceived during Union membership, as compared with
those (7.1 percent) conceived before or after it. Exposure to
sulfur, zinc, cobalt and arsenic was considered possible for workers
of a metallurgical plant. Seven spontaneous abortions were
recorded, giving a frequency of 21 percent of all pregnancies.
Scheme 2 involved analysis of occupations of women and their
husbands in a community with metallurgical industry. The rate of
spontaneous abortions was higher for all economically active women
as compared with all the women in the community. The wives of
industrial workers did not deviate from all the women in the
community in the rate of spontaneous abortions. The wives of the
workers employed at the metallurgical factory had somewhat more
spontaneous abortions than the wives of all industrial workers. In
scheme 3, the frequency of spontaneous abortions was analysed in
relation to the occupation of the woman and her husband as stated in
the census taken at the end of 1975. One group of female metal
workers (welders) had an abortion rate of 9.5 percent as compared
with 8.2 percent for all industrial workers.

INTRODUCTION

It has been estimated that up to 50 percent of human pregnancies terminate in spontaneous abortion (Miller et al., 1980). Most of the early spontaneous abortions can only be recognized with the help of hormonal pregnancy tests. In retrospective interview studies, the cited frequencies of spontaneous abortions range between 5 percent and 15 percent of the pregnancies in reference populations (Hemminki et al., 1979, Sever, 1981; Strobino et al., 1978; Sullivan and Barlow, 1979). A large proportion of the abortion specimens, particularly in the early part of pregnancy, display chromosomal aberrations (Carr, 1977; Stein et al., 1975). Thus, because of its frequency and partial genetic etiology, spontaneous abortion has been recommended for environmental health surveillance (Kline et al., 1977; Hemminki et al., 1979). The difficulty in recognizing a spontaneous abortion has, however, been of serious concern in the instances when it has been applied in environmental surveillance.

We have used a nation-wide hospital discharge register to identify cases of spontaneous abortion. The frequency of hospitalized spontaneous abortions has been studied in relation to occupational determinants (Hemminki et al., 1980a,b,c; Hemminki and Niemi, 1982; Hemminki et al., 1982). In this communication, we present three study schemes for the application of the spontaneous abortion register in relation to metal workers and exposure to metals. Both maternal and paternal exposures are considered.

HOSPITAL DISCHARGE REGISTER

The Finnish National Board of Health maintains a computerized hospital discharge registry which includes all the patients discharged from general hospitals. From the registry we obtained information on all the Finnish women who had been treated either for spontaneous abortion (diagnoses numbers 643 and 645) or for induced abortions (diagnoses numbers 640-642). We also collected data about women who gave birth (diagnoses numbers 650-662). The diagnoses were based on the 8th revised version of the International Classification of Diseases. Patients who had been discharged from the hospital twice within a short time, and whose diagnosis was number 645 in connection with either spontaneous or induced abortion on each occasion were excluded from study. The information has been collected from years 1973 - 1979 covering 42,639 spontaneous abortions, 115,062 induced abortions, and 412,580 births. The regulations for induced abortions are liberal in Finland. The number of suspected illegal abortions is small, as indicated by infrequent hospitalization with diagnosis number 644 (febrile abortion).

The number of spontaneous abortions was related to the number of pregnancies (births + induced abortions + spontaneous abortions) referred to as the rate of spontaneous abortions, and to the number of births, referred to as the ratio of spontaneous abortions. Two different proportions for spontaneous abortions were calculated because of the large number of induced abortions in Finland. However, where the rates and the ratios agree well with one another, only the rates are given. In many cases, the frequency of induced abortions was also analysed, to assure that induced abortions were not misclassified as spontaneous abortions.

The general coverage of the hospital discharge register has been described (Hemminki et al., 1980c). The register includes 91 percent of all hospitalized spontaneous abortions, 83 percent of induced abortions and 93 percent of births. An ad hoc quality control study in a large hospital has indicated that the diagnoses in the hospital discharge register agreed with hospital journals in about 90 percent of the cases (Niemi et al., 1983). The mean gestational age of the hospitalized spontaneous abortions was 2 to 3 months (Niemi et al., 1983). Although regional differences in the frequency of hospitalized spontaneous abortions exist, the distance between the place of residence and the nearest hospital with a gynecological department does not correlate with the frequency of spontaneous abortions (Niemi et al., 1983).

Our experience with the hospital discharge register is positive relating to the efficiency of case retrieval and reliability of the data. Of course, the use of the register depends critically on the large degree of hospitalization of spontaneous abortions, which is the case in Finland. Somewhat more numbers of spontaneous abortions can usually be identified by personal interviews, as compared to the hospital discharge register. Yet the reporting bias may be very difficult to avoid in interview studies, defeating the gain in numbers.

SPONTANEOUS ABORTIONS OF UNION MEMBERS

In a previous study, we analysed the frequency of spontaneous abortions among female members of the Union of Metal Workers covering the years 1973 - 1976 (Hemminki et al., 1980c). The rate and the ratio of spontaneous abortions were somewhat higher than those of all Finnish women (Table 1). Among the main branches, the frequency of spontaneous abortions were increased in electronics, focusing on a chapter whose members were employed by a radio and television manufacturer. The particular risk group there, as investigated in collaboration with the company's health personnel, appeared to be solderers exposed to the vapors of solder resin. This particular study was too small to identify a sufficient number of pregnancies for women with exposure to metals.

Table 1   Rate and Ratio of Spontaneous Abortions among the Finnish
          Metal Workers between 1973 and 1976

Branch of Employment	Number of Spontaneous Abortions	Rate of Spontaneous Abortions[a]	Rate of Spontaneous Abortions[b]
Electronics	58	9.22	16.48***
Section mainly in radio and television production	24	12.44**	20.87**
Manufacturing of machinery	46	6.70	12.40
Manufacturing of other metal objects	25	8.20	13.09
Shipbuilding	23	7.32	14.20
Manufacturing of household machinery	11	9.91	15.94
Manufacturing of iron and steel	9	10.00	17.65
Manufacturing of transport equipment	6	5.56	8.00
Manufacturing of precious metal objects	4	15.38	33.33
Mining	3	12.00	25.00
Other branches of metal industry	10	6.21	9.90
All Union members	195	7.82	13.79***
All Finnish women	24,107	7.34	10.34

[a]Rate = spontaneous abortions x 100/pregnancies
[b]Ratio = spontaneous abortions x 100/births
* $p < 0.05$
** $p < 0.01$
*** $p < 0.001$

To increase the power of detection, the study among the female members of the Union of Metal Workers was repeated in 1982. The records of hospitalized spontaneous abortions were collected from years 1973 - 1979; the analysis also included women who had resigned from the Union. The new study was comprised of 1100 spontaneous abortions. The age-standardized rate of spontaneous abortions was 7.8 percent for pregnancies conceived during membership, as compared to a rate of 7.1 percent for pregnancies conceived before or after membership (p < 0.10, Mantel-Haenszel test). Older age groups mainly contributed to the difference (Figure 1).

The Union branches, where exposure to metals is possible, were analyzed in Table 2. It is of interest to compare individual branches with all Union members, as well as the pregnancies conceived during the membership to those conceived before or after the membership. Although variation was seen in the rates, no differences reached the level of statistical significance. However, the branches are still wide categories, and they are likely to be rather uninformative as far as true exposures are concerned.

Further analysis was carried out with individual chapters where exposure to metals is possible. The types of chapters included those mainly involved in metal smelting, where exposure to sulfur, zinc, arsenic, cobalt and copper is possible. In two chapters, to which melters belong, the crude rate of spontaneous abortions was increased. In one chapter, the rate of spontaneous abortions was 21

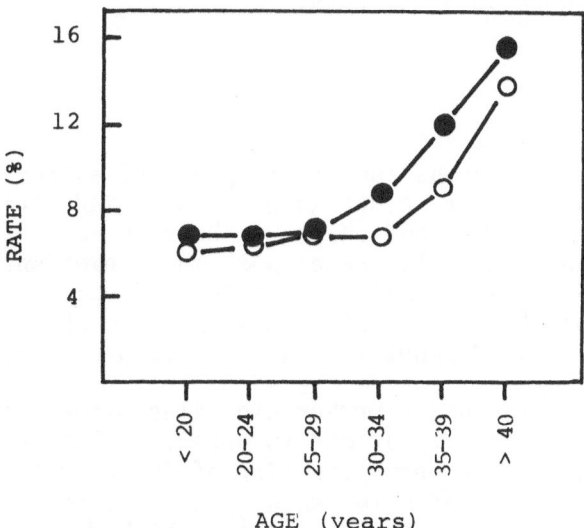

Figure 1   Rate of spontaneous abortions among female metal workers for pregnancies conceived during membership (—— • ——), and before or after it (—— o ——).

Table 2   Age-Standardized Rate of Spontaneous Abortions among Female
          Members of the Union of Metal Workers According to the
          Branch in which Exposure to Metals is Possible

Branch	Conception during Membership		Conception before/after Membership	
	Number Spontaneous Abortions	Rate: %	Number Spontaneous Abortions	Rate: %
Manufacturing of metal objects	91	8.5	55	6.5
Shipbuilding	77	7.5	73	9.2
Manufacturing of iron and steel	24	8.4	23	11.1
Mining*	5	8.8	3	7.5
Foundry*	7	4.9	8	6.1
All Union	665	7.8	476	7.1

*Women aged 15 - 35 years.

percent, with 7 spontaneous abortions ($p < 0.05$ as compared with all
Union members; $p < 0.10$ as compared with local industrial workers,
binomial test); in the second chapter, the rate was 15 percent with
3 spontaneous abortions. The rates were much lower when the
pregnancies were conceived before or after the Union membership. A
closer inspection of the largest metals smelting chapter will
follow, when the second scheme of analysis is presented.

As a summary, the Union membership files offer an efficient way
to focus on the type of employment in question. However, they are
not usually adequate for identification of individual exposures, and
special inquiries are needed for such specific information. The use
of the union records requires a reasonably high degree of
unionization and good management of the membership files. In
Finland, the degree of unionization is high, over 90 percent in most
branches. Membership files are well maintained as the membership
register is used for the collection of fees.

SPONTANEOUS ABORTIONS IN A COMMUNITY WITH METALLURGICAL INDUSTRY

The second scheme used in the analysis of spontaneous abortions was a community study. Information on spontaneous abortions and pregnancies was obtained from years 1974 - 1977. Information on women, their family conditions, occupation and husband's occupation was collected from the population and housing census taken at the end of 1975. These data were obtained for 83 percent of the women. Most of the cases for whom data were not available had probably either moved from the community before the census was taken, or moved to it after the census had been taken. We collected a sample of 15 percent of the persons we could not trace. The analysis of the data on these persons showed that they had a higher rate of spontaneous abortion (12.7 percent) than the persons whose data were available from the census (9.8 percent).

The major employer in the community was a metallurgical factory producing zinc and cobalt. In addition to these metals, the workers would be exposed to sulfur dioxide, hydrogen sulfide, arsenic, and to a smaller extent cadmium and mercury. Approximately one fourth of the men and many women of the community's population were employed at the metallurgical plant. The main employment for women was in the textile industry.

The rate of spontaneous abortions was significantly higher ($p < 0.001$) for all economically active women as compared with all the women in the community (Table 3). The rate for industrial production workers exceeded that for all economically active women, but it was lower than the rate for textile workers. It is possible that excretion may contribute to the results, but it does not explain the high rate of spontaneous abortions of some occupational groups discussed later. The wives of industrial workers did not deviate from all the women in the community in the rate of spontaneous abortions. The wives of the workers employed at the metallurgical factory had somewhat more spontaneous abortions than the wives of all industrial workers. Not enough pregnancies were recorded for female workers at the metallurgical plant for evaluation. Thus, the data derived from the Union records, covering more years, were more useful in this respect (the Union members from the above metallurgical factory had 7 spontaneous abortions and 33 pregnancies: rate = 21 percent).

The occupations of the men whose wives had spontaneous abortions were analyzed in more detail (Table 4). The wives of smelters had 19 spontaneous abortions and a rate of 11.5 percent, slightly above all employees. The wives of the machine repairmen had a rate of 12.7 percent. The wives of the men belonging to the category "other occupations" also had a high rate, 12.5 percent. This group included administrative and office personnel, where extensive exposure to metals was unlikely. Thus, the job titles did not appear to provide evidence on any particular risk group.

Table 3 Frequency of Spontaneous Abortions According to Some Women's and Husbands' Occupations in the Industrial Community in 1974 - 1977

Occupation	Woman Number Spontaneous Abortions	Rate: %	Husband Number Spontaneous Abortions	Rate: %
Industrial production	56	12.2	104	9.3
Metallurgical industry	-	-	41	10.4
Sewer in textile industry	31	12.9	-	-
Economically active women	194	11.4	-	-
Economically inactive women	63	6.3	-	-
Community total	257	9.5	210	9.8

        The possible modifying effect of the husband's occupation on the frequency of spontaneous abortions was analyzed in Table 5. When a woman employed in the textile industry was married to a man employed at the metallurgical factory, the rate of spontaneous abortion was 21.7 percent, as compared with a rate of 8.4 percent for women employed in other industries. The rate for a textile worker married to a man not employed in the metallurgical factory was 11.1 percent showing that the combination: a woman in the textile industry married to a man at the metallurgical factory, was unique. One possible reason for the interaction, in addition to chance, may be a selectional one, for instance, a social effect. Another possibility is a paternal effect caused by an occupational exposure to metals or other agents at the metallurgical plant.

        The experience of the community study showed that detailed information on occupation and employment may be obtained from the available data sources, e.g. the files of the population and housing census. Access to such sources of data would be a particular asset

Table 4 Spontaneous Abortions of Wives of Men Employed at the
Metallurgical Plant

Husband's Occupation	Number Spontaneous Abortions	Rate: %
Engineer, technician	4	10.3
Laboratory staff	4	9.8
Smelter worker	19	11.5
Machine repairman	7	12.7
Welder	2	6.9
Other manual worker	13	8.8
Other occupations	10	12.5
All employees	59	10.5

Table 5 Modification of the Frequency of Spontaneous Abortions
According to the Husbands' Employment

Woman	Husband	Number Spontaneous Abortions	Rate: %	Odds Ratio
Textile industry	Metallurgical factory	20	21.7	
				3.0[a]
Other industries	Metallurgical factory	22	8.4	
Textile industry	Other factories	23	11.1	
				0.9
Other industries	Other factories	94	11.9	

[a]p-value for homogeneity of odds ratios, $p < 0.01$.

if employment records were unavailable or unreliable. However, the numbers may turn out to be very small in a community-based study.

SPONTANEOUS ABORTIONS IN RELATION TO OCCUPATION STATED IN CENSUS

The data of the population and housing census, as applied above, may be used on a national basis to overcome the problem of small numbers. In the present application, scheme three, the frequency of hospitalized spontaneous abortions in years 1973 - 1976 was analyzed in relation to the occupation of the woman and her husband as stated in the census taken at the end of 1975.

The analysis covered a few hundred occupational titles. Some occupations, where exposure to metals is possible, are presented in Table 6. The rate of spontaneous abortions for all female workers in industry was 8.2 percent. Welders had 28 spontaneous abortions and a rate of 9.5 percent. The regional distribution of the female welders suggested that many of them were employed in shipbuilding. Female smelter workers did not have enough pregnancies for any conclusion to be drawn. The rate for the foundry workers was below that of all industrial workers. The husbands' occupations were also analysed but no significant differences were seen from all industrial workers.

The population and housing census covering the entire nation provides important background information for occupational studies. It may be used to generate hypotheses and to collect groups of workers for further studies. Another advantage is the availability of data on the paternal occupation. However, the occupational information is not specific enough in most cases to reconstruct exposures.

CONCLUSIONS

Three different study designs were introduced to study the effect of occupational factors on spontaneous abortions. Some preliminary results were presented using exposure to metals as a model. This is not an easy model, as pregnant women are infrequently employed in operations where extensive exposure to metals is possible. Thus, the numbers observed tend to be small. Even in Finland, where the proportion of women employed in industry is relatively high, few pregnant women are found as smelter workers or welders, who may be exposed. Many more men are found in these occupations, but it may be that clinically-recognized spontaneous abortions are less sensitive to effects transmitted through male exposure as compared to direct effects during pregnancy. Even as a test for mutation in experimental animals, the dominant-lethal test in which males are exposed, is considered relatively insensitive.

Table 6   Spontaneous Abortions Classified by the Women and their
          Husbands' Occupations Stated in Census

Occupation	Women Number Spontaneous Abortions	Rate: %	Husband Number Spontaneous Abortions	Rate: %
Smelter worker	1	3.4	39	6.2
Foundry worker	5	5.9	36	6.1
Welder	28	9.5	317	6.1
All industrial workers	2260	8.2	6049	6.7

In spite of the exploratory nature of the studies described,
some interesting leads appeared to emerge. Studies on smelter
workers, possibly exposed to sulfur compounds, arsenic, cobalt, zinc
and cadmium, suggested ill effects through maternal and paternal
exposure. It is important to increase the size of the studies, and
to confirm the likelihood of exposure. Interestingly, many types of
reproductive ill effects transmitted through maternal and paternal
exposure, have been reported in a Swedish copper smelter (Nordstrom
et al., 1978; 1979a,b); the reported exposures include arsenic and
lead. In view of the many types of reproductive ill effects
elicited by metals in experimental animals (Wilson, 1977; Hemminki,
1980), it is important to pursue reproductive studies among exposed
workers.

REFERENCES

Carr, D.H., 1977, Detection and evaluation of pregnancy wastage,
    in "Handbook of Teratology", Vol. 3, J.G. Wilson and F.C.
    Fraser, eds., pp. 189-213, Plenum Press, New York.
Hemminki, K., 1980, Occupational chemicals tested for
    teratogenicity, Int. Arch. Occup. Environ. Health 47:191-208.
Hemminki, K. and Niemi, M.-L., 1982, Community study of
    spontaneous abortions: Relation to occupation and air pollution
    by sulfur dioxide, hydrogen sulfide and carbon disulfide, Int.
    Arch. Occup. Environ. Health (in press).
Hemminki, K., Sorsa, M. and Vainio, H., 1979, Genetic risks
    caused by occupational chemicals, Scand. J. Work Environ.
    Health 5:307-327.

Hemminki, K., Franssila, E. and Vainio, H., 1980a, Spontaneous
     abortions among female chemical workers in Finland, Int. Arch.
     Occup. Environ. Health 45:123-126.
Hemminki, K., Niemi, M.-L., Saloniemi, I., Vainio, H. and
     Hemminki, E., 1980b, Spontaneous abortions by occupation and
     social class in Finland, Int. J. Epidemiol. 9:149-153.
Hemminki, K., Niemi, M.-L., Koskinen, K. and Vainio, H., 1980c,
     Spontaneous abortions among women employed in the metal
     industry in Finland, Int. Arch. Occup. Environ. Health 47:53-60.
Hemminki, K., Niemi, M.-L., Kyyronen, P., Kilpikari, I. and
     Vainio, H., 1982, Spontaneous abortions and reproductive
     selection mechanisms in rubber and leather industry in Finland,
     Brit. J. Ind. Med. (in press).
Kline, J., Stein, Z., Strobino, B., Susser, M. and Warburton, D.,
     1977, Surveillance of spontaneous abortions. Power in
     environmental monitoring, Am. J. Epidemiol. 106:345-350.
Miller, J.F., Williamson, E., Glue, J., Gordon, Y.B.,
     Grudzinskas, J.G. and Sykes, A., 1980, Fetal loss after
     implantation. A prospective study, Lancet 2:554-556.
Niemi, M.-L., Hemminki, K. and Sallmen, M., 1983, Application of
     hospital discharge register for studies on spontaneous
     abortions, in "Occupational Hazards and Reproduction", K.
     Hemminki, M. Sorsa, and H. Vainio, eds., Hemisphere Publishing
     Co., Washington DC, in press.
Nordstrom, S., Beckman, L. and Nordenson, I., 1978, Occupational
     and environmental risks in and around a smelter in Northern
     Sweden. III. Frequencies of spontaneous abortions, Hereditas
     88:51-54.
Nordstrom, S., Beckman, L. and Nordenson, I., 1979a, Occupational
     and environmental risks in and around a smelter in Northern
     Sweden. V. Spontaneous abortions among female employees and
     decreased birth weight in their offspring, Hereditas 90:291-296.
Nordstrom, S., Beckman, L., and Nordenson, I., 1979b,
     Occupational and environmental risks in and around a smelter in
     Northern Sweden. VI. Congenital malformations, Hereditas
     90:297-300.
Sever, L.E., 1981, Reproductive hazards of the workplace, J.
     Occup. Med. 23:685-689.
Stein, S., Susser, M., Warburton, D., Wittes, J. and Hine, J.,
     1975, Spontaneous abortion as a screening device: The effect of
     fetal survival on the incidence of birth defects, Am. J.
     Epidemiol. 102:275-290.
Strobino, B.R., Kline, J. and Stein, Z., 1978, Chemical and
     physical exposures of parents: Effects on human reproduction
     and offspring, Early Human Develop. 1:371-399.
Sullivan, F.M. and Barlow, S.M., 1979, Congenital malformations
     and other reproductive hazards from environmental chemicals,
     Proc. R. Soc. Lond. B. 205:91-110.
Wilson, J.G., 1977, Environmental chemicals, in "Handbook of
     Teratology", Vol. 1, J.G. Wilson, and F.C. Fraser, eds.,
     pp. 357-385, Plenum Press, New York.

METAL-INDUCED CONGENITAL MALFORMATIONS

Vergil H. Ferm and David P. Hanlon

Department of Anatomy
Dartmouth Medical School
Hanover, New Hampshire

ABSTRACT

Certain heavy metals induce specific patterns of developmental malformations in the hamster model. These metals are indium, cadmium, mercury, copper and arsenic (as arsenate) listed in order of increasing dose required to provoke a teratogenic response. The hamster model is well suited to teratogenic investigations by reason of its short gestation period and remarkably condensed period of organogenesis in addition to the fact that maternal toxicity is not a problem at teratogenic doses. Each of the metal teratogens causes a characteristic response in the form of a particular pattern of fetal abnormalities. These characteristic responses can be modified by the presence of certain other metals or genetic and environmental factors. Non-teratogenic metals cross the hamster placenta with ease. In contrast, heavy metal teratogens concentrate in the placenta and only small amounts are deposited in the embryo. These data imply the presence of a placental barrier to heavy metals; further studies with cadmium have suggested that this barrier is a cadmium-binding protein. Future studies on heavy metal teratogenesis should focus on the potential effect of chronic low-level exposure to these metals, genetic factors influencing teratogenic response, and identification of possible environmental factors which can modify heavy metal teratogens.

INTRODUCTION

The mammalian embryo occupies a unique ecological niche among vertebrate systems. It is isolated from the external and maternal environments by a barrier of its own making, the placenta. It is

completely dependent for growth and survival on the maternal system
for energy and nutrients. The developing embryo is thus in a very
dependent position of compromise as toxic agents available to the
maternal system could gain access to the embryonic system.

The embryonic unit, including both the embryo/fetus and the
placenta, undergoes a continuum of development from the moment of
fertilization to the late stages of development. Few mammalian
tissues change as dramatically as the placenta during its short life
span. These changes include gross and microscopic morphologic
features as well as biochemical and physiological phenomena. During
its development a whole range of events proceeds stepwise, many of
which are limited in time to a particular period which may be as
brief as a few minutes or hours. Each of these sequential events is
probably biochemically controlled and could include enzymatic
reactions, peculiar to development, which are metal sensitive.
Within the developing embryo, the maximum sensitivity to
malformation-causing stimuli occurs during the critical stages of
organogenesis and is very time-limited in all species. Finally, the
developing mammalian embryo is genetically different from the
maternal environment in which it develops.

All of these factors - the enzymatic events proceeding at the
time of organogenesis, the changing structure and function of the
placenta at the same period, and the genetic constitution of the
embryo - are important factors in any teratological event.

ANIMAL MODEL

Almost all teratogenic studies concerned with heavy metals have
used rodent models with an intact materno-uterine-embryonic unit.
The animal model we have used is the pregnant hamster. Almost all
of our data are derived from one strain of that animal making
comparisons among the teratogenic metals more realistic than
comparisons between species. The virtues of our animal model are;
1) the short gestation period (16 days), 2) the reliability and ease
of obtaining accurately-timed matings, 3) the large litter size
(average 12), 4) the remarkably condensed but consistent period of
organogenesis which occurs over a 24-hour interval from day 8 to day
9 of gestation (Ferm, 1967). This period corresponds to the 10-day
period between the 18th day and 28th day of human gestation.

METAL TERATOGENS

For the past 12 years we have been investigating the effects of
heavy metals on embryonic development. We have identified five
metals, which, in their ionic state, induce specific patterns of
congenital abnormalities in the embryos of pregnant hamsters if

administered during the critical phase of organogenesis. Metals are
in one sense ideal teratogens for they cannot be degraded and are
easily traced in the materno-embryonic unit with a variety of
quantitative techniques. The biomedical literature concerning the
toxic effects of metals on embryos is varied and growing. The
recent excellent review by Mottet (1981) on this subject is highly
recommended.

    Certain metal ions, for example zinc and magnesium, are
essential for life processes. Others such as copper are also
required by the living system, but are very toxic at slightly higher
concentrations. On the other hand, most of our metal teratogens
play no vital role and display increasing degrees of toxicity with
increasing concentrations in most biological systems; this is also
true of the metalloid, arsenic. Teratogenicity, like toxicity, must
depend in part on the physico-chemical properties of agents since
these properties dictate not only the nature of the specific sites
attacked, but also the accessibility of the sites to each teratogen.
Accessibility in turn depends on the distribution and chemical status
of a teratogen. By "chemical status" we mean that fraction of the
total metal ion which is bound to high molecular weight or low
molecular weight chelators and thereby sequestered to some degree,
as well as that fraction which is "free", i.e., not bound to other
molecules or bound so weakly that it is readily available to enter
into other reactions.

    Neither the mechanism of action nor the sites of action are
known for metal teratogens. While critical sites of action could be
in the maternal system and produce teratogenic effects indirectly,
it is far more likely that the specific sites are located in the
embryo and/or the placental tissues.

    Most of the abnormalities caused by metal ions are reductive in
nature, which is to say, the normal pattern of embryonic development
is subverted; limb buds do not form, critical tissue closures are
not made, etc. This points to the inhibition of some process at a
critical time during organogenesis. Hanlon and Ferm (1974) have
suggested some likely modes of teratogenic insult by metal ions at
the biochemical level. These include inhibition of one or more
critical enzyme reactions, destabilization of a cell membrane system
and/or interference with the transport of specific factors across
the nuclear membrane.

MODIFYING FACTORS IN METAL TERATOGENESIS

    1) Co-metal effects. It is apparent from some of our later
studies that the exposure of pregnant animals to certain combinations
of heavy metals results in different patterns of malformations
(synergism) as compared to single metal exposure alone. On the

other hand, certain combinations of metals may reduce significantly
the expression of the teratogenic effect of a single metal
(protection).

2) Genetic factors affecting the expression of heavy metal
teratogenesis. There are as yet few indications that the genotype
of the embryo affects the expression of heavy metal teratogenesis
but some initial studies in our animal model suggest that such
factors may be important (vida infra).

3) Environmental factors affecting the expression of heavy
metal teratogenesis. Modifications of teratogenic response to
chemicals, drugs, etc., by manipulation of the maternal environment
during organogenesis, has received very little attention. We have
shown in our animal model (vida infra) that maternal hyperthermia
induced by an increase in environmental temperature enhances the
teratogenic effect of certain metals.

LEAD

Our first studies of the teratogenic effects of metals in the
hamster model were with lead. This metal when injected into pregnant
hamsters on the 8th day of gestation caused a highly site-specific
and consistent malformation in a high percentage of embryos (Ferm
and Carpenter, 1967). This malformation was localized at the caudal
end of the vertebral column and consisted of tail abnormalities and
sacral vertebral anomalies (see Table 1). Subsequently, a study of
the histogenesis of this lesion from its earliest expression to the
final malformation (Carpenter and Ferm, 1977) revealed a sequence of
localized edema, blisters and hematomas. The resulting lesions
(dysgenesis or agenesis) of the vertebrae and tail buds may have
been the result of disruptive steps in development and/or repair
mechanisms which followed the teratogenic event. It is important to
note that lead administered at different times during the
organogenetic period did not cause any significantly different
patterns of malformation; only caudal malformations developed (Ferm
and Ferm 1971).

Co-metal Effects. There is an interesting teratogenic
lead-cadmium synergism which will be discussed below.

Genetic Factors. Gale and Layton (1978) treated five inbred
strains and one non-inbred strain of hamsters with lead. Three of
the inbred strains and the non-inbred strain were equally
susceptible to the teratogenic effects of lead. Two other inbred
strains were more resistant to lead-caused effects. These
differences also appeared in an analysis and comparison of the
frequency of the specific defect. The authors speculated that there
may be a difference in the rate at which lead penetrates the

placenta in these strains during the critical period of organogenesis.

   Environmental Factors.   No environmental factors affecting lead teratogenicity have as yet been identified.

CADMIUM

   Cadmium is the most intriguing and probably the best studied of all the teratogenic metals in the hamster model. Administration of this metal during the critical stages of development induces a specific pattern of malformations. Unlike lead, cadmium affects different organ systems depending upon the time that it is administered during the 24-hour period (Ferm, 1970). The characteristic and severe facial clefts induced by cadmium in the hamster have been studied by Mulvihill et al. (1970) who correlated these facial clefts with an apparent deficiency in the supportive mesenchyme in the region of the lesions on day 12 of gestation. This mesenchymal defect has been noted in other species treated with cadmium. Ferm and Layton (1979) studied the effect of pretreatment of the pregnant hamster with a single exposure to cadmium 24-48 hours prior to injection of the normally teratogenic dose of cadmium on day 8, the sensitive teratogenic period. This phenomenon had been reported also in mice (Semba et al., 1977). The results showed that the developing embryo was significantly protected when the mother was pretreated with cadmium. They postulated that this protective effect might be due to the maternal synthesis of a metal-binding protein, possibly a metallothionein. As a further example of this phenomenon, Layton and Ferm (1980) reported that pregnant C57BL/6J mice, which respond to cadmium with a high degree of limb malformations in the fetus, can also be protected from cadmium teratogenesis by pretreatment of the mother with either cadmium or mercury. In this species, the protective effect of pretreatment with cadmium extended to a prepregnancy period of three weeks. This protective effect of cadmium against cadmium may explain the lack of definitive evidence that cadmium is a serious human teratogenic threat. These results also show that the effect of pretreatment with a teratogen and its subsequent effect on teratogenicity, may be important criteria in the design and evaluation of teratogenic testing in animal systems.

   Co-metal Effects.   The teratogenic effect of cadmium can be affected by the presence of other metals during the time of teratogenesis. For example, the teratogenic effect of cadmium in our animal model can be almost completely inhibited by the simultaneous administration of an equivalent dose of zinc (Ferm and Carpenter, 1967). This protection diminishes when the zinc is administered 6 hours after the cadmium treatment and disappears completely after 12 hours. Zinc by itself is non-teratogenic in our

Table 1   The Organ Specificity of Teratogenic Metals in the Golden Hamster[a]

	In	Cd	Hg	Cu	As	Pb
CNS					++++	
HEART		+		+++		
URO-GENITAL					++++	
LIMBS	++++[b]					
RIBS		++++	+		+	+
FACIAL		++++				
TAIL	+	+				++++
EDEMA			+++			

[a]Metals listed in order of increasing doses (μMoles per kg/dam) required to provoke a teratogenic response (Reading L > R).
[b]Digits only.

animal model. We have also shown that zinc does not prevent the placental transfer of cadmium during the critical stages of embryogenesis (Ferm et al., 1969), nor does cadmium prevent the placental transfer of zinc during the same time period (Ferm and Hanlon, 1974a). These points will be considered later.

Likewise, the simultaneous administration of teratogenic doses of cadmium and lead considerably changes the teratogenic outcome (Ferm, 1969; Hilbelink, 1980). Following combined dosage, the facial malformations induced by cadmium alone are reduced in frequency and severity. On the other hand, the caudal malformations induced by the cadmium-lead combination are much more severe. They range from minor abnormalities of the sacral vertebrae to complete fusion of the lower extremities (symmelia). These malformations of the caudal region are much more severe than those seen with lead alone; for some reason, the presence of cadmium potentiates the effect of lead. However, the reverse is not true since lead does not increase the frequency or severity of those malformations attributable to cadmium.

Genetic Factors. Using the same five inbred and one non-inbred strain of hamsters as in the lead experiments described above, Gale and Layton (1980) reported the inter-strain variation to cadmium-induced teratogenesis was not as striking as it was in the comparable lead studies. Layton and Layton (1979) examined the comparative teratogenic effects of cadmium in six inbred strains of mice. Three of these strains carried a gene cdm which confers resistance (in the homozygous recessive state) to cadium-induced testicular damage (Taylor et al., 1973). The Layton studies revealed that the strains which were resistant to the cadmium-induced testicular damage were significantly more sensitive to the teratogenic effect of cadmium than were the other three testicular-sensitive strains.

Environmental Factors. There are as yet no known environmental factors which affect cadmium teratogenesis.

ARSENIC

The metalloid, arsenic, in the form of arsenate, is teratogenic in the hamster model and shows a site-specific effect on the developing embryo. A very high percentage of fetuses recovered from mothers treated on the 9th day of gestation demonstrate neural tube defects (Ferm and Carpenter, 1968b). Most of these neural tube lesions are confined to the head region and most frequently in the mid-brain area (Table 1). Histopathologic studies by Willhite (1981) revealed that areas of cellular necrosis in the cephalic mesenchyme could be found some 10 to 12 hours after treatment with arsenate, suggesting that the closure of the neural tube was prevented by some deficiency in the underlying cephalic mesoderm. Burk and Beaudoin (1977) demonstrated a remarkable site-specificity of arsenate on the embryonic rat uro-genital system. Uro-genital malformations, including renal agenesis, uterine malformations, and ureteral anomalies apparently resulted from a primary defect on the developing mesonephric duct of the rat embryo.

In the hamster, the pattern of malformations varies depending upon the time during organogenesis when the arsenic is administered (Ferm et al., 1971). Arsenic is more teratogenic than arsenate, but the methylated metabolites of inorganic arsenic, methylarsonic acid and dimethylarsinic acid, are not nearly as teratogenic as the inorganic form in this animal model (Willhite, 1981).

Co-metal Effects. The simultaneous administration of selenium
with a teratogenic dose of arsenate reduces the teratogenicity of
arsenic to a considerable degree. Selenium is not a significant
teratogen in the hamster (Holmberg and Ferm, 1969).

Genetic Factors. There is no experimental evidence to date to
suggest that genetic factors affect the expression of
arsenic-induced teratogenesis.

Environmental Factors. Because the central nervous system
lesions induced by arsenate in the hamster are so similar to those
lesions induced by exposure of the dam to short-term hyperthermia
(39.5°C for one hour), we examined the possible synergistic action
of maternal hyperthermia and sodium arsenate. We found that exposure
of the pregnant hamster to 50 minutes in an environment at 39.5°C
caused the maternal core body temperature to rise to 40°C at the end
of the 50-minute period and then return to normal within one hour
post treatment. This exposure resulted in a very low percentage
(<10 percent) of central nervous system anomalies (a baseline
effect). When one-half the ambient teratogenic dose of arsenate was
administered prior to the hyperthermic treatment, the number of
central nervous system malformations increased considerably (Ferm
and Kilham, 1977).

INDIUM

The teratogenic effect of indium on the hamster embryo is
almost exclusively limited to the developing limb buds, although a
few other minor anomalies occur (Table 2). The limb bud defects are
usually confined to the digits and take the form of syndactyly,
polydactyly or missing digits (Ferm and Carpenter, 1970). McCord et
al. (1942) reported that the histopathology of lesions induced in
adult animals was the same following intravenous or subcutaneous
administration of indium. After parenteral administration to
hamsters, the maximum levels of indium were found in bone, muscle,
and skin, a possible clue to its site-specific teratogenicity (Smith
et al., 1960). Germanium and gallium are not significant teratogens
in the animal model.

Co-metal Effects. Because others had noted the protective
effect of ferric dextran in the severe hepatic damage caused by
indium in rats, we studied the possible interaction of indium and
ferric dextran in the hamster model (Ferm, 1970). Both the fetal
resorption rate and the malformation rate are reduced by the
simultaneous administration of ferric dextran and indium. The fact
that ferric dextran stimulates the formation of a PAS-stainable
material wherever it is deposited in tissues could suggest the
mechanism of protection against the teratogenic effect of indium.
On the other hand, Gabbiani et al. (1962) reported that ferric

Table 2   The Distribution of Metal Teratogens in Three Compartments of the Hamster Materno-Embryonic Unit 24 Hours After a Bolus Teratogenic Dose Given on Day 8 of Gestation

Teratogen	Acute Teratogenic Dose	Embryos	Placentas	Maternal Blood
Cd	7.80[a]	0.357	2.11	0.185
Hg	12.4	0.562	12.0	4.34
AsO$_4$	64.1	0.719	1.97	0.863
Pb	151	2.17	17.5	8.84

[a]Numerical values expressed as micromoles/kg.

dextran is only one agent out of many examined which protects against the indium-induced hepatic lesions in rats.

Genetic Factors.   At this time there are no known genetic factors influencing indium teratogenicity.

Environmental Factors.   Because the teratogenic end-points of indium and maternal hyperthermia in the hamster model are so different, we thought it might be possible to use these two teratogenic agents to determine if maternal hyperthermia is a sensitizing agent to other teratogens.   Our preliminary results have shown that, indeed, the digital malformations are increased in number when indium-treated mothers are exposed to a minimal teratogenic hyperthermic stress.   On the other hand, this combined treatment did not result in an increase in those CNS malformations typically found when mothers are exposed to hyperthermia alone. This suggests that a hyperthermic event in early pregnancy may well potentiate the effects of certain teratogens including at least two of the metals studied to date, arsenic and indium.

COPPER

Copper is teratogenic in the hamster (Ferm and Hanlon, 1974b). DiCarlo (1980) has studied the teratogenic effect of copper citrate on the developing hamster embryonic heart.   He showed that a common and consistently-induced malformation was a double outlet right ventricle associated with an inter-ventricular septal defect (Table 1).   This suggests that these cardiac anomalies arise from a common pathogenetic basis. Copper in the chelated form (citrate) is more teratogenic in this model than copper sulfate (Ferm and Hanlon, 1974b).

Co-metal Effects. No other metals are known to alter copper teratogenicity.

Genetic Factors. Scheinberg and Sternlieb (1975) have reviewed 18 cases of human pregnancy in patients with Wilson's disease; some of these patients were on penicillamine therapy. No abnormal infants at term were encountered, although the authors mention that miscarriages are common in untreated Wilson's disease.

Environmental Factors. Intrauterine devices containing copper inhibited implantation in the hamster but no conclusions could be drawn concerning a teratogenic effect of this metal (Chang et al., 1970). Intrauterine devices containing copper release free copper ions which presumably account for their contraceptive effect. There is no published evidence to show that copper-containing IUD's are associated with congenital malformations in the human.

MERCURY

Both inorganic and organic mercurial compounds are relatively non-specific teratogens in the hamster model system (Gale and Ferm, 1971). Maternal toxicity is characterized by weight loss, diarrhea, tremor, and somnolence. Fetuses examined near term showed a generalized edema and were small-for-date (Table 1). These findings are simlar to those described by Mottet (1974) for rats.

Co-metal Effects. There is evidence to suggest that treatment of pregnant mice with mercury prior to the sensitive teratogenic period decreases the teratogenic effect of cadmium in this species (Layton and Ferm, 1980).

Genetic Factors. No genetic factors affecting mercury teratogenicity have been documented.

Environmental Factors. The potential damage that mercury might do to the developing central nervous system of the human embryo is well documented in the Minimata Bay exposure (Harriss and Hohenemser, 1978).

THE DISTRIBUTION AND CHEMICAL STATUS OF METAL AND METALLOID TERATOGENS IN THE PREGNANT HAMSTER

Our studies of the distribution of metal ions in the pregnant hamster, while less revealing than a combination of distribution and chemical status data, have provided some useful insights. For example, non-teratogenic essential ions such as zinc and manganese cross the placenta with ease and are distributed in approximately equal concentrations in placental tissues and embryos (Ferm and Hanlon, 1974a; Hanlon et al., 1975). In contrast, the heavy metal teratogens, mercury (Gale and Hanlon, 1976), cadmium (Ferm et al., 1969) and lead (Hanlon and Ferm, 1981) are concentrated in the placental tissues 24 hours after the injection of optimal teratogenic doses of each (Table 2). Very small, but detectable, amounts of each are deposited in the embryos. The ratios of metal ion concentrations in 9-day placentas/embryos are 21, 5, and 15 for mercuric ion, cadmium ion and lead ion, respectively. When the relative masses of placental tissues and embryos are considered, virtually all of the total embryonic system load of each of the metal ion teratogens (greater than 98 percent) is contained within the placenta.

The metalloid arsenic, in the form of arsenate, also crosses the hamster placenta during organogenesis (Hanlon and Ferm, 1977). The placenta is less of a barrier to arsenate than it is to the metal ion teratogens. The pattern of arsenate distribution is the same in maternal and embryonic tissues following a teratogenic dose or a trace dose of [^{74}As]arsenate. Thus, arsenate is partitioned in identical fashion for doses of teratogen differing by more than 2100 times. Constancy in the pattern of arsenate distribution over a wide concentration range implies that very little teratogen is bound to macromolecules or other tissue components. This observation is entirely consistent with the chemical nature of arsenate, which is far more similar to phosphate ion than to heavy metal ions per se. On the other hand, the distribution of lead ion at teratogenic and trace doses, while indicating a selective loading of the placenta relative to the embryos at both doses, shows a concentration dependency which strongly suggests that most of the lead ion present in the placental tissues is bound to macromolecules (Hanlon and Ferm, 1981). Our cadmium ion distribution data (Ferm et al., 1969) for the hamster animal model also indicates that a significant fraction of the heavy metal ion load of placental tissue is sequestered, probably in the form of a macromolecular chelate complex (see below). A comparison of the cadmium ion concentrations in the embryos of hamsters sacrificed 24 hours after injection of a bolus teratogenic dose with those sacrificed 96 hours after injection shows a sixty-fold decrease of cadmium in embryos, nearly all of which could be accounted for by changes in the mass of the embryos. This dilution of cadmium ion in embryonic tissues is entirely consistent with the existence of a cadmium ion barrier in the placenta which prevents a continuous passage of the teratogen into the embryos.

What is the chemical status of the cadium ion barrier Our study (Hanlon et al., 1982) of the chemical status of cadmium in the hamster placenta 24 hours after administration of a teratogenic dose provides some answers. Syrian hamsters were injected with 7.8 micromoles of cadmium ion, radiolabelled with ^{109}Cd, per kg dam on day 8 of pregnancy. The animals were sacrificed after 24 hours and the chorioallantoic placentas collected. Homogenates of the placentas were prepared and centrifuged. The cadmium ion status of the supernatant fractions was determined by gel filtration chromatography. Most of the soluble cadmium ion fraction was accounted for in two peaks. A single ^{109}Cd peak, containing 20 percent of the ^{109}Cd applied to the column, was eluted in the volume expected for macromolecules having weights between 12,000 and 15,000 daltons. Most of the remaining radioactivity emerged near the excluded volume and probably reflects cadmium ion binding to larger proteins (molecular weights greater than 100,000 daltons) or to fragments of cell debris not removed by centrifugation. Virtually all of the ^{109}Cd put on the column was accounted for in elution volumes which would indicate the absence of unbound cadmium ions in the system. The shape and location of the peak containing the low molecular weight fraction of the placenta suggests that it could be a metallothionein. We do not know whether the cadmium-binding molecule is of parental origin and transported to the placenta or has been synthesized in the placenta.

Metallothioneins are known to be synthesized in a wide variety of animals as a response to a cadmium challenge; such could be the case here. On the other hand, our studies on the early SWV mouse placenta imply that a similar cadmium-binding molecule probably does not function primarily as a means to sequester exogenous cadmium (Hanlon et al., 1982).

DIRECTION OF FUTURE INVESTIGATIONS OF HEAVY METAL TERATOGENESIS

We have shown that a number of heavy metals qualify as molecular probes and as such should offer new and interesting techniques for analysis of both normal and abnormal embryogenetic events. The ultimate goal of such studies should be directed toward an understanding of the basic cellular mechanisms of metal-induced malformations.

Very little attention has been paid in the past to the potential teratogenic threat of low-level chronic exposures to heavy metals. Most of the information concerning the teratogenicity of heavy metals is based on experimental data derived from acute, usually bolus, exposure. It is most probable that the manner in which the human embryo would be exposed to heavy metals is through chronic low-level exposure. Thus, techniques for testing the teratogenic threat of chronic exposure must be developed. Further studies should be done to determine quantitatively the amounts of heavy metals within the placenta and embryo needed to provoke a teratogenic response under conditions of both acute and chronic conditions.

It is clear from some of the studies cited that the genotype of the embryo may play an important part in determining sensitivity to the teratogenic effects of metals, and thus, investigations concerning heavy metal teratogenesis should consider genetic factors.

The growing evidence that maternal hyperthermia during gestation is a teratogenic factor in animals (Edwards, 1974; Kilham and Ferm, 1976) and humans, (Smith et al., 1978) as well as the recent evidence that maternal hyperthermia can enhance the teratogenic effect of certain heavy metals as cited above, suggests that there might well be other environmental factors which can modify the effects of these metals on the embryonic system.

Finally, future research in heavy metal teratogenesis should be designed to define with greater precision the possible public health threat of these metals to the human embryo.

REFERENCES

Burk, D. and Beaudoin, A.R., 1977, Arsenate-induced renal agenesis in rats, Teratology 16:247-260.

Carpenter, S.J. and Ferm, V.H., 1977, Embryopathic effects of lead in the hamster: A morphological analysis, Lab. Invest. 37:369-385.

Chang, C.C., Tatum, H.J. and Kincl, F.A., 1970, The effect of intrauterine copper and other metals on implantation in rats and hamsters, Fertil. Steril. 21:274-278.

DiCarlo, F.J., 1980, Syndromes of cardiovascular malformations induced by copper citrate in hamsters, Teratology 21:89-101.

Edwards, M.J., 1974, The effects of hyperthermia on pregnancy and prenatal development, Exp. Embryol. Terat. 1:90-133.

Ferm, V.H., 1967, The use of the golden hamster in experimental teratology, Lab. Anim. Care 17:452-462.

Ferm, V.H., 1969, The synteratogenic effect of lead and cadmium, Experientia 25:56-57.

Ferm, V.H., 1970, Protective effect of ferric dextran on the embryopathic action of indium, Experientia 26:633-634.

Ferm, V.H., 1971, Developmental malformations induced by cadmium: A study of timed injections during embryogenesis, Biology of the Neonate 19:101-107.

Ferm, V.H. and Carpenter, S.J., 1967, Developmental malformations resulting from the administration of lead salts, J. Exp. Mol. Pathol. 7:208-213.

Ferm, V.H. and Carpenter, S.J., 1968a, The relationship of cadmium and zinc in experimental mammalian teratogenesis, Lab Invest. 18:429-432.

Ferm, V.H. and Carpenter, S.J., 1968b, Malformations induced by sodium arsenate, J. Reprod. Fertil. 17:199-201.

Ferm, V.H. and Carpenter, S.J., 1970, Teratogenic and embryopathic effect of indium, germanium and gallium, Toxicol. Appl. Pharm. 16:166-170.

Ferm, V.H. and Ferm, D.W., 1971, The specificity of the teratogenic effect of lead in the golden hamster, Life Sciences 10:35-39.

Ferm, V.H. and Hanlon, D.P., 1974a, Placental transfer of zinc in early embryogenesis, J. Reprod. Fertil. 39:49-52.

Ferm, V.H. and Hanlon, D.P., 1974b, Toxicity of copper salts in hamster embryonic development, Biol. Reprod. 11:97-101.

Ferm, V.H. and Kilham, L., 1977, Synergistic teratogenic effect of arsenic and hyperthermia in the hamster, Env. Res. 14:483-486.

Ferm, V.H. and Layton, W.M., Jr., 1979, Reduction in cadmium teratogenesis by prior cadmium exposure, Env. Res. 18:347-350.

Ferm, V.H., Hanlon, D.P. and Urban, J., 1969, The permeability of the hamster placenta to radioacative cadmium, J. Embryol. Exp. Morph. 22:107-113.

Ferm, V.H., Saxon, A. and Smith, V.W., 1971, The teratogenic profile of sodium arsenate in the golden hamster, Arch. Env. Health 22:577-560.

Gabbiani, G., Selye, H. and Tuchweber, B., 1962, Prevention of indium intoxication by ferric dextran, Br. J. Pharmac. 19:508-512.

Gale, T.F. and Ferm, V.H., 1971, Embryonic effects of mercuric salts, Life Sciences 10:1341-1347.

Gale, T.F. and Hanlon, D.P., 1976, The permeability of the Syrian hamster placenta to mercury, Env. Res. 12:26-31.

Gale, T.F. and Layton, W.M., Jr., 1978, A variable embryotoxic response to lead in different strains of hamsters, Env. Res. 17:325-333.

Gale, T.F. and Layton, W.M., Jr., 1980, The susceptibility of inbred strains of hamsters to cadmium-induced embryotoxicity, Teratology 21:181-186.

Hanlon, D.P. and Ferm, V.H., 1974, Possible mechanisms in metal-induced teratogenesis, Teratology 9:18-19.

Hanlon, D.P. and Ferm, V.H., 1977, Placental permeability of arsenate ion during early embryogenesis in the hamster, Experientia 33:1221-1222.

Hanlon, D.P. and Ferm, V.H., 1981, The distribution of plumbous ion in the materno-fetal unit of the Syrian hamster, Anat. Rec. 199:105A.

Hanlon, D.P., Gale, T.F. and Ferm, V.H., 1975, Permeability of the Syrian hamster placenta to manganous ion during early embryogenesis, J. Reprod. Fertil. 44:109-112.

Hanlon, D.P., Specht, C. and Ferm, V.H., 1982, The chemical status of cadmium ion in the placenta, Env. Res. 27:89-94.

Harriss, R.C. and Hohenemser, C., 1978, Mercury, measuring and
    managing the risk, Environment 20:25-36.
Hilbelink, D.R., 1980, Caudal dysplasia: An animal model in the
    cadmium-lead treated golden hamster, Teratology 21:44A.
Holmberg, R.E. and Ferm, V.H., 1969, Inter-relationships of
    selenium, cadmium and arsenic in mammalian teratogenesis, Arch.
    Env. Health 18:873-877.
Kilham, L. and Ferm, V.H., 1976, Exencephaly in fetal hamsters
    following exposure to hyperthermia, Teratology 14:323-326.
Layton, W.M., Jr. and Layton, M.W., 1979, Cadmium induced limb
    defects in mice: Strain associated differences in sensitivity,
    Teratology 19:229-236.
Layton, W.M., Jr. and Ferm, V.H., 1980, Protection against
    cadmium-induced limb malformations by pre-treatment with
    cadmium or mercury, Teratology 21:357-360.
McCord, C.P., Meek, S.J., Harold, G.C. and Heussner, C.E., 1942,
    The physiologic properties of indium and its compounds, J. Ind.
    Hyg. 24:243-254.
Mottet, N.K., 1974, Effects of chronic low-dose exposure of rat
    fetuses to methylmercury hydroxide, Teratology 10:173-189.
Mottet, N.K., 1981, Biochemical mechanisms of trace element
    teratogenesis, in "The Biochemical Basis of Chemical
    Teratogenesis", M.R. Juchau, ed., pp. 201-246, Elsevier/North
    Holland, New York.
Mulvihill, J.E., Gamm, S.H. and Ferm, V.H., 1970, Facial
    malformation in normal and cadmium-treated golden hamsters, J.
    Embryol. Exp. Morph. 24:393-403.
Scheinberg, H. and Sternlieb, I., 1975, Pregnancy in
    penicillamine-treated patients with Wilson's disease,
    N. Engl. J. Med. 293:1300-1302.
Semba, R., Yamamura, H. and Murakami, U., 1977, Effect of cadmium
    pretreatment and fetolethality of cadmium, Okajimas Folia Anat.
    Jpn. 54:282-288.
Smith, G.A., Thomas, R.G. and Scott, J.K., 1960, The metabolism of
    indium after administration of a single dose to the rat by
    intratracheal, subcutaneous, intramuscular and oral injection,
    Health Phys. 4:101-108.
Smith, D.W., Clarren, S.K. and Harvey, M.A.S., 1978, Hyperthermia
    as a possible teratogenic agent, J. Ped. 93:878-883.
Taylor, B.A., Heiniger, H.J. and Meier, H., 1973, Genetic analysis
    of resistance to cadmium-induced testicular damage in mice,
    Proc. Soc. Exptl. Biol. Med. 143:629-633.
Willhite, C.C., 1981, Arsenic-induced axial skeletal (dysraphic)
    disorders, Exper. Molec. Pathol. 34:145-158.

EMBRYOTOXICITY AND TERATOGENICITY OF NICKEL COMPOUNDS

F. William Sunderman, Jr., Marilyn C. Reid,
Samuel K. Shen and Catharine B. Kevorkian

Departments of Laboratory Medicine and Pharmacology
University of Connecticut School of Medicine
Farmington, Connecticut

ABSTRACT

Three experiments are described that illustrate the effects of nickel compounds upon the progeny of Fischer rats. In the first experiment, administration of $Ni(CO)_4$ to pregnant dams by intravenous injection (11 mg Ni/kg) on day 7 of gestation caused increased fetal mortality, diminished body weight of live pups, and 16 percent incidence of fetal malformations, including anophthalmia, microphthalmia, cystic lungs, and hydronephrosis. In the second experiment, a dominant lethal mutation test in male rats, administration of $Ni(CO)_4$ by inhalation (0.05 mg Ni/litre/15 min) 2 to 6 weeks prior to breeding did not impair fertilization rates or reproductive yields; under the same conditions, administration of $Ni(CO)_4$ by intravenous injection (22 mg Ni/kg) diminished the number of live pups in litters sired during the fifth week, consistent with chromosomal damage during the meiotic stage of spermatogenesis. In the third experiment, administration of Ni_3S_2 to female rats by intrarenal injection (30 mg Ni/kg) one week prior to breeding produced intense erythrocytosis in the dams but did not cause erythrocytosis in the pups; on the contrary, pups from Ni_3S_2-treated dams had diminished blood hematocrits at two weeks postpartum. In light of previous reports that Ni_3S_2-induced erythrocytosis is mediated by increased renal production of erythropoietin, the present observations suggest that increased erythropoietin activity in maternal serum does not stimulate erythropoiesis in the fetus. The discussion section of this paper presents comprehensive tabulations of the literature on embryotoxicity and teratogenicity of nickel compounds.

399

INTRODUCTION

Three nickel compounds with dissimilar physical and chemical properties have been tested in our laboratory for embryotoxicity and teratogenicity in rodents (Sunderman et al., 1978, 1979, 1980; Kuehn and Sunderman, 1982). Nickel carbonyl, Ni(CO)$_4$, a volatile liquid that readily traverses lipid membranes and is practically insoluble in water, was administered by inhalation to pregnant rats on day 7 or 8 of gestation, and to pregnant hamsters on day 4 or 5 of gestation. In both species, Ni(CO)$_4$ exposure induced frequent fetal malformations (Sunderman et al., 1979, 1980). In rats, the predominant anomalies were anophthalmia and microphthalmia (Sunderman et al., 1979); in hamsters, the anomalies included exencephaly, cystic lungs, anophthalmia and cleft palate (Sunderman et al., 1980). Nickel chloride, NiCl$_2$, an ionic water-soluble compound, was administered to pregnant rats by intramuscular injection on day 8 of gestation; NiCl$_2$ reduced the mean litter size, diminished the mean body weight of pups, but did not cause any congenital deformities (Sunderman et al., 1978). Nickel subsulfide, Ni$_3$S$_2$, a crystalline mineral that slowly dissolves in body fluids,* was administered to pregnant rats by intramuscular injection on day 6 of gestation; Ni$_3$S$_2$ reduced the mean litter size but did not affect the body weight of pups or produce any malformations (Sunderman et al., 1978). A two-year transplacental carcinogenesis test of Ni$_3$S$_2$ in rats did not yield increased incidence of tumors in the progeny (Sunderman et al., 1981), despite the induction of metastasizing sarcomas in all of the Ni$_3$S$_2$-treated dams (Sunderman, 1974).

The present article describes three hitherto unreported experiments in our laboratory, including: (a) intravenous administration of Ni(CO)$_4$ to pregnant rats on day 7 of gestation to test for embryotoxicity and teratogenesis; (b) exposure of male rats to Ni(CO)$_4$ by inhalation or intravenous injection to test for dominant lethal mutations; and (c) administration of Ni$_3$S$_2$ to virgin female rats by intrarenal injection prior to mating, in order to assess the effects of erythropoietin-mediated maternal polycythemia upon body weight and hematocrit of the progeny. The discussion section of this article summarizes the scientific literature on embryotoxicity and teratogenicity of nickel compounds in experimental animals.

MATERIALS AND METHODS

Nickel carbonyl, Ni(CO)$_4$, was obtained from Pressure Chemical Co., Pittsburgh, PA; nickel subsulfide, αNi$_3$S$_2$, median particle

---

*After intramuscular injection in rats, the dissolution half-time of Ni$_3$S$_2$ is 24 days (Kuehn and Sunderman, 1982).

diameter < 2 μm, was provided by INCO Ltd., Toronto, Ontario, Canada. Albino rats of the Fischer-344 strain were purchased from Charles River Breeding Laboratories, Wilmington, MA. The rats were housed singly in polypropylene cages; they were given tap water and rat chow (Ralston Purina Co., St. Louis, MO) ad libitum.

The embryotoxicity and teratogenicity test of intravenous $Ni(CO)_4$ involved 13 virgin female rats (mean body weight = 156 g ± 15 S.D.). Breeding was performed by placing two or three of the females into the cage of a male rat from 4 p.m. until 8 a.m.. This procedure was repeated on successive nights until copulation was confirmed by the presence of sperm in a vaginal smear (day 0 of gestation). At 9 a.m. on day 7 of gestation, $Ni(CO)_4$ was administered intravenously at a dosage of 25 μl/kg body weight (equivalent to 11 mg Ni/kg body weight) as previously described (Hackett and Sunderman, 1967; Hui and Sunderman, 1980), by injection with a 5 μl syringe (Hamilton Corp., OH) into a polyethylene catheter that had been inserted in a tail vein. There were 8 dams in the $Ni(CO)_4$-treated group and 5 dams in a control group that received an intravenous injection of NaCl solution (0.14 mol/litre, 25 μl/kg body weight). The dams were anesthetized with diethyl ether on day 20 of gestation and the fetuses were delivered by Caesarean section. The numbers of live and stillborn fetuses, early and late resorptions, and corpora lutea were recorded; each fetus was weighed. Half of the fetuses in each litter were fixed in Bouin's solution and sliced in serial sections (1 mm thickness) for detection of malformations by the method of Wilson (1965); the remaining fetuses were fixed in absolute ethanol, cleared in glycerol, and stained with alizarin S for detection of skeletal anomalies by the method of Murphy (1965).

Dominant lethal tests of $Ni(CO)_4$ involved 40 male rats (mean body weight = 273g ± 42 S.D.). The $Ni(CO)_4$-treated groups comprised (a) 8 rats that received an intravenous injection of $Ni(CO)_4$ in a dosage of 50 μl/kg body (equivalent to 22 mg Ni/kg body weight), and (b) 10 rats that were placed individually in an all-glass chamber (20 litre volume) for a single 15-minute exposure to inhalation of $Ni(CO)_4$ vapor (0.16 mg/litre/15 min, equivalent to 0.05 mg Ni/litre/15 min), as previously described (Kincaid et al., 1953; Baselt et al., 1977). The control groups comprised (a) 12 rats that received an intravenous injection of NaCl solution (0.14 mol/litre, 50 μl/kg body weight), and (b) 10 rats that were placed individually in the exposure chamber for 15 minutes but were exposed to air instead of $Ni(CO)_4$. The males were caged with 2 mature females each week during the second to sixth weeks after the injection or inhalation exposure. The females were subjected to Caesarian section on the eleventh day after separation from the male; the numbers of live and stillborn fetuses, early and late resorptions, and corpora lutea were recorded.

The study of Ni_3S_2-induced polycythemia involved 14 female rats (mean body weight = 196g ± 6 S.D.) The Ni_3S_2 group comprised 7 females that received an intrarenal injection of Ni_3S_2 (10 mg/rat in 0.1 ml of NaCl solution, equivalent to 30 mg Ni/kg body weight), as previously described (Jasmin and Solymoss, 1975; Morse et al., 1977). Each rat was anesthesized with diethyl ether, and the right kidney was exposed by subcostal lumbar incision. Using a tuberculin syringe with 25 gauge needle, 0.1 ml of Ni_3S_2 suspension was slowly injected into the upper pole of the kidney. The musculature was sutured and the skin incision was closed with surgical clips. The control group comprised 7 females that received an intrarenal injection of 0.1 ml of NaCl vehicle under the same experimental conditions. Each female was caged with a male beginning 7 days after the intrarenal injection; vaginal plugs were found in each female at 8-10 days after the intrarenal injection. Hematocrits of the pregnant dams were measured on the 21st and 56th days after intrarenal injection (i.e., on days 11-13 of gestation and days 25-27 postpartum). In all dams, gestation lasted 21-22 days; parturition occurred 29-32 days after the intrarenal injection. On day 3 postpartum, the number of live pups in each litter was recorded, and the litters were culled to 6-8 pups. The pups were fed rat chow after days 15-18 postpartum. The pups were weighed at 13-14 days and at 25-27 days postpartum, and blood samples (40 µl) were collected from the tips of the tails by means of heparinized microhematocrit capillary tubes. Blood hematocrits were determined by centrifugation (Strumia et al., 1954).

Statistical analyses of the experimental data were performed according to recommendations of Gaylor (1978) and Vollmar (1977); two-tailed p-values were computed, as appropriate, by (a) Fisher's exact test; (b) Chi-square test with Yates's correction; (c) Student's t-test; or (d) Mann-Whitney U-test (Siegel, 1956).

RESULTS

Administration of $Ni(CO)_4$ to pregnant rats by intravenous injection on day 7 of gestation caused embryotoxicity and produced the same congenital malformations that were previously reported in rats and hamsters exposed to inhalation of $Ni(CO)_4$ (Sunderman et al., 1979; 1980). As indicated in Table 1, intravenous injection of $Ni(CO)_4$ caused: (a) increased fetal mortality; (b) diminished mean body weight of live pups; and (c) 16 percent incidence of fetal malformations, including anophthalmia, microphthalmia, hydronephrosis, and cystic lungs. Four progeny of $Ni(CO)_4$-treated dams had hemorrhages into body cavities (peritoneal and subdural spaces), such as were previously observed in progeny of $Ni(CO)_4$-exposed hamsters (Sunderman et al., 1980).

Table 1   Teratogenesis Test of Intravenous $Ni(CO)_4$ in Rats

Observations	Controls	$Ni(CO)_4$-treated
Number of litters	5	8
Live fetuses/litters[a]	9.2 ± 4.0	7.1 ± 3.9
Live fetuses/corpora lutea/litter[a]	0.74 ± 0.31	0.67 ± 0.37
Dead fetuses/implants	1/47	13/70[b]
Dead fetuses/implants/litter[a]	0.02 ± 0.04	0.20 ± 0.34
Weights of live fetuses/litter (g)[a]	3.3 ± 0.2	2.8 ± 0.5[c]
Litters with malformed fetuses	0/5	6/8[d]
Live fetuses with malformations	0/46	9/57[b]
Ocular anomalies	0	4[e]
Hydronephrosis	0	4[f]
Cystic lung	0	2
Live fetuses with hemorrhages	0/46	4/57
Intraperitoneal	0	3
Subdural	0	1

[a]Mean ± SD.
[b]$p < 0.01$ by Chi-square test.
[c]$p < 0.05$ by t-test.
[d]$p < 0.02$ by Fisher's exact test.
[e]Includes 1 pup with bilateral anophthalmia, 1 pup with
   bilateral microphthalmia, 1 pup with unilateral
   microphthalmia, and 1 pup with anophthalmia (right) and
   microphthalmia (left).
[f]One pup with hydronephrosis also had unilateral
   microphthalmia.

Dominant lethal tests of $Ni(CO)_4$ in male rats are summarized in Table 2. Since no significant differences were observed between the two control groups, the data for these groups were pooled. Administration of $Ni(CO)_4$ by inhalation or intravenous injection produced respiratory symptoms (dyspnea, tachypnea) that lasted 7 to 10 days, as previously described (Hackett and Sunderman, 1967). Sires that were exposed to inhalation of $Ni(CO)_4$ did not have impaired rates of fertilization nor did their progeny sustain increased pre-implantation or post-implantation losses. Sires that received intravenous injection of $Ni(CO)_4$ had diminished fertilization rates (especially during the second week); this observation may reflect failure to copulate, owing to inanition that occurs after acute $Ni(CO)_4$ toxicity (Sunderman, 1981a). Litters that were sired during the fifth week following intravenous injection of $Ni(CO)_4$ sustained significantly increased fetal wastage, attributable in large part to post-implantation losses. The occurrence of fetal losses during the fifth week after injection

Table 2   Dominant Lethal Test of $Ni(CO)_4$ in Male Rats

Observations	Controls	$Ni(CO)_4$ Inhalation	$Ni(CO)_4$ Injection
Number of sires	22	10	8
Fertilization rate[a]			
week 2	36/44	19/20	3/16[c]
week 3	27/42	17/20	9/16
week 4	35/44	17/20	9/16
week 5	32/44	17/20	7/16
week 6	34/44	19/20	9/16
weeks 2-6	164/218	89/100	37/80
Live fetuses/litter [b]			
week 2	8.9 ± 2.3	9.2 ± 1.3	9.3 ± 0.6
week 3	8.5 ± 2.1	7.5 ± 3.4	7.5 ± 3.5
week 4	8.6 ± 2.4	8.9 ± 2.2	7.7 ± 4.7
week 5	9.1 ± 2.0	8.8 ± 2.1	4.3 ± 4.1[d]
week 6	9.0 ± 2.4	8.6 ± 2.0	8.0 ± 2.3
weeks 2-6	8.8 ± 2.2	8.6 ± 2.3	7.2 ± 3.7[e]
Live fetuses/corpora lutea/dam[b]			
week 2	0.85 ± 0.21	0.91 ± 0.09	0.88 ± 0.12
week 3	0.84 ± 0.18	0.75 ± 0.32	0.70 ± 0.30
week 4	0.80 ± 0.22	0.83 ± 0.18	0.68 ± 0.41
week 5	0.85 ± 0.18	0.82 ± 0.17	0.42 ± 0.38[d]
week 6	0.84 ± 0.20	0.84 ± 0.17	0.70 ± 0.20
weeks 2-6	0.84 ± 0.20	0.83 ± 0.20	0.66 ± 0.33[d]
Dead fetuses/implants			
week 2	6/327	5/180	1/29
week 3	13/242	1/129	11/79[f]
week 4	25/327	2/154	26/96[c]
week 5	12/305	11/161	21/51[c]
week 6	5/311	8/171	6/78[f]
weeks 2-6	61/1521	27/795	65/333[c]
Dead fetuses/implants/litter[b]			
week 2	0.03 ± 0.07	0.03 ± 0.07	0.03 ± 0.06
week 3	0.05 ± 0.09	0.01 ± 0.03	0.16 ± 0.30
week 4	0.08 ± 0.16	0.01 ± 0.03	0.28 ± 0.39
week 5	0.04 ± 0.08	0.09 ± 0.23	0.35 ± 0.46
week 6	0.02 ± 0.06	0.04 ± 0.06	0.06 ± 0.10
weeks 2-6	0.04 ± 0.11	0.04 ± 0.12	0.19 ± 0.32

[a]Number of fertilized dams/number of dams used.
[b]Mean ± SD.
[c]$p < 0.001$ by Chi-square test.
[d]$p < 0.001$ by t-test.
[e]$p < 0.05$ by t-test.
[f]$p < 0.01$ by Chi-square test.

of $Ni(CO)_4$ is consistent with chromosomal damage during the meiotic stage of spermatogenesis (Epstein and Rohrborn, 1971).

Intrarenal administration of Ni_3S_2 to adult rats causes intense stimulation of erythropoiesis, due to increased renal production of erythropoietin (Jasmin and Riopelle, 1976; Solymoss and Jasmin, 1978; Hopfer et al., 1978; 1979; 1980). An experiment was performed to test whether or not intrarenal injection of Ni_3S_2 in female rats prior to breeding stimulates erythrocytosis in the progeny. As indicated in Table 3, erythrocytosis developed in the Ni_3S_2-treated dams, but not in their offspring; these findings suggest that increased maternal erythropoietin production does not stimulate erythropoiesis in the fetus. On the contrary, pups from Ni_3S_2-treated dams had diminished hematocrits at 2 weeks postpartum. The neonatal anemia apparently was caused by deficiency of iron or other nutrient, since the hematocrit values promptly became normal when the pups began to consume rat chow. At 2 and 4 weeks postpartum, the body weights of pups from Ni_3S_2-treated dams were significanly less than the weights of pups from control dams.

Table 3   Effect on Progeny of Intrarenal Injection of Ni_3S_2 in Rats

Observations	Controls[a]	Ni_3S_2-Treated[a]
Hematocrit of dams (%)		
21 days post-injection	48 ± 3 (7)	71 ± 4 (7)[b]
56 days post-injection	50 ± 2 (7)	80 ± 2 (7)[b]
Live pups/litter	9.3 ± 1.4 (7)	10.1 ± 1.9 (7)
Hematocrit of pups (%)		
13-14 days postpartum	38 ± 4 (55)	32 ± 5 (55)[b]
25-27 days postpartum	40 ± 5 (54)	41 ± 4 (54)
Weight of male pups (g)		
13-14 days postpartum	18.2 ± 2.4 (26)	14.9 ± 1.8 (26)[b]
25-27 days postpartum	44.2 ± 6.5 (26)	36.1 ± 5.8 (26)[b]
Weight of female pups (g)		
13-14 days postpartum	18.0 ± 2.5 (29)	14.2 ± 2.4 (29)[b]
25-27 days postpartum	39.9 ± 6.3 (28)	34.2 ± 6.5 (28)[c]

[a]Mean ± SD; N is given in parentheses.
[b]$p < 0.001$ by t-test.
[c]$p < 0.01$ by t-test.

Table 4   Studies of Embryotoxicity and Teratogenicity of Nickel Compounds

Authors and Date	Ni Compound, Route[a], and Dosage	Species and Period of Gestation	Experimental Observations
Phatak and Patwardhan, 1950	$NiCO_3$ (po) 0.25– 1 g Ni/kg of food	Rat, throughout gestation	Normal litter size, normal body weight, increased Ni content of pups at 0.5 and 1 g Ni/kg dosages
Ridgway and Karnofsky, 1952	$NiCl_2$ (ys,ca), 0.05–0.08 mg Ni/egg	Chick, days 4, 8	LD_{50} = 0.05 mg Ni/egg (ys, da 4); 0.08 mg Ni/egg (ca, day 8)
Schroeder and Mitchener, 1971	Ni II (po) 5 mg Ni/litre of water	Rat, throughout life	Increased runts and neonatal deaths in 3 generations
Ferm, 1972	$NiCH_3COOH$ (iv), 2–30 mg Ni/kg body wt	Hamster, day 8	General malformations
Ambrose et al., 1976	$NiSO_4$ (po), 0.25– 1 g Ni/kg of food	Rat, throughout life	Increased stillbirths in first generation; decreased body weight of pups in 3 generations
Sunderman et al., 1978	$NiCl_2$ (im), 8–16 mg Ni/kg body wt; Ni_3S_2(im), 30 mg Ni/kg	Rat, days 6, 8	Increased fetal wastage, diminished body weight, no malformations
Nadeenko et al., 1979	$NiCl_2$ (po), 0.01– 10 mg Ni/litre of water	Rat, throughout gestation	Increased fetal wastage, fetal cyanosis and hemorrhages, no malformations

Reference	Compound and dose	Species and days	Effects
Lu et al., 1979	$NiCl_2$ (ip), 1-7 mg Ni/kg body wt	Mouse, days 7-11	Increased resorptions, decreased fetal weight, cerebral, ocular, palatine, and skeletal anomalies
Sunderman et al., 1979	$Ni(CO)_4$ (inh) 0.03-0.1 mg Ni/litre/15 min	Rat, days 7,8	Intrauterine deaths, decreased fetal weight, ocular anomalies in 28 percent of fetuses
Sunderman et al., 1980	$Ni(CO)_4$ (inh) 0.02 mg Ni/litre/15 min	Hamster, days 4,5	Malformations (CNS, ocular, lung, and palate) in 29 percent of fetuses; hemorrhages into serous cavities
Gilani and Marano, 1980	$NiCl_2$ (as) 0.02-0.7 mg Ni/egg	Chick, days 0-4	Microphthalmia, exencephaly, everted viscera, ectopia cordis, skeletal anomalies and hemorrhages
Weischer et al., 1980	NiO (inh) 1,3-2.5 mg Ni/m^3 for 21 days	Rat, throughout gestation	Decreased fetal weight; hematocrit and hemoglobin normal in pups, but increased in dams
Storeng and Jonsen, 1980	$NiCl_2$ (in culture medium, 0.6-18 mg Ni/litre	Mouse embryo in vitro, day 2,3	Growth inhibition at 0.6 mg Ni/litre on day 2 and 18 mg Ni/litre on day 3
Storeng and Jonsen, 1981	$NiCl_2$ (ip), 5 mg Ni/kg body wt	Mouse, days 1-6	Increased resorptions and deaths, decreased body weight, fetal anomalies (exencephaly), frequent hematomas

[a]Abbreviations: as, air sac; ca, chorioallantoic membrane; im, intramuscular; ip, intraperitoneal; iv, intravenous; po, oral; ys, yolk sac.

DISCUSSION

    A clear pattern of nickel embryotoxicity and teratogenicity can
be discerned from a survey of the literature (Table 4), as well as
the the results of the present study. First, evidence of nickel
embryotoxicity has been obtained in a dozen investigations,
involving a wide assortment of nickel compounds in four test
species, - chick, mouse, hamster, and rat. Second, rats seem to be
resistant to the teratogenic effects of water-soluble nickel
compounds (e.g., $NiCl_2$, $NiSO_4$, $NiCO_3$). Fetal malformations
have been found in chicks, mice, and hamsters following exposures to
soluble nickel compounds during organogenesis; such anomalies have
been notably absent in rats treated with soluble nickel compounds.
Third, nickel carbonyl, $Ni(CO)_4$, is the most potent teratogen
among the nickel compounds that have been studied to date. Exposure
of pregnant rats and hamsters to inhalation of $Ni(CO)_4$ causes
frequent fetal malformations. The present study shows that similar
teratogenic effects are produced in rats by intravenous injection of
$Ni(CO)_4$ during early gestation. The propensity of $Ni(CO)_4$ to
induce fetal anomalies probably reflects its lipid solubility
(Sunderman, 1981a), which may facilitate transport of $Ni(CO)_4$
across placental and fetal membranes. Moreover, $Ni(CO)_4$ slowly
decomposes to liberate carbon monoxide (Sunderman, 1981a), which may
augment the teratogenic effects of nickel. Fourth, nickel compounds
induce internal bleeding in fetuses. Subcutaneous hematomas and
extravasations of blood into peritoneal, pleural, pericardial, or
subdural spaces have been observed in fetal chicks (Gilani and
Marano, 1980), mice (Storeng and Jonsen, 1981), rats (Nadeenko et
al., 1979), and hamsters (Sunderman et al., 1980) following
exposures to $NiCl_2$ or $Ni(CO)_4$. The hematomas and hemorrhages
may be caused by congenital aneurysmal defects in fetal blood
vessels; alternatively, they may reflect toxic effects of nickel on
platelets or coagulation factors in fetal blood. Such hematomas and
hemorrhages have not been reported in adult animals following
treatment with nickel compounds (Sunderman, 1977; 1981a).

    Investigations listed in Table 5 show that Ni[II] traverses
maternal-fetal barriers and enters mouse and rat fetuses throughout
gestation. Olson and Jonsen (1979) demonstrated uptake of ^{63}Ni
[II] by mouse embryos as early as day 5 of gestation. Accumulation
of ^{63}Ni in mouse fetuses was greatest on day 16, presumably
related to the onset of renal function on day 17 of gestation (Olsen
and Jonsen, 1979). Jacobsen et al. (1978) reported that ^{63}Ni
concentrations were generally higher in fetal organs than in
maternal organs of mice following injection of ^{63}NiCl_2 on day 18
of gestation. Sunderman et al. (1978) found that ^{63}Ni[II] crossed
the rat placenta on day 18 of gestation; ^{63}Ni accumulated in the
fetal kidney, and to a lesser degree, in other organs.

    Nickel concentrations in human products of conception are

summarized in Table 6.   McNeely et al. (1971) observed that serum
nickel concentrations are approximately equal in cord blood samples
from full-term infants and in venous blood samples from their
mothers at parturition.   Stack et al. (1976) showed that nickel
occurs in relatively high concentrations in enamel and dentine of
teeth from human fetuses.   Karp and Robertson (1977) measured nickel
concentrations in human placentas.   Schneider et al. (1980) reported
that nickel concentrations in human embryos at 10 to 16 weeks of
gestation average 3.6 µg/g (dry weight), which is 2.2 times the
corresponding nickel concentration of 1.6 µg/g in human fetuses at
20 to 28 week of gestation.   Casey and Robinson (1978) found that
nickel concentrations in kidney from human fetuses at 22 to 25 weeks
of gestation average 0.9 µg/g (dry weight), which is significantly
higher than the corresponding mean concentration of 0.4 µg/g in
kidneys from full-term infants.   These data indicate that nickel can
traverse the human placenta and enter the fetus throughout
gestation; they also suggest that nickel concentrations in human
fetuses are highest during early prenatal development.

Jacquet and Mayence (1982) reported that intraperitoneal
administration of nickel nitrate (12 mg Ni/kg) to male mice reduces
the fertilization rate 3 to 4 weeks after treatment, but does not
produce clastogenic effects.   In contrast, the present study shows
that intravenous $Ni(CO)_4$ causes pre-implantation and
post-implantation loss of fetuses conceived 5 weeks after treatment
of male rats.

There is practically no clinical or epidemiological evidence
that nickel compounds are embryotoxic or teratogenic in humans.   The
only possible exception is the description by Schneider et al.
(1980) of a malformed infant that died 12 days after delivery.
Nickel concentrations in ribs and kidneys of this infant were 27 and
5 µg/g (dry weight), respectively, which correspond to 5-times and
3-times the corresponding mean concentrations of nickel in ribs and
kidneys of 18 control infants that died from various causes during
the first year of life.   Schneider et al. (1980) did not state
whether the mother of the malformed infant was exposed to nickel
compounds during pregnancy.

The molecular pathogenesis of nickel embryotoxicity and
teratogenesis is unknown.   Investigations of nickel toxicity in
adult animals suggest several avenues that might be used to explore
the molecular mechanisms of nickel embryotoxicity and teratogenesis.
Exposure of rats to $Ni(CO)_4$ results in Ni-binding to DNA and
chromatin and inhibition of DNA and RNA synthesis in liver and
kidney (Sunderman and Esfahani, 1968; Beach and Sunderman, 1969,
1970; Hui and Sunderman, 1980).   Administration of $NiCO_3$ to rats
induces DNA-protein cross-links, and DNA strand-breaks in kidney
(Ciccarelli et al., 1981).   In vitro exposure of cultured mammalian
cells to certain nickel compounds produces morphological

Table 5   Studies of Transplacental Movement of Nickel in Rodents

Authors and Date	Ni Compound, Route and Dosage[a]	Species and Day of Gestation	Time from Injection	Analytical Techniques	Observations
Sunderman et al., 1978	63NiCl2 (im), 12 mg Ni/kg body wt	Rat, days 8, 18	24 hours	Autoradiography and scintillation counting	63Ni in membrane, placenta, fetus, and amniotic fluid
Jacobsen et al., 1978	63NiCl2 (ip), 0.14 mg Ni/kg body wt	Mouse, day 18	2 days	Scintillation counting	63Ni conc. in fetal fetal tissues: kidney bone brain heart liver
Lu et al., 1979	NiCl2 (ip), 4.6 mg Ni/kg body wt	Mouse, day 8	4 hours	Atomic absorption	Ni in fetal tissue
Olson and Jonsen, 1979	63NiCl2 (ip), 50 Ci/dam[a]	Mouse, days 2-20	15 min-3 days	Autoradiography	Fetal uptake of 63Ni on days 5-16
Bergman et al., 1980	63NiCl2 (iv), 0.5 mg Ni/kg body wt	Mouse, day not specified	16 hours-2 days	Autoradiography	Fetal uptake of 63Ni, especially in cartilage
Lu et al., 1981	NiCl2 (ip) 4.6 mg Ni/kg body wt	Mouse, day 16	2-48 hours	Atomic absorption	Maximum Ni conc. in placenta at 2 hrs and fetus at 8 hrs

[a]The dosage of 63NiCl2 (as mg Ni/kg) was not specified.

Table 6 Nickel Concentrations in Human Products of Conception

Authors and Date	Analytical Technique	Tissue and Time of Gestation	Nickel Concentration
McNeely et al., 1971	Atomic absorption	Cord-blood, full-term infant	3.0 ± 1.2 (12) µg/litre
Stack et al., 1976	Atomic absorption	Teeth, stillbirth	23 ± 7 (12) µg/g (dry weight)
Karp and Robertson, 1977	Not specified	Placenta, full-term pregnancy	6 ± 6 (58) µg/g (dry weight)
Casey and Robinson, 1978	Atomic absorption	Fetal tissue, 22-43 weeks gestation	
		liver	0.7 ± 0.5 (39) µg/g (dry weight)
		brain	0.4 ± 0.3 (28) µg/g
		heart	0.7 ± 0.6 (19) µg/g
		lung	0.4 ± 0.3 (24) µg/g
		muscle	0.2 ± 0.2 (22) µg/g
		bone	0.4 ± 0.2 (31) µg/g
Schneider et al., 1980	Spectro-photometry	Entire fetus	
		3-4 months	3.6 ± 0.9 (5) µg/g (dry weight)
		5 months	1.6 ± 0.7 (5) µg/g
		6-7 months	1.6 ± 0.3 (5) µg/g

Mean $\pm$ SD; N is given in parentheses.

transformation (Beach and Sunderman, 1970; DiPaolo and Castro, 1979; Costa et al., 1979; Ciccarelli et al., 1981) and chromosomal aberrations (Basrur and Gilman, 1967; Swierenga and Basrur, 1968; Nishimura and Umeda, 1979; Saxholm et al., 1981). In vitro exposure of human lymphocytes to nickel compounds increases the incidence of sister-chromatid exchanges (Wulf, 1980; Larramendy et al., 1981; Swierenga and Basrur, 1968). For reviews of biochemical and cytological effects of nickel compounds that may be pertinent to teratogenesis, mutagenesis, and carcinogenesis, readers are referred to recent articles (Sunderman, 1979, 1981b; Leonard et al., 1981; Raithel and Schaller, 1981).

ACKNOWLEDGEMENTS

This work was supported by DOE Grant EV-03140 and NIEHS Grant ES-01337.

REFERENCES

Ambrose, A.M., Larson, P.S., Borzelleca, J.F. and Hennigar Jr., G.F., 1976, Long term toxicologic assessment of nickel in rats and dogs, J. Food Sci. Tech. 13:181-187.

Baselt, R.C., Sunderman Jr., F.W., Mitchell, J.M. and Horak, E., 1977, Comparisons of antidotal efficacy of sodium diethyl-dithiocarbamate, d-pencillamine, and triethylenetetramine upon acute toxicity of nickel carbonyl in rats, Res. Commun. Chem. Pathol. Pharmacol. 18:677-688.

Basrur, P.K. and Gilman, J.P.W., 1967, Morphologic and synthetic response of normal and tumor muscle cultures to nickel subsulfide, Cancer Res. 27:1168-1177.

Beach, D.J. and Sunderman Jr., F.W., 1969, Nickel carbonyl inhibition of ^{14}C-orotic acid incorporation into rat liver RNA, Proc. Soc. Exp. Biol. Med. 131:321-322.

Beach, D.J. and Sunderman Jr., F.W., 1970, Nickel carbonyl inhibition of RNA synthesis by a chromatin-RNA polymerase complex from hepatic nuclei, Cancer Res. 30:48-50.

Bergman, B., Bergman, M., Magnusson, B, and Soremark, R., 1980, The distribution of nickel in mice: An autoradiographic study, J. Oral Rehabil. 7:319-324.

Casey, C.E. and Robinson, M.F., 1978, Copper, manganese, zinc, nickel, cadmium and lead in human foetal tissues, Brit. J. Nutr. 39:639-646.

Ciccarelli, R.B., Hampton, T.H. and Jennette, K.W., 1981, Nickel carbonate induces DNA-protein crosslinks and DNA strand breaks in kidney, Cancer Letters, 12:349-354.

Costa, M., Nye, J.S., Sunderman Jr., F.W., Allpass, P.R. and Gondos, B., 1979, Induction of sarcomas in nude mice by implantation of Syrian hamster fetal cells exposed in vitro to nickel subsulfide, Cancer Res. 19:3591-3597.

DiPaolo, J.A. and Castro, B.C., 1979, Quantitative studies of in vitro morphological transformation of Syrian hamster fetal cells by inorganic metal salts, Cancer Res. 39:1008-1013.

Epstein, S.S. and Rohrborn, G., 1971, Recommended procedures for testing genetic hazards from chemicals, based on the induction of dominant lethal mutations in mammals, Nature 230:459-460.

Ferm, V.H., 1972, The teratogenic effects of metals on mammalian embryos, Adv. Teratol. 5:51-75.

Gaylor, D.W., 1978, Methods and concepts of biometry applied to teratology, in "Handbook of Teratology", vol. 1, J.G. Wilson and F.C. Fraser, eds., pp. 429-444, Plenum Press, New York.

Gilani, S.H. and Marano, M., 1980, Congenital abnormalities in chick embryos, Arch. Environ. Contam. Toxicol. 9:17-22.

Hackett, R.L. and Sunderman Jr., F.W., 1967, Acute pathological reactions to administration of nickel carbonyl, Arch. Environ. Health 14:604-613.

Hopfer, S.M., Sunderman Jr., F.W., Morse, E.E. and Fredrickson, T.N., 1978, Nickel-induced erythrocytosis: Efficacies of nickel compounds and susceptibilities of rat strains, Ann. Clin. Lab. Sci. 8:396-402.

Hopfer, S.M., Sunderman Jr., F.W., Fredrickson, T.N. and Morse, E.E., 1979, Increased serum erythropoietin activity in rats following intrarenal injection of nickel subsulfide, Res. Commun. Chem. Pathol. Pharmacol. 23:155-170.

Hopfer, S.M., Sunderman Jr., F.W., Fredrickson, T.N. and Morse, E.E., 1980, Effects of intrarenal injection of nickel subsulfide in rodents, Ann. Clin. Lab. Sci. 10:54-64.

Hui, G. and Sunderman Jr., F.W., 1980, Effects of nickel compounds on incorporation of [^{3}H]-thymidine into DNA in rat liver and kidney, Carcinogenesis 1:297-304.

Jacobsen, N., Alfheim, I. and Jonsen, J., 1978, Nickel and strontium distribution in some mouse tissues; passage through placenta and mammary glands, Res. Commun. Chem. Pathol. Pharmacol. 20:571-584.

Jacquet, P. and Mayence, A., 1982, Application of the in vitro embryo culture to the study of the mutagenic effects of nickel in male germ cells, Toxicol. Lett. 11:193-197.

Jasmin, G. and Solymoss, B., 1975, Polycythemia induced in rats by intrarenal injection of nickel subsulfide, Ni$_3$S$_2$, Proc. Soc. Exp. Biol. Med. 148:774-776.

Jasmin, G. and Riopelle, J.L., 1976, Renal carcinomas and erythrocytosis in rats following intrarenal injection of nickel subsulfide, Lab. Invest. 35:71-78.

Karp, W.B. and Robertson, A.F., 1977, Correlation of human placental enzymatic activity with trace metal concentration in placentas from three geographical locations, Environ. Res. 13:470-477.

Kincaid, J.F., Strong, J.S. and Sunderman, F.W., 1953, Nickel
    poisoning. I. Experimental study of the effects of acute and
    subacute exposure to nickel carbonyl. Arch. Indust. Hyg.
    8:48-60.
Kuehn, K. and Sunderman Jr., F.W., 1982, Dissolution half-times of
    nickel compounds in water, rat serum, and renal cytosol, J.
    Inorg. Biochem. 17:29-39.
Larramendy, M.L., Popescu, N.C. and DiPaolo, J.A., 1981, Induction
    by inorganic metal salts of sister chromatid exchanges and
    chromosome aberrations in human and Syrian hamster cell
    strains, Environ. Mutagen. 3:597-606.
Leonard, A., Gerber, G.B. and Jacquet, P., 1981, Carcinogenicity,
    mutagenicity, and teratogenicity of nickel, Mutat. Res. 87:1-15.
Lu, C.-C., Matsumoto, N. and Iijima, S., 1979, Teratogenic effects
    of nickel chloride on embryonic mice and its transfer to
    embryonic mice, Teratology 19:137-142.
Lu, C.-C., Matsumoto, N. and Iijima, S., 1981, Placental transfer
    and distribution of nickel chloride in pregnant mice, Toxicol.
    Appl. Pharmacol. 59:409-413
McNeely, M.D., Sunderman Jr., F.W., Nechay, M.W. and Levin, H.,
    1971, Abnormal concentrations of serum nickel in myocardial
    infarction, stroke, hepatic cirrhosis, and burns, Clin. Chem.
    17:1123-1128.
Morse, E.E., Lee, T.Y., Reiss, R.F. and Sunderman Jr., F.W., 1977,
    Dose-response and time-response study of erythrocytosis in rats
    after intrarenal injection of nickel subsulfide, Ann. Clin.
    Lab. Sci. 7:17-24.
Murphy, M.L., 1965, Factors affecting teratogenic responses to
    drugs, in: "Teratology, Principles and Techniques", J.G. Wilson
    and J. Warkany, eds., pp. 145-161, University of Chicago Press,
    Chicago.
Nadeenko, V.G., Lenchenko, V.G., Arkhipenko, T.A., Saichenko, S.P.
    and Petrova, N.N., 1979, Embryotoxic effect of nickel ingested
    in drinking water, Gig. Sanit. 6:86-88.
Nishimura, M. and Umeda, M., 1979, Induction of chromosomal
    aberrations in cultured mammalian cells by nickel compounds,
    Mutation Res. 68:337-349.
Olsen, I. and Jonsen, J., 1979, Whole-body autoradiography of
    ^{63}Ni in mice throughout gestation, Toxicology 12:165-175.
Phatak, S.S. and Patwardhan, V.N., 1950, Toxicity of nickel, J.
    Sci. Indust. Res. 9B:70-76.
Raithel, H.J. and Schaller, K.H., 1981, Toxicity and
    carcinogenicity of nickel and its compounds: A review of the
    current status, Zbl. Bakt. Hyg. I. Abt. Orig. B. 173:63-91.
Ridgeway, L.P. and Karnofsky, D.A., 1952, The effects of metals on
    the chick embryo: Toxicity and production of abnormalities in
    development, Ann. N.Y. Acad. Sci. 55:203-215.
Saxholm, H.J.K., Reith, A. and Brogger, A., 1981, Oncogenic
    transformation and cell lysis in C3H/10T 1/2 cells and
    increased sister chromatid exchange in human lymphocytes by
    nickel subsulfide, Cancer Res. 41:4136-4139.

Schneider, H.J., Anke, M. and Klinger, G., 1980, The Ni-status of
human beings, in "Nickel", M. Anke, H.J. Schneider, and C.
Bruckner, eds., pp. 277-284, Karl-Marx-Univ. Press, Leipzig.
Schroeder, H.A. and Mitchener, M., 1971, Toxic effects of trace
elements on the reproduction of mice and rats, Arch. Environ.
Health 23:102-106.
Siegel, S., 1956, "Nonparametric Statistics for the Behavioral
Sciences", pp. 1-312, McGraw-Hill, New York.
Solymoss, B. and Jasmin, G., 1978, Studies on the mechanism of
polycythemia induced in rats by Ni₃S₂, Exp. Hemat. 6:43-47.
Stack, M.V., Burkitt, A.J. and Nickless, G., 1976, Trace metals in
teeth at birth, Bull. Environ. Contamin. Toxicol. 16:764-766
Storeng, R. and Jonsen, J., 1980, Effect of nickel chloride and
cadmium acetate on the development of preimplantation mouse
embryos in vitro, Toxicology 17:183-187.
Storeng, R. and Jonsen, J., 1981, Nickel toxicity in early
embryogenesis in mice, Toxicology 20:45-51.
Strumia, M.M., Sample, A.B. and Hart, E.D., 1954, An improved
microhematocrit method, Amer. J. Clin. Pathol. 24:1016-1024.
Sunderman Jr., F.W., 1974, Carcinogenicity and
anti-carcinogenicity of metal compounds, in: "Environmental
Carcinogenesis", P. Emmelot and E. Kriek, eds., pp. 165-192,
Elsevier/North-Holland Biomedical Press, Amsterdam.
Sunderman Jr., F.W., 1977, A review of the metabolism and
toxicology of nickel, Ann. Clin. Lab. Sci. 7:377-398.
Sunderman Jr., F.W., 1979, Mechanisms of metal carcinogenesis
Biol. Trace Element Res. 1:63-86.
Sunderman Jr., F.W., 1981a, Nickel, in: "Disorders of Mineral
Metabolism", vol. 1, F. Bronner and J.W. Coburn, eds., pp.
201-230, Academic Press, New York.
Sunderman Jr., F.W., 1981b, Recent research on nickel
carcinogenesis, Environ. Health Perspect. 40:131-141.
Sunderman Jr., F.W. and Esfahani, M., 1968, Nickel carbonyl
inhibition of RNA polymerase activity in hepatic nuclei, Cancer
Res. 28:2565-2567.
Sunderman Jr., F.W., Shen, S.K., Mitchell, J.M., Allpass, P.R. and
Damjanov, I., 1978, Embryotoxicity and fetal toxicity of nickel
in rats, Toxicol. Appl. Pharmacol. 43:381-390.
Sunderman Jr., F.W., Allpass, P.R., Mitchell, J.M., Baselt, R.C.
and Albert, D.M., 1979, Eye malformations in rats: Induction by
prenatal exposure to nickel carbonyl, Science 203:550-553.
Sunderman Jr., F.W., Shen, S.K., Reid, M.C. and Allpass, P.R.,
1980, Teratogenicity and embryotoxicity of nickel carbonyl in
Syrian hamsters, Teratogen. Carcinogen. Mutagen. 1:223-233.
Sunderman Jr., F.W., McCully, K.S. and Rinehimer, L.A., 1981,
Negative test for transplacental carcinogenicity of nickel
subsulfide in Fischer rats, Res. Commun. Chem. Pathol.
Pharmacol. 31:545-554.
Swierenga, S.H.H. and Basrur, P.K., 1968, Effect of nickel on
cultured rat embryo muscle cells, Lab. Invest., 19:663-674.

Vollmar, J., 1977, Statistical problems in mutagenicity tests, Arch. Toxicol. 38:13-25.

Weischer, C.H., Kordel, W. and Hochrainer, D., 1980, Effects of NiCl$_2$ and NiO in Wistar rats after oral uptake and inhalation exposure respectively, Zbl. Bact. Hyg. I. Abt. Orig. B. 171:336-351.

Wilson, J.G., 1965, Embryological considerations in teratology, in: "Teratology, Principles and Techniques", J.G. Wilson and J. Warkany, eds., pp. 251-277, University of Chicago Press, Chicago.

Wulf, H.C., 1980, Sister chromatid exchanges in human lymphocytes exposed to nickel and lead, Danish Med. Bull. 27:40-42.

THE INFLUENCE OF WEIGHT AND OTHER PHYSIOLOGICAL CHANGES DURING PREGNANCY AND LACTATION ON THE TOXICITIES OF MERCURY AND CADMIUM

Laszlo Magos and Michael Webb

Toxicology Unit
MRC Laboratories
Carshalton, Surrey, United Kingdom

ABSTRACT

Weight and other physiological changes during pregnancy and lactation may alter the target organ, the elimination rate, and the whole body concentration of a toxic metal and also confound the use of weight loss as a toxic response. Such changes and interactions are illustrated by the toxic effects of cadmium, mercury and methylmercury. At the end of pregnancy, the target organ for cadmium is changed and acute toxicity is increased. The change in the toxicity of cadmium in late pregnancy can be related in part to an increase in the placental accumulation of this metal. Lactation accelerates whole body elimination of methylmercury and improves the clinical condition of lactating female rats without a decline either in the brain concentration of methylmercury or in cerebellar damage.

When weight loss is used as a response versus dose, non-pregnant animals seem to be more sensitive to the toxic effect of methylmercury than pregnant ones because the effect on weight (e.g. on food consumption) is imposed on very different weight curves. However, when coordination disorders are compared with the body concentration of methylmercury in virgin rats (which lose more body weight and thus concentrate their body burden in a smaller body volume), coordination disorders occur at higher body concentrations than in pregnant rats.

INTRODUCTION

In fertility, teratogenicity and foetotoxicity experiments, maternal toxicity is an important factor. Suter (1975), for

example, found that the administration of 2.0 mg $HgCl_2$/kg to
female rats, one-half to four days before mating, increased the
incidence of dead implants. Whether this increase was the
consequence of the direct toxic effect of mercuric chloride on the
genetic material, or was the result of severe renal damage inflicted
on the mother, remained open. In general, toxic changes in the
maternal organism are important reference points when a heavy metal
is tested for effects on fertility and for teratogenic or foetotoxic
potential in experimental animals, or when the sensitivity of a
pregnant woman is compared with the sensitivity of her foetus.
Thus, in follow-up studies from Japan (Harada, 1978) and Iraq (Marsh
et al., 1977; Amin-Zaki et al., 1979), special attention was paid to
the relationships between maternal exposure, maternal toxicity and
developmental defects in the offspring. Foetal sensitivity not only
can be higher than the sensitivity of adult females, but also may
appear higher if pregnancy decreases the sensitivity of the mother.
This latter possibility was one of the reasons why a comparative
study on the sensitivity of virgin, pregnant and lactating rats to
methylmercury was included in our research programme. These
comparative studies, together with others on the teratogenicity and
foetotoxicity of $CdCl_2$ and $HgCl_2$, made us realize that the
physiological changes in pregnant and lactating rats cause inherent
difficulties in the interpretation of results and even in the
selection of dose. This presentation is limited to these three
compounds and, even within these limits, is not comprehensive
because our aim at the time of the experimental work differed from
the aim of this lecture and, unfortunately, the literature is too
scanty to fill the gaps.

Pregnancy is associated with the development of an extra
compartment and both pregnancy and lactation are associated with
physiological weight changes. Toxicity may be influenced by the
presence of the placental-foetal unit, or by a shift in relative
organ weights. For example, as Table 1 shows, the relative liver
weight of female rats does not show any consistent change during
pregnancy, but it suddenly increases with parturition. There is a
further increase in relative liver weight during suckling, while in
non-lactating mothers the change is in the opposite direction. The
absolute increase in liver weight during gestation and the relative
increase after parturition may have toxicological significance for
methylmercury or cadmium because the liver stores a significant part
of the body burden. A toxic metal may interact with liver in many
ways, and, after the administration of a toxic dose of mercuric
chloride, relative liver weight declines.

Weight change, which can be caused by the physiological
condition or by the toxic metal, can affect the concentration of the
metal even without any change in elimination rate. Thus,
post-treatment weight gain causes a progressive decrease and weight
loss causes a progressive increase in concentration. When one of

Table 1   Relative Liver Weight of Female Rats in Different
          Physiological Conditions with or without Treatment with
          Mercurials

Condition	Relative Liver Weight	Effect of Treatment on Relative Liver Weights	
		Multiple Doses of MeHg	Single Dose of Hg^{2+}
Virgin	1.0	none	decrease
15-21 Gestation Days	1.0	none	decrease
Zero Parturition Day	1.26	-	-
18 Days after Parturition:			
Lactating	1.40	none	-
Non-Lactating	1.08	none	-

the toxic effects is loss of appetite, virgin rats may be already in
negative weight balance, whereas in pregnant rats only the weight
gain declines. Negative weight balance, in addition to
concentrating the body burden in a smaller body volume, may
accelerate the progression of intoxication or diagnosis: abnormal
gait, flailing reflex, or hind leg crossing may be observed in
weaker animals earlier than in stronger ones. Finally, maternal
toxicity may be influenced by the placental-foetal unit, not only as
a compartment which retains a certain part of the body burden, but
by the toxic damage inflicted on this unit.

     The following survey is an attempt to illustrate the problem of
maternal toxicity during pregnancy and lactation. Before the
detailed discussion it seems necessary to list the relevant toxic
characteristics of these three compounds (see Table 2). The choice
of treatment schedules in our experiments was dictated by these
characteristics. When the main pathological damage is proximal
tubular necrosis, as is the case with mercuric chloride, the
rational way to compare toxicities is after a single treatment,
because regenerating kidneys accumulate mercuric mercury more slowly
than normal kidneys (Tandon and Magos, 1980), and - at least until
they regenerate - are tolerant to the tubulotoxic effect of further

Table 2   The Relevant Toxic Characteristics of $HgCl_2$, $CdCl_2$ and MeHgCl

Toxic Characteristics	$HgCl_2$	$CdCl_2$	$MeHgCl_2$
Number of Doses Required to Produce Main Pathological Lesion	single	single	multiple
Main Pathological Effects:			
in non-pregnant rats	renal	haemorrhage in lung, congestion and necrosis in liver	neural
in pregnant rats	renal	placental transport defect or haemorrhage, kidney damage	neural
Weight Change with Sub-Lethal Treatment	slight	none	pronounced
Placental Barrier	yes	yes	no
Foetotoxicity	linked to maternal death	linked to placental damage	direct
Teratogenicity	linked to maternal intoxication	linked to placental transport disorder	direct

doses (Tandon et al., 1980). In contrast to mercuric chloride, mutiple doses of methylmercury are required to produce typical and comparable clinical and morphological signs. Table 2 also shows that the main pathological effects of the two mercurials, $HgCl_2$ and MeHgCl, are not influenced by pregnancy. The main toxic effects of $CdCl_2$ in pregnant rats, however, are dominated by defects in the functional and morphological integrity of the placenta. After a single dose of $CdCl_2$, placental damage, like traumatic shock (Oliver et al., 1951), may be the causative factor in the development of renal damage (Samarawickrama and Webb, 1979, 1981). For the inorganic mercury and cadmium compounds, the placenta forms an efficient barrier (Mills and Davies, 1979). The foetotoxicity and teratogenicity of the three compounds, according to their passage through or their toxic effect on the placenta, are different.

METHYLMERCURY TOXICITY AND PREGNANCY

The weight curves of virgin and pregnant rats are distinctly different with or without methylmercury treatment, as Figure 1 shows. Depressed weight gain or weight loss is one of the first toxic effects of methylmercury in the rat (Hunter et al., 1939; Magos and Butler, 1972). In relation to appropriate controls, weight gain is depressed in approximately the same proportion in virgin and pregnant rats, but with very different consequences. Figure 1 shows that in non-pregnant rats methylmercury can result in a negative weight balance, whilst pregnant rats submitted to the same treatment continue to gain weight. Because after the longer treatment period both groups lose weight, their body concentrations of mercury remain fairly constant in the first seven post-treatment days, in spite of the steady decrease in total body burden (Magos et al., 1980a). Table 3 shows the initial body weight, the total dose, body burden and whole body concentration for those groups given ten doses of methylmercury. It can be seen that, because of differences in weight change during and after the treatment period, total dose and body burden at the last treatment day in these experiments were higher in the pregnant than in the virgin rats; virgin rats received 12 mg mercury (= 47.8 mg Hg/kg initial body weight) and pregnant rats 13.1 mg (= 50.8 mg Hg/kg initial body weight). Probably this difference in dose in relation to initial body weight contributed to the lack of detectable difference in the brain concentration of mercury or in clinical and morphological signs of methylmercury intoxication in the two groups, despite higher body concentrations in the virgin animals. That the brain reacts to changes in body burden, and to concentration changes outside the brain with a considerable delay, will be discussed later in connection with lactation.

Another group of pregnant rats included in this experiment was treated with the same total dose per initial body weight as the

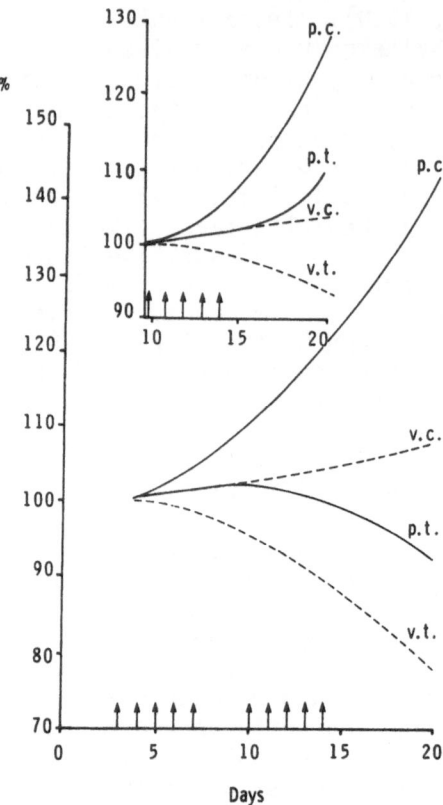

Figure 1   Weight curves of virgin (v) and pregnant (p) rats with
            (t) and without (c) methylmercury treatment.
            Methylmercury was given by gastric gavage in a dose of 5
            mg Hg/kg five or ten times. Days of administration are
            marked by arrows (Magos et al., 1980a).

virgin rats. This particular dosing schedule reflected the
uncertainty of a "comparable" dose in pregnant rats. Since the
brain weight of pregnant rats does not increase with body weight
during gestation, it seemed possible that their brains might take up
disproportionately more mercury than expected from the dose.
Results presented in the section on liver and kidney uptake of
$CdCl_2$ and $HgCl_2$ indicate that the kidney uptake of mercuric
mercury is accelerated in pregnant rats in the early accumulation
phase, which has a special significance for the renotoxicity of this
heavy metal (Magos, 1981). However, when pregnant rats were dosed
according to the weight of virgins, they accumulated less mercury in
their brains than the other groups, and the development of
coordination disorders was delayed. It must be pointed out that the
brains of male rats, like those of pregnant rats, are smaller in

Table 3   Data on Weight, Total Dose and Body Burden of Methylmercury-Treated Virgin and Pregnant Rats. Methylmercury was administered ten times in a dose of 5.0 mg Hg/kg as shown in Figure 1

	Virgin	Pregnant
Initial body weight (g)	251	259 (+3%)
Total dose (mg)	12	13.1 (+9%)
Body burden at the end of treatment (mg)	10.6	11.5 (+8.5%)
Concentration in whole body at the end of treatment (μg/g)	50.0	46 (-13%)
Concentration on the 5th post-treatment day (μg/g)	52	44 (-15%)
Loss of body burden in the first 5 post-treatment days (%)	10	10 (0%)

relation to body weight than those of virgin females and accumulate disproportionately less mercury after methylmercury administration than the brains of virgin females (Magos, 1981).

Finally, it is necessary to consider the effect of the placental-foetal unit as a compartment on the maternal toxicity of methylmercury. Table 4 indicates that the placental-foetal unit can cause a noticeable effect on the maternal body burden only at term. This table also illustrates the rapidity of foetal development in relation to the distribution of body burden between the maternal and foetal parts. It can be seen that while the contribution of the liver to total body burden decreases only slightly from day 18 to day 20 of gestation, the contribution of the litters trebles within the same 48-hour period, because the litter weight increases three-fold without a change in the concentration of mercury. Thus, the ability of the placental-foetal unit to withdraw methylmercury from the maternal body is so limited in time that its effect is undetectable when mothers are treated for ten days from the third gestation day. The effect of pregnancy on the brain uptake of methylmercury is slight though demonstrable after a single dose, when toxic changes do not interfere with distribution. Thus, a decrease in the brain uptake of methylmercury with the progression

Table 4   Mercury Concentration in the Litters or Livers of Pregnant Rats on the 18-20 days of Gestation.   Methylmercury was administered by gastric gavage on the 10-14 days of gestation in a dose of 5 mg Hg/kg/day

Day of Gestation	Number of Foetuses	Hg Concentration µg/g		Total Hg in % of Body Burden	
		in Litter	in Liver	in Litter	in Liver
18	6	21.6	28.4	2.7	5.3
"	12	21.1 21.8	17.8 25.0	5.5 4.1	3.7 4.9
"	11	22.8	28.7	4.2	5.7
19	11	18.1	20.3	4.0	4.7
"	12	22.5	24.2	7.4	6.6
"	8	23.7 21.8	21.0 21.4	4.0 6.2	4.2 4.7
"	14	20.2	22.3	8.2	4.1
"	13	24.0	19.0	7.5	4.1
20	13	20.4 19.7	19.1 20.0	12.3 12.8	3.9
"	13	19.0	20.8	13.2	4.5 4.2

of pregnancy (King et al., 1976) or in pregnant versus virgin rats (Null et al., 1973) has been reported.

THE LIVER AND KIDNEY UPTAKE OF THE CATIONS OF CADMIUM AND MERCURY AND TOXICITY

One of the most striking differences in the distribution of cadmium and mercury after acute exposure is that mercury mainly accumulates in the kidneys and cadmium in the liver. Figure 2 compares the kidney and liver storage of these metals after their intravenous injection to male rats. It can be seen that, within the dose range used, cadmium has no effect on relative organ weights at 48 hours, whereas mercury caused a significant increase in kidney weight and a slight decrease in the relative liver weight. Of these changes, the increase in kidney weight has toxicological significance because, in addition to loss of mercury with desquamated tubular cells (Magos and Clarkson, 1977), increased kidney weight contributes to the decline of the renal concentration of mercury after a peak value is reached. The accumulation of cadmium within the first two days is very much less in the kidneys than in the liver, which at 48 hours contains approximately 50 percent of the dose. The hepatic concentration of this metal is similar to the concentration of mercury in kidneys and three times higher than the liver concentration of mercury. This accumulation pattern is responsible for the involvement of liver in the toxic reactions to acute doses of cadmium.

Table 5 shows that on day 20 of gestation, kidneys and livers of pregnant rats accumulate slightly less cadmium than the livers and kidneys of non-pregnant rats. The table also shows that between 30 minutes and 24 hours the concentration of cadmium remains constant in these organs. As cadmium accumulation in the kidneys of pregnant rats at 20 days of gestation is not more, but less than in non-pregnant rats and the weight of kidneys remains unchanged, the increased incidence of renal damage at this gestational age cannot be the consequence of the direct effect of cadmium on this organ.

In contrast to cadmium, the liver mercury concentration declines from 30 minutes onward, though even at 30 minutes the renal concentration is four times greater. As the amount of mercury distributed outside the kidneys is determined by the efficiency of the renal mercury accumulation process, it is to be expected that an increase in body weight during pregnancy and, therefore, the increase of dose in relation to the weight of the kidney, may increase the uptake of mercury by this organ. Figure 3 shows that this is the case, but when renal uptake is expressed as percent of dose, pregnant animals do not accumulate more mercury than non-pregnant ones. However, as the toxicity of mercury depends on the concentration of mercury, one may expect that pregnancy

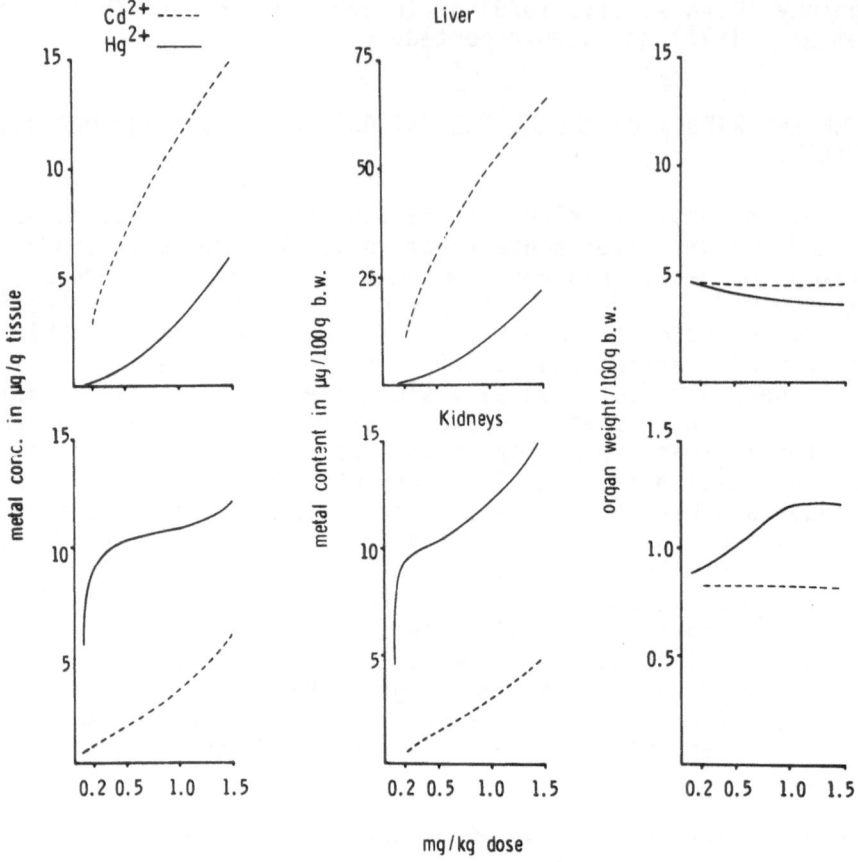

Figure 2   The concentrations and contents of cadmium and mercury in
            the kidneys and livers and relative weights of these
            organs in male rats 48 hours after intravenous injection
            of CdCl$_2$ or HgCl$_2$.

increases the tubular toxicity of inorganic mercury, though no
difference in mercury uptake can be detected between the 12th and
19th gestation days. Actually, Table 6 shows that the LD$_{50}$ of
HgCl$_2$ does not change during gestation. However, it must be
pointed out that in inorganic mercury intoxication there is a
correlation between mercury accumulation and damage in the proximal
tubular cells (Taugner et al., 1966), but there is no correlation
between proximal tubular damage and acute renal failure (DiBona et
al., 1971; Dunnill, 1974), which is the cause of death.

Table 5 The Liver and Kidney Accumulation of Cd^{2+} and Hg^{2+} in Pregnant and Non-Pregnant Rats after the Administration of 1.58 mg Cd/kg (as $CdCl_2$) or 0.79 mg Hg/kg (as $HgCl_2$). Pregnant rats were in the 20 (Cd) and 19 (Hg) days of gestation

	Ratio of Tissue Concentration to Dose[a]							
	in Pregnant				in Non-Pregnant			
Time after	Liver		Kidneys		Liver		Kidneys	
Injection	Cd	Hg	Cd	Hg	Cd	Hg	Cd	Hg
30 min	14	8	2.8	40	17	10	3.5	41
60 min	14	7	2.8	57	16	8	4.6	49
2 hr	-	5	-	66	-	8	-	53
4 hr	13	5	3.0	72	16	8	4.9	63
6 hr	-	4	-	76	-	7	-	64
8 hr	16	-	2.9	-	17	-	5.2	-
24 hr	15	3	2.6	30	17	5	5.2	47

[a]Concentration in μg/g per dose in μg/g.

Unlike mercuric chloride, the acute toxicity of cadmium chloride is significantly increased at the end of pregnancy (see Table 6). This change in the sensitivity of pregnant rats to $CdCl_2$ was first described by Parizek (1969) who noted that the removal of placentae, but not the foeti only, restored sensitivity to the original level.

PLACENTAL ACCUMULATION AND MATERNAL TOXICITY

The frequency of placental haemorrhage at toxic cadmium doses increases from the 12th gestational day onward, and at 20 days, vaginal bleeding and massive placental haemorrhage are always present with renal tubular degeneration, vacuolation and dilation (Samarawickrama and Webb, 1981). As the renal accumulation of

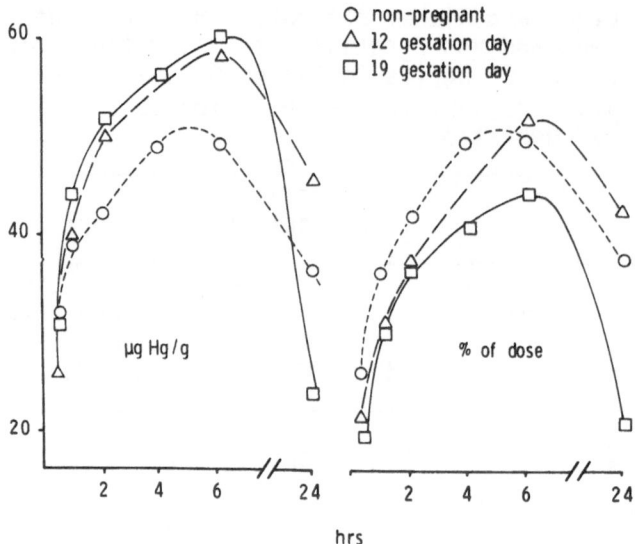

Figure 3   Renal concentration and content of mercury in
            non-pregnant and pregnant rats at the 12th and 19th
            gestation days, 24 hours after intravenous injection of
            790 µg Hg/kg as HgCl₂. (D. Holt and M. Webb,
            unpublished observations.)

cadmium is not increased, it is reasonable to suggest that as
traumatic shock is able to cause acute renal failure, placental
haemorrhage and not renal cadmium is responsible for the kidney
damage in the late gestation period.

        The concentration of mercury after the intravenous injection of
metallic mercury (Clarkson et al., 1972; Greenwood et al., 1972) or
after methylmercury treatment is similar in the foetus and placenta;
but after the administration of inorganic mercury (Suzuki et al.,
1967) and cadmium (Levin and Miller, 1980), the placenta contains 10
and 35 times higher concentrations than the foeti. Table 7 shows
that the placenta usually accumulates less mercury or cadmium than
does maternal liver and that liver accumulates approximately five
times more cadmium than mercury, though their placental accumulation
is very similar. The placental accumulation of cadmium is
influenced by dose and gestational age. Figure 4 shows placental
accumulation to be highest at the end of pregnancy and, therefore,
the placental toxicity of cadmium is associated with an increase in
placental accumulation. However, the placental uptake of cadmium
alone cannot explain the sudden increase in toxicity. At the time
of maximum sensitvity, the placental concentration of cadmium 6

Table 6   Acute Toxicities of $CdCl_2$ and $HgCl_2$ During Gestation

Gestation Age days	Cd^{2+} LD_{50} (mg/kg)	Hg^{2+} LD_{50} (mg/kg)
0	1.8 (1.4 - 2.2)	1.0 (0.8 - 1.2)
4	2.2 (1.8 - 2.8)	-
8	2.2 (1.8 - 2.8)	1.0 (0.9 - 1.1)
12	2.5 (1.9 - 3.3)	-
16	2.5 (1.9 - 3.3)	1.2 (1.0 - 1.4)
20	1.2 (1.2 - 1.2)	1.0 (0.9 - 1.1)

[a]from Samarawickrama and Webb (1981)
[b]D. Holt and M. Webb, personal communication

hours after the intravenous injection of the LD_{50} dose was only 5.1 µg/g, while after the very much higher LD_{50} at the 16th day of gestation, the concentration of cadmium was as high as 7.1 µg/g (Samarawickrama and Webb, 1981). Besides cadmium concentration, another factor can be the shift from histriotrophic nutrition to haematotrophic nutrition, which begins to be established at about 11 days of gestation and reaches a critical level after the disappearance of the parietal layer of the yolk sac at 16 days (Beck, 1976). This shift is associated with the hypertrophy of the chorioallantoic placenta, sudden increase in foetal weight (see Table 4) and probably with other placental changes which makes this tissue more vulnerable to cadmium.

Nevertheless, placental cadmium accumulation is an important factor in the placental toxicity of cadmium. Why only cadmium, but not mercury, produces severe placental haemorrhage may be explained by differences in their placental molar concentrations. From Tables 6 and 7, it can be calculated that at late gestation the molar concentration of cadmium in the placenta is twice the molar concentration of mercury at equivalent toxic doses, and is four times higher at and before 16 gestation days. It is impossible to produce a mercury molar concentration equivalent to the cadmium molar concentration at the LD_{50} level, because the preferential renal mercury accumulation process not only renders this organ the target of mercury toxicity, but also protects others against direct

Table 7 The Placental and Liver Accumulation of Cd^{2+} and Hg^{2+}
on Different Gestation Days

Metal	Gestation Day	Dose in mg/kg	Ratio of Tissue Concentration to Dose		Reference
			Placenta	Liver	
Hg^{2+}	12	0.79(i.v.)	1.1	3.2	Holt and Webb (personal communication)
Hg^{2+}	19	0.79(i.v.)	1.8	3.0	"
Hg^{2+}	19	0.24(s.c.)	3.7	3.7	Parizek et al. (1969)
Cd^{2+}	13	0.50(i.p.)	0.84	14	Rohrer et al. (1978)
Cd^{2+}	13	1.50(i.p.)	1.4	14	Rohrer et al. (1978)
Cd^{2+}	18	4.5 (s.c.)	2.8	-	Levin and Miller (1980)
Cd^{2+}	20	1.58(i.v.)	2.7	15.4	Samarawickrama and Webb (1981)

toxic effects (Magos, 1973). As far as placental toxicity is concerned, this protective effect works not only at late gestation, but also earlier, when cadmium inhibits placental zinc transport without placental haemorrhage (Webb and Samarawickrama, 1981). Although zinc transport can be inhibited by mercuric mercury, inhibition is appreciable only at doses which produce severe renal damage and only when renal damage is already present (D. Holt and M. Webb, personal communication).

LACTATION AND METHYLMERCURY INTOXICATION

In pregnancy the nutrition of the foeti through the yolk sac and placenta is unable to influence the course of maternal methylmercury intoxication, because the contribution of the

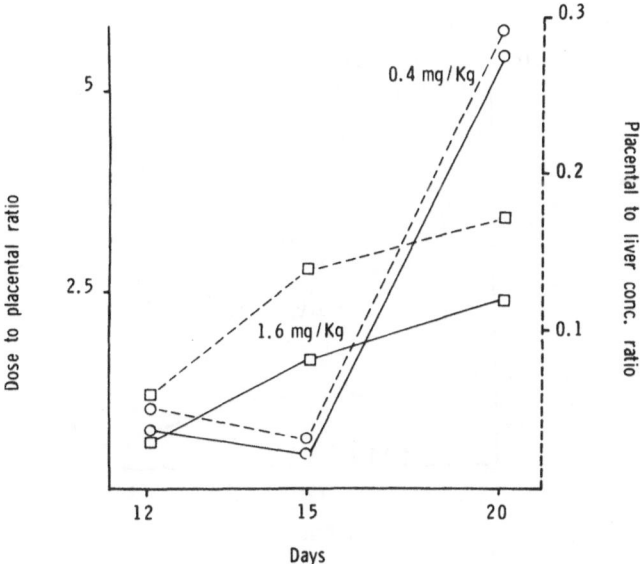

Figure 4   The placental accumulation of cadmium at different
            gestational days 24 hours after the intravenous injection
            of 0.4 mg Cd/kg or 1.6 mg Cd/kg given as $CdCl_2$. Values
            are calculated from the data of Sonawane et al. (1975) on
            the assumption of 270 g body weight at 1 gestation day
            and the weight curve presented for untreated rats in
            Figure 1.

placental-foetal unit to the total body burden throughout most of
the gestation time is too small (Magos et al., 1980a). However, on
the 20th day of gestation there is a sudden upsurge in foetal
development, which raises the contribution of foeti to more than ten
percent of the total body burden (see Table 3). After parturition,
there is a possibility that this nutritional transfer of
methylmercury from the mother to the offspring can influence the
development of intoxication in the mother. It has been demonstrated
that this transfer process can influence the clearance of
methylmercury in women and mice (Greenwood et al., 1978) and, in the
rat, can decrease the maternal body burden to a degree which has a
profound effect on the health of the mother (Magos et al., 1980b).

     Figure 5 shows the weight curves of lactating mothers,
non-lactating mothers and virgin rats of identical age. It can be
seen that, after five doses of 8.0 mg Hg/kg given as methylmercury
on consecutive days, weight loss starts earlier in non-lactating
than in lactating mothers and is more pronounced in non-lactating

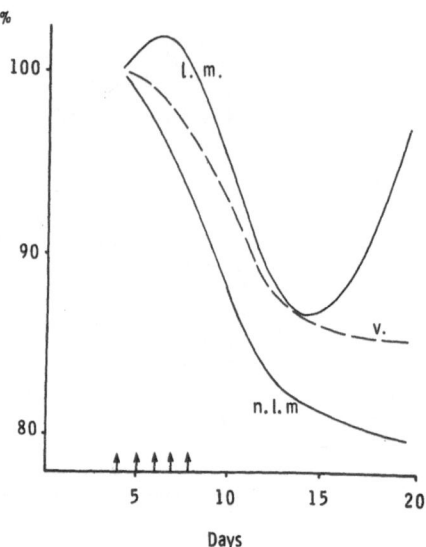

Figure 5 Weight curves of virgin (v), lactating (l.m.) and non-
lactating (n.l.m) mothers. Methylmercury was given by
gastric gavage in a dose of 8 mg Hg/kg as methylmercury
to rats of identical age on days marked by arrows (Magos
et al., 1980b).

mothers than in virgin rats. The most likely explanation of the
difference between the weight loss of non-lactating mothers and
virgin rats is that the former lose some additional weight gained
during pregnancy. However, after the 7th post-treatment day, the
difference between lactating and non-lactating rats becomes
significant; lactating rats start to gain weight, and at the 12th
post-treatment day they have nearly regained their original weight.
While during this 12-day period virgin rats clear about 20 percent
of the mercury body burden, lactating animals eliminate about 46
percent. The clinical course of intoxication in lactating and
non-lactating rats reflects these differences in whole body
clearance. While the coordination of non-lactating animals
continuously deteriorates, lactating animals do not show any
deterioration from the third day onward.

The brain concentration of methylmercury starts to decline only
about 10 days after the last treatment (Magos and Butler, 1976), but
in rats treated with dimercaptosuccinic acid, the brain concentration
decreases nearly as fast as the body burden (Magos et al., 1978).
It is surprising, therefore, that lactation, inspite of the
significantly accelerated whole body clearance, does not affect the

brain concentration of mercury. In agreement with the absence of any noticeable effect on brain mercury, lactation does not appear to mitigate the severity of granular layer damage in the cerebellum. Thus, the effect of lactation on methylmercury intoxication is far from straightforward; it can accelerate whole body clearance without accelerating clearance from the brain and it can prevent clinical deterioration without preventing cerebellar granular layer damage. Therefore, it seems that changes connected with reproduction are not powerful enough to influence every effect of methylmercury, but compared with pregnancy, lactation is able to reduce at least the body burden of methylmercury and the intensity of coordination disorders.

SUMMARY

It is usual to relate a toxic response either to dose or to the concentration of a toxic metal in the critical organ or an index medium (Nordberg, 1976). In animal experiments, when the toxic metal is labelled with a gamma emitter, the index medium can be the whole body and this technique permits the estimation of whole body burden and whole body concentration at any time. In dose-response curves, dose, body burden and concentration are convertible, but physiological changes during pregnancy and lactation may change the dose response curve for these convertibles differently or can change the response. The reason for this may be: a) a change in the target organ; b) a change in elimination rate; or c) the interaction between physiological and toxic weight changes which confounds the use of weight loss as a response and also can affect the whole body concentration of the toxic metal.

Such changes and interactions have been illustrated in the present discussion on the toxic effects of cadmium, mercury and methylmercury. At the end of pregnancy, the target organ for cadmium is changed and acute toxicity is increased. No such change occurs with inorganic mercury, although there is some indication that in pregnancy the renal uptake of this metal is accelerated. The change in the toxicity of cadmium in late pregnancy can be related at least partly to an increase in the placental accumulation of this metal, but probably the changing role of the placenta in late gestation is also a contributory factor. The same placental changes are probably responsible for the significant shift of the maternal body burden of methylmercury into the foeti around the 20th day of gestation. However, as a result of the less acute nature of methylmercury intoxication and the restriction of this shift to a very short time, neither the maternal toxicity nor the brain concentration of mercury is affected in an appreciable way.

Lactation accelerates the elimination of methylmercury from the whole body and improves the clinical condition of lactating female rats without either a decline in the brain concentration of methylmercury or in cerebellar damage. The slow reaction of brain clearance to a significant loss of total burden probably exemplifies that the relatively short time span of treatment, dictated by the duration of lactation (or pregnancy), prevents the change in body burden (or whole body concentration) from reaching the brain.

One of the first effects of methylmercury intoxication is on weight gain. When weight loss is used as a response versus dose, non-pregnant animals seem to be more sensitive to the toxic effects of methylmercury than pregnant ones and non-lactating mothers are more sensitive than virgin rats, because the toxic effect on weight (e.g. on food consumption) is imposed on very different weight curves. However, when coordination disorders are compared with the body-concentration of methylmercury, in virgin rats which lose more body weight and thus concentrate their body burden in a smaller body volume, coordination disorders occur at higher body concentrations than in pregnant rats.

REFERENCES

Amin-Zaki, L., Majeed, M.A., Elhassani, S.B., Clarkson, T.W., Greenwood, M.R., and Doherty, R.A., 1979, Prenatal methylmercury poisoning: clinical observations over five years, Amer. J. Dis. Child. 133:172-177.

Beck, F., 1976, Comparative placental morphology and function, Environ. Health Perspectives 18:6-12.

Clarkson, T.W., Magos, L., and Greenwood, M.R., 1972, The transport of elemental mercury into fetal tissues, Biol. Neonate 21:239-244.

DiBona, G.F., MacDonald, F.D., Flamenbaum, W., Dammin, G.J., and Oken, D.E., 1971, Maintenance of renal function in salt loaded rats despite severe tubular necrosis induced by $HgCl_2$, Nephrol. 8:205-220.

Dunnill, M.S., 1974, A review of the pathology and pathogenesis of acute renal failure due to acute tubular necrosis, J. Clin. Pathol. 27:2-13.

Greenwood, M.R., Clarkson, T.W., Doherty, R.A., Gates, A.H., Amin-Zaki, L., Elhassani S.B., and Majeed, M.A., 1978, Blood clearance half-times in lactating and non-lactating members of a population exposed to methylmercury, Environ. Research 16:48-54.

Greenwood, M.R., Clarkson, T.W., and Magos, L., 1972, Transfer of metallic mercury into foetus, Experientia 28:1455-1456.

Harada, M., 1978, Congential minamata disease: intrauterine methylmercury poisoning, Teratology 18:285-290.

Hunter, D., Bomford, R.R., and Russel, D.S., 1939, Poisoning by
    methylmercury compounds, Quart. J. Med. 35:193-213.
King, R.B., Robkin, M.A., and Shepard, T.H., 1976, Distribution
    of ^{203}Hg in pregnant and fetal rats, Teratology 13:275-280.
Levin, A.A., and Miller, R.K., 1980, Fetal toxicity of cadmium in
    the rat: maternal vs fetal injections, Teratology 22:1-5.
Magos, L., 1973, Factors affecting the uptake and retention of
    mercury by kidneys in rats, in: "Mercury, Mercurials and
    Mercaptans", M.W. Miller and T.W. Clarkson, eds., pp. 167-186,
    Charles C. Thomas, Springfield.
Magos, L., 1981, Metabolic factors in the distribution and half
    time of mercury after exposure to different mercurials, in:
    "Industrial and Environmental Xenobiotics", I. Gut, M. Cikrt
    and G.L. Plaa, eds., pp. 1-15, Springer-Verlag, Berlin.
Magos, L., and Butler, W.H., 1972, Cumulative effects of
    methylmercury dicyandiamide given orally to rats, Food Cosmet.
    Toxicol. 10:513-517.
Magos, L., and Butler, W.H., 1976, The kinetics of methylmercury
    administered repeatedly to rats, Arch. Toxicol. 35:25-39.
Magos, L., and Clarkson, T.W., 1977, Renal injury and urinary
    excretion, in: "Reactions to Environmental Agents", D.K. Lee,
    ed., pp. 503-512, American Physiological Society, Bethesda.
Magos, L., Peristianis, G.C., and Snowden, R.T., 1978, Postexposure
    preventive treatment of methylmercury intoxication in rats with
    dimercaptosuccinic acid, Toxicol. Appl. Pharmacol. 45:463-475.
Magos, L., Peristianis, G.C., Clarkson, T.W., Snowden, R.T., and
    Majeed, M.A., 1980a, Comparative study of the sensitivity of
    virgin and pregnant rats to methylmercury, Arch. Toxicol.
    43:283-291.
Magos, L., Peristianis, G.C., Clarkson, T.W., and Snowden, R.T.,
    1980b, The effect of lactation on methylmercury intoxication,
    Arch. Toxicol. 45:143-148.
Magos, L., Peristianis, G.C., Clarkson, T.W., Brown, A., Preston,
    S., and Snowden, R.T., 1981, Comparative study of the
    sensitivity of male and female rats to methylmercury, Arch.
    Toxicol. 48:11-20.
Marsh, D.O., Myers, G.J., Clarkson, T.W., Amin-Zaki, L., and
    Tikriti, S., 1977, Fetal methylmercury poisoning: new data on
    clinical and toxicological aspects, Transactions Amer. Neurol.
    Assoc. 102:1-3.
Mills, C.F., and Davies, N.T., 1979, Perinatal changes in the
    absorption of trace elements, in: "Development of Mammalian
    Absorptive Processes", Ciba Foundation Symposium 70, Exerpta
    Med., pp. 247-266, Amsterdam.
Nordberg, G.F., ed., 1976, "Effects and Dose-Response Relationships
    of Toxic Metals", Elsevier, Amsterdam.
Null, D.H., Gartside, P.S., and Wei, E., 1973, Methylmercury
    accumulation in brains of pregnant, non-pregnant and fetal
    rats, Life Sciences 12:65-72.

Oliver, J., MacDowell, M., and Tracy, A., 1951, The pathogenesis acute renal failure associated with traumatic shock and toxic injury. Renal ischemia, nephrotoxic damage and the ischemuric episode, J. Clin. Invest. 30:1307-1351.

Parizek, J., 1969, Influence of trace amounts of metals on the reproductive function, Yearbook of the Czechoslovak Academy of Sciences, pp. 111-126, Prague.

Parizek, J., Babicky, A., Ostadalova, I., Kalouskuva, J., and Pavlik, L., 1969, The effect of selenium compounds on cross-placental passage of ^{203}Hg, in: "Radiation Biology of the Fetal and Juvenile Mammal", M.R. Sikov and D.D. Mahlum, eds., pp. 137-143, U.S. Atomic Energy Commission, Washington.

Rohrer, S.R., Shaw, S.M., Born, G.S., and Vetter, R.J., 1978, The maternal distribution and placental transfer of cadmium in zinc deficient rats, Bull. Environ. Contam. Toxicol. 19:556-563.

Samarawickrama, G.P., and Webb, M., 1979, Acute effects of cadmium on the pregnant rat and embryo-fetal development, Environ. Health Persp. 28:245-249.

Samarawickrama, G.P., and Webb, M., 1981, The acute toxicity and geratogenicity of cadmium in pregnant rats, J. Appl. Toxicol. 1:264-269.

Sonawane, B.R., Nordberg, M., Nordberg, G.F., and Lucier, G.W., 1975, Placental transfer of cadmium in rats: Influence of dose and gestational age, Environ. Health Persp. 12:97-102.

Suter, K.E., 1975, Studies on the dominant-lethal and fertility effects of the heavy metal compounds methylmercury hydroxide, mercuric chloride and cadmium chloride in male and female mice, Mutation Res. 30:365-374.

Suzuki, T., Matsumoto, N., Miyama, T., and Katsunumua, H., 1967, Placental transfer of mercuric chloride, phenyl mercury acetate and methyl mercury acetate in mice, Indust. Health (Japan) 5:149-155.

Tandon, S.K., and Magos, L., 1980, Effect of kidney damage on the mobilization of mercury by thiol-complexing agents, Brit. J. Indust. Med. 37:128-132.

Tandon, S.K., Magos, L., and Cabral, J.R.P., 1980, Protection against mercuric chloride by nephrotoxic agents which do not induce thionein, Toxicol. Appl. Pharmacol. 52:227-236.

Taugner, R.K., Winkel, K., and Iravani, J., 1966, Zur Lokalization der Sublimatanreicherung in der Rattenniere. Virchows, Arch. Pathol. Anat. Physiol. 340:369-383.

Webb, M., and Samarawickrama, G.P., 1981, Placental transport and embryonic utilization of essential metabolites in the rat at the teratogenic dose of cadmium, J. Appl. Toxicol. 1:270-277.

ULTRASTRUCTURAL AND BIOCHEMICAL ALTERATIONS OF CELLULAR ORGANELLES BY PRENATAL EXPOSURE TO TOXIC TRACE METALS

Bruce A. Fowler

Laboratory of Pharmacology
NIEHS, National Institutes of Health
Research Triangle Park, North Carolina

ABSTRACT

There are relatively few studies concerning either the ultrastructural or biochemical effects of toxic elements on subcellular organelles. Ultrastructural studies which show cellular vesiculation, mitochondrial damage and cellular necrosis have been reported for lead and arsenate. Ultrastructural/biochemical data are available for the effects of methylmercury on fetal organisms. These studies show cellular vesiculation of hepatocytes, decreased synthesis of protein and DNA associated with inhibition of mitochondrial biogenesis and respiratory function. One, or a combination of these effects, appears to be responsible for the known reduction in fetal size at doses of methylmercury below which overt teratogenic or maternal toxicity are observed.

INTRODUCTION

It has been known for many years that high-dose prenatal exposure to toxic trace elements such as arsenic, cadmium, mercury, lead and indium (see review by Ferm and Hanlon, this volume) will produce gross fetal malformations. The biochemical and organelle system alterations which underly these effects have received relatively little attention and there are currently no published mechanistic data available to explain these teratogenic changes. Furthermore, there are even fewer studies involving the effects of prolonged low-dose maternal exposure to these agents on developing subcellular systems in the fetal at dose levels below which gross morphological changes occur.

437

The present review examines the literature pertaining to the effects of various metals on organelle systems and uses data from our laboratory to illustrate how prenatal exposure to methylmercury, at subtoxic doses in maternal rats, resulted in changes in fetal liver mitochondrial structure and biochemical function which resulted in apparent biochemical defects in this organelle later in life.

REVIEW OF LITERATURE CONCERNING SUBCELLULAR EFFECTS OF TOXIC TRACE METALS

Arsenic

Morrissey and Mottet (1983) have demonstrated a failure of closure of the rhombencephalon in fetal mice of dams injected with arsenate (45 mg/kg) on day 8 of pregnancy. They observed cell necrosis, mitochondrial damage and an increase in small, clear vesicles as prominent ultrastructural changes in neural tube cells.

Lead

DeGennaro (1978) studied the morphological effects of lead nitrate on the developing nervous system of chick embryos. By electron microscopy, he observed extensive cellular vacuolization and disorganization of the endoplasmic reticulum as most prominent early manifestations of toxicity in the central nervous system. Little morphological alteration of mitochondrial structure was observed, although biochemical dysfunction characterized by uncoupling of oxidative phosphorylation of brain mitochondria has been reported (Holtzman and Hsu, 1976) in suckling rats.

Methylmercury

Of the toxic trace elements, the in utero effects of methylmercury have been most well-studied with respect to the ultrastructural/biochemical effects of this agent in fetal and developing animals. Several studies with methylmercury (Mottet, 1974; Spyker and Spyker, 1977; Chen et al., 1979) have reported decreased birthweights and growth/development patterns in rodents exposed in utero to methylmercury. This finding is similar to that observed in infants exposed in utero to methylmercury in Iraq (Amin-Zaki et al., 1979). The underlying mechanism of this effect is not totally known but a number of studies in recent years (Fowler and Woods, 1977; Chang et al., 1977; Olson and Massaro, 1977; Robbins et al., 1978; Chen et al., 1979) have clearly demonstrated both ultrastructural and/or biochemical changes in rodents exposed to methylmercury which suggest several interrelated hypotheses. A central feature of several of these studies (Fowler and Woods, 1977; Olson and Massaro, 1977; Chen et al., 1979) is the decreased incorporation of amino acids and at higher dose levels (Chen et al., 1979) ^{3}H-thymidine into fetal organs yielding decreased protein and DNA content. There are a number of possible mechanisms to explain these phenomena.

Olson and Massaro (1977) examined protein synthesis in fetuses of maternal mice injected subcutaneously with 5 mg Hg/kg of methylmercury on day 12 of gestation and measured incorporation of [^{3}H] leucine after 3, 6, 12 or 24 hours. They found a 22 percent decrease in total fetal protein content, while DNA content was unaltered. They concluded, on the basis of pulse-labeling studies, that decreased fetal protein synthesis was responsible for decreased fetal protein content which seemed to be, in part, related to reduced plancental/fetal transfer of amino acids and that this occurred prior to changes in DNA synthesis. Chen et al. (1979) administered 25 ppm methylmercury in drinking water to pregnant rats from days 1 through 20 of pregnancy. This treatment resulted in reduction of whole organ protein and DNA content of livers and kidneys, which appeared to be related to fewer cells per organ rather than reduced cell size as the predominant factor. They concluded that decreased fetal organ size was due to fewer cells in the organs due to the decreased proliferative activity.

The study from our laboratory (Fowler and Woods, 1977) employed both ultrastructural morphometry and biochemical techniques to study the effects of methylmercury on fetal liver mitochondrial structure and function. Our work was based on the preliminary observation of Ware et al. (1974) that in utero exposure to a single small dose of this compound produced swollen mitochondria in livers of fetal rats. The following discussion reviews the in utero transplacental effects of methylmercury on fetal hepatic mitochondrial biogenesis and the subsequent effects on respiratory function in mitochondria isolated from newborn, weanling and adult rats as an index of subcellular toxicity. A brief description of the experiment is given below.

Treatment of animals. Female Charles River CD rats were divided into four groups of 20 each in a series of five replicate experiments (Fowler and Woods, 1977). The animals were given access to deionized drinking water containing 0, 3, 5, or 10 ppm of mercury as methylmercury hydroxide for 4 weeks prior to mating with untreated males. All animals were fed laboratory chow and housed in barrier isolation rooms. Once impregnated, the animals were continued on their respective dose regimens through day 19 of pregnancy at which time they were sacrificed by decapitation and the fetuses were removed. In order to obtain a sufficient sample size for assessment of the various biochemical and analytical parameters, livers in all fetuses in each dam at every dose level were pooled for each replicate experiment.

Morphologic procedures. Liver tissue from the first fetus in the right uterine horn of each dam in the first replicate experiment was cut into blocks of approximately 1 cu mm in volume and fixed in a glutaraldehyde-formaldehyde fixative and processed for electron microscopy as previously described (Fowler and Woods, 1977).

Morphometric analyses were conducted on three randomly-selected blocks from five fetal livers at each methylmercury dose level. Five photographs were consistently taken in the upper left corner of the first five grid spaces which contained sectioned tissue. This random selection procedure was used in order to compare more accurately ultrastructural findings with biochemical studies in mitochondria from liver homogenates of the same animals. Initial plate magnification was x5,586 and final print magnification was x16,758. The microscope was calibrated by photographing a carbon grating replica with 28,500 lines per inch prior to each photographic session throughout the study. Magnification was found to vary by less than 5 percent. The relative volume densities of lysosomes, mitochondria, nuclei and vacuoles were determined by contact printing a multipurpose grid containing 168 test points onto each micrograph and these were evaluated according to established stereologic methods.

In addition, morphometric analyses for mitochondrial diameter (D), length (L), volume (V) of a "standardized" mitochondria and estimated number (N) of these "standardized" mitochondria per unit volume of cytoplasm were made using the method of Loud et al. (1965), making the arbitrary assumption that the mitochodria are right cylinders with a diameter to length ratio (ϵ) of 0.6 (Lang and Herbener, 1972).

Mitochondrial respiration studies. The respiratory function of fetal liver mitochondria from control dams and dams treated with 0, 3, 5, or 10 ppm methylmercury hydroxide was performed as previously described (Fowler and Woods, 1977). In addition, pilot respiratory function studies were conducted using this same system in liver mitochondria isolated from newborn, weanling and 12-week-old adult male rats from dams treated with 0, 5, or 10 ppm methylmercury hydroxide to determine if prenatal effects in this organelle system persisted into later phases of life.

Results. As previously reported (Fowler and Woods, 1977), the dosages of methylmercury hydroxide used in these studies produced no changes in either weight gain or water consumption of the dams before or during pregnancy relative to controls, thus indicating that this dose regimen did not produce overt maternal toxicity. There was also no observed increase in fetal resorptions or obvious gross teratologic effects in the fetuses.

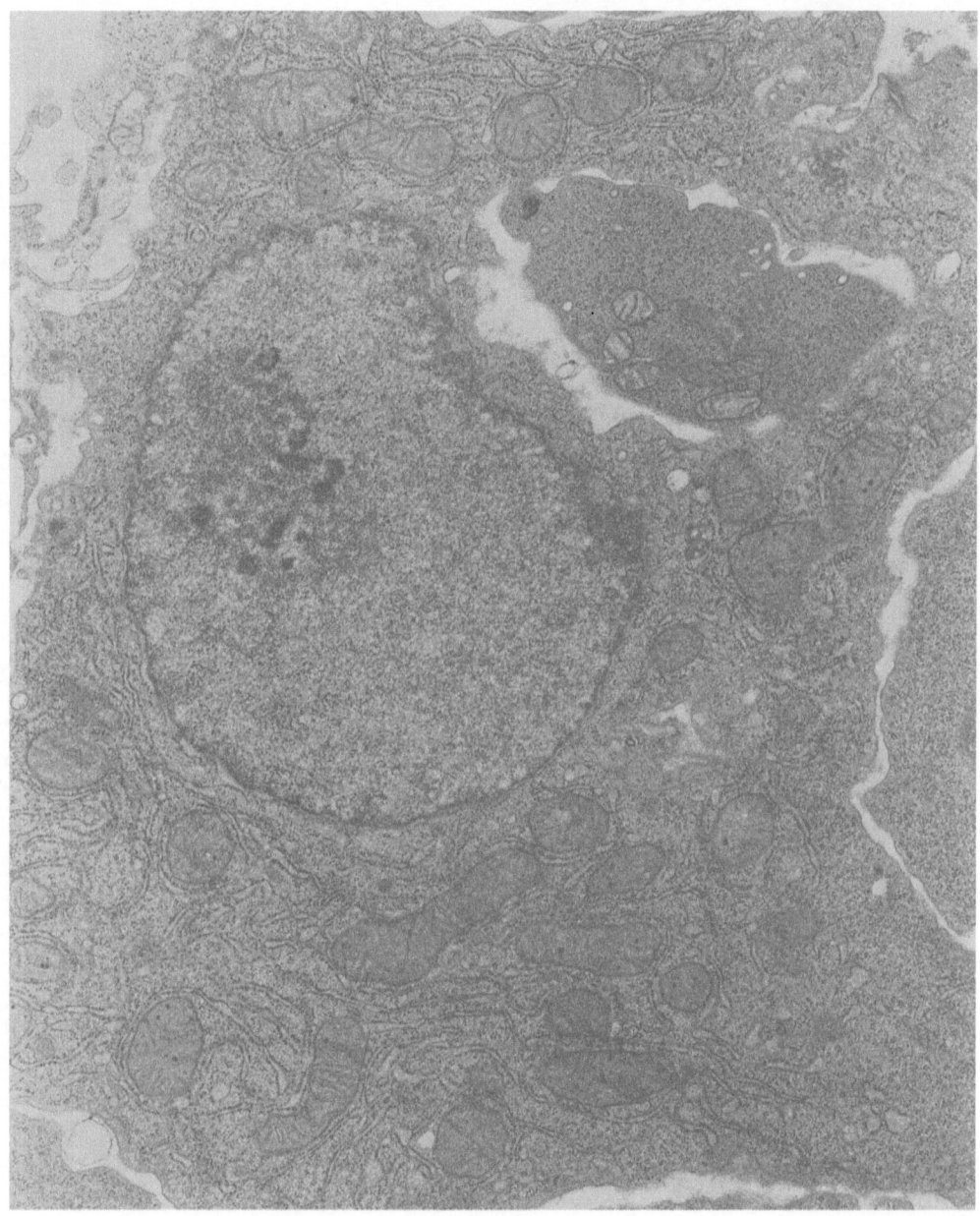

Figure 1   Hepatocytes from a day 19 control fetal rat showing
            normal cellular architecture.   x16,758.

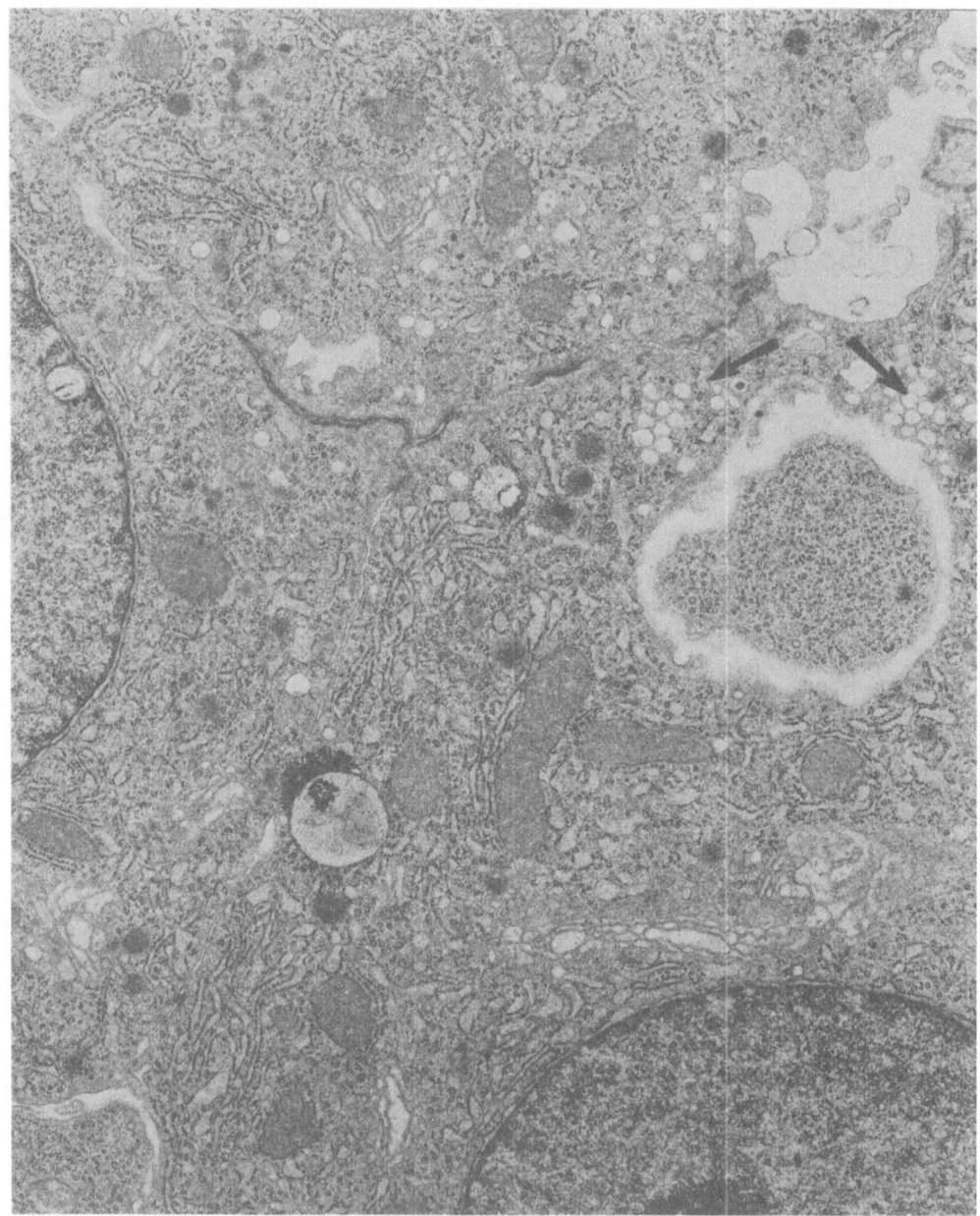

Figure 2   Hepatocytes from a day 19 fetal rat from a dam exposed to
           10 ppm methylmercury hydroxide in drinking water showing
           numerous small vesicles (arrows) adjacent to rudimentary
           bile canaliculus.   x16,758.

Ultrastructural morphometric studies. As previously reported (Fowler and Woods, 1977), the only major obvious ultrastructural change in fetal hepatocytes was an increase in clear vacuoles which were most conspicious near rudimentary bile caniculi (Figures 1 and 2). Morphometric analyses showed a highly significant (p < 0.01) dose-related increase in the relative volume density of vacuoles and decrease in that of the mitochondrial compartment. In order to determine if this decrease in the volume density of the mitochondrial compartment was due to a change in the number or dimensions of the mitochondria, further morphometric analyses were conducted (Table 1). In Table 1, statistical analysis was performed to determine if there were any significant trends present among dimensions for the treatments and control. There are significant decreases (p < 0.05) in mitochondrial dimensions with increasing dose levels. In addition, there is no significant difference (p < 0.31) in estimated number of mitochondria among the treated and control groups. This information, along with the volume fraction results, seems to indicate that it is the size of the mitochondria and not the number present which decreases with increasing dose of methylmercury hydroxide.

Biochemical studies. Among the parameters of mitochondrial function which were measured in fetal mitochondria, respiratory function was found to be among the most markedly affected (Table 2). In liver mitochondria isolated from fetal rats in the 5 and 10 ppm methylmercury hydroxide dose groups, state 3 respiration was abolished and state 4 respiration showed an overall, significant inhibition (p < 0.05) relative to controls.

Evaluation of respiratory function in mitochondria isolated from newborn, weanling and 12-week-old adult male rats (Tables 3, 4 and 5) also shows inhibitory effects with decreases in respiratory control ratios (RCR) as the only alteration relative to controls. The point to be made here is that structural/biochemical changes produced during fetal mitochondrial biogenesis persisted postnatally. We have not been able to produce similar biochemical changes in hepatic mitochondria of weanling male rats exposed to the above methylmercury hydroxide dose regimen for 6 weeks (Fowler and Woods, unpublished observations), supporting the idea that the observed respiratory changes in hepatic mitochondria of postnatal animals exposed to methylmercury hydroxide prenatally results from this in utero exposure. This finding is also somewhat similar to that reported by Robbins et al. (1978) for hepatic cytochrome P-450-dependent monooxygenase systems of adult male rats exposed in utero to methylmercury at similar dose levels to those used in the above study. These authors observed significant decreases in cytochrome P-450 content, ethylmorphine N-demethylase, benzo(a)pyrene hydroxylase, aniline hydroxylase and NADPH-cytochrome c reductase activities at 26 or 35 weeks of age but not 3 or 8 weeks. Taken together, the two above studies support the concept of a biochemical

Table 1   Estimated Dimensions of Average Mitochondria and Mitochondrial Numerical Density (N_V) Per Unit Volume of Cytoplasm in 19-day Fetal Rats[a] Exposed <u>in utero</u> to Methylmercury

Dimensions Mean ± SEM	Methylmercury Treatment[b]				Dose Response Test[c]
	0	3	5	10	
X̄ Diameter (μ)	0.93 ± 0.02	0.94 ± 0.02	0.84[d] ± 0.01	0.84[d] ± 0.02	$p < 0.05$
X̄ Length (μ)	1.56 ± 0.03	1.57 ± 0.03	1.41[d] ± 0.02	1.41 ± 0.02	$p < 0.05$
X̄ Volume (μ³)	1.08 ± 0.08	1.11 ± 0.06	0.79[d] ± 0.03	0.80 ± 0.04	$p < 0.05$
X̄ No./100 (μ³) cytoplasm	8.15 ± 0.35	7.01 ± 0.33	7.98 ± 0.23	8.58 ± 0.32	NS

a N = 5 rats per group (see Fowler and Woods, 1977).
b mg Hg/l deionized drinking water.
c Jonckheere's test for trends (one-tailed).
d Differs from control $p < 0.05$ Mann-Whitney U test (one-tailed).

Table 2A Respiratory Parameters[a] of Liver Mitochondria from 19-Day Fetal Rats Exposed to Methylmercury _in utero_

Methylmercury Dose Level	State 4[b]	State 3[b]	RCR	ADP:0
0	29.54	57.67	1.50	0.85
3	27.85	57.85	-	-
5	33.24	-	-	-
10	28.34	-	-	-

Table 2B Respiratory Data for Methylmercury Treatment Groups Expressed as Mean $\pm$ SEM Percent of Control[c]

Methylmercury Dose Level	State 4	State 3
3	66 $\pm$ 16	73 $\pm$ 15
5	96 $\pm$ 12	
10	72 $\pm$ 10	
Significance of overall difference[d]	$p < 0.05$	NS

[a] Succinate as substrate.
[b] μg atoms O_2 consumed/min/g protein.
[c] N = 5 determinations.
[d] Jonckheere's test.

Table 3A Respiratory Parameters[a] of Liver Mitochondria from
          Newborn Male Rats Exposed to Methylmercury _in utero_

Methylmercury Dose Level	State 4[b]	State 3[b]	RCR	ADP:O
0	85.0	144.5	10.00	2.0
5	57.5	129.0	2.56	1.6
10	91.0	143.0	2.76	1.5

Table 3B Respiratory Data for Methylmercury Treatment Groups
          Expressed as Mean ± SEM Percent of Control[c]

Methylmercury Dose Level	State 4	State 3	RCR	ADP:O
5	104 ± 36	114 ± 25	38 ± 12	72 ± 07
10	118 ± 11	131 ± 44	46 ± 18	72 ± 03

[a] Succinate as substrate.
[b] μg atoms O_2 consumed/min/g protein.
[c] N = 2 determinations of 3 pooled livers per group.

Table 4A Respiratory Parameters[a] of Liver Mitochondria from Weaning Male Rats Exposed to Methylmercury in utero

Methylmercury Dose Level	State 4[b]	State 3[b]	RCR	ADP:O
0	45.3	149.4	9.0	2.0
5	46.6	144.3	6.8	2.0
10	37.9	113.8	7.5	2.0

Table 4B Respiratory Parameters for Methylmercury Treatment Groups Expressed as Mean ± SEM Percent of Control[c]

Methylmercury Dose Level	State 4	State 3	RCR	ADP:O
5	88 ± 15	94 ± 03	66 ± 09	97 ± 03
10	97 ± 13	88 ± 12	72 ± 11	95 ± 06

[a] Succinate as substrate.
[b] μg atoms O_2 consumed/min/g protein.
[c] N = 2 determinations of 3 pooled livers per group.

Table 5A Respiratory Parameters[a] of Liver Mitochondria from
          12-week-old Male Rats Exposed to Methylmercury _in utero_

Methylmercury Dose Level	State 4[b]	State 3[b]	RCR	ADP:O
0	47.6	146.0	2.60	2.0
5	41.0	164.0	2.80	2.0
10	43.0	130.0	1.80	1.9

Table 5B Respiratory Parameters for Methylmercury Treatment Groups
          Expressed as Mean ± SEM Percent of Control[c]

Methylmercury Dose Level	State 4	State 3	RCR	ADP:O
5	88 ± 02	111 ± 02	95 ± 14	98 ± 02
10	94 ± 04	95 ± 06	76 ± 05	95 ± 02

[a] Succinate as substrate.
[b] μg atoms O_2 consumed/min/g protein.
[c] N = 2 determinations of 3 pooled livers per group.

shift in metabolic capacity of the liver in adult animals as a result of in utero exposure to methylmercury at dosages below which overt maternal toxicity or gross fetal malformations occur. The overall impact of such shifts in hepatic biochemical function on mitochondrial metabolism of carbohydrates and porphyrins, and the effective generation of ATP or microsomal metabolism of steroids, carcinogens or other xenobiotics is presently unknown.

GENERAL DISCUSSION

The results of the above studies with arsenic, lead and methylmercury indicate that these agents are capable of producing ultrastructural damage to a number of different organelle systems in utero. Only in the case of methylmercury are there any correlative biochemical data for these effects or evidence of continuing postnatal biochemical dysfunction at dose levels below which overt maternal toxicity or fetal malformations occur.

A common finding in fetal animals whose mothers were exposed to methylmercury is lower birth and organ weight associated with decreased tissue protein content (Olson and Massaro, 1977; Chen et al., 1979) which appears to stem from decreased protein synthesis (Fowler and Woods, 1977; Olson and Massaro, 1977; Chen et al., 1979). Given these mutually supportive findings with respect to decreased protein synthetic activity, what are the possible mechanisms for such a phenomenon? Chen et al. (1979) have suggested five possible mechanisms for the observed effects: 1) lengthened cell cycle; 2) decreased dividing cell fractions; 3) increased rate of necrosis; 4) reduction in biosynthesis of cellular materials; and 5) reduction in biosynthesis of extracellular materials.

In their study, these authors observed a decreased number of kidney and liver cells and a reduction in incorporation of ^{3}H-thymidine, indicating a reduction of active cellular proliferation in support of numbers 1 and 2 above. Cellular necrosis (3) was not observed in their study or in that from our laboratory (Fowler and Woods, 1977). Possibility number 5 has never been studied but evidence for specific inhibition of intracellular materials (4) is confirmed by the dose-related decrease in mitochondrial structural (acid insoluble) proteins but not (acid soluble) proteins synthesized outside the mitochondria (Fowler and Woods, 1977). Attendant diminution of mitochondrial structure and biochemical function with respect to respiration (Fowler and Woods, 1977) appears to occur as a result of this rather selective effect on mitochondrial membrane protein biosynthesis. The impact of inhibition of mitochondrial biogenesis of cellular ATP needs some consideration with respect to the observed reduction of cellular proliferation since intracellular generation of ATP is essential to this process (Bass et al., 1978). Studies with thiamphenicol (Bass et al., 1978) have demonstrated inhibition of embryonic development similar to that observed with methylmercury and suggested that measured decreases in mitochondrial respiratory function with attendant reduction of embryonic ATP levels played a central role. The main point here is that mitochondrial structure and energy-producing systems also undergo development during the embryonic period in both animals (Jakovcic et al., 1971; Mackler et al., 1971, 1973) and humans (Cammer and Moore, 1972) and as such are highly sensitive to chemical perturbation with resultant reduction in embryonic energy balance leading to changes in many other cellular processes such as membrane transport of nutrients and electrolytes or DNA biosynthesis. In other words, disruption of mitochondrial biogenesis with subsequent inhibition of cellular ATP levels could readily explain the observed effects of in utero methylmercury exposure on overall fetal/organ development.

Another possible mechanism which may play a role in reduced protein synthesis by fetal organisms exposed to methylmercury is partial inhibition of energy-dependent placental/fetal transport of amino acids as suggested by Olson and Massaro (1977). It should be noted, however, that the measurement of relatively high concentrations of methylmercury in the fetal organisms (Fowler and Woods, 1977; Chen et al., 1979) coupled with the selective effect of incorporation of amino acids into mitochondrial structure but not mitochondrial enzymatic protein synthesis strongly suggests that a direct in utero effect in the fetus is also operating.

Finally, it is entirely possible that all or a number of the above effects occur, depending upon the dose-level administered and that what is ultimately observed as reduction in fetal weight and development represents a summation of biochemical injuries sustained at different organelle and molecular sites. The task at hand is to delineate which of these injuries occurs at the earliest time point and lowest dose level.

REFERENCES

Amin-Zaki, L., Majeed, M.A., Elhassani, S.B., Clarkson, T.W., Greenwood, M.R. and Doherty, R.A., 1979, Prenatal methylmercury poisoning: clinical observations over 5 years, Am. J. Dis. Child. 133:172-177.

Bass, R., Oerter, D., Krowke, R. and Spielmann, H., 1978, Embryonic development and mitochondrial function. III. Inhibition of respiration and ATP generation in rat embryos by thiamphenicol, Teratology 18:93-102.

Cammer, W. and Moore, C.L., 1972, Biochemical properties of human fetal mitochondria, Biol. Neonate. 21:259-267.

Chang, L.W., Reuhl, K.R. and Lee, G.W., 1977, Degenerative changes in the developing nervous system as a result of in utero exposure to methylmercury, Environ. Res. 14:414-423.

Chen, W.-J., Body, R.L. and Mottet, N.K., 1979, Some effects of
    continuous low-dose congenital exposure to methylmercury on
    organ growth in the rat fetus, Teratology 20:31-36.
DeGenaro, L.D., 1978, The effects of lead nitrate on the central
    nervous system of the chick embryo. I. Observations of light
    and electron microscopy, Growth 42:141-155.
Fowler, B.A. and Woods, J.S., 1977, The transplacental toxicity
    of methylmercury to fetal rat liver mitochondria: morphometric
    and biochemical studies, Lab. Invest. 36:122-130.
Holtzman, D. and Hsu, J.S., 1976, Early effects of inorganic lead
    on immature rat brain mitochondrial respiration, Pediat. Res.
    10:70-75.
Jakovcic, S., Haddock, J., Getz, G.S., Rabinowitz, M. and Swift,
    H., 1971, Mitochondrial development in liver of fetal and
    newborn rats, Biochem. J. 121:341-347.
Lang, C.A. and Herbener, G.H., 1972, Quantitative comparison of
    the mitochondrial populations in livers of newborn and weanling
    rats, Develop. Biol. 29:176-182.
Loud, A.V., Barany, W.C. and Pack, B.A., 1965, Quantitative
    evaluation of cytoplasmic structures in electron micrographs,
    Lab. Invest. 14:258-263.
Mackler, B., Grace, R. and Duncan, H.M., 1971, Studies of
    mitochondrial development during embryogenesis in the rat,
    Arch. Biochem. Biophys. 144:603-610.
Mackler, B., Grace, R., Haynes, B., Bargman, G.J. and Shephard,
    T.H., 1973, Studies of mitochondrial energy systems during
    embryogenesis in the rat, Arch. Biochem. Biophys. 158:662-666.
Morrissey, R.E. and Mottet, N.K., 1983, Arsenic-induced
    exencephalopathy in mice: studies of lesions occurring during
    neurulation, Teratology (in press).
Mottet, N.K., 1974, Effects of chronic low-dose exposure of rat
    fetuses to methylmercury hydroxide, Teratology 10:173-189.
Olson, F.C. and Massaro, E.J., 1977, Effects of methylmercury on
    murine fetal amino acid uptake, protein synthesis and palate
    closure, Teratology 16:187-194.
Robbins, M.S., Hughes, J.A., Sparber, S.B. and Mannering, G.J.,
    1978, Delayed teratogenic effect of methylmercury on hepatic
    cytochrome P-450-dependent monooxygenase systems of rats, Life
    Sci. 22:287-294.
Spyker, D.A. and Spyker, J.M., 1977, Response model analysis for
    cross-fostering studies: prenatal versus postnatal effects on
    offspring exposed to methylmercury dicyandiamide, Toxicol.
    Appl. Pharmacol. 40:511-527.
Ware, R.A., Chang, L.W. and Burkholder, P.M., 1974, Ultrastructural
    evidence for fetal liver injury induced by in utero exposure to
    small doses of methylmercury, Nature 251:236-237.

453

CRITICAL PROCESSES IN CNS DEVELOPMENT AND THE PATHOGENESIS OF EARLY INJURIES

Patricia M. Rodier

Department of Anatomy
University of Rochester
School of Medicine and Dentistry
Rochester, New York

ABSTRACT

Though mercury and lead exposure are known to be more injurious to developing CNS than mature CNS, the nature of the difference is not understood. If the only difference is in accumulation or retention of the toxic agents, then it should be possible to apply the same tests of toxicity, no matter when exposure occurs. On the other hand, if developing tissue responds to metals in ways that mature tissue does not, then the nature of the injury may be different in subjects exposed at different times. In this case, the measures best suited to detect adult toxicity might be inappropriate to detect toxicity after early exposure. One way to evaluate whether metals interfere with development is to test the integrity of processes which occur only in developing CNS. There is already some evidence that mercury and/or lead alter several such processes. Neuron proliferation, formation of glia and myelin, cell migration, development of connections, and differentiation of transmitter characteristics all have been reported to be affected by early exposure to metals. Interruption of these developmental events by other teratogens has been shown to cause permanent alterations in nervous system form and function. The experimental paradigms necessary to demonstrate failures in developmental processes are not necessarily the same as those used in general toxicity testing. Therefore, it would be useful to apply more varied experimental approaches to the questions surrounding metal effects on developing nervous system.

INTRODUCTION

One of the most compelling clinical findings in cases of mercury poisoning is a differential effect on mature vs. developing brain. The difference in degree of impairment is obvious. Harada (1977) and Harada (1978) reported severe neurological symptoms and retardation in children exposed in utero, even though their mothers were asymptomatic during pregnancy. At higher doses, sufficient to produce maternal toxicity, effects on offspring were still greater in magnitude than effects on the mother (Amin-Zaki et al., 1974). In the case of lead, also, there is general agreement that the same exposure has more serious toxic consequences in young individuals (e.g. Pentschew and Garro, 1966).

The reasons for these differences remain unclear, and they may be important. For example, if young organisms are more affected only because they accumulate more of the metal, either because more reaches the brain, or because less is cleared from the brain, then we need to focus our research attention on accurate predictions of body burdens from exposure levels, but the measures of CNS structure and function used to assess toxicity in adults should be adequate to assess early injuries. If, on the other hand, metals have qualitatively different effects on developing vs. mature brain, then our attention must turn to the biological differences that determine the differential effects. If brain tissue at different ages actually responds differently to metals, then early injuries could have different effects, and even different mechanisms. Thus, it is not merely an academic question whether metals have special effects on developing brain; it is a central issue in selecting methods of toxicity testing and, ultimately, in setting safety standards.

Several lines of evidence suggest that some metals may present special hazards to the developing CNS aside from the toxic effects exerted in adults. For example, the potential of mercury compounds and lead to cause gross malformations (reviewed by Ferm and Hanlon, this volume) is an indication that these agents can interfere with developmental processes, as well as the biologic processes of mature organisms. Several pathological findings in humans exposed to methylmercury in utero are consonant with the hypothesis that the exposure altered brain development. That is, heterotopic neurons (Choi et al., 1978) and resting ventricular matrix cells (Takeuchki and Eto, 1977) could not arise in adult tissue. These conditions suggest interference with cell migration and/or differentiation, processes which do not occur in mature brain. Further, it has been suggested that early exposure may be associated with pathologic effects in regions of the brain different from those affected by adult exposure (Choi et al., 1978).

The idea that developing brain and mature brain may be affected differentially by some agents or conditions is hardly new. In fact,

some of the best known CNS teratogens are not toxic to mature CNS.
For example, rubella and x-irradiation are innocuous to the mature
nervous system yet devastating to the immature nervous system. The
discrepancy arises because these agents interfere with development
itself. If we wish to know whether metals have the same capacity to
disrupt development, then we need to ask: What processes are
characteristic of the developing nervous system? Which are subject
to interference? What agents or conditions are already known to
disrupt these processes? What properties do these teratogens share
with metals?

     The purpose of this chapter is to review some features of
nervous system development that may determine the kinds of pathology
likely to occur after early injury. The first section will provide
a very general overview of the gross development of the nervous
system and the second will focus on specific biologic processes that
occur during development. The closing section will be an attempt to
relate developmental data to evaluations of early injury.

GENERAL OVERVIEW

     Most of the nervous system is derived from the ectodermal cells
of the neural plate, which early in development folds into a tube,
internalizing the nervous system. Post-mitotic neurons first appear
around the time of neural tube closure. Since closure failures are
a common malformation, it is important to know the time of closure
if one is interested in CNS teratology. In the human, closure
occurs during the fourth week of gestation. In the mouse, closure
occurs at about 9-1/2 days. The production, migration and
differentiation of neurons then begin in wave-like patterns in which
various sets of cells, or whole CNS regions, develop at different
times and at different rates. The gross appearance of the mammalian
brain over development suggests that the spinal cord forms very
early, as does the medulla (see Figure 1). The midbrain and pons
also appear disproportionately large in embryos, because of their
relatively early development. The diencephalon and corpus striatum
enlarge, followed by cortical structures - cerebral cortex,
olfactory bulbs, hippocampus, and cerebellum. In the human, the
most rapid growth occurs just before birth and late-forming
structures, such as the cerebellum, more than double their weight
postnatally (Dobbing and Sands, 1973).

     The sequence of expansion of the various regions of the CNS, of
course, represents only one measure of development - increase in
tissue volume - and this measure is dependent on many separable
developmental events. In general, neuron production per se does not
underlie the periods of most rapid size increases. Young neurons
are small, and often closely packed. It is the subsequent growth of
the axons and dendrites of these cells, the addition of glia and

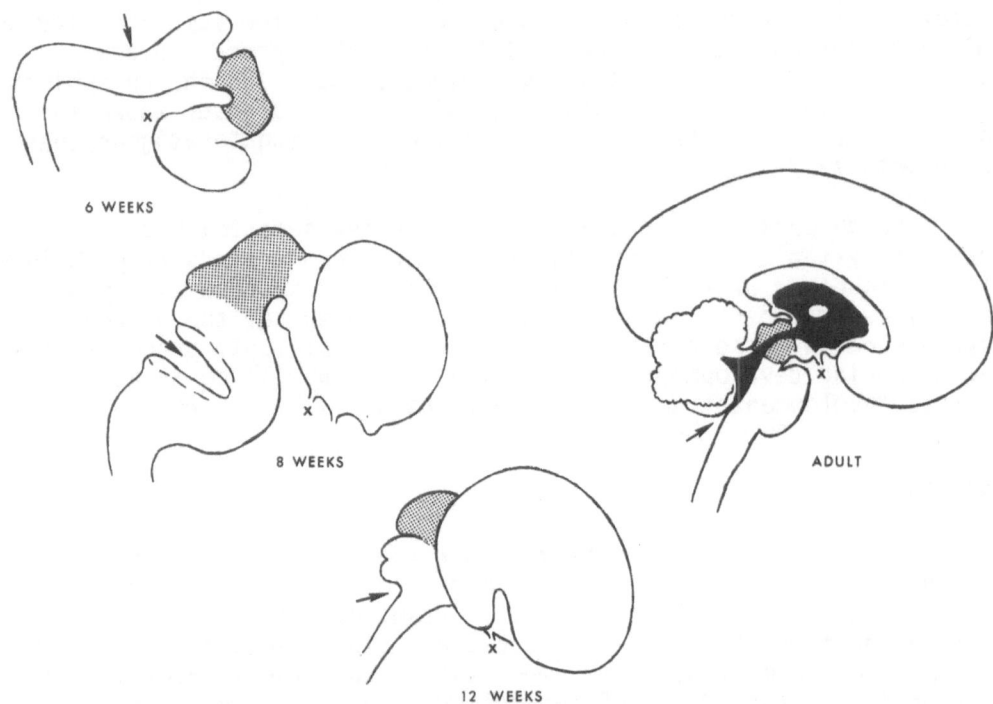

Figure 1   Relative growth in the developing CNS. This figure
           describes the development of the cephalic end of the
           neural tube but does not represent the overall enlargement
           from the embryo to maturity. Rather, the relative size of
           brain regions is emphasized. The stippled area is the
           midbrain. Since it is formed early, it appears to be
           quite large in the early stages. At maturity, it is small
           in proportion to the later-forming cerebral hemispheres
           and cerebellum. The arrow marks the pontine flexure, just
           caudal to the developing cerebellum, and the x marks the
           site of the pituitary stalk. As the tube grows and folds
           on itself, its proportions are altered so drastically that
           regions like the midbrain and diencephalon are covered by
           the expansion of the cerebrum. Thus, the adult brain must
           be presented in sagittal section to allow a view of the
           basic component parts, which were externally visible
           earlier.

myelin and increases in vascular elements that coincide with maximum changes in tissue volume.

In contrast to organs like the liver, in which a small number of different cell types develop, the nervous system produces neurons of many different types, distinguishable by morphologic, biochemical, and physiologic characteristics. Both the spatial arrangement of these cells and their connections to one another are highly organized. A normal, mature nervous system requires not just the production of a large mass of tissue, but rather the production of a large number of specific elements which must be properly arranged, connected and supported by non-neuronal tissue. The timing of these events, while orderly, is quite different from one region of the nervous system to another. Thus, teratogenic insults may affect different regions at different stages of development. For example, if a teratogen affects a process completed in some regions, active in others, and not yet begun in others, then only those regions in which the process is active will be susceptible to damage. At other times, other regions pass through their own periods of susceptibility.

While it is often convenient to picture the development of a particular part of the nervous system as beginning with neuron production, followed by migration, then by differentiation of distinguishing characteristics, and, finally by the addition of glia and other surrounding tissue, we know that the sequence does not characterize all regions of the nervous system. For example, some presumptive neurons migrate and then reenter the cell cycle (granule cells of cerebellum - Miale and Sidman, 1961), and some develop the ability to produce their characteristic transmitter before undergoing a second round of mitotic activity (neurons of sympathetic ganglia - Rothman et al., 1978). While neurons may form connections quickly, some appear to add or subtract connections over a period of months or years (e.g. the visual system - Hubel et al., 1975). Thus, it is an empirical problem to put the most basic processes in order for a given set of cells, much less identify the time when they occur in disparate regions and in different species.

Perhaps because so many steps are involved in the development of the nervous system, the time course from the earliest neuron production to mature form and function is considerably longer than that seen in most organ systems. This may be one reason why congenital brain damage is more common than other malformations - i.e. to the extent that the course of development can be interrupted, accidents should be more frequent in those organs in which mature form and function develop slowly, because these organs are vulnerable to interference over a longer period than rapidly developing structures.

DEVELOPMENTAL PROCESSES

It has long been known that the effects of toxic agents may vary between adults and developing organisms. In some cases, adults are at greater risk. For example, anoxia is injurious to mature or immature brain, but prenatal animals can survive on much less oxygen than adults, and neonates retain some resistance to anoxia (Fazekas et al., 1941; Glass and Snyder, 1942). The difference is explained by the different metabolic requirements which characterize the brain at different stages of life. On the other hand, a virus such as rubella, which affects proliferating cells preferentially (Naeye and Blanc, 1965), is more damaging in young animals than in mature ones. No one can identify all the processes and products subject to injury in the developing nervous system, but some are obvious possibilities, and some have already been demonstrated to be susceptible to teratogens.

a. neuron proliferation - The most obvious, and most studied, process that distinguishes immature nervous system is the production of neurons. Interference with cell proliferation in general is a common feature of many known teratogens (Wilson, 1973). Some agents interrupt the cell cycle in such a way that mitosis is prevented (e.g. colchicine - Borisy and Taylor, 1967) while others disrupt dividing cells in such a way that they die soon after exposure (e.g. azacytidine - Langman and Shimada, 1971). Methylmercury has been shown to be antimitotic in vitro (Imura et al., 1980) and in vivo (Sager et al., 1982). At most stages of development, the ability of the organism to compensate for a loss of neurons appears to be poor (Andreoli et al., 1973) and, therefore, such losses tend to be permanent (e.g., Rodier and Gramann, 1979).

The final effects of interference with proliferation are dependent on the stage of development when cell production is decreased. During embryogenesis, such an injury can cause gross malformations. Until all neuron production is complete, the structure and function of the nervous system can be altered by agents that preferentially attack dividing cells. The location of damage and the behavioral outcome differ with the time of exposure. For example, Figure 2 shows the times of production for various neuron types in the developing mouse brain (Rodier, 1980). Experimental reduction of proliferation at a variety of stages of mouse development has demonstrated that regions of significant reductions in the brains of subjects sacrificed as adults are correlated with those regions where proliferation is rapid at the time of experimental intervention (Rodier and Reynolds, 1977; Rodier and Gramann, 1979). While it is difficult to predict the behavioral effects of these lesions, there is a definite relationship between areas injured and behaviors affected. For example, exposure

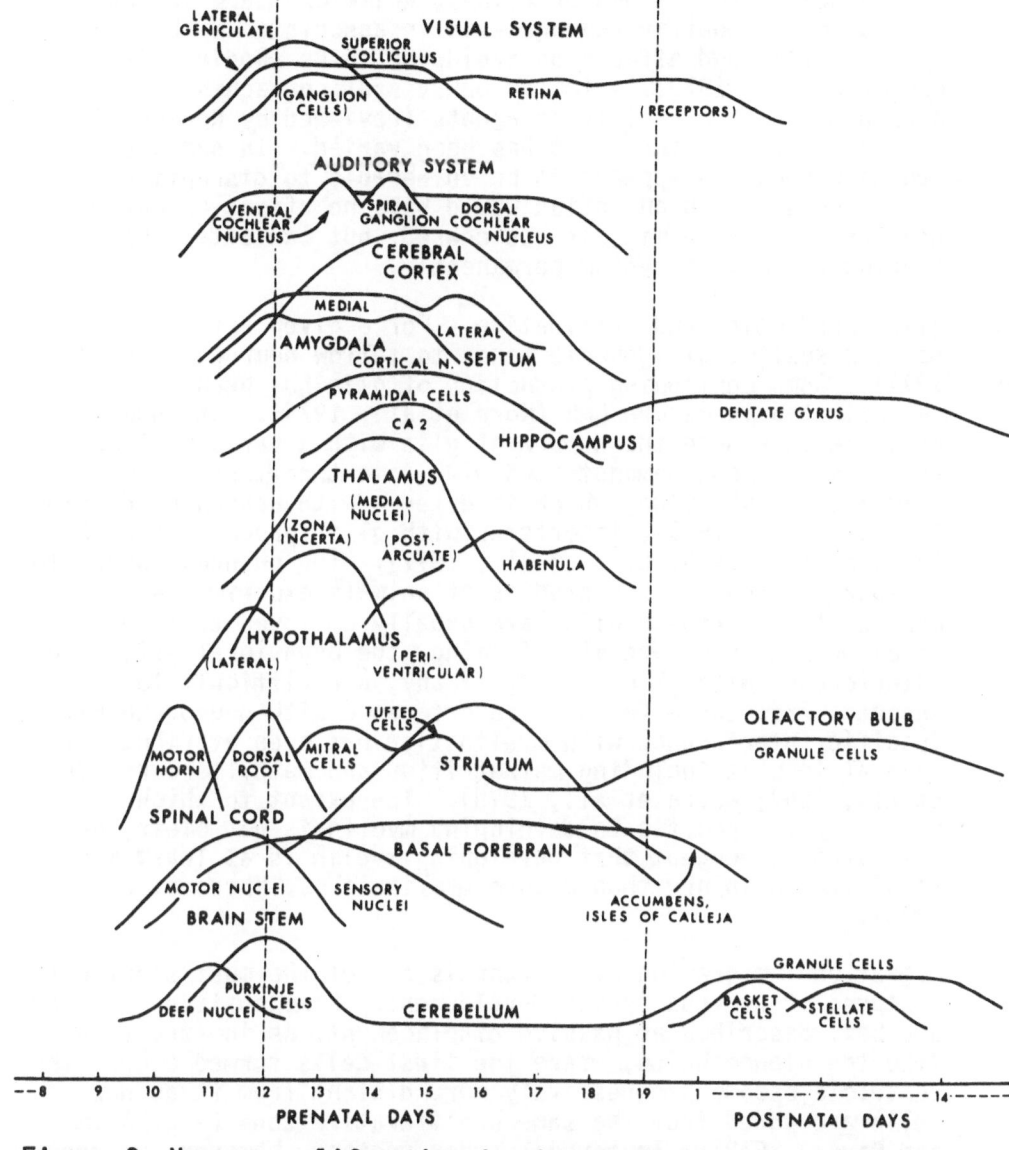

Figure 2 Neuron proliferation in the mouse CNS. The bursts of
cell production that create the CNS are represented as
curves. The abcissa indicates the time course of
development. The ordinate is arbitrary and used only to
display a variety of neuron populations. The vertical
line on day 12 of gestation marks the end of the period
when mice are highly susceptible to teratogenesis, as
indicated by gross malformations. The vertical line on
day 19 marks the day of birth.

during production of cerebellar neurons is associated with
reflex delays and locomotor delays, while exposure in between
periods of cerebellar neurogenesis is associated with
hyperactivity and effects on avoidance tasks (Rodier, 1976;
Rodier et al., 1979). Similar behavioral consequences have
been noted with a variety of agents (reviewed by Rodier, 1980)
for which time of treatment has been varied. In summary,
neuron production appears to be vulnerable to disruption by
many agents. Such an action would have no effect on mature
neurons, for which mitosis has ceased, but can alter the
developing nervous system permanently.

b.   glial production and myelination - For a given area of the
nervous system, gliogenesis tends to follow neurogenesis (Das,
1977). Some continuing production of glia has been
demonstrated in mature CNS (Korr et al., 1975). It should be
possible to reduce the number of glia with a variety of agents
and this has been demonstrated with some treatments. For
example, malnutrition, which interferes with neuron production
(Lewis et al., 1975), interferes with glial production as well
(Bass et al., 1970; Clos et al., 1977). The changes appear to
be long-lasting. Since studies of animals experimentally
manipulated to reduce glia have usually employed treatment
times when neurons are also forming, the behavioral effects of
interference with gliogenesis, if any, are difficult to
separate from the effects of interference with neurogenesis.
Specific interference with myelination has been attributed to
several insults including malnutrition and methylmercury (Chase
et al., 1967; Khera et al., 1975). The extent to which
pathology is specific to developing myelin is not clear, but
some studies suggest that developing myelin is at least more
sensitive to injury than mature myelin (e.g., Khera et al.,
1975).

c.   migration - Migration of neurons is one of the most spectacular
features of nervous system development. Some position changes
are best described as passive displacement, as in structures
like the diencephalon, where the first cells formed around the
ventricle become progressively more distant from it as new
cells are added from the same proliferative zone (e.g. Altman
and Bayer, 1978). In several other regions, however, neurons
travel great distances through layers of earlier-formed cells
to reach their final locations. In the cerebral cortex, each
new wave of neuroblasts is deposited more distally, until the
last burst of proliferation produces the neurons of the
outermost layers (Berry and Rogers, 1965). In the cerebellum,
the last neurons to form in the external germinal layer on the
pial surface travel deep into the cerebellum, passing other
neurons to reach their proper position (e.g. Miale and Sidman,
1961). In the autonomic nervous system, the neurons of

sympathetic and parasympathetic ganglia arise in the neural crest, and migrate to their final destinations in the sympathetic chain, paraaortic ganglia, gut wall, etc. (e.g. LeDouarin and Teillet, 1973). Migration in the CNS may be involved with formation of connections along the route. In the case of autonomics, the migration route seems to play a role in cell differentiation, bringing neurons near inductive influences at critical stages of development (e.g. Cohen, 1972). Whatever the reasons that migration has evolved, it is a common phenomenon and one that appears to be subject to disruption. Migration failures are seen after a variety of teratogenic insults. For example, postnatal treatment of rodents with 5-FUdR (Langman et al., 1972), or x-irradiation (Altman et al., 1968) leads to cell rests of granule cells in the cerebellar molecular layer. Yet cells exposed to FUdR can migrate away from the DNA synthetic zone of the rhombic lip even when they are severely injured (Webster et al., 1973). Thus, it may be that some cases of interference with migration do not arise from direct effects on the migrating cells themselves. One possibility is that the cells cannot migrate because of injury to or loss of the neighboring glial processes which are thought to act as "guides" in some long distance migration (Rakic, 1971, 1972). On the other hand, agents such as colchicine amd methylmercury, with their actions on the cytoskeleton, may have the potential to alter migration directly. Choi (this volume) has focused attention on the effects of methylmercury on migration because migration failures were characteristic of the brains of the children exposed in utero in Iraq.

d.   growth of processes and connections - The elaboration of cell processes and connections is thought to continue throughout life and has been observed in aging brain (Buell and Coleman, 1981). Much of the growth of immature brain reflects development of the extensive network of projections characteristic of many groups of neurons. Some basic pathways are operational very early although they may undergo many changes as development proceeds. For example, chick motor horn cells can operate their muscle targets within a few days of their final mitoses (Oppenheim, 1974). On the other hand, some parts of monkey cerebral cortex do not exhibit mature function for several years after birth (Alexander and Goldman, 1978) despite the fact that cortical neurons of this species form by midgestation (Rakic, 1977). Extension of processes is clearly related to the availability of target tissue, and abnormal processes have been reported after manipulation of target cells (e.g. Altman and Anderson, 1971). It is often difficult to separate such indirect effects on processes from direct effects, but several agents have been reported to be candidates for influencing dendritic development directly. Nerve growth factor promotes axonal growth (Levi-Montalcini et al., 1954).

Hyperthyroidism increases dendritic development and hypothyroidism decreases it (Lewis et al., 1976; Clos et al., 1974). Experimentally-induced hyperphenylalaninemia reduces the length of dendrites in the pyramidal cells of motor cortex, but not in stellate cells (Hogan and Coleman, 1981a) and reduces the area of the dendritic tree of Purkinje cells (Hogan and Coleman, 1981b), suggesting that the forces responsible for dendritic elaboration may be somewhat different in different neurons. Decreased dendritic branching has been reported after early exposure to lead (Averill and Needleman, 1980; Krigman et al., 1974). All the agents mentioned have been shown to alter nervous system function, so early insults to developing connections appear to have important functional consequences.

e. level and turnover of neurotransmitters - Changes in levels and turnover rates of transmitters in adult animals have been observed after a variety of early injuries. Such changes would be expected as secondary effects of neuron loss, connection failures, etc., as has been shown after treatment with methylazoxymethanol (Johnston and Coyle, 1979; Johnston et al., 1979). In other cases, however, investigators have suspected a direct effect on transmitter development. For example, recent studies in the peripheral nervous system demonstrate that both the qualitative and quantitative transmitter characteristics of developing neurons can be altered independently of the factors that influence neuron production and connectivity (reviewed by Black, 1982). That means that it is possible to have a teratogen which affects transmitter content or activity of neurons which would not be recognized as injurious by assay of cell numbers and connections.

Among the metals, lead is known to interfere with catecholamine, acetylcholine, and GABA transmission in vitro (reviewed by Silbergeld and Hruska, 1980). In vivo, persistent changes in transmitter activity have been observed after early exposure to lead (Jason and Kellogg, 1977). Whether such changes are specific to exposure during development, or occur after exposure of adult brain as well, is not known. However, some agents with transient psychotrophic effects in mature brain have been shown to have lasting functional effects when introduced during brain development (e.g. Vorhees et al., 1979), so it is possible that lead has similar actions.

Another consideration related to neurotransmitters is the fact that these substances are thought to act as inducers, not only in nervous system development (Lauder and Krebs, 1978) but possibly in development of other systems as well. At least, neurotransmitters can be detected in embryos and blastulas before any neurons are formed (McMahon, 1974). Since interference with transmitters is an obvious mechanism for

toxic effects in the mature nervous sytem, it is interesting to
speculate that such an action could have more widespread and
unpredictable effects in early embryos, where the normal
function of these compounds is poorly understood.

DEVELOPMENTAL PROCESSES AND TOXICITY TESTING

Despite the wealth of data on toxic effects of heavy metals on
the CNS, the number of studies that address developmental issues is
small. There are many reports of injury after treatment during
development, but few that compare exposure at different ages or
examine the effects of metals on specific developmental processes.
Even the most basic familiarity with events in the developing nervous
system suggests some experimental strategies which might prove useful
if we wish to separate developmental effects from general toxic
effects.

Perhaps the most valuable addition to traditional evaluations
would be more experiments in which developing tissue is studied at
the time of injury and at selected times thereafter. For example,
if an agent reduces the number of neurons or glia, it is difficult
to tell from adult tissue whether the cells degenerated or failed to
form. Yet in developing brain, it is easy to measure the rate of
mitosis and to check for specificity of cytotoxic actions. Does the
agent affect only proliferating cells, only cells with a particular
transmitter, only migrating cells   Such information not only speaks
to issues of mechanism of action, it also can direct our attention
to more definitive studies of adult tissue. For example, if we can
establish that a particular set of cells is preferentially affected
during development, and we know where to find those cells in the
adult, then we can focus our attention on restricted parts of the
nervous sytem, at a great savings of time and effort. From a purely
practical point of view, it is important to note that samples of
developing nervous system appear to be less variable in cell numbers
and other features than mature nervous system. This means that it
is often possible to get the same information with fewer animals in
a developmental study.

The value of testing at a variety of times is not restricted to
morphological studies. Because some behaviors vary greatly with the
age of the animal, there may be times when functional differences are
difficult to detect and other times when they are obvious. For
example, adult animals with motor handicaps may appear normal on very
easy tasks, such as righting from a supine position, but the same
animals may be deficient on this measure if tested neonatally, when
the righting reflex first appears. Conversely, some tests that
require mature CNS function, such as delayed-response tasks, are
unlikely to discriminate brain-damaged animals until they are fully
mature.

Because the nervous system differs so much from one stage of development to another, and its state at the time of injury plays such an important role in the outcome of an injury, studies that vary the time of injury can often provide valuable information. Many studies of metals have involved chronic exposures, for obvious reasons. First, chronic exposure is the best model for typical human exposure patterns. Second, the slow elimination of metals makes very brief exposures impossible. However, for studies of mechanisms of action, restriction of exposure periods is often a critical element of appropriate experimental designs. For example, we can never address the question of whether exposure causes permanent deficits with data collected from animals whose exposure continued during the test period. Similarly, we cannot assess whether a metal interferes directly with connectivity if the tissue was exposed while neighboring cells formed, changing their number. Thus, for many purposes, acute exposures offer some interpretive advantages. Finally, because so many teratologic studies are acute, we have more background data from other agents to which metals can be compared if we follow traditional paradigms. This is not to say that acute studies are "better" than chronic ones, only that no one paradigm can answer all questions.

A recent example of the efficacy of short-term exposures in studies of metals is the series by Eccles and Annau (1982a,b). The results demonstrate differences in behavioral effects after single-dose exposures to methylmercury at different stages of gestation. Such findings support the hypothesis that some metals may interfere with brain development, rather than acting solely through the same general cytotoxic mechanisms thought to account for their effects in mature CNS. The results also can be related to those obtained with other CNS teratogens (e.g. x-ray - Furchtgott and Echols, 1958).

In addition to treatment and testing schedules that focus on developmental injuries, a final requisite for more powerful experiments in this area is the use of measures known to be altered by interference with developmental processes. It is possible that early exposure to metals affects the nervous system in ways that are unique but it seems more likely that metals affect some of the processes subject to interference by other teratogens. There are already some data to suggest that this is the case, yet answers to some of the most basic questions are missing. This is true despite the fact that methods are available for testing all the processes mentioned in the previous section.

While the overriding concern of toxicity and teratology is to make decisions about the relative safety of various exposure levels, our ability to make such judgments is dependent on appropriate measures of effect. In the absence of data on the effects of metals on the processes specific to the developing CNS, our choice of measures is necessarily based on observations of a relatively small number of clinical cases. It is possible that the behavioral and morphologic symptoms exhibited by those cases represent the aspects of function and anatomy most sensitive to damage, but it is also possible that better measures can be found. For example, if methylmercury has a consistent effect on cell migration at levels of exposure below those that produce consistent behavioral effects, it may be appropriate to use migration effects to determine safety levels. If neurotransmitter turnover effects of early lead exposure are more stable than nerve conduction effects, measures of turnover would allow us to make better judgments about hazardous levels of lead.

Unless toxicologists are willing to borrow the information and techniques of developmental neurobiology, important toxic effects of metals could be overlooked. It is clear from the information presently available that the hypothesis that metals interfere with development of the CNS cannot be dismissed without a series of direct tests.

REFERENCES

Alexander, G.E. and Goldman, P.S., 1978, Functional development of the dorsolateral prefrontal cortex: An analysis utilizing reversible cryogenic depression, Brain Res. 143:223-249.

Altman, J. and Anderson, W.J., 1971, Irradiation of the cerebellum in infant rats with low level x-ray: histological and cytological effects during infancy and adulthood, Exper. Neurol. 30:492-509

Altman, J. and Bayer, S.A., 1978, Development of the diencephalon in the rat. I. Autoradiographic study of the time of origin and settling patterns of neurons of the hypothalamus, J. Comp. Neurol. 182:945-972.

Altman, J., Anderson, W.J. and Wright, K.A., 1968, Gross morphological consequences of irradiation of the cerebellum in infant rats with repeated doses of low level x-ray, Exper. Neurol. 21:69-91.

Andreoli, J., Rodier, P.M. and Langman, J., 1973, The influence of a prenatal trauma on formation of Purkinje cells, Am. J. Anat. 137:87-102.

Amin-Zaki, L., Elhassani, S., Majeed, M.A., Clarkson, T.W., Doherty, R.A. and Greenwood, M., 1974, Intrauterine methylmercury poisoning in Iraq, Pediatrics 54:587-594.

Averill, D.R. and Needleman, H.L., 1980, Neonatal lead exposure retards cortical synaptogenesis in the rat, in: "Low Level Lead Exposure: The Clinical Implications of Current Research", H.L. Needleman, ed., pp. 201-210, Raven Press, New York.

Bass, M.A., Netsky, M.G., Young, E., 1970, Effect of neonatal malnutrition on developing cerebrum, I. Microchemical and histologic study of cellular differentiation in the rat, Arch. Neurol. 23:289-302.

Berry, M. and Rogers, A.W., 1965, The migration of neuroblasts in the developing cerebral cortex, J. of Anat. 99:691-709.

Black, I.B., 1982, Stages of neurotransmitter development in autonomic neurons, Science 215:1198-1204.

Borisy, G.G. and Taylor, E.W., 1967, The mechanism of action of colchicine. Colchicine binding to sea urchin eggs to the mitotic apparatus, J. Cell Biol. 34:535-548.

Buell, S.J. and Coleman, P.D., 1981, Quantitative evidence for selective dendritic growth in normal human aging but not in senile dementia, Brain Res. 214:23-41.

Chase, H.P., Dorsey, J. and McKhann, G.M., 1967, The effect of malnutrition on the synthesis of a myelin lipid, Pediatrics 40:551-559.

Choi, B.H., Lapham, L.W., Amin-Zaki, L. and Saleem, T., 1978, Abnormal neuronal migration, deranged cerebral cortical organization and diffuse white matter astrocytosis of human fetal brain: a major effect of methylmercury poisoning in utero, J. Neuropath. and Exp. Neurol. 37:719-733.

Clos, J., Crepel, F., Legrande, C., Legrande, J., Rabie, J. and Vigourouz, E., 1974, Thyroid physiology during the postnatal period in the rat: A study of the development of thyroid function and of the morphogenetic effects of thyroxine with special references to cerebellar maturation, Gen. Comp. Endocrinol. 23:178-192.

Clos, J., Favre, C., Selme-Matrat, M. and Legrande, J., 1977, Effects of undernutrition on cell formation in the rat brain and specially on cellular composition of the cerebellum, Brain Res. 123:13-26.

Cohen, A.M., 1972, Factors direcing the expression of sympathetic nerve traits in cells of neural crest origin, J. Exp. Zool. 179:167-182.

Das, G.D., 1977, Gliogenesis during embryonic development in the rat, Experientia 33:1648-1649.

Dobbing, J. and Sands, J., 1973, Quantitative growth and development of human brain, Arch. Dis. Child. 48:757-767.

Eccles, C.U. and Annau, Z., 1982a, Prenatal methylmercury exposure: I. Alterations in neonatal activity, Neurobehav. Tox. and Terat. 4:371-376.

Eccles, C.U. and Annau, Z., 1982b, II. Alterations in learning and psychotropic drug sensitivity in adult offspring, Neurobehav. Tox. and Terat. 4:377-382.

Fazekas, J.R., Alexander, F.A.D. and Himwich, H.E., 1941, Tolerance of the newborn to anoxia, Am. J. Physiol. 134:281-287.

Furchtgott, E. and Echols, M., 1958, Activity and emotionality in pre- and neonatally x-irradiated rats, J. Comp. Physiol. Psych. 51:541-545.

Glass, H. and Snyder, F.F., 1942, The increased tolerance to anoxia of animals born prematurely, Anat. Rec. 82:465-466.

Harada, Y., 1977, Congenital Minamata disease, in: "Minamata Disease", K. Tsubaki and K. Irukayama, eds., pp. 209-239, Elsevier, Amsterdam/New York.

Harada, M., 1978, Congenital Minamata disease: intrauterine methylmercury poisoning, Teratology 18:285-288.

Hogan, R.N. and Coleman, P.D., 1981a, Experimental hyperphenylalaninemia: Dendritic alterations in motor cortex of rat, Exp. Neurol. 74:218-233.

Hogan, R.N. and Coleman, P.D., 1981b, Experimental hyperphenylalaninemia: Dendritic alterations in cerebellum of rat, Exp. Neurol., 74:234-244.

Hubel, D.H., Wiesel, T.N. and LeVay, S., 1975, Functional architecture of area 17 in normal monocularly deprived macaque monkeys, Cold Spring Harbor Symp. Quant. Biol. 15:581-590.

Imura, N., Miura, K., Inokawa, M. and Nakada, S., 1980, Mechanism of methylmercury cytotoxicity: By biochemical and morphological experiments using cultured cells, Toxicol. 17:244-254.

Jason, K. and Kellogg, C., 1977, Lead effects on behavioral and neurochemical development in rats, Federation Proc. 36:1008.

Johnston, M.V. and Coyle, J.T., 1979, Ontogeny of neurochemical markers for noradrenergic, GABA ergic and cholinergic neurons in neocortex lesioned with methylazoxymethanol acetate, J. Neurochem. 34:1429-1441.

Johnston, M.V., Grzanna, R. and Coyle, J.T., 1979, Methylazoxymethanol treatment of fetal rats results in abnormally dense noradrenergic intervation of neocortex, Science 203:369-371.

Khera, K.S., Iverson, F., Hierlihy, L., Tanner, R. and Trivitt, G., 1975, Toxicity of methylmercury in neonatal cats, Teratology 10:69-76.

Korr, H., Schultz, B. and Maurer, W., 1975, Autoradiographic investigations of glial proliferation in the brain of adult mice, II. Cycle time and mode of proliferation of neuroglia and endothelial cells, J. Comp. Neurol. 160:477-490.

Krigman, M.R., Druse, J.J., Taylor, T.D., Wilson, M.H., Newell, L.R. and Hogan, E.L., 1974, Lead encephalopathy in the developing rat: Effect on cortical ontogenesis, J. Neuropath. Exp. Neurol. 33:671-686.

Lauder, J.M. and Krebs, H., 1978, Serotonin as a differentiation signal in early neurogenesis, Dev. Neurosci. 1:15-30.

Langman, J. and Shimada, M., 1971, Cerebral cortex of mouse after a prenatal chemical insult, Am. J. Anat. 132:355-374.

Langman, J., Shimada, M. and Rodier, P.M., 1972, Floxuridine (5 FUdR) and its influence on postnatal cerebellar development, Ped. Res. 6:758-764.

LeDouarin, N.M. and Teillet, M.A., 1973, The migration of neural crest cells to the wall of the digestive tract in avian embryo, J. Embryol. Exp. Morphol. 30:31-48.

Lewis, P.D., Balazs, R., Patel, A.J. and Johnson, A.L., 1975, The effect of undernutrition in early life on cell generation in the rat brain, Brain Res. 83:235-247.

Lewis, P.D., Patel, A.J., Johnson, A.L. and Balazs, R., 1976, Effect of thyroid hormone deficiency on cell acquisition in the postnatal rat brain: A quantitative histological study, Brain Res. 104:49-62.

Levi-Montalcini, R., Meyer, H. and Hamburger, V., 1954, In vitro experiments on the effects of mouse sarcoma 180 and 37 on the spinal and sympathetic ganglia of the chick embryo, Cancer Res. 14:49-57.

McMahon, D., 1974, Chemical messengers in development: A hypothesis, Science 185:1012-1021.

Miale, I.L. and Sidman, R.L., 1961, An autoradiographic analysis of histogenesis in the mouse cerebellum, Exper. Neurol. 4:277-296.

Naeye, R.L. and Blanc, W., 1965, Pathogenesis of congenital rubella, J. Am. Med. Assn. 194:1277-1283.

Oppenheim, R.W., 1974, The ontogeny of behavior in the chick embryo, in: "Advances in the Study of Behavior", D.S. Lehrman, J.S. Rosenblatt, R.A. Hinde, and E. Shaw, eds., pp. 133-171, Academic Press, New York.

Pentschew, A. and Garro, F., 1966, Lead encephalomyelopathy of suckling rats and its implications on the porphyrinopathic nervous diseases, Acta Neuropathol. 6:266-278.

Rakic, P., 1971, Neuron-glia relationship during granule cell migration in developing cerebellar cortex: A Golgi and electromicroscopic study in Macacus rhesus, J. Comp. Neurol. 141:283-312.

Rakic, P., 1972, Mode of cell migration to the superficial layers of fetal monkey cortex, J. Comp. Neurol. 145:61-84.

Rakic, P., 1977, Prenatal development of the visual system in rhesus monkey, Phil. Trans. of the Roy. Soc. London Series B 378:245-260.

Rodier, P.M., 1976, Critical periods for behavioral anomalies in mice, Env. Health Persp. 18:79-83.

Rodier, P.M., 1980, Chronology of neuron development: Animal studies and their clinical implications, Devel. Med. Child Neurol. 22:525-545.

Rodier, P.M. and Reynolds, S.S., 1977, Morphological correlates of behavioral abnormalities in experimental congenital brain damage, Exp. Neurol. 57:81-93.

Rodier, P.M. and Gramann, W.J., 1979, Morphologic effects of interference with CNS development in the early fetal period, Neurobehav. Toxicol. 1:129-135.

Rodier, P.M., Reynolds, S.S. and Roberts, W.N., 1979, Behavioral consequences of interference with CNS development in the early fetal period, Teratology 19:327-336.

Rothman, T.P., Gershon, M.D. and Holtzer, H., 1978, The relationship of cell division to the acquisition of adrenergic characteristics by developing sympathetic ganglion cell precursors, Dev. Biol. 65:322-341.

Sager, P., Doherty, R.A. and Rodier, P.M., 1982, Effects of
    methylmercury on developing mouse cerebellar cortex, Exp.
    Neurol. 77:179-193.
Silbergeld, E.K. and Hruska, R.E., 1980, Neurochemical investigations
    of low level lead exposure, in: "Low Level Exposure: The
    Clinical Implications of Current Research", H.L. Needleman,
    ed., pp. 135-157, Raven Press, New York.
Takeuchi, T. and Eto, K., 1977, Pathology and pathogenesis of
    Minamata disease, in: "Minamata Disease", K. Tsubaki, and K.
    Irukayama, eds., pp. 103-141, Elsevier, Amsterdam/New York.
Vorhees, C.V., Brunner, R.L. and Butcher, R.E., 1979, Psychotropic
    drugs as behavioral teratogens, Science 205:1220-1225.
Webster, W.S., Shimada, M. and Langman, J., 1973, Effect of
    fluorodeoxyuridine, colcemid, and bromodeoxyuridine on
    developing neocortex of the mouse, Am. J. Anat. 137:67-86.
Wilson, J.G., 1973, "Environment and Birth Defects", Academic Press,
    New York.

EFFECTS OF PRENATAL METHYLMERCURY POISONING UPON GROWTH AND

DEVELOPMENT OF FETAL CENTRAL NERVOUS SYSTEM

Ben H. Choi

Division of Neuropathology, Department of Pathology
California College of Medicine
University of California, Irvine, California

ABSTRACT

Analysis of neuropathological findings in human infants poisoned by maternal ingestion of methylmercury-contaminated food during pregnancy reveals that the principal histopathologic changes are represented by the outcome of disturbance in brain development, more specifically abnormal neuronal migration, deranged cortical differentiation and exuberant white matter astrocytosis. Although these changes are by no means specific, the striking similarity of the pathologic anatomy of the brain of all infants reported in Japan and Iraq and the detailed account of clinical and toxicological data is highly suggestive of a common pathogenetic link to methylmercury poisoning in utero. Thus, the critical periods of vulnerability of developing CNS for sublethal exposure to methylmercury appear to be the late embryonic and fetal periods when neuronal migration and histogenetic development of brain are taking place actively. In order to test this hypothesis, experimental studies using cultures of human fetal brain cells were carried out. Using time-lapse cinematography, phase and electron microscopy and immunocytochemistry, we have been able to observe the cessation of migratory activity of cultured human fetal neurons and astrocytes due to cytotoxic actions of methylmercury. Methylmercury not only caused rapid disruption and degeneration of membranes but also caused specific damage to microtubules in neurons and astrocytes in culture. We have also demonstrated inhibitory effect of methylmercury on DNA synthesis of human fetal astrocytes by radioautography and showed beneficial effect of meso-2,3-dimercaptosuccinic acid on methylmercury-damaged human fetal astrocytes by time-lapse cinematography. Studies of developing mouse brain revealed significant reduction in dendritic arborization of

Purkinje cells and a delay in the proliferative activity of external granule cells of cerebellum following in utero methylmercury intoxication. These changes were only demonstrable after application of special procedures such as Golgi methods and radioautography, indicating the value of correlative morphological approach in bringing out some of the more subtle effects of methylmercury upon the developing CNS. For better understanding of the pathogenesis of methylmercury effects on developing CNS, however, more work is needed to clarify the normal sequence of neuroembryological events, both at the molecular and at the cellular level. Until the uncertainties regarding neurogenesis are resolved, therefore, it will be difficult to ascertain precisely the molecular mechanisms and stages of development that are applicable to methylmercury poisoning in utero.

INTRODUCTION

Since the first report by Engleson and Herner (1952) of psychomotor retardation in children suspected to have been poisoned by methylmercury in utero in Sweden, there has been ample clinical evidence to indicate the vulnerability of the human fetal central nervous system (CNS) to the toxic effects of methylmercury. Subsequent experiences in Japan (Harada, 1968) and Iraq (Amin-Zaki et al., 1974, 1976) have clearly demonstrated that severe methylmercury intoxication of pregnant mothers may lead to fetal death, while lesser degrees of intoxication may lead to some form of cerebral palsy accompanied by mental retardation. Furthermore, there is evidence to suggest that, following poisoning in utero, an infant may appear completely normal at birth, only to develop psychomotor deficits as the nervous system matures (Amin-Zaki et al., 1974, 1976, 1978; Marsh et al., 1980). Thus, the sensitivity of the human fetal CNS to the toxic effects of methylmercury in utero appears to be well established.

In the meantime, there have been numerous reports of experimental studies designed to elucidate the prenatal effects of methylmercury poisoning and to establish the neurotoxic nature of methylmercury poisoning in utero. These studies have shown that transplacental passage of methylmercury readily occurs in man and experimental animals (Amin-Zaki et al., 1974, 1976; Fujita, 1969; Garrett et al., 1972; Mansour et al., 1974; Nakamura and Saeki, 1967; Wannag and Skjerasen, 1975), and that, once across the placenta, methylmercury may have a greater affinity for the fetal than the adult CNS (Berlin and Ulberg, 1963; Null et al., 1968; Yang et al., 1972). In a variety of animal species, investigators have demonstrated embryotoxic and fetotoxic effects of methylmercury (Chen et al., 1979; Dial, 1976, 1978; Fujimoto et al., 1979; Fuyuta et al., 1978; Murakami, 1969, 1972) and have found effects ranging from fetal resorption, gross organ defects, or growth retardation to

subtle behavioral abnormalities that become manifest only in adult
life, depending upon the species and strains of animals used, the
timing of the insults, and the duration and dosage of administration
(Bornhausen et al., 1980; Fuyuta et al., 1979; Harris et al., 1972;
Khera, 1973; Mottet, 1974; Musch et al., 1978; Rosenthal and
Sparber, 1972; Schalock et al., 1981; Spyker and Smithberg, 1972; Su
and Okita, 1976a,b). In spite of all of these efforts, however, our
knowledge of the nature of the CNS tissue and cellular abnormalities
responsible for clinical neurological dysfunction in methylmercury-
affected children is extremely limited.

    In adults and in postnatal children, the signs and symptoms of
methylmercury intoxication of the nervous system typically commence
with sensory disturbances of extremities, lips and tongue followed
by tremor, ataxia, constriction of the visual fields and impaired
hearing. Although the mode of pathogenesis and the morphological
sequence of events are not known, the resulting changes in the brain
tend to be similar. Selective damage to the visual cortex and
precentral gyrus of the cerebrum and to the granule cells of the
cerebellum have been described as being characteristic of
methylmercury intoxication in human adults (Hunter and Russell,
1954; Takeuchi, 1968). The histopathology is characterized by
degeneration and death of nerve cells and their axons and myelin
sheaths, accompanied by neuroglial hyperplasia and scarring.

    On the other hand, our understanding on the neuropathology of
methylmercury poisoning in the developing CNS is rather poor.
Although there have been occasional clinical reports of human fetal
poisoning by methylmercury in recent years (Afonso and DeAlvarez,
1960; Amin-Zaki et al., 1976; Bakir et al., 1973; Engleson and
Herner, 1952; Harada, 1968; Snyder, 1971), detailed neuropathological
descriptions of the fetal CNS following maternal ingestion of
methylmercury-contaminated food are limited to the reports by
Matsumoto et al. (1965) and by Choi et al. (1978). The majority of
experimental studies of prenatal methylmercury intoxication have
been directed primarily toward reproductive, embryocidal and gross
teratogenic effects, without sufficient regard for the
histopathological changes. A review of the handful of reports in
the experimental literature that deal with fetal or neonatal
neuropathology following maternal methylmercury-intoxication during
pregnancy (Chang and Reuhl, 1977; Chang et al., 1977a,b; Khera and
Tabacover, 1973; Matsumoto et al., 1967; Morikawa, 1961; Murakami,
1972; Nonaka, 1969) reveals that many of the descriptions are too
superficial and lacking in detail to permit an adequate understanding
of the effects of methylmercury poisoning upon the developing fetal
CNS.

    The purpose of this review is threefold; first, to describe in
detail the neuropathological findings in human infants poisoned by
maternal ingestion of methylmercury-contaminated food during

pregnancy, and to characterize specific features of such poisoning in the developing CNS; secondly, to correlate the changes observed with embryological events that are taking place in the developing CNS at the time of methylmercury exposure; and third, to present briefly a few of the experimental studies that have been carried out in our laboratory in an attempt to elucidate some of the cellular and subcellular mechanisms involved.

NEUROPATHOLOGICAL FINDINGS IN MAN FOLLOWING METHYLMERCURY INTOXICATION IN UTERO

The following descriptions of the neuropathology of prenatal intoxication of methylmercury in human infants are based on reports by Matsumoto et al. (1965) of two cases from Minamata, Japan and by Choi et al. (1978) of two autopsied newborn infants from Iraq.

The infants described by Matsumoto et al. (1965) were born to mothers who had consumed large quantities of methylmercury-contaminated fish throughout gestation. Although the infants had not been fed contaminated fish, the possibility of postnatal exposure during the breast-feeding period could not be excluded. Death occurred at 6-1/4 and 2-1/2 years, respectively, after a course characterized by severe cerebral palsy and repeated seizures.

Grossly, the brains of the two infants were severely diminished in weight and showed narrowing of gyri, marked reduction in the thickness of the corpus callosum, and hypoplasia of the basal ganglia and cerebellum, changes that were attributed to neuronal degeneration with hyperplasia of neuroglial cells. The histopathological findings, which were identical in the two cases, were said to be "very similar in type and distribution to those found in adult patients suffering from Minamata disease... hence the name "Fetal Minamata Disease." However, detailed analysis of the description (Takeuchi, 1968) reveals that, in both of their cases, there was evidence of brain maldevelopment which in fact represented a considerable departure from the findings in adult cases of Minamata disease. Many heterotopic neurons were identified in the cerebral and cerebellar white matter, as well as the persistence of matrix cell remnants along the walls of the ventricles and in the deeper regions of the diencephalon. In addition, disordered cerebral cortical architecture, as evidenced by abnormal intermingling of large and small neurons and irregularities of neuronal alignment, was also noted. Thus, although foci of neuronal degeneration were described in the cerebral cortex and in the granular layer of the cerebellum, it is obvious that abnormal developmental features were present throughout the brain.

The cases that we have examined were derived from a disastrous outbreak of methylmercury poisoning in Iraq, resulting from

consumption of home-made bread prepared from the seed grain of wheat
that had been treated with fungicide containing methylmercury.

Each infant was the product of a full-term gestation and an
uncomplicated, in-hospital labor and delivery. Both showed slight
reduction in birth weight, without dysmorphic features or obvious
neurological abnormalities. Both were bottle fed. One infant had
an episode of fever and diarrhea for which she was treated with
antibiotics with good response. She died unexpectedly on the 33rd
hospital day with interstitial pneumonitis, which was confirmed at
autopsy. The blood levels of mercury during life ranged from 442 to
658 ng/ml. The second infant had a rather high blood mercury level
at birth (1,568 ng/ml), requiring exchange transfusion. During the
procedure, she developed pallor and bradycardia, requiring
resuscitation. Despite these measures, she died approximately seven
hours after birth.

Both brains were smaller than normal, weighing approximately
250 grams (the normal weight of a neonatal human brain being about
330 grams). Grossly, the external surfaces of both brains were
characterized predominantly by irregularities in gyral configuration
and width.

Microscopically, the two brains were remarkably similar in
appearance. The principal findings consisted of the presence of
large numbers of heterotopic neurons in cerebral and cerebellar
white matter and of disorganization of cerebral cortical
architecture. Heterotopic neurons were noted both singly and in
groups deep within the cerebral white matter. Most of the neurons
were well differentiated pyramidal forms, but there were also groups
of immature neurons, particularly in the subependymal regions and in
the perivascular spaces of the deep white matter and of basal ganglia
(Figure 1). The laminar pattern of the cerebral cortex was disturbed
in many places. The upper cortical layers showed irregular
undulations and contained admixtures of large and small neurons.
Irregular grouping and columnar arrangement of cortical neurons were
prominent in the frontal and temporal regions (Figure 2). In many
areas as the neurons were abnormally oriented, their apical dendrites
pointing upward at various angles to the perpendicular (Figure 2).
The deeper nuclear structures of the basal ganglia and the thalamus
were within normal limits.

The overall architectural pattern of the cerebellum was
preserved. However, there were large numbers of heterotopic neurons
throughout the folial and medullary white matter; many of them were
large and of pyramidal configuration, presumably representing
heterotopic Purkinje cells (Figure 3), but there were also clusters
of small granular cells (Figure 4). The thickness and pattern of
formation of both the external and internal granular layers varied
from place to place. There were scattered foci of heterotopic grey

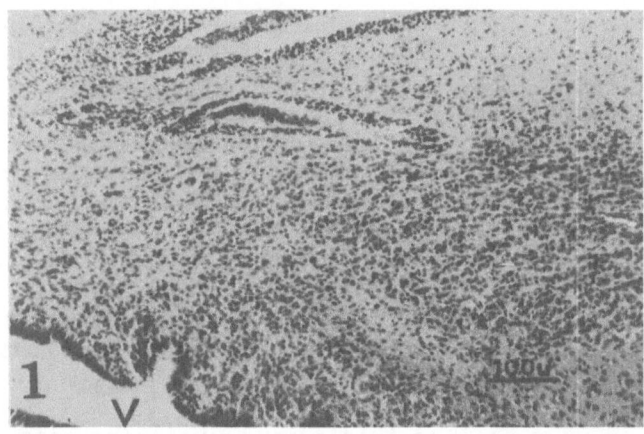

Figure 1   Heterotopic small granular neurons in the subventricular
zone of the cerebrum. Note perivascular localization of
immature neurons in addition to nodular collection of
neurons in the white matter. V: lateral ventricle.

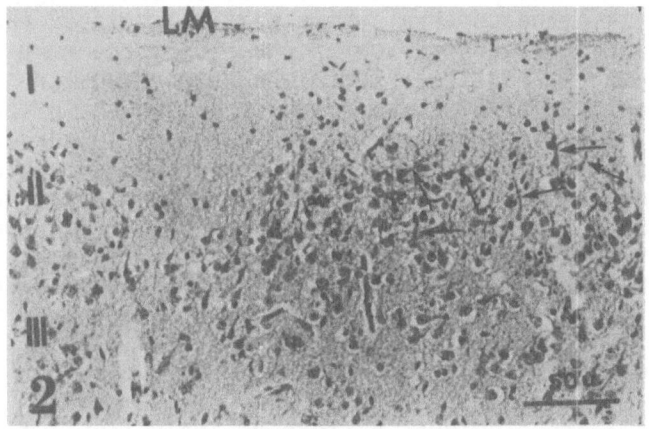

Figure 2   Irregular laminar cortical layering of the cerebrum. Note
clumps of large pyramidal neurons in the upper layers of
the cortex with abnormal alignment of apical dendrites
(arrows). LM: leptomeninges. I-III: cortical layers.

matter in the cerebral leptomeninges which contained both neurons and glial cells (Figure 5). Scattered foci of melanosis were also noted in the cerebral and cerebellar leptomeninges. An additional prominent feature in the white matter of both cerebrum and cerebellum was the presence of numerous gemistocytic astrocytes containing large amounts of eosinophilic cytoplasm and an abundance of glial fibrils (Figure 6). These astrocytes were not associated with either tissue necrosis or reactive microglia or macrophages. The axons in the white matter were intact. There was a paucity of myelin in the cerebral and cerebellar white matter.

The nature of the pathologic changes observed in these two newborn infants and in the Japanese cases represents the outcome of disturbances in brain development, more specifically abnormal neuronal migration and derangement in the basic structuring of grey matter. These findings contrast greatly with the pathologic changes observed in adult cases of methylmercury intoxication in which focal degeneration of neurons in selective regions of the brain is prominent.

The clinical features observed in the Japanese cases differ somewhat from those of our cases. The mothers of our cases exhibited the signs and symptoms of severe methylmercury intoxication, and the infants, though seemingly normal at birth, died during early postnatal life. In the Japanese cases, on the other hand, the mothers were asymptomatic except for minor sensory disturbances, and the infants, who lived for 6 years, 3 months and 2 years, 6 months, respectively, suffered from severe cerebral palsy accompanied by repeated convulsions. It is possible that the Japanese infants may have shown additional effects related to continued postnatal exposure, but the underlying basic pathology related to methylmercury exposure during pregnancy appears to be similar in nature to that of our two cases. Certainly the histopathologic findings were remarkably similar in all four cases.

Taking into account the clinical features, toxicological data, and histopathological findings in the two Iraqi infants and two Japanese children, it seems reasonable to conclude that the characteristic neuropathological alterations resulting from methylmercury intoxication in utero are attributable to disturbed neuronal migration, deranged cortical organization and differentiation, and exuberant white matter astrocytic reaction. It should be realized, at the same time, that heterotopia and heterotaxia of neurons and disordered cortical organization are by no means specific. They are seen in a variety of conditions in man (Brzustowicz and Kernohan, 1952; Crome, 1952; Hanaway et al., 1968; Norman, 1966; Rorke et al., 1968; Terplan et al., 1966; Volpe and Adamas, 1972) and in a number of experimental disorders (Caviness and Sidman, 1973; Hicks et al., 1968; Langman and Shimada, 1971; Webster et al., 1973). It should be further realized that not all

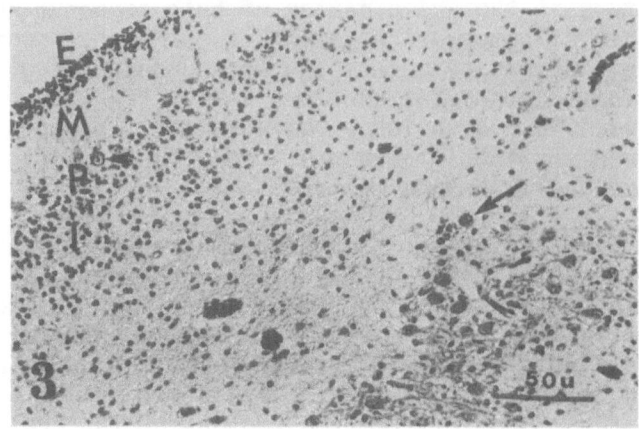

Figure 3   Heterotopic Purkinje cells (arrow) in the white matter of
           the cerebellum.   E: External granular layer.   M:
           Molecular layer.   P: Purkinje cell layer.   I: Internal
           granular layer.

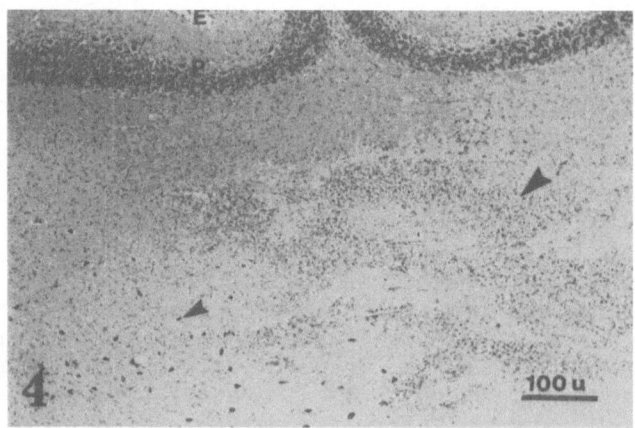

Figure 4   Heterotopic neurons in the cerebellar white matter.   Note
           groups of small granular neurons (large arrow head) and
           large pyramidal neurons (small arrow head).   E: External
           granular layer.   P: Purkinje cell layer.

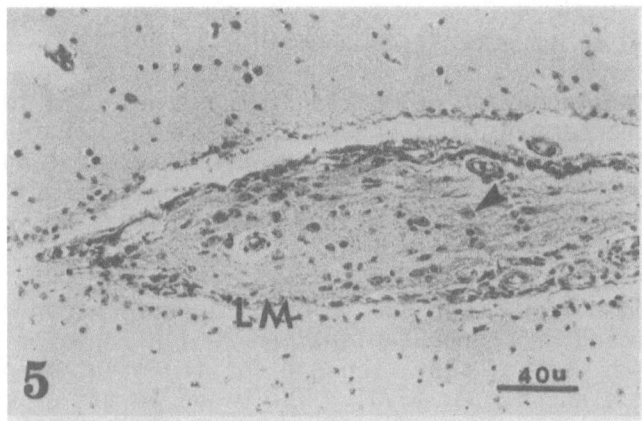

Figure 5 Heterotopic grey matter in the subarachnoid space of
cerebrum. It is composed of both neurons (arrow head) and
glial cells. LM: Leptomeninges.

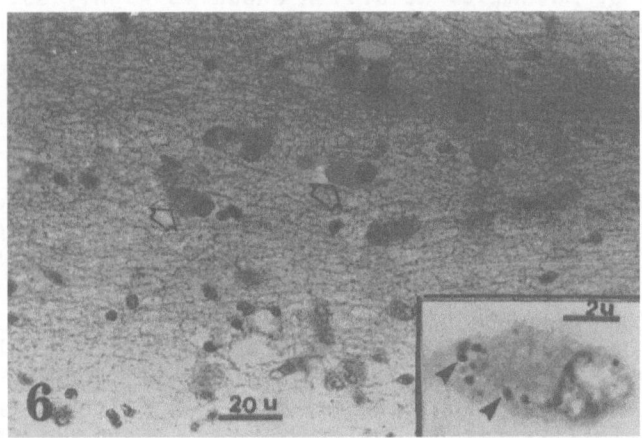

Figure 6 Gemistocytic astrocytosis of the white matter of
cerebrum. Note abundant amount of cytoplasm (empty
arrows) of the astrocytes. Inset shows photoemulsion
histochemical demonstration of mercury grain (arrow heads)
in the cytoplasm of astrocyte.

cases of cerebral palsy with or without mental retardation will be accompanied by demonstrable morphological changes. Mulamud (1964) found that 61 percent of 1410 mentally defective children had some demonstrable anatomic defect of the brain at autopsy, whereas the remainder showed no structural abnormalities. Jellinger (1972) reported that the proportion of brains showing no lesions among the mentally retarded to be approximately 12.1 percent of a total of 1,050 cases. The compensatory power of the brain, particularly in young individuals, must also be considered when attempting to correlate anatomical defects with mental dysfunction. Conversely, the presence of gross anomalies of the brain may not necessarily be associated with defective mentation.

In the Iraqi cases, exposure to methylmercury occurred during the critical period of neuronal migration, which normally begins at about the seventh week of gestation and continues into the third trimester (Sidman and Rakic, 1973). The blood levels of mercury and the postmortem brain levels of mercury were much above those expected in normal infants, and the blood and hair levels of mercury in their mothers were also markedly elevated during pregnancy. In the Japanese cases, exposure to methylmercury occurred throughout gestation. Although blood levels of mercury were unknown, the mercury levels in hair of both mothers and children were elevated above control levels at the time of autopsy. The striking similarity of the pathologic anatomy of the brain of our two infants and to those reported by Matsumoto et al. in Japan is highly suggestive of a common pathogenetic link to methylmercury poisoning in utero.

CRITICAL PERIODS OF CNS VULNERABILITY TO PRENATAL METHYLMERCURY EXPOSURE

It is customary to divide human gestation into embryonic and fetal periods. The embryonic period lasts until the end of the eighth week of gestation; the fetal period starts from the eighth week and lasts until the time of birth. The susceptibility to teratogenesis and the products of teratogenic insults vary according to the period of embryogenesis during which exposure to the adverse influence occurs. In general, teratogenic insults during the early embryonic period, i.e., from fertilization to implantation, result in embryonic lethality but do not cause gross organ defects. Susceptibility to gross organ defects reaches maximum during the late embryonic period, when organogenesis is taking place very rapidly. Toxic insults during this period may also cause some embryonic lethality. Starting from the late embryonic period through the remainder of the fetal period, histogenesis and functional maturation occurs in various organs. The fetus is relatively resistant to lethality or gross organ defects but may develop subtle histogenetic abnormalities and functional disturbances which may become manifest only at a subsequent stage of development. It should be recognized also that susceptibility to teratogenesis depends upon the genotype of the conceptus and the manner in which the agent interacts with that genotype.

The developing human brain undergoes a programmed series of developmental events during its protracted ontogenesis. Organogenesis is complete at three months, and a full quotient of nerve cells is attained by the time of birth or beyond, after which there is no further numerical increase. The structure of the brain is more complex than that of any other organ and undergoes profound changes during neurogenesis. Cellular events during neurogenesis are also varied and complex. These include proliferation of germinal cells to produce neurons and glial cells at the ventricular and subventricular zones, migration of neurons to their final destinations, aggregation of neurons to form organized nuclear groups or to form cortical plates, elongation of axons and dendrites with establishment of synapses, programmed cell death, and, finally, differentiation and maturation. It should also be realized that the brain is not a homogeneous organ but is composed of many distinctly different structures with different functions. Thus, the degree of individual variability at certain periods of growth and development must be well understood before proper assessment of any alleged deviation can be made.

It is probable that methylmercury causes developmental deviations in fetal brain through diverse pathogenetic mechanisms, such as mitotic interference, chromosomal defects, enzyme inhibition or altered energy sources. It is possible that the same pathogenetic mechanism may not be operative at all stages of gestation. The teratogenic effects may appear immediately and result in cell death or embryonic death, or they may appear much later and be ascertainable only in the postpartum or adult period. Undoubtedly, the duration and level of exposure to methylmercury at different developmental stages contribute significantly to the eventual outcome. Cell death may be minimally important at one stage, for example, because of the ability to replace damaged or dead cells. At another stage, however, cell death may be of great importance, resulting in permanent cell depletion in a critical area of the brain. The type of cells undergoing active proliferation at the time of the insult is also important.

In view of the foregoing, a simple generalization regarding vulnerability of the prenatal CNS to methylmercury poisoning is difficult to formulate. However, much of the clinical and toxicologial data, and, particularly, the neuropathological findings in children affected by prenatal methylmercury poisoning is Japan and Iraq, indicate that the critical periods for severe, sublethal CNS exposure to methylmercury appear to be the late embryonic and fetal periods. As stated earlier, teratogenic insults during the period of histogenesis and functional maturation tend to produce

subtle abnormalities which may cause behavioral disturbances without
causing grossly appreciable defects in the brain.

Our hypothesis is that abnormal neuronal migration, disturbed
cortical differentiation, and white matter astrocytosis represent
the major effects of severe sublethal methylmercury poisoning in
utero, and that the critical periods for such exposure, as far as
the developing CNS is concerned, are the late embryonic and fetal
periods.

As with other teratogenic agents, methylmercury appears to have
relatively imperceptible effects prior to the blastocytst stage. In
general, exposures to toxic agents during the period of gametogenesis
results in death of the sperm or egg, chromosomal defects, or
embryonic death leading to abortion. There have been reports of
methylmercury-induced polypoidy in the root cells of plants (Ramel,
1969), XXY nondisjunction in the fruit fly (Ramel and Magnusson,
1969) and chromosomal breakage in lymphocytes of methylmercury-
exposed humans (Skerfving et al., 1970). At the molecular level,
interaction of methylmercury with microtubule proteins may be of
fundamental importance. We have shown that methylmercuric chloride
exerts profound effects upon the neurotubules of human fetal neurons
and astrocytes in cultures (Choi et al., 1981a). Others have also
described the effects of methylmercury upon mitotic spindle fibers
in certain types of neural tumors (Koerker, 1980; Miura et al.,
1978). Whether or not methylmercury may also act on the mitotic
apparatus of germ cells is not known at the present time.

Although no reliable data are available from those fetuses
aborted during the Japanese or Iraqi epidemics, gross CNS defects or
multiple organ defects do not appear to be a prominent feature of
human fetal methylmercury poisoning.

EXPERIMENTAL STUDIES OF THE EFFECTS OF METHYLMERCURY UPON THE
DEVELOPING FETAL BRAIN IN OUR LABORATORY

Effects of Methylmercuric Chloride on Migration of Human Fetal
Neuron In Vitro

1.   Time-lapse cinematographic studies of neuronal migration in
      vitro.

Nerve cells of the developing CNS are generated exclusively
within the ventricular zone and subsequently migrate outward to
their final destinations. Use of tritiated thymidine radioautography
in pregnant animals has provided a considerable amount of information
concerning the time of origin and the pattern of migration of neurons
in certain laboratory animals. The use of radioactive label for

experiments of this kind in humans is not possible. Tissue culture
techniques, however, provide a convenient means for observing the
growth and development of living human fetal brain cells. Although
there are certain inherent limitations, tissue culture permits
precise control of environmental factors and allows direct
observation of developmental phenomena within living human cells.
It has been amply demonstrated that many of the developmental events
which occur in normal fetal brain are recapitulated in culture.

Using time-lapse cinematography, phase and electron microscopy,
and immunocytochemistry, we have been able to observe the migratory
activity of cultured human fetal neurons. The processes of neurons
and astrocytes are seen at the edges of brain tissue explants within
48-72 hours. Shortly thereafter, astrocytes begin to emigrate and
to proliferate around the periphery of the explants. Small dark
neurons migrate outward in rapid succession. The sequence of
neuronal movements is rather orderly. First, the pulsating tips of
neurites anchor themselves to the processes or cytoplasm of
astrocytes and to other neurons. While thus securely fastened,
translocation of nerve cell somata is effected by movement of their
nuclei into the extended neuritic processes and by subsequent
withdrawal toward the cell body of the trailing neurites. Neurons
or groups of neurons frequently follow the same pathways, using
astroglial processes as guides. A remarkable phenomenon during
neuronal migration is the intimate association between neuronal cell
bodies and astrocytic cytoplasm or processes. Neurons often cluster
along astroglial processes during migration, and groups of neurons
may then be carried away to more distant locations as the astrocytes
move about.

There are several viewpoints concerning the mode of neuronal
migration in the developing vertebrate CNS. One theory, the
so-called karyokinesis theory (Berry and Rodgers, 1965) proposes
movement of the nuclei of postmitotic neurons of the ventricular
zone within extended cytoplasmic cylinders. Another theory proposes
that postmitotic neurons migrate along glial processes (Rakic, 1972;
Choi, 1979). Our experiments have shown that both of these phenomena
take place in cultures of human fetal brain cells. Detailed
ultrastructural analysis of organotypic cultures of human fetal
cerebrum have also demonstrated that a special type of junctional
complex develops between elongated neurites and astrocytic membranes
(Choi and Lapham, 1976). Although the functional significance of
these complexes is unclear, their presence constitutes additional
evidence of the importance of astrocytes in neurogenesis. The close
association between neurons and astrocytes both in vivo and in vitro,
the beneficial effects of astrocytes upon the survival of immature
neurons in culture (Choi and Lapham, 1976) and possible production
of a nerve growth factor-like substance by astrocytes (Varon and
Somjen, 1979), strongly support the concept that nerve cell-astrocyte
interaction is critical to the development of the vertebrate CNS.

2.   Effects of methylmercury on human fetal neurons and astrocytes.

       To test the effects of methylmercuric chloride upon neuronal
migration under these experimental conditions, explants of human
fetal cerebral tissue were exposed to various concentrations of
methylmercuric chloride in complete medium (Choi et al., 1981b).
Addition of methylmercuric chloride caused abrupt cessation of cell
movement in these cultures. With the aid of time-lapse
cinematography, we have observed the rapid development of severe
cytotoxic damage, first to thin neurites and neuronal cell bodies
and subsequently to astrocytes. Exposure to 0.1 mM methylmercuric
chloride results in irreversible damage to neurons within 20
minutes, while exposure to 0.2 mM methylmercuric chloride caused
damage within 10 minutes. The initial site of injury appeared to be
neuritic membrane, particularly in the vicinity of the growth cones.
By electron microscopy, in addition to disruption and separation of
membranes, there was degeneration and disappearance of neuritic
neurotubules as well as of the cytoplasm. Another striking finding
was the presence of astrocytes in metaphase arrest, associated with
a complete lack of mitotic spindle fibers.

       Thus, it would appear that the methylmercuric chloride-exposed
neurons failed to extend their neurites not only because of membrane
damage but also because of the lack of neurotubules necessary for
structural support as well as axoplasmic transport. Damage occurred
most rapidly and most severely to thin neurites and neuronal cell
bodies while damage to astrocytes developed somewhat later, although
eventually both types of cells were irreversibly injured. However,
following exposure to 0.01 mM methylmercuric chloride for 30 to 40
minutes, the progression of damage to astrocytes could be halted by
placing the cells in normal culture media, after which a slow
recovery to normal was observed. Any neurons which survived the
initial insult in the explant proper, could start to migrate out
again in an orderly manner as described.

       There is probably more than one mechanism by which methylmercury
interferes with neuronal migration. It will, therefore, be important
to characterize sequentially and individually the specific and
nonspecfic effects of methylmercury upon filopodial motion,
elongation of neurites, transport of materials within neurites,
etc., using time-lapse cinematography in conjunction with a variety
of morphologic techniques. Direct comparisons can be made to
alterations induced by agents known to influence specific subcellular
organelles, e.g., colchicine (microtubules) and cytochalasin B
(microfilaments). Determination of the effects of methylmercury
upon the cytoskeletal components of astrocytes as well as of neurons

may be also of value in elucidating the manner in which methylmercury influences neuronal motility and survival.

Evaluation of the role of astroglia during neurogenesis and their response to methylmercury exposure during development will be of considerable interest in future investigations of methylmercury toxicity. We have carried out a number of experiments using monolayer cultures of human fetal astrocytes. The immature neurons eventually degenerate in organotypic cultures. However, astrocytes continue to proliferate and can be maintained in long-term culture which can be used for various experimentations. The pattern of DNA synthesis within human fetal astrocytes was investigated using radioautographic technique. The result showed that levels above 2.99×10^{-3} mM methylmercuric chloride profoundly inhibited DNA synthesis, whereas at levels below 1.19×10^{-3} mM methylmercuric chloride, there was no demonstrable inhibition (Choi et al., 1981a).

Meso-2,3-dimercaptosuccinic acid (DMSA) is known to be effective in decreasing body burden and brain content of mercury in experimental animals. This compound has also been found to be much less toxic than agents such as BAL or penicillamine. Experiments with secondary monolayer cultures of human fetal astrocytes demonstrated that the addition of 0.01 mM methylmercuric chloride caused rapid retraction and coagulative cell membrane damages under time-lapse cinematography. After 30 to 40 minutes of methylmercuric chloride exposure, cultures were washed and replaced with complete media containing 1.0 mM DMSA. The damaged cells reformed smooth membrane with active filopodial motion and ruffling. Exposures to DMSA alone in cultures over a 12-hour period did not cause damage at least on phase microscopic observation. DMSA and methylmercuric chloride in combination likewise prevented cellular damage under similar experimental conditions (Choi and Lapham, 1981). DMSA treatment also restored polymerization of neurotubules in these astrocytes within a short period of time.

Although the results of tissue culture experiments cannot be interpreted literally as phenomena that are occurring in the living organism, the system allows in-depth analysis of molecular events taking place between living human fetal brain cells and methylmercuric chloride under precisely controlled conditions. Many questions remain unanswered. What are the mechanisms involved in the damaging and reparative phenomena seen in these experiments How is the damaged membrane put together to form a new membrane with the addition of the complexing agent What is the pattern of methylmercury localization before and after the addition of complexing agents These are some of the questions that must be addressed in future investigations.

Effects of Methylmercuric Chloride on Development of Cerebellum in Mice

Recently our laboratory has carried out a number of experiments designed to provide insight into the effects of methylmercury upon specific regions of developing CNS in the mouse. Cerebellar development in mice is primarily a postnatal phenomenon. The cerebellum has a specific architecture composed of specific cell types, and its normal growth and development have been studied extensively. Moreover, the cerebellum has been a favored site of pathological changes following methylmercury intoxication in humans as well as in experimental animals.

Newborn mice (C57BL/6J) were injected subcutaneously once a day on postnatal days 3, 4, and 5 with 5.0 mg/kg body weight of methylmercuric chloride labeled with 203-mercury (totaling 15 mg/kg body weight in each animal). Control animals received physiological saline in place of methylmercuric chloride. The animals were sacrificed on postnatal day 15.

Grossly, brains of the two groups were not remarkable. Hematoxylin and eosin-stained 6 micron paraffin-embedded sections and 1.0 micron epon-embedded sections stained with toluidine blue did not show any apparent abnormalities. Using Golgi methods and electron microscopy, however, two significant findings were noted in the cerebella of the mice. The first was demonstrated by the rapid Golgi method and consisted of greatly simplified dendritic arborization of many Purkinje cells in methylmercury-treated animals, even though the overall number of Purkinje cells and the general architectonic pattern of the cerebellar cortex were maintained. Extensive survey of electron micrographs revealed marked swelling of the cytoplasm of pericapillary astroglia. The cytoplasm of endothial cells was electron-dense and attentuated (Choi et al., 1981c).

The mechanism by which methylmercury lead to the incomplete differentiation of Purkinje cell dendrites remains unknown. The changes in astroglia and vascular endothelium were of a regressive nature and may not bear any relation to dendritic differentiation but may indicate an important role for astroglia and the vascular system in overall cerebellar development in toxic injury.

In another study, a single injection of methylmercuric chloride labeled with 203-mercury was given intraperitoneally on day 16 of gestation in pregnant mice. Control animals received physiological saline. Animals were allowed to come to term, and the offspring were sacrificed on postnatal days 5, 10 and 20. Whole body count of radioactivity of mothers during the period of gestation and during lactation following delivery were made daily in a gamma counter. One day prior to the time of sacrifice, 1.0 microcurie/ml of tritiated thymidine was injected intraperitoneally into the offspring (both control and experimental).

The clearance half-time of radioactivity in lactating mothers was 8.7 days, indicating a relative increase of clearance in lactating mothers as compared to controls which is approximately 10 to 14 days (Greenwood et al., 1978). Relatively high radioactivity was retained in the brains of methylmercuric chloride-treated offspring. A statistically significant reduction of body weight in methylmercury-treated litters was noted. Preliminary Golgi surveys of the cerebellum showed marked reduction in differentiation of dendritic arborization of Purkinje cells in methylmercury-treated animals on all days of sacrifice.

Radioautographic analysis of tritiated thymidine uptake in the external granular cells of the vermis showed an apparent delay of proliferative activity in the methylmercury-treated group as indicated by high index of tritiated thymidine labeling. The control animals appeared to have begun completion of proliferative activity at the external granular layer, indicated by progressive decline of labeling index from postnatal day 5 to postnatal day 10. The methylmercury-group showed a labeling index of 9.3 percent on postnatal day 5 (control, 8.6 percent) and 18.1 percent on postnatal day 10 (control, 6.2 percent), indicating continued proliferative activity in the methylmercury-group, prior to migration of external granule cells into the internal granular layer.

The results of this study, which indicate a delay in dendritic differentiation of Purkinje cells and a delay in the proliferative activity of external granular cells following in utero methylmercury intoxication, clearly illustrate the value of a correlative morphological approach in bringing out some of the more subtle effects of methylmercury upon the developing CNS.

A word of caution must be expressed at this time. The morphological studies described in the literature must be interpreted with a thorough understanding on the degree of individual variability during growth and development of CNS. Often, subtle changes that have been described using various histopathological techniques are esoteric and unreliable and may be too subjective and limited in scope. Frequently, what has been described as abnormal may simply be nonspecific or artifactious and may not bear any relationship to the functional and neurological derangements or behavioral abnormalities observed. In fact, in some instances, the effects may be too subtle for morphological delineation, using currently available techniques.

For a better understanding of the effects of methylmercury upon the developing CNS, however, more work is needed to clarify the normal sequence of neuroembryological events, both at the molecular and at the cellular level. For example, during the histogenesis of the developing CNS, it is generally believed that larger neurons are generated first, followed by intermediate neurons and finally small

neurons (Jacobson, 1978). However, there are still many
uncertainties regarding the time of origin of different types of
neurons and glial cells in various regions of the developing human
CNS. Contrary to the general belief that neuronal development
precedes glial development (Fujita, 1963, 1967), our studies (Choi,
1981) and those of others (Levitt et al., 1980, 1981) suggest the
likelihood of concomitant generation of both types of cells in the
early developing human embryo. Until these and other uncertainties
regarding neurogenesis are resolved, therefore, it will be difficult
to ascertain precisely the molecular mechanisms and stages of
development that are applicable to methylmercury poisoning in utero.

ACKNOWLEDGMENTS

The author wishes to express his deep appreciation for help
given by Dr. Ronald C. Kim during the preparation of this manuscript.
He also wishes to express thanks to J. Neuropath. Exp. Neurol.
(Editor-in-Chief: Dr. John Moosey) for presentation of cases
published in that Journal. (Supported in part by NIEHS Grants RO1
ES 02928 and ES 01247.)

REFERENCES

Alfonso, J. and DeAlvarex, R., 1960, Effects of mercury on human
    gestation, Am. J. Obst. Gynecol. 80:145-154.
Amin-Zaki, L., Elhassani, S., Majeed, M.A., Clarkson, T.W., Doherty,
    R.A. and Greenwood, M.R., 1974, Intra-uterine methylmercury
    poisoning in Iraq, Pediat. 54:587-595.
Amin-Zaki, L., Elhassani, S., Majeed, M.A., Clarkson, T.W., Doherty,
    R.A., Greenwood, M.R. and Giovanoli-Jakubezak, T., 1976,
    Perinatal methylmercury poisoning in Iraq, Am. J. Dis. Child.
    130:1070-1076.
Amin-Zaki, L., Elhassani, S., Majeed, M.A., Clarkson, T.W. and
    Greenwood, M.R., 1978, Methylmercury poisoning in Iraqi
    children: clinical observations over two years, Brit. Med. J.
    1:597-606.
Bakir, F., Damluji, S.F., Amin-Zaki, L., Murtadha, M., Khalidi, A.,
    Al-Rawi, N.Y., Takiriti, S., Chahir, H.I., Clarkson, T.W.,
    Smith, J.C. and Doherty, R.A., 1973, Methylmercury poisoning in
    Iraq, Science 181:230-240.
Berlin, M. and Ullberg, S., 1963, Accumulation and retention of
    mercury in the mouse brain: A comparison of exposure to
    mercury vapor and intravenous injection of mercuric salt, Arch.
    Environ. Health 12:33-42.
Berry, M. and Rodgers, A.W., 1965, The migration of neuroblasts in
    the developing cerebral cortex, J. Anat. 99:691-709.

Bornhausen, M., Musch, H.R. and Greim, H., 1980, Operant behavior performance changes in rats after prenatal methylmercury exposure, Tox. Appl. Pharmacol. 56:305-310.

Brzustowicz, R.J. and Kernohan, J.W., 1952, Cell rests in the region of the fourth ventricle, Arch. Neurol. Psychiat. 67:585-591.

Caviness, V.S. and Sidman, R.L., 1973, Time of origin of corresponding cell clones in the cerebral cortex of normal and reeler mutant mice: An autoradiographic analysis, J. Comp. Neurol. 148:141-152.

Chang, L.W. and Reuhl, K., 1977, Ultrastructural study of the latent effects of methylmercury on the nervous system after prenatal exposure, Environ. Res. 13:171-185.

Chang, L.W., Reuhl, K.R. and Lee, G.W., 1977a, Degenerative changes in the developing nervous system as a result of in utero exposure to methylmercury, Environ. Res. 14:414-423.

Chang, L.W., Reuhl, K.R. and Spyker, J.M., 1977b, Ultrastructural study of the latent effects of methylmercury on the nervous system after prenatal exposure, Environ. Res. 13:171-185.

Chen, W., Body, R.L. and Mottet, K.N., 1979, Some effects of continuous low-dose congential exposure to methylmercury on organ growth in the rat fetus, Teratol. 20:31-36.

Choi, B.H., 1979, Mechanism of neuronal migration in human foetal cerebrum in vitro, Yonsei Med. J. 20:92-104.

Choi, B.H., 1981, Radial glia of developing human fetal spinal cord: Golgi, immunohistochemical and electron microscopic study, Dev. Brain Res. 1:249-267.

Choi, B.H. and Lapham, L.W., 1976, Interactions of neurons and astrocytes during growth and development of human fetal brain in vitro, Exp. Mol. Pathol. 24:110-125.

Choi, B.H. and Lapham, L.W., 1981, Effects of meso-2,3-dimercaptosuccinic acid on methylmercury injured human fetal astrocytes in vitro, Exp. Mol. Pathol. 34:25-33.

Choi, B.H., Lapham, L.W., Amin-Zaki, L. and Saleem, T., 1978, Abnormal neuronal migration, deranged cerebral cortical organization, and diffuse white matter astrocytosis of human fetal brain: A major effect of methylmercury poisoning in utero, J. Neuropath. Exper. Neurol. 37:719-733.

Choi, B.H., Cho, K.H. and Lapham, L.W., 1981a, Effects of methylmercury on DNA synthesis of human fetal astrocytes in vitro, Brain Res. 202:238-242.

Choi, B.H., Cho, K.H. and Lapham, L.W., 1981b, Effects of methylmercury on human fetal neurons and astrocytes in vitro: A time-lapse cinematographic, phase and electron microscopic study, Environ. Res. 24:61-74.

Choi, B.H., Kudo, M. and Lapham, L.W., 1981c, A Golgi and electron microscopic study of cerebellum in methylmercury-poisoned neonatal mice, Acta Neuropath. (Berl.) 54:233-237.

Crome, L., 1952, Microgyria, J. Pathol. Bact. 64:479-495.

Dial, N.A., 1976, Methylmercury: Teratogenic and lethal effects in frog embryos, Teratol. 13:327-334.

Dial, N.A., 1978, Methylmercury: Some effects on embryogenesis in the Japanese Medaka, Oryzias Latipes, Teratol. 17:83-92.

Engleson, G. and Herner, T., 1952, Alkylmercury poisoning, Acta Paediatr. Scand. 41:289-294.

Fujimoto, T., Fuyuta, M., Kiyofuji, E. and Hirata, S., 1979, Prevention by Tiopronin (2-mercaptopropionoyl glycine) of methylmercuric chloride-induced teratogenic and fetotoxic effects in mice, Teratol. 20:297-302.

Fujita, S., 1963, The matrix cell and cytogenesis in the developing central nervous system, J. Comp. Neurol. 120:37-42.

Fujita, S., 1967, Quantitative analysis of cell proliferation and differentiation in the cortex of the postnatal mouse cerebellum, J. Cell Biol. 32:277-287.

Fujita, E., 1969, Experimental studies of organic mercury poisoning. The behavior of the Minamata disease-causing agent in maternal bodies, and its transfer to their infants via either placenta or breast milk, J. Kumamoto Med. Soc. 43:47-57.

Fuyuta, M., Fujimoto, T. and Hirata, S., 1978, Embryotoxic effects of methylmercury chloride administered to mice and rats during organogenesis, Teratol. 18:353-366.

Fuyuta, M., Fujimoto, T. and Kiyofuji, E., 1979, Teratogenic effects of a single oral administration of methylmercuric chloride in mice, Acta Anat. 104:356-362.

Garrett, N.E., Burrises, J., Garrett, B. and Archdeacon, J.W., 1972, Placental transmission of mercury to the fetal rat, Tox. Appl. Pharmacol. 22:649-654.

Greenwood, M.R., Clarkson, T.W., Doherty, R.A., Gates, A.H., Amin-Zaki, L., Elhassani, S. and Majeed, M.A., 1978, Blood clearance half-times in lactating and non-lactating members of a population exposed to methylmercury, Environ. Res. 16:48-54.

Hanaway, J., Lee, S.I. and Netsky, M.G., 1968, Pachygyria: Relation of findings to modern embryologic concepts, Neurol. 18:791-799.

Harada, Y., 1968, Congenital (or fetal) Minamata disease, in "Minamata Disease", Study group of Minamata disease. pp. 93-117, Kumamoto Univ. Japan.

Harris, S.B., Wilson, J.G. and Printz, R.H., 1972, Embryotoxicity of methylmercuric chloride in golden hamsters, Teratol. 6:139-142.

Hicks, S.P., D'Amato, C.J., Coy, M.A., O'Brien, E.D., Thurston, J.S. and Joftes, D.L., 1968, Migrating cells in the developing central nervous system studied by radiosensitivity and tritiated thymidine uptake, Brookhaven Symp. Biol. 14:246-304.

Hunter, D. and Russell, D.S., 1954, Focal cerebral and cerebellar atrophy in a human subject due to organic mercury compounds, J. Neurol. Neurosurg. Psychiat. 17:235-241.

Jacobson, M., 1978, "Developmental Neurobiology". Plenum Press, New York.

Jellinger, K., 1972, Neuropathological features of unclassified mental retardation, in "The Brain in Unclassified Mental Retardation", J.B. Cavanaugh, ed., pp. 293-312, Churchill Livingston, London.

Khera, K.S., 1973, Teratogenic effects of methylmercury in the cat. Note on the use of this species as a model for teratogenicity studies, Teratol. 8:293-304.

Khera, K.S. and Tabacover, S.A., 1973, Effects of methylmercuric chloride on the progeny of mice and rats treated before or during gestation, Fd. Cosmet. Toxicol. 11:245-254.

Koerker, R., 1980, The cytotoxicity of methylmercuric hydroxide and colchicine in cultured mouse neuroblastoma cells, Toxicol. Appl. Pharmacol. 53:485-469.

Langman, J. and Shimada, M., 1971, Cerebral cortex of the mouse after prenatal chemical insult, Am. J. Anat. 132:355-374.

Levitt, P. and Rakic, P., 1980, Immunoperoxidase localization of glial fibrillary acidic protein in radial glial cells and astrocytes of the developing rhesus monkey brain, J. Comp. Neurol. 193:417-448.

Levitt, P., Cooper, M.L. and Rakic, P., 1981, Coexistence of neuronal and glial precursor cells in the cerebral ventricular zone of the fetal monkey: An ultrastructural immunoperoxidase analysis, J. Neuroscience 1:27-39.

Mulamud, N., 1964, Neuropathology, in "Mental Retardation", H.A. Stevens and R. Heber, eds., pp. 429-452, Univ. of Chicago Press, Chicago, Illinois.

Mansour, M.M., Dyer, N.C., Hoffman, L.H., Davies, J. and Brill, A.B., 1974, Placental transfer of mercuric nitrate and methylmercury in the rat, Am. J. Obst. Gynecol. 119:557-562.

Marsh, D.O., Myers, G.J., Clarkson, T.W., Amin-Zaki, L., Tikiriti, S. and Majeed, M.A., 1980, Fetal methylmercury poisoning: Clinical and toxicological data on 29 cases, Ann. Neurol. 7:348-353.

Matsumoto, H., Koya, G. and Takeuchi, T., 1965, Fetal Minamata Disease, J. Neuropath. Exp. Neurol. 24:563-574.

Matsumoto, H., Suzuki, A. and Morita, C., 1967, Preventive effect of penicillamine on the brain defect of fetal rat poisoned transplacentally with methylmercury, Life Sci. 6:2321-2326.

Miura, K., Suzuki, K. and Imura, N., 1978, Effects of methylmercury on mitotic mouse glioma cells, Environ. Res. 17:453-471.

Morikawa, N., 1961, Pathological studies on organic mercury poisoning, Kumamoto Med. J. 14:87-93.

Mottet, N.K., 1974, Effects of chronic low-dose exposure of rat fetuses to methylmercury hydroxide, Teratol. 10:173-190.

Musch, H.R., Bornhausen, M., Kriegel, H.,, and Breim, H., 1978, Methylmercury chloride induces learning deficits in prenatally treated rats, Arch. Tox. 40:103-108.

Murakami, U., 1969, Toxicity of organic mercury compounds in prefetus embryo, Japanese Med. Assoc. 61:1059-1073.

Murakami, U., 1972, The effect of organic mercury on intrauterine life, Acta Exp. Med. Biol. 27:301-336.

Nakamura, K. and Saeki, S., 1967, Preventive effect of penicillamine on the brain defect of fetal rat poisoned transplacentally with methylmercury, Life Sci. 6:2321-2326.

Nonaka, I., 1969, An electron microscopical study on the experimental congenital Minamata disease in rat, Kumamoto Med. J. 22:27-39.

Normon, R.M., 1966, Neuropathological findings in trisomes 13-15 and 17-18 with special reference to the cerebellum, Develop. Med. Child Neurol. 8:170-177.

Null, D.H., Gartside, R.S. and Wei, E., 1968, Methylmercury accumulation in brains of pregnant, non-pregnant and fetal rats, Life Sci. 12:65-72.

Rakic, P., 1972, Mode of cell migration to the superficial layers of fetal monkey neocortex, J. Comp. Neurol. 145:61-84.

Ramel, C., 1969, Methylmercury as a mitosis disturbing agent, J. Jpn. Med. Assoc. 61:1072-1077.

Ramel, C. and Magnusson, J., 1969, Chromosome segregation in Drosophila melanogaster, Hereditas 61:231-254.

Rorke, L.B., Fogelson, M.H. and Riggs, H.E., 1968, Cerebellar heterotopia in infancy, Dev. Med. Child Neurol. 10:644-650.

Rosenthal, E. and Sparber, S.B., 1972, Methylmercury dicyandiamide: Retardation of detour learning in chicks hatched from injected eggs, Science 11:883-892.

Schalock, R.L., Brown, W.J., Kark, R.A.P. and Menon, N.K., 1981, Perinatal methylmercury intoxication: Behavioral effects in rats, Dev. Psychobiol. 14:213-219.

Sidman, R.L. and Rakic, P., 1973, Neuronal migration, with special reference to developing human brain: A review, Brain Res. 62:1-35.

Skerfving, S., Hansson, K. and Lidsten, J., 1970, Chromosome breakage in human exposed to methylmercury through fish consumption, Arch. Environ. Health 21:133-139.

Snyder, R.D., 1971, Congenital mercury poisoning, N. Eng. J. Med. 284:1014-1016.

Spyker, J.M. and Smithberg, M., 1972, Effects of methylmercury on prenatal development in mice, Teratol. 5:181-190.

Su, M. and Okita, G., 1976a, Behavioral effects on the progeny of mice treated with methylmercury, Tox. Appl. Pharmacol. 38:195-205.

Su, M. and Okita, G., 1976b, Embryocidal and teratogenic effects of methylmercury in mice, Tox. Appl. Pharmacol. 38:207-216.

Takeuchi, T., 1968, Pathology of Minamata Disease, in "Minamata Disease. Study group of Minamata Disease", Kumamoto Univ. Japan.

Terplan, K.L., Sandberg, A.A. and Aceto, Jr., T., 1966, Structural anomalies in the cerebellum in association with trisomy, JAMA 197:129-140.

Varon, S.S. and Somjen, G.G., 1979, Neuron-glia interactions. Neurosciences Research Program Bulletin, 17:80-86.

Volpe, J.J. and Adamas, R.D., 1972, Cerebro-hepato-renal syndrome of Zellweger: An inherited disorder of neuronal migration, Acta Neuropathol. 20:175-198.

Wannag, A. and Skejerasen, J., 1975, Mercury accumulation in
    placenta and fetal membranes. A study of dental workers and
    their babies, Environ. Physiol. Biochem. 5:348-352.
Webster, W., Shimada, M. and Langman, J., 1973, Effects of
    fluorodeoxyaridine on developing neocortex of the mouse, Am. J.
    Anat. 137:67-86.
Yang, M.G., Krawford, K.S., Garcia, J.D., Wang, J.H.C. and Lei,
    K.Y., 1972, Deposition of mercury in fetal and maternal brain,
    Proc. Soc. Exp. Biol. 141:1004-1007.

NEUROBEHAVIORAL CONSEQUENCES OF EARLY EXPOSURE TO LEAD IN RHESUS

MONKEYS: EFFECTS ON COGNITIVE BEHAVIORS

Nellie K. Laughlin, Robert E. Bowman, Edward D. Levin,
and Philip J. Bushnell*

Psychology Primate Laboratory
University of Wisconsin
Madison, Wisconsin

INTRODUCTION

The present paper reports on a series of studies of rhesus
monkeys exposed to low levels of lead administered daily throughout
the first year of life. These lead-treated monkeys have provided an
animal model directed at understanding childhood lead toxicity. The
results to be described here focus on a cognitive test paradigm,
reversal learning (RL), in which a reliable, lead-associated
performance deficit was elicited and studied in several successive
experiments. The emphasis of this report is on investigations of
the RL test procedure designed to discover task parameters which
elicited, enhanced, or sustained the lead-associated RL deficit, and
which might identify the nature of the cognitive dysfunction
responsible for the deficit.

GENERAL EXPERIMENTAL PROCEDURES

The monkeys (Macaca mulatta) in these studies all were
separated from their mothers within 78 hours of birth and reared in
individual cages in a primate nursery according to procedures
developed by Blomquist and Harlow (1961). Soft muslin diapers were
available in the home cage for at least six months postpartum and
social interaction with age peers was provided 5 days per week
during most of the first year of life.

---

*Now at New York University Medical Center, Institute of
Environmental Medicine, New York, NY.

A commercial milk formula (Similac with Iron, Ross Laboratories, Columbus, OH) was fed to all animals daily from birth to one year postpartum. Purina Monkey Chow (12 percent protein, Ralston Purina Co., St. Louis, MO) was introduced at about 30 days of age. Chronic lead exposure was imposed from birth to one year of age by adding lead acetate to the daily milk formula. Lead dosage was controlled in one of two ways. In some studies, lead doses were adjusted weekly as necessary to maintain blood lead levels at approximately 50 µg/100 ml (low-dose groups) or 80 µg/100 ml (high-dose groups). In other studies, lead was given at daily levels which were held constant throughout the year of exposure, and which also produced blood lead levels of about 50 µg/100 ml or 80 µg/100 ml. Control animals were given no added dietary lead and maintained mean blood lead levels of 5 µg/100 ml in all experiments. Lead content of Similac and monkey chow has been reported to be 20 µg/l (D. Benton, Ross Laboratories, personal communication) and 1 µg/g, respectively (Cohen et al., 1974). Adventitious lead intake from chow and Similac, given the average daily food intake by the infants, was therefore approximately 50 µg/day. This calculation of adventitious intake agrees well with an estimate based on extrapolations to baseline of the regression of blood lead on lead dosage (unpublished data). Food consumption and weight gain were monitored regularly and were normal for all animals. Blood was obtained weekly during lead exposure and periodically thereafter for analysis of several measures, including the blood lead level. A variety of behavioral functions, including the cognitive tasks to be reported here, were assessed at various times during and following the year of lead exposure.

COGNITIVE TEST PROCEDURE

Most of the tests of cognitive function employed in this project have been conducted in the Wisconsin General Test Apparatus (WGTA). The WGTA was developed by Dr. Harry Harlow at the University of Wisconsin Psychology Primate Laboratory (Harlow and Bromer, 1938). It is a reliable and versatile apparatus, widely used for studying a large variety of cognitive tasks over a broad age range in primates. The present paper reports on investigations of reversal learning (RL) sets in the WGTA. RL is a cognitive paradigm which has proven sensitive to early, chronic lead treatment in rhesus monkeys (Bushnell and Bowman, 1979a,b). More generally, the RL paradigm has been of major importance in documenting effects including ontogeny, aging and brain lesions on learning and memory in the monkey (e.g., Harlow, 1959; Mahut, 1971; Bartus et al., 1979). In addition, RL tests have proven applicable not only in monkeys, but also in rats, humans and other species (e.g., Kendler, et al., 1960; Bitterman, 1965).

The standard WGTA test situation is depicted in Figure 1. Animals are allowed to move freely in a test cage which is adjacent to a table containing a movable stimulus tray. The stimulus tray is moved into and out of the subject's reach by a human tester. For the RL tasks, two stimuli were displayed on the tray. Each stimulus covered a shallow recess or food well, one of which contained a small bit of food. The animal was allowed to respond to one stimulus per trial (non-correction procedure). Response to the correct stimulus revealed the bit of food which was available to the monkey as a reward. An opaque screen was interposed between the subject and the stimulus array between each trial to prevent the animal from seeing which stimulus was being baited. A second opaque screen concealed the tester and thereby reduced tester-animal interaction which might have either distracted the animal or provided inadvertent cues. The second screen was equipped with a one-way mirror allowing the tester to view the response of the subject. Animals generally worked in this fashion for over 50 food treats a day without the necessity of food deprivation.

The RL tasks were categorized according to the stimulus dimension associated with food reward. In Spatial RL tests one spatial position (left or right) was consistently rewarded. Once a criterion for learning had been met (original learning), the opposite spatial position was rewarded on subsequent trials (Reversal 1). When the monkey had performed Reversal 1 to criterion, the reward contingency was shifted back to the side

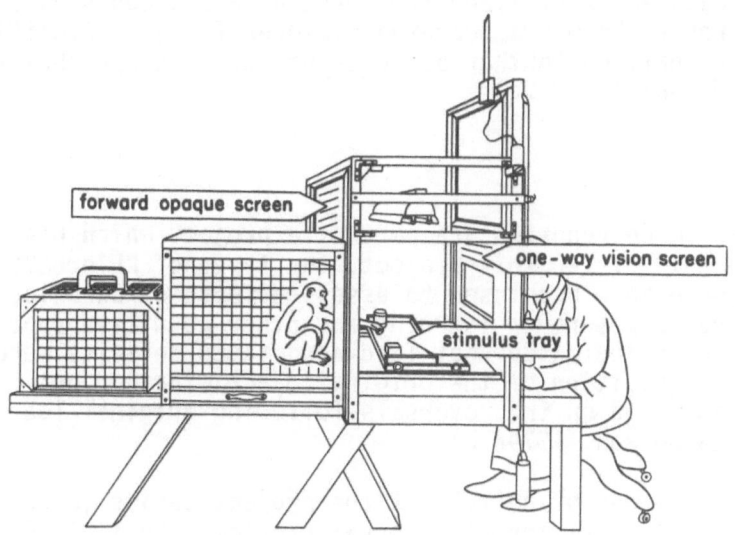

Figure 1 Wisconsin general test apparatus. From Harlow, 1949. Reprinted by permission.

correct during original learning (Reversal 2). As many reversals as
desired could be administered in this manner. Two types of learning
criteria were employed: 1) standard criterion which was 9 correct
responses in 10 consecutive trials; and 2) strict criterion which
was at least 90 correct responses in 100 consecutive trials.
Training to the strict criterion can be regarded as overtraining.
The potential effects of overtraining on subsequent reversal
learning have provided an additional parameter for analysis.

The stimulus items in Spatial RL tasks usually were identical
and provided information neither about the correct solution nor
irrelevant cues which would distract the animal from solving the
problem. In other types of RL problems, the stimuli were not
identical and object cues rather than position cues were used as the
relevant dimension. For example, the monkey was presented with two
objects of the same color which differed only in shape (e.g., a
cylinder and a cube as in Figure 1), or with two objects of the same
shape which differed only in color (e.g., a red cylinder and a green
cylinder). The animal was required to respond to one of the two
shapes in the first case (Shape RL) and to one of the two colors in
the second (Color RL) to obtain reward. In some cases,
two-dimensional or planometric stimuli were used. These stimuli
were 7.5 cm cardboard squares on which were printed colored patterns.

RL performance was assessed by analysis of variance (ANOVA) of
trials to criterion, and frequency of errors and balks (failures to
respond on a trial) recorded on original learning and on each
reversal. Each ANOVA utilized treatment as a between subjects
factor and reversals was a repeated measures factor. Significant
effects were analyzed further by post hoc test, as appropriate (see
Bushnell and Bowman, 1979a).

BACKGROUND

Studies to be reported are part of a project which has been
ongoing since 1973. In this project, the types of RL problems
described above have been used to assess effects of chronic, early,
low-level lead exposure on learning and other cognitive processes.
Previous results indicated that lead-associated deficits were not
seen during acquisition of the original discrimination but
frequently appeared on the reversals following original learning
(Bushnell and Bowman, 1979a,b).

The first group of animals of the project series (Experiment I)
was tested on three different reversal problems, Spatial, Color and
Size RL tasks beginning at about 2 months of age (Bushnell and
Bowman, 1979a). These monkeys had been exposed to high (1.02
mg/kg/day), low (0.33 mg/kg/day) and control (no added lead) levels
of lead. High lead animals required more trials to reach criterion

and balked more frequently than low lead and control animals on the reversal immediately following original learning (Reversal 1). Likewise, high lead animals made significantly more errors than control animals on Reversals 1 and 2. Low lead animals were intermediate in errors on these reversals and did not differ significantly from either the high lead or the control groups. This pattern indicated a dose-related effect of lead on this task. It is unlikely that these deficits resulted from perceptual or motor impairment, since the lead animals performed at control levels on original learning and on reversals late in the series.

Subsequent studies with other monkeys exposed to similar doses of lead (Experiment II of the project series) replicated this reversal deficit and indicated that the deficit did not reflect motivational impairment, was not specific to working for a food reward, was apparent at different ages of testing and stages of lead exposure, and could be demonstrated even three years after termination of lead intake (Bushnell and Bowman, 1979a,b). At this later age of testing, both high and low lead groups were significantly worse than controls on Reversal 1 of the first problem and the high lead animals were also worse than controls on the succeeding reversals. In these studies, the reversal deficit was overcome by practice, but usually could be reinstated by suitable test procedures such as changing the stimulus dimension associated with reward, changing the type of stimuli or by imposing a period of inactivity on RL tests (Bushnell and Bowman, 1979a). Finally, a lead-induced reversal deficit has also been observed in another laboratory using a different species of macaque, Macaca fascicularis (Rice and Willes, 1979; Rice, this volume).

In summary, a reversal-learning deficit sensitive to low-level, chronic lead exposure was demonstrated and replicated across several different test parameters. The results suggested that an underlying cognitive dysfunction arose during the period of early lead exposure and persisted in some form for at least several years postexposure. Subsequent research was designed to characterize the conditions under which the dysfunction would most likely be displayed. Accordingly, the series of studies reported below employed the RL technique and manipulated various task parameters to determine those which would elicit, reinstate or sustain the RL deficits.

OVERTRAINING

An overtraining reversal effect has been described for rats (Turrisi, 1973), in which overtraining facilitated learning of the subsequent reversal. Since the reversal deficits reported for lead-treated monkeys had been seen only on reversals following overtraining, Bushnell and Bowman (1979a) considered the hypothesis that overtraining may have been a necessary prerequisite for the deficit. This hypothesis was tested in a new cohort of lead-exposed and control monkeys.

The design called for administering overtraining on Reversal 3 but not on the original learning immediately preceding Reversal 1. A lead-associated deficit on Reversal 4 but not on Reversal 1 would clearly implicate the role of overtraining, whereas a deficit on Reversal 1, whatever the effect on Reversal 4, would indicate that overtraining was not the essential factor in producing the effect.

The animals used in these experiments were designated as Experiment III in the project series. Lead treatment of these animals is described in more detail by Bushnell and Bowman (1979c). Briefly, two groups of four monkeys each were intubated daily with lead during weeks 5 and 6 postpartum so as to produce blood lead levels peaking between 250 and 300 µg/100 ml. One of these groups was also given dietary lead daily from birth to one year postpartum at a dose adjusted weekly to produce a blood lead level of approximately 80 µg/100 ml (pulse-chronic group). The second group received no additional lead (pulse-only group). A third group of four monkeys received daily dietary lead adjusted weekly as for the pulse-chronic group, but was not given the lead pulse treatment (chronic-only group), and a fourth group of four was given no added lead (control group). Chronic lead intake for each animal of the chronic-only and pulse-chronic groups averaged over the year of treatment was approximately 0.5 mg/kg/day.

Testing on reversal learning began at 12 months of age when mean blood lead levels were 55.0, 53.4, 8.6 and 3.4 µg/100 ml for the pulse-chronic, chronic-only, pulse-only and control groups, respectively. Animals were tested on object reversal problems using color, size and shape, respectively, as the relevant discrimination. Each problem consisted of original learning and nine reversals. Original learning and each reversal were trained to standard criterion (9 correct responses in 10 consecutive trials). Fifty trials of overtraining were given on Reversal 3 of the first problem and on original learning for each of the next three problems.

The first problem in the series proved to be much more difficult than in previous studies in which overtraining had been administered on original learning. Performance of all animals was seriously impaired and many required extensive training (even including reshaping of the basic response) to reach criterion, particularly on the first reversal. Within group variance was high and no significant group differences were observed on this problem or on any of the three subsequent problems in the series. The absence of overtraining on the initial discrimination of this series appears to have been very disruptive and may have accounted for the lack of a difference between lead and control animals in reversal learning performance. Further, the lack of an effect on Reversal 4 did not eliminate overtraining as a critical determinant of the lead associated deficit since the unexpectedly extensive practice obtained in reaching criterion on Reversals 1 and 2 could have precluded the effect. Earlier studies have reported lack of lead-associated reversal deficits after extensive RL training (Bushnell and Bowman, 1979a).

PLANOMETRIC STIMULI

The absence of a reversal deficit in the first RL series administered to the Experiment III animals suggested two possibilities. The lead treatments administered to these animals may not have been sufficient to produce a lead-associated cognitive dysfunction similar to that obtained in the Experiment I and II animals, and/or the RL task reported above may have been sufficiently different from earlier studies to have obscured a lead effect in Experiment III. Assuming the latter possibility, a second RL series was administered to the Experiment III monkeys. The second series utilized overtraining on original learning since original learning had been overtrained in every problem on which an RL deficit had previously been obtained. In addition, the second series used two-dimensional stimuli since such stimuli had been effective in reinstating a lead-associated RL deficit in other RL-experienced monkeys (Bushnell and Bowman, 1979a). As a final challenge, the difficulty of the third problem in the series was further enhanced by retaining the relevant stimulus dimension of Problem 2 as an irrelevant dimension in Problem 3.

Immediately upon completion of the first series, each monkey was administered the second series consisting of Color (blue vs. red square), Size (6.5 vs. 2 cm diameter circle) and Spatial (left vs. right) RL problems in that order. Stimuli for the Spatial RL problem were yellow octagons similar in size to the two circles used in the previous Size RL task. The two octagons were presented in a random sequence over the left and right food-wells and hence were irrelevant to the solution of the Spatial RL problem. Each of the three reversal problems consisted of original learning and nine reversals, with overtraining (strict criterion) on original learning. Animals were about 16 months old at the beginning of testing, at which time the group mean blood lead level was 30.2, 29.5, 7.8 and 4.0 µg/100 ml for the pulse-chronic, chronic-only, pulse-only and control animals, respectively.

No group differences were observed for trials to criterion on the first or second planometric RL problems. However, the third problem yielded a significant main effect of treatment, $F(3,11) = 7.62$, $p < .005$, and a treatment x reversal interaction, $F(27,99) = 1.89$, $p < 0.025$ (Figure 2). Further tests indicated that significant group differences were specific to the first reversal. The

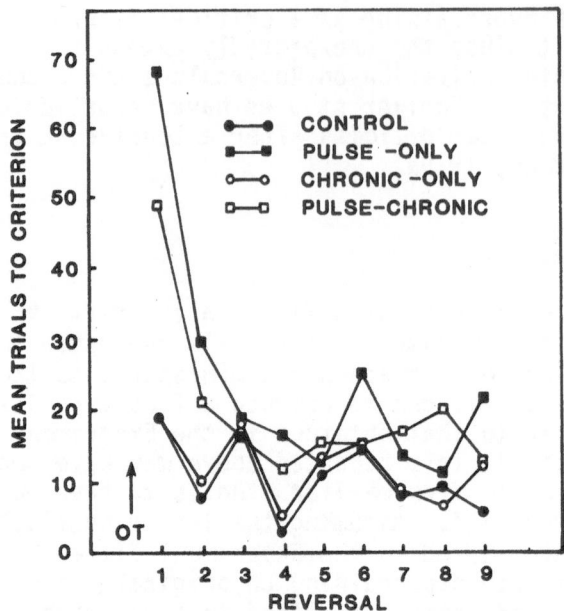

Figure 2 Mean trials to criterion on each reversal of a Spatial
         Reversal Learning Task using two-dimensional stimuli for
         the control, pulse-only, chronic-only and pulse-chronic
         groups of Experiment III.

pulse-only and pulse-chronic groups required more trials to reach
criterion on Reversal 1 than the chronic-only and control groups.
The chronic-only and control groups did not differ from each other.

     The behavioral deficit observed in this series was associated
with an early high lead pulse and indicated another pattern of lead
exposure which could produce a reversal learning deficit.
Furthermore the results suggest an enduring effect of early lead
treatment, since blood lead levels for the pulse-only group had
averaged below 10 μg/100 ml for several months prior to these
behavioral tests.

     The lack of a reversal deficit associated with chronic lead
exposure was not necessarily inconsistent with previous findings of
a deficit associated with chronic lead exposure, since several
conditions were different between the present and previous chronic
lead experiments. In the first place, the chronic lead intake in
Experiment III was only a little above that of the low lead
conditions in Experiments I and II and may have been too low to
produce a reversal deficit. Secondly, several task parameters
incorporated into the Experiment III RL series were different from
those under which RL deficits were observed in Experiments I and II.

These differences, described above, may have decreased the sensitivity of the RL paradigm to detect deficits, particularly at such a low level of chronic lead exposure.

IRRELEVANT CUES

The results of the second series of testing of the Experiment III animals suggested that irrelevant cues could be an important parameter in eliciting a lead-associated reversal deficit. Effects of irrelevant cues on RL learning were further examined using shape as an irrelevant cue in a Spatial RL series. Stimuli were a blue cylinder and cube. The shape was irrelevant to the solution of the problem (i.e. shape was randomly associated with rewarded postion). Original learning and 10 reversals were trained to standard criterion. Overtraining to the strict criterion was administered on original learning as in earlier experiments and also at Reversal 5.

The monkeys tested in this study were designated as Experiment V of the project series. Eight monkeys were given lead at a dose of 1.0 mg/kg/day from birth to one year of age (lead group) and eight were given no added lead (control group). In addition, since certain dietary constituents which occur in milk have been implicated in biological responses to lead, half of the animals in each group were fed milk ad lib (up to 600 cc per day) and half were given milk at levels which were gradually restricted to 100 cc per day. Monkey chow was supplied to all animals ad lib. Testing began at 22 months of age when blood lead levels were about 30 μg/100 ml for both of the lead groups and 5 μg/100 ml for both of the control groups.

The differential milk diets had no effect on any phase of this task and lead treatment had no effect on performance in the original learning or overtraining phases. However, analysis of trials to criterion on the reversal phase, using a square root transformation to reduce heterogeneity of variance, yielded a significant lead treatment x reversal interaction $F(9,108) = 2.32$, $p < .025$ (Figure 3). Further analysis indicated that lead-treated animals required significantly more trials than the control animals to reach criterion on both Reversals 3 and 4 and that trials to criterion were significantly elevated on Reversal 6 relative to Reversal 5 for control but not for lead-treated monkeys.

The irrelevant cues used in this study clearly increased the difficulty of the Spatial RL task and appear to alter the pattern of reversal learning for both lead and control monkeys. Control animals did not demonstrate an advantage over lead animals immediately following overtraining at Reversal 1 as in previous studies, and performance of lead animals was impaired for more reversals than usual. One of the possible explanations for these

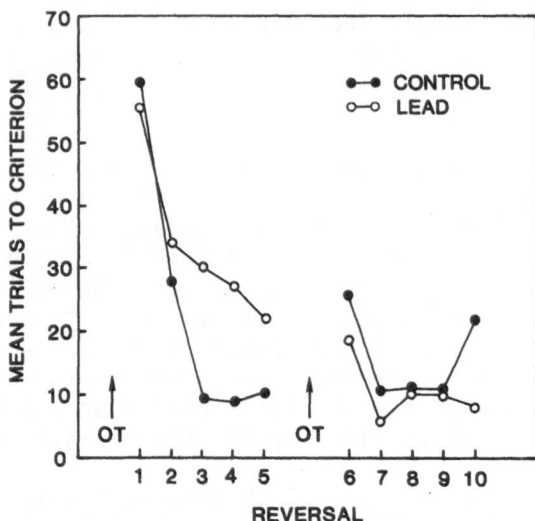

Figure 3   Mean trials to criterion on each reversal of a Spatial
           Reversal Learning task for the control and lead animals of
           Experiment V.   The reversals were performed in the
           presence of irrelevant stimulus cues.   OT indicates
           placement of overtraining.

results is that lead-treated animals are in general more
distractable than controls, and this distractability was enhanced by
the presence of irrelevant cues in this task.   This interpretation
would be in agreement with reports by Needleman et al. (1979) of
lead-associated distractability in children.   In addition,
overtraining on Reversal 5 transiently disrupted control performance
in a manner similar to that seen for both lead and control animals
by Rice and Willes (1979).   The task in the Rice and Willes study
was a simple RL discrimination series using no irrelevant cues.   In
the present study, overtraining in the middle of the series may also
have disrupted performance of lead-treated animals, since without
overtraining on Reversal 5 performance might have reached asymptotic
levels on Reversal 6.   Alternatively, overtraining on Reversal 5 may
have facilitated performance of the lead-treated animals by reducing
the distraction provided by the irrelevant cues.   This latter
interpretation would be consistent with the attentional model
proposed by Turrisi (1973) as the basis of the advantage provided by
overtraining for subsequent reversal learning.   Thus, the lead
animals reached asymptotic performance for the first time on
Reversal 7, possibly as a benefit of the second overtraining.

SUPPLEMENTAL CUES

Since lead-related effects had been observed in association
with the use of irrelevant cues, other cue relationships were
analyzed; the addition of relevant cues was examined next. A series
of studies was designed in collaboration with Dr. Mark Heironimus as
a complement to other studies using irrelevant cues to assess
toxicity of polychlorinated biphenyls (Heironimus et al., 1981).
The series consisted of two successive RL problems. The first
problem was a Spatial RL task using two identical yellow cubes as
stimuli. Animals were overtrained on original learning (strict
criterion). Original learning was followed by 20 consecutive reversals, each trained to standard criterion. Problem 1 was designed to
establish stable RL performance prior to the introduction of the new
stimuli in Problem 2. Stimuli for the second problem were a red and
an orange cube. The schedule of reversals on spatial positions was
maintained in phase with the previous problem with red always
presented in the correct spatial position and orange always
presented in the incorrect position. Thus, the new stimuli provided
supplemental color cues which were redundant with the spatial cue.
Eight spatial reversals were given in this manner, each to standard
criterion. Given the difficulty shown by the lead animals in the
previous experiment in the presence of irrelevant cues, lead-exposed
animals might be expected to show similar difficulties in the
presence of the supplemental color cues in Problem 2.

A new set of WGTA-naive monkeys, Experiment VI of the project
series was tested on these problems. In addition to the usual
postnatal lead administration, these animals were also exposed to
lead throughout gestation. For prenatal exposure, lead acetate was
added to the daily drinking water of the mothers beginning two
months prior to mating and continuing until birth. Maternal lead
intake during pregnancy was 5.6 + 1.28 mg/kg/day and blood lead
level was 59.9 + 6.89 µg/100 ml (mean + S.E.). Offspring were
separated from their mothers at birth and continued to be exposed to
lead in milk formula at an initial dose of 0.3 mg/kg/day. This dose
was increased to 0.5 mg/kg/day at 23 weeks of age to maintain blood
lead levels in the range of 40 to 60 µg/100 ml. Control animals
were treated identically except neither they nor their mothers were
given added lead. There were five animals in each group. Testing
of the offspring began at about 19 months of age, 32 weeks after
termination of lead exposure. Blood lead levels (mean + S.E.) at
the beginning of testing were 15.6 + 1.9 µg/100 ml for the lead
group and 4.8 + 0.59 µg/100 ml for the control group.

There were no significant group differences between the lead
and control groups on Problem 1. All monkeys mastered the
discrimination readily, both the lead and control groups averaged
about three errors to criterion on Reversals 5 to 20. In Problem 2,
lead-treated animals made more errors than controls early in the
problem as indicated by a significant treatment x reversals

interaction, F(7,56) = 3.25, p < 0.01. Further analysis indicated
that lead-treated animals were significantly worse than controls on
Reversals 1 and 2. The effect on Problem 2 was considered in
conjunction with performance on the final three reversals of Problem
1 (Figure 4). With the addition of the supplemental cue in Problem
2, the performance of control monkeys immediately improved to zero
or one error to criterion and was maintained essentially at this
level thereafter. Lead animals did not achieve such asymptotic
performance until two reversals later. This delay in cue
utilization apparently did not result from a delay in cue detection
since respose latencies were similarly affected by the change of
stimuli for both control and lead animals (Table 1). Analysis of
these latencies yielded a significant effect for reversals,
F(3,24) = 6.80, p < 0.005. Further tests revealed that latencies on
Reversal 1 of the second problem were significantly different from
all other reversals. Latencies for both the lead and control groups
were equivalently longer on this reversal. This increase in
response latency suggests that the change in stimuli coincident with
Reversal 1 was observed by all animals.

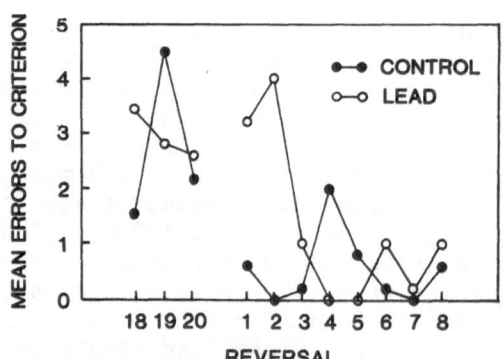

Figure 4 Mean errors to criterion on the last three reversals of
          Problem 1 and each reversal of Problem 2 for the control
          and lead animals of Experiment VI. Both problems were
          part of a Spatial Reversal Learning series. Problem 1
          used identical stimuli. In Problem 2, new stimuli were
          introduced and the correct position was indicated by a
          nonreversing color cue.

Table 1   Mean Latency ($\pm$ S.E.) to Respond to Trial 1 on the Last Two Reversals of Problem 1 and on the First Two Reversals of Problem 2

	Problem 1		Problem 2	
	Reversal			
Group	19	20	1	2
Control	3.5 $\pm$ 0.65	4.3 $\pm$ 1.16	7.0 $\pm$ 1.66*	1.39 $\pm$ 4.5
Lead	3.5 $\pm$ 0.74	5.3 $\pm$ 1.48	9.8 $\pm$ 2.79*	4.2 $\pm$ 1.02

*Reversal 1 is significantly different from all other reversals for both groups ($p < 0.01$).

The absence of a reversal deficit on Problem 1 is generally in agreement with results obtained in Experiments I and II for animals dosed comparably postpartum (low-lead groups) and tested at approximately the same age (Bushnell and Bowman, 1979a). Apparently, the additional prenatal lead exposure employed in the Experiment VI animals did not enhance effects of postnatal lead exposure at this low-dose. Results of Problem 2 suggested that, as predicted, control animals utilized the information provided by the supplemental cues more quickly than did the lead animals. This result complements the outcome of the irrelevant cue problem discussed above. On the one hand, lead monkeys were slower to learn reversals in the presence of irrelevant cues; on the other hand, they failed to utilize supplemental cues as readily as did controls.

DELAYED SPATIAL ALTERNATION

Most recently, a somewhat different RL paradigm has been found to yield a continuous deficit over a prolonged period of testing. This paradigm is the Delayed Spatial Alternation (DSA) task and has been a standard procedure for assessing effects of such variables as brain lesions and pharmacological treatment in the monkey (e.g. Goldman et al., 1971; Brazowski et al., 1979). It can be considered as an example of the general reversal paradigm taken to the minimum limit of one trial per reversal. That is, the rewarded position was reversed on every trial rather than after a criterion level of responding was reached. Delays of 5, 10, 20, and 40 seconds were interposed between trials in a counterbalanced order as contrasted with the constant 10 sec intertrial interval typical of the previous RL testing. The use of several different intertrial delays is a standard procedure to vary problem difficulty and assess memory function. The stimulus objects were identical red cubes. Each animal was tested for 50 sessions of 32 trials each.

Animals from Experiment III, described earlier, served as subjects. Attrition extraneous to the lead treatment had resulted in the loss of all but three subjects in the pulse-chronic group and two subjects in the control group. The monkeys were six years old at the beginning of testing and had previous extensive training on RL discriminations and in other tests conducted in the WGTA. Blood lead levels at the beginning of DSA testing were 3.5 ± 0.5 µg/100 ml and 4.0 ± 1.15 µg/100 ml for the control and lead groups, respectively ($X \pm$ S.E.).

Percent correct scores in the DSA task, averaged over blocks of 10 sessions, are shown in Figure 5. Analysis of variance yielded a significant main effect of lead treatment, $F(1,3) = 23.70$, $p < 0.025$. As can be seen in Figure 5, both lead and control groups improved with repeated testing but the lead-associated deficit remained relatively constant across blocks of trials. Analysis with respect to intertrial delays yielded a treatment x trials interaction, $F(3,9) = 12.30$, $p < .05$ (Table 2). The lead deficit was more pronounced at the 5, 10 and 20 second delays than at the 40 second delay.

These results indicate that neonatal lead exposure resulted in a profound deficit in DSA in monkeys tested as young adults. This deficit persisted over 50 sessions of testing and was much more stable than any of the previous RL deficits observed. Previous RL tests were sensitive in detecting a lead-induced deficit, but after the first few reversals, the deficit usually disappeared and could be reinstated only by changing the task. The stable nature of the DSA deficit allows repeated testing without loss of the deficit. This will permit studies on these animals using drug probes, to help elucidate mechanisms which might account for the lead-behavioral effect. We are presently investigating this approach, using selected drugs to study the involvement of the dopaminergic system with lead effect.

The lead-induced deficit was most pronounced at the short delays. This suggests that the lead deficit was not in memory retention but instead reflected other processes, such as attentional effects. The stability of the DSA deficit will also permit investigation of these behavioral parameters.

Finally, these results are important because they were found in 6-year-old monkeys which were last exposed to lead at 1 year of age. At 6 years of age, these monkeys were young adults, indicating that their lead-induced cognitive deficit was long lasting and possibly permanent.

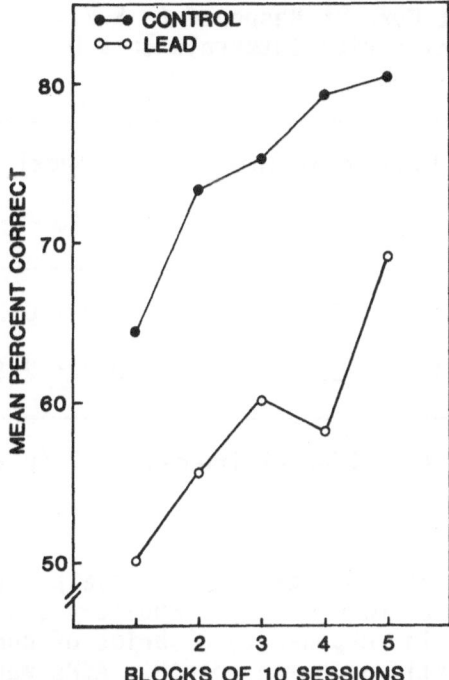

Figure 5   Mean percent correct responses on each 10-session block of
           Delayed Spatial Alternation for the control and lead
           (pulse-chronic group) animals of Experiment III.   Correct
           responses are averaged over all delays.

AUDITORY EVOKED POTENTIALS

Finally, data are presented here on a quite different line of
cognitive research than the above. This research is being done in
collaboration with Dr. Dennis Molfese of Southern Illinois
University and Dr. Philip Morse of the University of Wisconsin.
Scalp-recorded evoked potentials are being studied. Evoked
responses are portions of the EEG which are time locked to the
occurrence of specific stimulus events. Evoked potentials were
obtained for monkey subjects in this study in the context of
investigating the ontogeny of perceptual mechanisms. Specifically,
these studies focused on the ability of nonhuman primates to
discriminate and categorize various human speech sounds and on the
cerebral laterality of these processes. Data are reported here from
the 5 lead-treated monkeys described earlier as Experiment VI in the
project series and 5 age-matched controls. Lead exposure in this
series was administered daily both prenatally and postnatally until
one year of age. The animals were 10 to 12 weeks old at the time of
the study and blood lead levels of the experimental animals were 35
to 45 μg/100 ml.

Table 2   Mean Percent Correct Response (+ S.E.) on 5, 10, 20 and
          40-Second Intertrial Intervals on a Delayed Spatial
          Alternation Task

Group	Intertrial Interval (seconds)			
	5	10	20	40
Control	83.2 + 1.22	79.3 + 1.12	77.3 + 0.25	59.3 + 1.14
Lead	60.3 + 3.32*	58.7 + 3.70*	60.8 + 2.50*	52.8 + 1.83

*Significantly different from control (p < 0.05).

        Electrodes were placed over temporal scalp sites of the left
and right hemisphere of each monkey. Auditory evoked responses
(AERs) were recorded in response to a series of consonant-vowel
syllables characteristic of human speech. AERs were digitized and
averaged over at least 16 repetitions of each stimulus for each
recording site for each animal and analyzed using principal
component analysis and ANOVA techniques described by Molfese
(1978). Results are presented for one stimulus set consisting of
the consonant-vowel syllables /bi, bæ, bɔ, gi, gæ, gɔ/. Analysis
yielded a significant treatment x consonant interaction, $F(1,8) =$
13.36, $p < .001$ (Figure 6). As can be seen in Figure 6, the
amplitude of the AERs was greater for control than for lead-treated
monkeys. More importantly, the waveforms differed between the two
consonant sounds for the control animals but not for the lead
animals. This difference in response reflected the contribution of
a component of the wave beginning 230 msec after stimulus onset for
which the controls exhibited an initial positive peak followed by a
negative peak at about 400 msec. The results for the control
monkeys were similar to those obtained with human subjects (Molfese,
1980). Waveforms for the control animals were different for the
consonant sounds /b/ and /g/ even though the acoustic frequency for
the transitions in these sounds changed when the consonants were
combined with different vowels. These are regarded as evidence for
discrimination of these different phoneme categories, /b/ and /g/
(Liberman, et al., 1967). Lead animals, however, did not make the
same distinctions. The two curves obtained for lead animals did not
differ and the second negative peak was absent in the lead animals.
The absence of this effect at this point in time does not reflect a
general inability of the lead animals to discriminate auditory
stimuli since there was evidence for discrimination of other
acoustic differences.

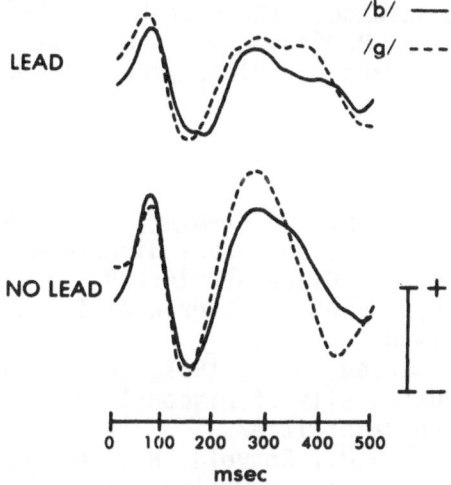

Figure 6   The average AERs elicited for the /b/ and /g/ syllables
collapsed across all vowel conditions for control and lead
groups. The calibration is 15 µV with positive up.

GENERAL CONCLUSIONS

Using a nonhuman primate model for childhood lead toxicity, we
have obtained evidence for cognitive dysfunction beginning during
the period of early lead exposure and persisting for many years
beyond the termination of lead exposure. The dysfunction had been
indicated by reversal learning deficits. Subsequent investigations
of test parameters of the reversal learning paradigm have revealed
several procedures which elicit or reinstate the learning deficit.
Lead-induced learning deficits have recently been found to be
especially protracted in a version of the reversal paradigm called
Delayed Spatial Alternation. This finding makes it practical to
conduct analytical studies in the monkey to characterize the
neurochemical and behavioral nature of the lead-induced
dysfunction. Finally, we have demonstrated that this primate model
can also reveal electrophysiological evidence for lead-induced
changes in auditory perceptual processing. These findings have
their counterparts in the clinical literature on childhood lead
toxicity and therefore emphasize the importance of the primate model
for studies of lead toxicity.

ACKNOWLEDGEMENT

This research was supported in part by U.S.P.H.S. grants
ES01062 and 5-T32-ES07015 from the National Institute of

Environmental Health Sciences, the Food Research Institute of the University of Wisconsin, Madison, Wisc., National Science Foundation grant BNS-8004429, and March of Dimes grant 12-13.

REFERENCES

Bartus, R.T., Dean III, R.L. and Fleming, D.L., 1979, Aging in the rhesus monkey: Effects on visual discrimination learning and reversal learning, J. Gerontol. 34:209.

Bitterman, M.E., 1965, Phyletic differences in learning, Am. Psychol. 20:396-410.

Blomquist, A.J., and Harlow, H.F., 1961, The infant rhesus monkey program at the University of Wisconsin Primate Laboratory, Proc. Animal Care Panel 11:57.

Brazowski, T.J., Brown, R.M., Rosvold, H.E. and Goldman, P.S. 1979, Cognitive deficit caused by regional depletion of dopamine in prefrontal cortex of rhesus monkey, Science 205:929-932.

Bushnell, P.J. and Bowman, R.E., 1979a, Reversal learning deficits in young monkeys exposed to lead, Pharmac. Biochem. Behav. 10:733-742.

Bushnell, P.J. and Bowman, R.E., 1979b, Persistence of impaired reversal learning in young monkeys exposed to low levels of dietary lead, J. Toxicol. Envir. Health 5:1015-1023.

Bushnell, P.J. and Bowman, R.E., 1979c, Effects of chronic lead ingestion on social development in infant rhesus monkey, Neurobehav. Toxicol. 1:207.

Cohen, N., Kneip, T.J., Ruson, V. and Goldstein, D.H., 1974, Biochemical and toxicological response of infant baboons to lead driers in paint, Environ. Health Perspect. 7:161-173.

Goldman, P.S., Rosvold, H.E., Vest, B. and Galkin, T.W., 1971, Analysis of the delayed-alternation deficit produced by dorsolateral prefrontal lesions in the rhesus monkey, J. Comp. Physiol. Psychol. 77:212-220.

Harlow, H.F., 1949, The formation of learning sets, Psychol. Rev. 56:51-65.

Harlow, H.F., 1959., The development of learning in the rhesus monkey, Am. Sci. 47:459-479.

Harlow, H.F. and Bromer, J.A., 1938, A test-apparatus for monkeys, Psychol. Rec. 2:434-436.

Heinronimus, M.P., Laughlin, N.K. and Bowman, R.E., 1981, Effects of early exposure to PCBs on learned irrelevancy of cues in rhesus monkeys: An incidental learning paradigm, Teratology 24:55A.

Kendler, T.S., Kendler, H.H. and Wells, D., 1960, Reversal and nonreversal shifts in nursery school children, J. Comp. Physiol. Psychol. 53:83-88.

Liberman, A.M., Cooper, F.S., Shankweiler, D.P. and Studdert-Kennedy, M., 1967, Perception of the speech code, Psychol. Rev. 74:431-461.

Mahut, H., 1971, Spatial and object reversal learning in monkeys with partial temporal lobe ablations, Neuropsychologia 9:409.

Molfese, D.L., 1978, Left and right hemisphere involvement in speech perception: Electrophysiological correlates, Perception and Psychophysics 23:237.

Molfese, D.L., 1980, The phoneme and the engram: Electrophysiological evidence for the acoustic invariant in stop consonants, Brain and Lang. 9:372.

Needleman, H.L., Gunnoe, C., Leviton, A., Reed, R., Peresie, H., Maher, C. and Barrett, P., 1979, Deficits in psychologic and classroom performance of children with elevated dentine lead levels, N. Engl. J. Med. 300:689-695.

Rice, D.C., and Willes, R.F., 1979, Neonatal low-level lead exposure in monkeys (Macaca fascicularis): Effect on two-choice nonspatial form discrimination, J. Envir. Path. Toxicol. 2:1195-1203.

Turrisi, F.D., 1973, Evidence for attentional explanation of the overtraining reversal effect, J. Exp. Psychol. 101:246-251.

CENTRAL NERVOUS EFFECTS OF PERINATAL EXPOSURE TO LEAD OR METHYLMERCURY IN THE MONKEY

Deborah C. Rice

Toxicology Research Division
Bureau of Chemical Safety, Food Directorate
Health Protection Branch, Health and Welfare Canada
Ottawa, Ontario, Canada

ABSTRACT

The behavioral consequences of chronic exposure to lead or methylmercury have been studied in monkeys (Macaca fascicularis). Monkeys exposed to lead from birth at a dose resulting in a blood lead level of 55 µg/dl preweaning and a steady state level of 33 µg/dl after weaning at 200 days of age produced impairment on a discrimination reversal task, as well as clear differences from control on an intermittent schedule of reinforcement, the fixed interval. Lead exposures to doses that produce blood levels in the range of 12-22 µg/dl results in performance outside of control range on these tasks for certain individuals. Monkeys exposed to methylmercury from birth at a dose resulting in a peak blood level of 1.2 ppm preweaning and .6-.9 ppm postweaning produced dificits in spatial visual function under conditions of both high and low luminance, while temporal visual function was superior in treated monkeys. Exposure to this same dose in utero plus postnatally resulted in two monkeys out of five exhibiting clinical signs, with monkeys exposed to half that dose apparently normal. Blood mercury levels of the infants at birth were considerably higher than those of the mother, and decreased to levels well below those of the mother over the course of several months. This was true despite the fact that infants were dosed from birth with the same dose the mothers had received. These monkeys were not severely impaired relative to controls on a series of discrimination reversal tasks, although some individuals failed to acquire the lever press response, so an easier operant had to be employed.

INTRODUCTION

A study has been ongoing since 1974 to determine the effects of chronic exposure to either lead or methylmercury in the macaque monkey (Macaca fascicularis). Monkeys exposed to lead were dosed from birth onward, while methylmercury was given either from birth or in utero plus postnatally. In the last several years, emphasis has been on testing for behavioral effects in these monkeys. This paper consists of some of these data, along with indications of body burden of the relevant metal.

All infants were separated from their mothers at birth and reared in a primate nursery (Willes et al., 1977). Infants were able to see and hear other monkeys at all times, and were exercised in large cages with their peers beginning at three weeks of age. This regimen allows the infant monkey to develop normally socially and intellectually (Harlow et al., 1971). Monkeys were dosed orally seven or (later in the study) five days per week. Infants were dosed by syringe, and older monkeys voluntarily consumed gelatin capsules containing the dose. Food consumption, weight gain, routine hematology, Serum Multiple Analyzer-18 (Technicon), and clinical neurological status were monitored routinely. With the exception of two monkeys exposed to methylmercury in utero plus postnatally, all monkeys were apparently normal.

BEHAVIORAL EFFECTS OF LEAD

It is been reported that excessive exposure to lead in children results in intellectual impairment of various forms, irritability, distractibility and short attention span, hyperactivity, and other behaviors that would make it difficult for the child to learn the skills needed to be successful in society (Beattie et al., 1975; de la Burde and Choate, 1975; Landrigan et al., 1975; Needleman et al., 1979; Winneke et al., 1981; Yule et al., 1981). The body burden of lead at which these deficits occur, and in some cases whether they occur at all, has been the subject of some controversy over the last several years. I therefore have concentrated my research program on trying to find monkey analogs to these human behaviors that may be tested in the laboratory, and to determine at what body burden impairment occurs.

Monkeys were exposed from birth to lead at doses equivalent to 0, 25, 50, 100, or 500 μg/kg/day. For all the treated groups, blood lead levels peaked by 100 days of age and decreased to a steady level after weaning from infant formula at 100 days of age (Figure 1). The highest dose of lead resulted in a blood level preweaning that is considered to be deleterious to children, while the postweaning blood lead is at a level for which the safety for children is presently a subject of controversy (Table 1). For the

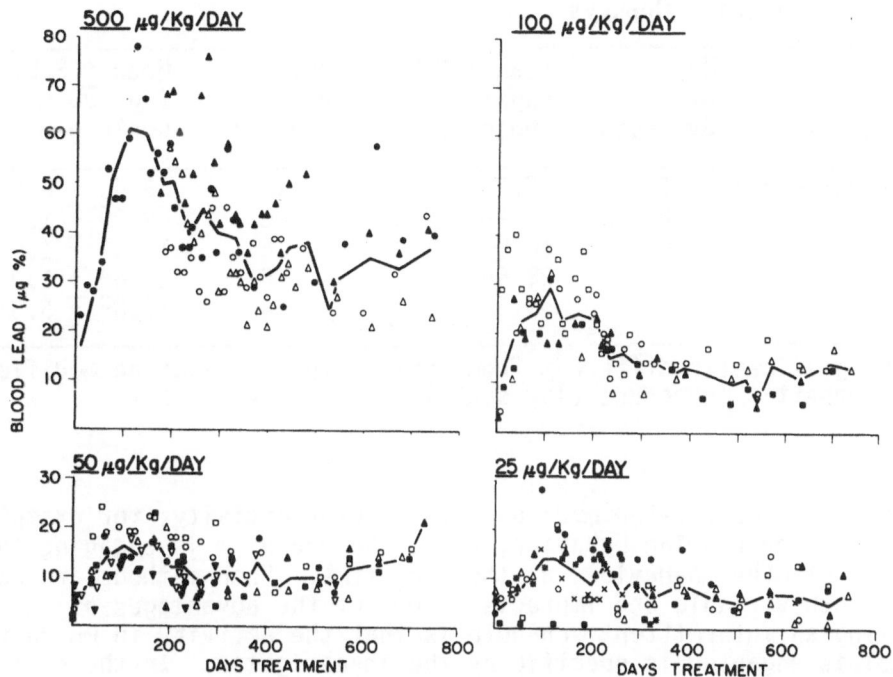

Figure 1   Blood lead levels vs. age of monkeys doses from birth with lead. Monkeys were weaned from infant formula at 200 days of age.

three lower doses, all levels are considered to be safe for children, and are found routinely in the general population. Blood lead levels of control monkeys were below those of most people in industrialized countries (below 5 µg/100 ml).

Monkeys in the 0, 50, 100, and 500 µg/kg/day dose groups have been tested on a variety of behavioral measures beginning at 2.5 to 3.0 years of age. Two of these experiments, which have been completed on all monkeys, will be discussed.

Fixed Interval Performance

The effect of lead has been examined on an intermittent schedule of reinforcement, the fixed interval (FI). (See Rice et al., 1979, for a report on the high dose group). Activity

Table 1   Mean Blood Lead Levels Before and After Weaning Lead
          Treated Monkeys

Dose (µg/kg/day)	No. of Subjects	Mean + S.E. (µg/100 ml whole blood)	No. of Subjects	Mean + S.E. (µg/100 ml whole blood)
0 (control)	5	2.2 + 0.4	10	3.4 + 0.8
25	8	9.9[a] + 2.0	6	9.2[a] + 1.5
50	8	16.0[a] + 2.4	6	11.8[a] + 1.9
100	5	22.4[a] + 2.2	5	11.6[a] + 1.3
500	4	55.3[a] + 6.7	4	32.8[a] + 5.3

[a]Significantly different from control (p < .01) using modified
Dunnett's procedure (log scale).

measures are most often made on a particular activity, for example,
locomotion or rearing behavior, while the organism is engaging in a
variety of other behaviors at the same time. Such methods are bound
to be both variable and imprecise. One of the advantages of
studying an intermittent schedule is that the activity in which the
animal is engaging is specific by the investigator. In the present
experiment, the monkey was required to press a lever once after
eight minutes had elapsed in order to receive fruit juice.
Responding before the eight minutes had no scheduled consequences.
Although only one response is required for reinforcement, FI
performance is characterized by responding throughout most of the
interval. The rate and pattern of response is characteristic of the
individual, since it is not specified by the schedule. The
performance of normal animals, as well as the effects of a wide
variety of psychoactive agents, have been well characterized for
this schedule.

     One way of examining the characteristics of the rate and
pattern of responding is to compile histograms of the time between
successive responses during a session. The interresponse time (IRT)
distributions for control and monkey exposed to 500 µg/kg/day of
lead is depicted in Figure 2. All of the treated monkeys had a
greater absolute number of responses than did controls, with three
of the four having a distribution skewed toward very short times
between successive responses. Thus three of the treated monkeys
were different from control in a manner similar to each other, while
the fourth was different from everyone else. This is an indication
of variability of response between treated animals, although at this
dose the performance of all the monkeys may be considered to be
affected by lead exposure.

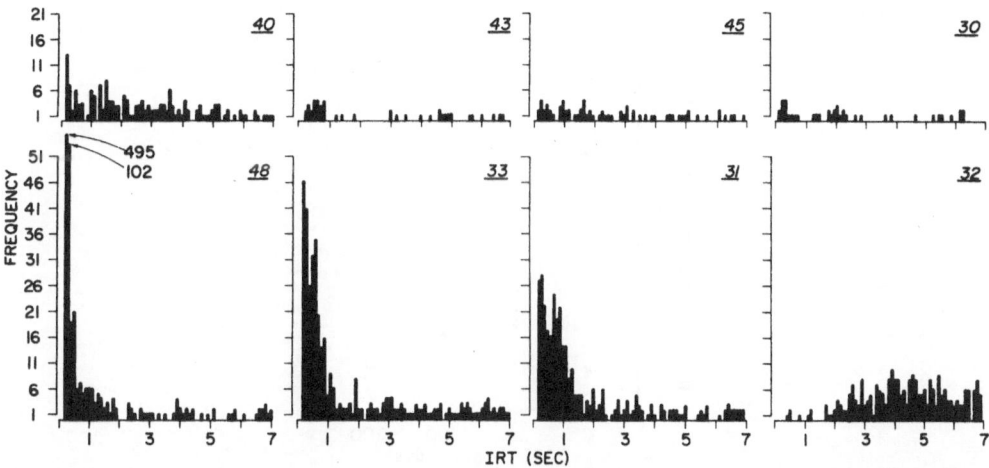

Figure 2   IRT absolute frequency distribution for one session of a
            fixed interval schedule for control (top) and monkeys
            exposed to 500 μmg/kg/day of lead (bottom). The division
            along the abscissa represent classes of time between
            successive responses, in 100 msec increments. The lead
            treated monkeys in general had a much higher absolute
            frequency of IRTs, and a distribution skewed toward shorter
            IRTs. Control and treated monkeys were statistically
            different on a variety of measure of FI performance, i.e.,
            FI run rate in sessions 1-20 and median of median IRT in
            sessions 1-20 (p < .05 by Mann-Whitney U test).

     A summary measure that may be derived from this kind of
analysis is the median IRT, which reflects the number of responses
emitted but omits much information concerning the pattern of
response. On this measure, there is a wide range of values for the
control monkeys (Figure 3). This is typical of fixed interval
performance, since the reinforcement density does not depend on rate
of response, within reasonable limits. With increasing lead dose,
the number of monkeys with longer median IRT's decreased, as did the
average median IRT for the group. Thus exposure to lead may shift
the behavior of the animal toward more activity.

     An additional set of parameters that may be analysed for this
type of schedule is variability of performance for an individual,
both within each session and across sessions (Figure 4). Note that
each symbol represents a measure of variability, rather than a
measure of performance. Normalized within session variability was
greater in the 50 and 100 μg/kg/day dose groups than in the
controls, while the response rate of the 500 μg/kg/day was as stable

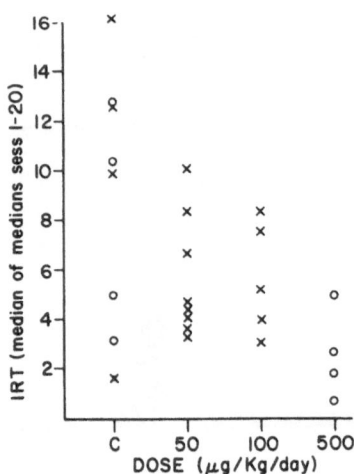

Figure 3   Median of median IRT for sessions 1-20 of a fixed interval
           schedule for monkeys exposed to 0, 50, 100, or 500
           µg/kg/day of lead from birth. Circles represent the 500
           µg/kg/day dose group and its controls, who are older and
           were tested at a different time than the others. Lead
           treated monkeys have shorter median IRT's than controls
           (0 vs 50, p < .05; 0 vs 100, p < .10; 0 vs 500, p < .025
           on a two-tailed t-test).

as (but at a higher rate than) controls. For the normalized between
sessions variability, there were individuals in the treated groups
whose performances were outside of control range. This increase in
variability, most apparent at the lower doses, may represent a
subtle effect of lead.

Discrimination Reversal

     A paradigm that examines a different set of behavioral skills
was also tested in this same group of monkeys. This experiment was
designed to test the monkey's ability to adapt to a change in the
effect its own behavior produced in its environment - specifically,
the ability of the monkey to respond in a manner opposite to a
previously learned response. The performance of the 500 µg/kg/day
group and its controls was examined (Rice and Willes, 1979) before
the lower dose groups were tested. The monkey faced two food wells,
one covered with a cube and the other with a triangle. Only the
well under the cube contained a raisin, and the monkey learned to

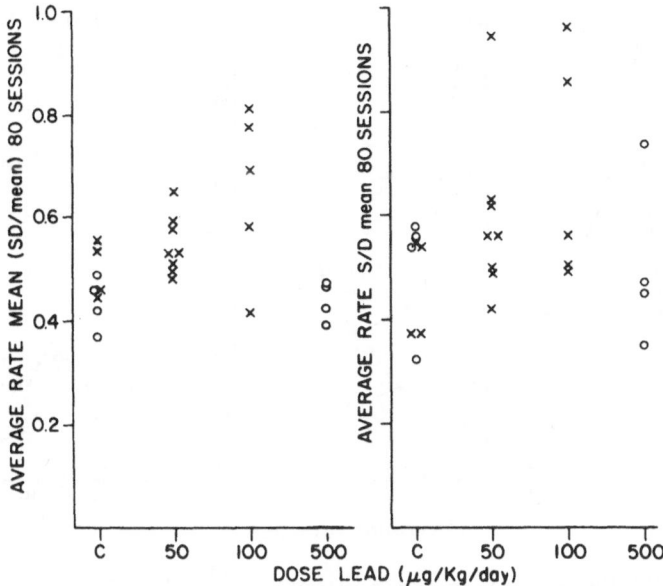

Figure 4   Variability of average response rate on an FI within
           session (left) and between sessions (right) for monkeys
           exposed to lead. Values are normalized. Symbols as in
           Figure 3. For within session variability, the 50 and 100
           µg/dl dose groups were significantly more variable than
           controls (.0039 and .0177, respectively, on test) (.67), a
           type of randomization test (Good, 1979). For between
           session variability results did not reach significance
           (.20 and .12, respectively) because of large within group
           variability in the treated groups.

knock the cube off either well to get the raisin. When each monkey
made nine correct choices out of ten trials, the raisin was placed
under the triangle instead of the cube, and the monkey had to learn
to respond to the formerly incorrect stimulus. A series of 20 such
reversals was performed. At two points in the experiment, the
monkey was given extra trials between reversals to see if the
performance of the lead-treated and control monkeys were disrupted
differentially. The lead-treated monkeys made more errors per
reversal, although their learning curves over successive reversals
paralleled that of the controls (Figure 5). Lead-treated and
control monkeys were disrupted to the same extent by the first
series of 150 extra trials. The second series of 500 extra trials
disrupted the performance of both sets of animals. These results
suggest that the lead-treated monkeys have a more difficult time
adapting their behavior to new circumstances than do controls, but

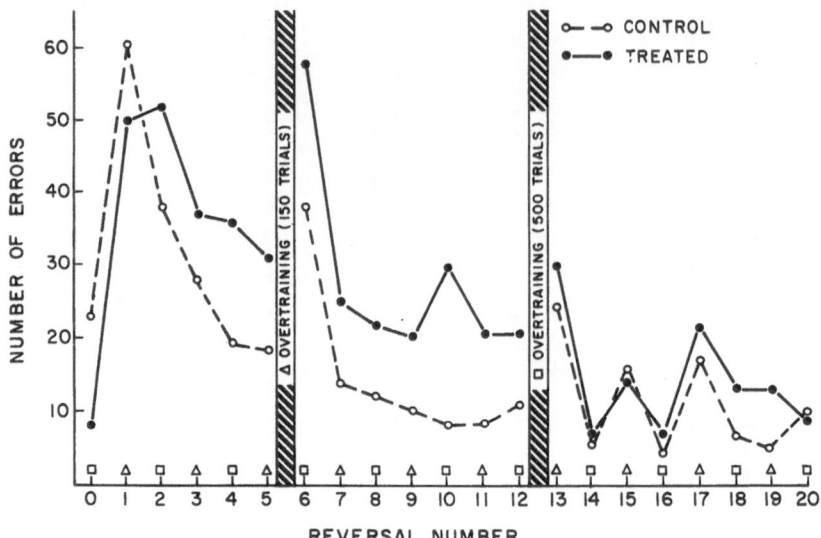

Figure 5   Mean number of unsuccessful trials to reversal criterion
on a form discrimination task. Ordinate represents the
mean number of trials for control (unfilled circles) and
monkeys dosed with 500 µg/kg/day lead (filled circles) to
satisfy the requirement of acquisition for each reversal.
Striped bars represent the points in the experiment where
monkeys were given extra trials before the next reversal.
Treated monkeys made statistically more errors than
controls before the second set of extra trials (ANOVA,
p < .05).

rather persevere in behaviors that are no longer appropriate to a
changed environment.

     A similar experiment was performed with the lower dose groups
and their controls, utilizing the computer for stimulus display as
well as experimental control and data acquisition. The monkey faced
a panel on which were two clear response disks and a tube for
delivery of apple juice. The disks were backlit with either red or
green, on which was superimposed either a two-dimensional square or
triangle. During one part of the experiment, one disk was backlit
with the square while the other was backlit with the triangle; the
position at which they appeared were chosen randomly from trial to
trial. The color of the surround was also varied randomly between
trials, independently of the forms, with one disk backlit with each
color. The monkey was required to attend to the form and ignore the
color of the surround; this followed a part in the experiment in
which the monkey has been required to attend to the color. When the

monkey learned to respond on the correct form using the same criterion as in the previous experiment (9 out of 10 correct), the previously negative stimulus became the correct one, for a total of 15 reversals. For the two treated groups, the number of errors to reach criterion on each reversal greatly exceeded those in the control range for certain individuals (Figure 6).

There was a tendency for there to be more "responders" to lead insult during the early reversals, and only one monkey in each group outside of the control range at the end of the experiment. For the 100 μg/kg/day dose, it was always the same monkey that was far outside of the control range during the last reversals, while for the 50 μg/kg/day group there were three individuals who showed aberrant behavior.

DISCUSSION

From the results of other behavioral tests as well as those described here, it seems that exposure to lead in a dose resulting in blood lead levels of 55 μg/dl preweaning and 33 μg/dl post-weaning behavioral impairment. Exposure to lead at the two lower doses produced some significant effects and was associated with an increase in variability between subjects and an increase in variability of behavior of individual monkeys. Such results have been reported by other investigators (see Cory-Slechta, 1982). There does not appear to be a dose-effect relationship, which is not surprising since the blood levels of the groups are so similar (22 or 16 μg/dl preweaning and 12 μg/dl for both postweaning). These blood levels are well within the limits of what is considered safe for children, and in fact span the range of values most commonly observed in children in industrialized nations.

EFFECTS OF METHYLMERCURY

Visual Function in Monkeys Treated Postnatally

One of the most consistent signs in adult methylmercury poisoning has been visual deficits, including constriction of visual fields and deficits in visual acuity (Sabelaish and Hilmi, 1976; Rustam and Hamdi, 1974). Human data suggest that the neonates exposed to methylmercury both prenatally and postnatally through the breast milk may be at greater risk than the adult (Amin-Zaki et al., 1974). The pattern of central nervous system, including visual cortex, damage may be different in the neonatally-exposed organism than in the adult (Chang, 1977).

In the present study, infant monkeys were separated from their mothers at birth and dosed with 50 μg/kg/day of mercury as

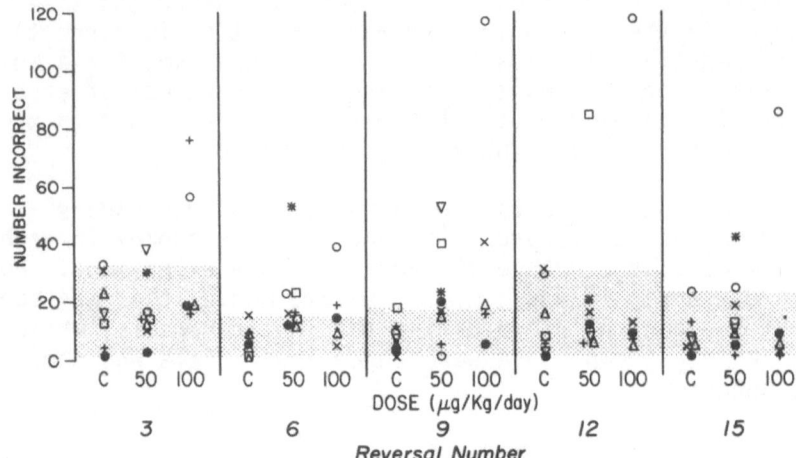

Figure 6   Number of errors before reaching reversal criterion for
           every third reversal for control and monkeys dosed with 50
           or 100 µg/kg/day of lead. Each symbol represents an
           individual monkey. Stippled areas represent the range of
           control values for each reversal.

methylmercury. The blood mercury levels of these monkeys peaked at
1.2 ppm preweaning and decreased to approximately 0.7 - 0.9 ppm
postweaning (Figure 7).

     When monkeys were approximately three years old, their ability
to see the various frequency components of objects was determined
(Rice and Gilbert, 1982). During testing, the monkey faced two
oscilloscopes; on one was a vertical sine wave grating, and on the
other was a blank field of equal average luminance (Figure 8). The
monkey pressed a lever corresponding to the scope displaying the
grating in order to receive a fruit juice reward. For each spatial
frequency, the contrast, which is a function of the difference in
luminance between the light and dark bars, was varied to determine
the value at which the monkey was unable to discriminate the sine
wave grating from the blank field. This was considered to be the
threshold for that frequency. A psychophysical function of
threshold vs. spatial frequency was generated for each individual.
The function for each monkey was determined at two luminance levels,
a high level (5 x 10^{-4} ft lamberti), and one that was very low
(5 ft lamberti), comparable to dim starlight. Testing at these
different luminances also allowed different functional components of
the visual system to be examined independently. As in human visual
testing, normal monkeys should produce functions virtually
superimposed one on the other (de Valois et al., 1974), so that
small decrements in visual function may be detected reliably.

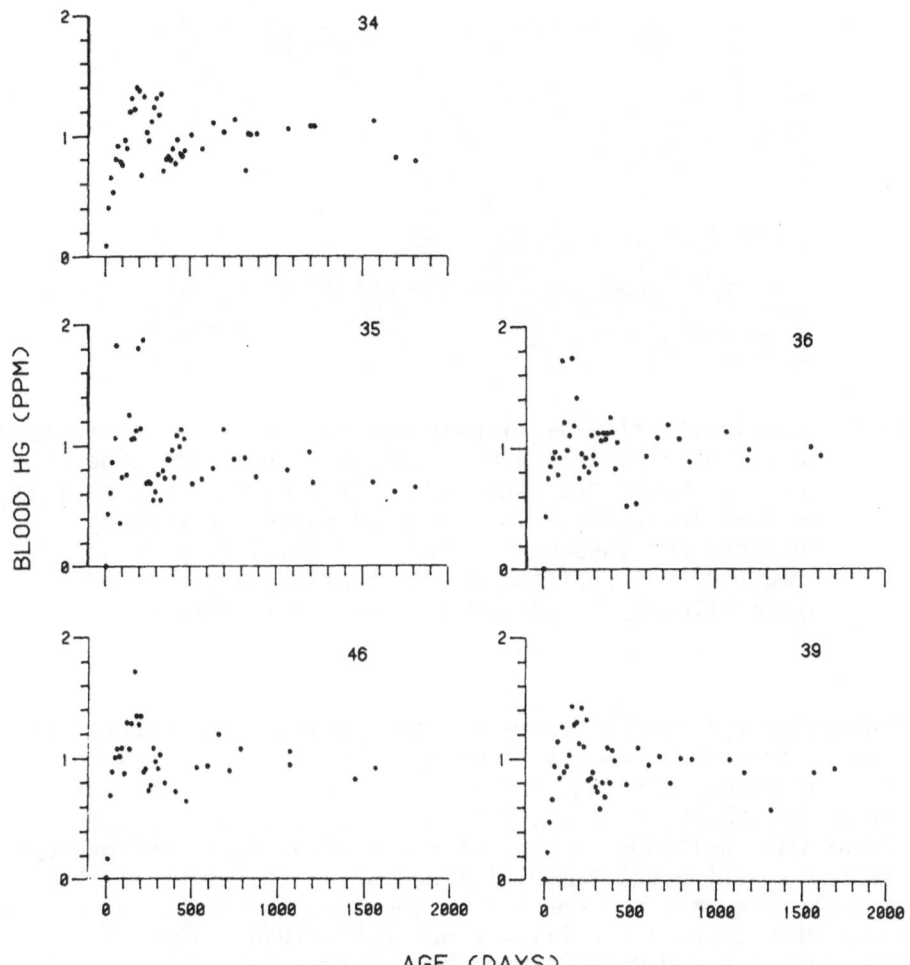

AGE (DAYS)

Figure 7   Total blood mercury levels for monkeys dosed with
           methylmercury from birth onward. Monkeys were weaned from
           infant formula at 20 days of age. Testing was begun when
           monkeys were approximately three years old.

     At the high luminance, two of the treated monkeys gave
performances indistinguishable from controls, two were impaired at
high spatial frequencies and somewhat impaired at middle frequencies,
and the fifth was severely impaired at all but very low spatial
frequencies (Figure 9). At the low luminance, all of the treated
monkeys were moderately impaired, with each individual monkey
showing a somewhat unique deficity.

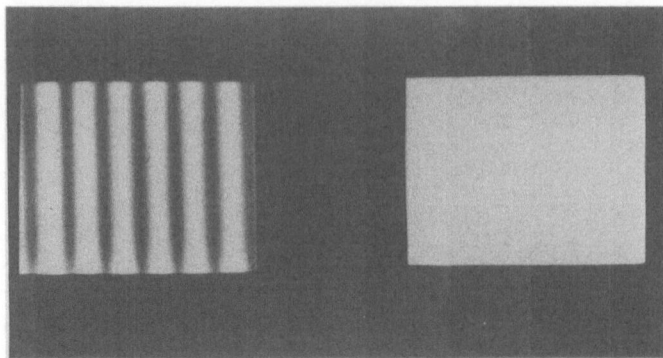

Figure 8 Example of stimulus display for testing of spatial visual
          function. The left scope contains a vertical sine wave
          grating, while the other scope is a blank field of equal
          average luminance. The scope on which the grating
          appeared was chosen randomly from trial to trial.
          Frequency and contrast of the grating were changed
          systematically to determine a threshold function.

        Following the evaluation of spatial vision, the temporal visual
function of these monkeys was examined. Instead of discriminating a
pattern, the monkey was required to choose the scope that was
flickering (blinking) from the one that was not. The design of the
experiment was analogous to that of the spatial task; the monkeys
were tested at different temporal frequencies (rates of flicker),
and at each frequency the modulation depth at which the monkey could
no longer discriminate the flicker was determined. The
methylmercury treated monkeys performed better than did control
monkeys under the same conditions (Figure 10). There is some
indication that the treated monkeys performed better than the
controls under the high luminance condition at the middle
frequencies. All but one treated monkey were clearly better than
controls under the low luminance condition, throughout the entire
range of frequencies.

        These results may be interpreted as resulting from the
plasticity of the nervous system of the young organism, and its
response to insult by methylmercury. Detection of high spatial
frequencies requires a relatively linear representation of neurons
from retina to cortex, in order to retain the necessary detailed
information. Temporal discrimination is subserved by a system that
would be made more sensitive by convergence of neurons between
retina and cortex; this would be truer under low luminance
conditions than high. It is well established that methylmercury
destroys visual cortex while sparing (relatively) other parts of the

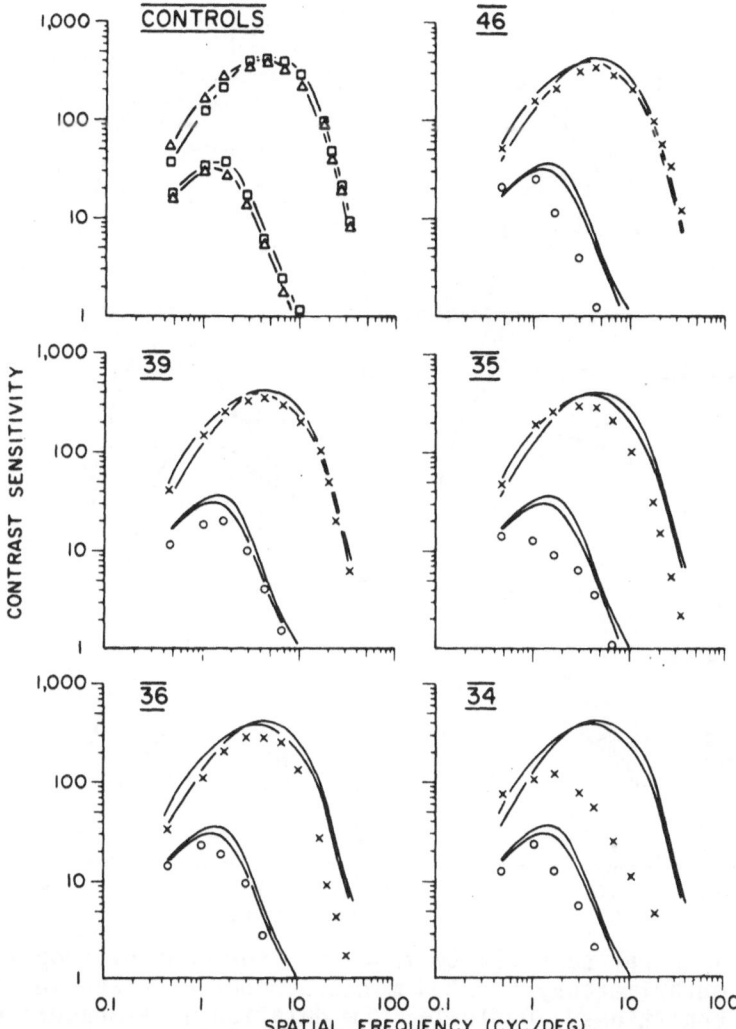

Figure 9 Spatial contrast sensitivity functions for two control (top left) and five methylmercury treated monkeys under high and low luminance conditions. Ordinate: contrast sensitivity = 100/contrast. For the control monkeys, the squares and triangles represent the individual animals. For each treated monkey, the x's represent threshold at each frequency under high luminance conditions, and circles the thresholds at low luminance conditions. Solid lines on each graph represent envelope of thresholds for control monkeys.

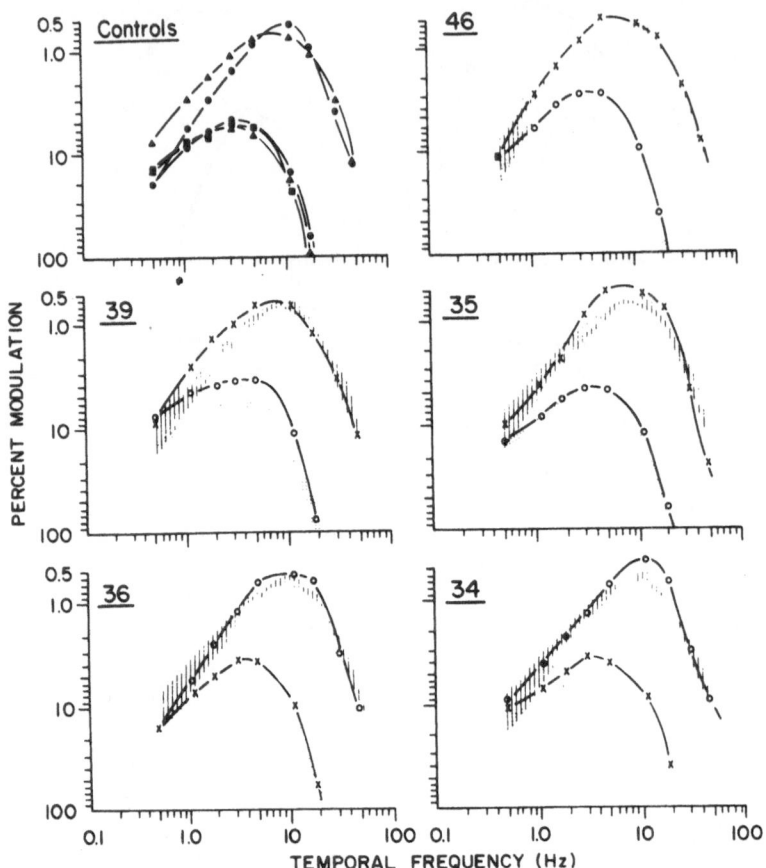

Figure 10   Temporal sensitivity functions for control (top left) and
            methylmercury treated monkeys under high and low luminance
            conditions. Ordinate: modulation is a measure of
            difference between the maximum and minimum luminance of
            the flicker. For the control monkeys, each symbol
            represents an individual. An additional control was
            added to the experiment but completed only the low
            luminance curve because of illness. For the treated
            monkeys, the symbols are as in Figure 9. Striped areas
            represent the envelope of control values under high
            luminance conditions, stippled areas represent low
            luminance values for controls.

visual system. It is becoming increasingly clear that the nervous
system continues to develop for a considerable period after birth,
with many more connections being formed than are present in the
adult, and which degenerate as the young organism matures. (For an
interesting discussion of nervous system development, see Clark,
1981). Such a mechanism may be used to explain the present
results. During the course of normal development, connection would
be made that would normally be "wrong" or superfluous and would
disappear later as the organism matured. As cells were lost from
visual cortex as a result of methylmercury exposure, "wrong"
connections would remain intact and perhaps new connections made to
remaining neurons. This would produce deficits in high frequency
spatial vision, because of the linear relationship needed to carry
such information would be lost. Temporal visual detection (for
broad fields) would be benefited, however, since convergence would
be increased. This hypothesis is obviously speculative, but it is
consistent with what is known about the effects of methylmercury and
the development of the nervous system.

In Utero Plus Postnatal Exposure

It is well established that methylmercury crosses the placenta
and can produce severe neurological and intellectual impairment in
the infant (Chang, 1977). A study was undertaken to determine the
potential hazard to the offspring of methylmercury ingestion by the
mother.

Fifteen cycling females (five at each level) were dosed until
their blood levels stabilized at an average of 1.5, 0.7 or .27 ppm
for doses of 50, 25 or 10 µg/kg/day, respectively (Figure 11). When
blood levels were stable, females were bred to untreated males. All
five of the high dose monkeys delivered live infants. Only three of
the ten monkeys from the two lower doses delivered live infants; one
delivered a dead infant and the remainder failed to get pregnant.
This is not atypical for the colony.

Infants were born with higher blood mercury levels than their
mothers (Figure 12). The relationship between infant blood mercury
level at birth and either mother's dose or mother's blood level did
not depart statistically from linearily (Figures 13 and 14). This
cannot be stated with certainty, however, since there are only a
total of three infants at the lower two doses. The infants' blood
levels decreased rapidly after birth to a steady state level lower
than that of the mothers: to approximately one-half of maternal
values in the case of the higher two doses. This was true even
though the infants were dosed from birth onwards at the same dose
the mothers had received.

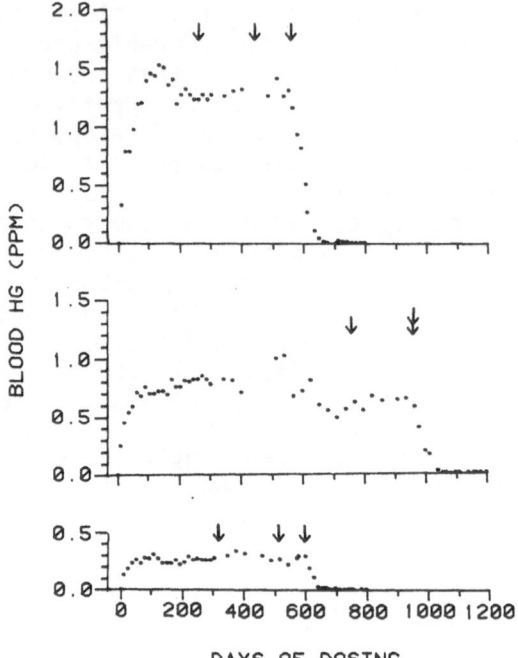

Figure 11   Sample total blood Hg curves for individual females dosed
             with (top to bottom) 50, 25 or 100 µg/kg/day of
             methylmercury. For each graph, the arrows indicate
             conception, delivery, and end of dosing, respectively.

        One of the infants in the high dose group was born with signs
similar to those seen in human fetal poisoning (Figure 15); this
infant's mother had the highest steady state blood mercury (1.8 ppm).

        The monkeys in the 25 and 50 µg/kg/day dose group and their
controls were tested on a discrimination paradigm and series of
reversals as infants (4-8 months old), excluding the monkey with
signs (monkey 110). Each infant was housed in a stainless steel
cage, and faced a panel on which were two push buttons and a tube
for delivery of infant formula. Sessions were 16 hours a day, and
infants received as much or more formula than those not being
tested. The infants were trained on the final discrimination by a
series of training procedures. As each monkey learned one step in
the procedure, the next step was introduced, until the monkey was
responding on the final pair of stimuli. Initially the monkey was
required to respond on the disk backlit with a red light rather than
the unlit disk in order to receive a reinforcement of infant
formula. When the infant had learned this task, a green light was

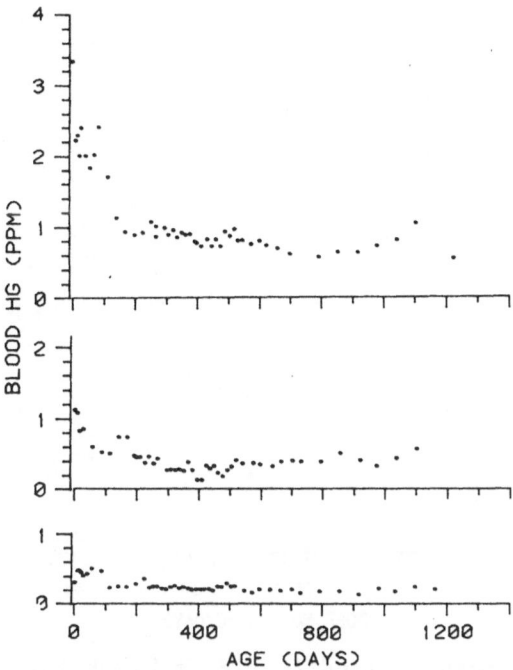

Figure 12   Sample total blood Hg curves for individual infants dosed
in utero plus postnatally with (top to bottom) 50, 25 or
10 μg/kg/day of methylmercury.

introduced as the negative stimulus. Two-dimensional forms (a cross
and triangle) were then superimposed on the colors, so that
cross-red was always correct, and triangle-green was incorrect.
Finally the colors were removed, and the infant was required to
respond on the cross and avoid the triangle. When the infant
performed to criterion on this task, a series of five reversals was
implemented to test the ability of the infant to reverse its
response choice from the previously correct stimulus to the
previously incorrect stimulus to the previous incorrect one. While
there is some indication that monkeys in the high dose group took
longer to learn the original discrimination (red-dark), treated
monkeys were certainly able to learn the task and performed as well
as controls on the series of reversals (Figure 16).

     Treated monkey 110 and a naive control were tested using
special apparatus beginning at nine months of age. There was a
feeder beneath each response level, and the monkey responded by
pressing with its nose. Both monkeys performed very well during the
first three stages of the acquisition of the task. The treated

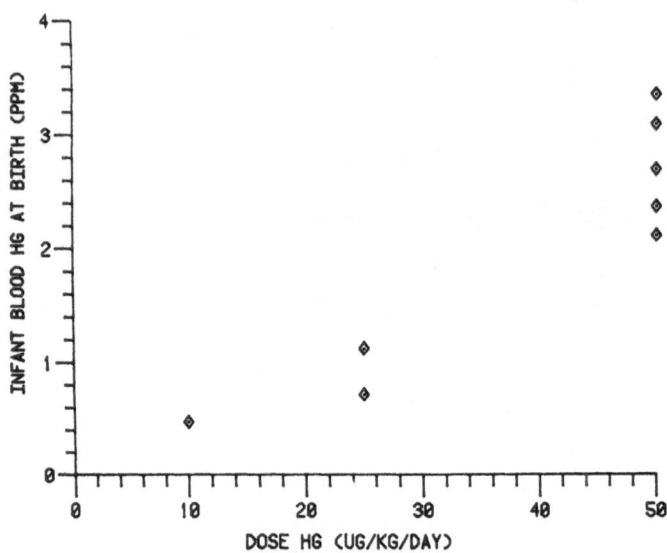

Figure 13   Total mercury blood levels at birth for infants as a
function of their mother's dose.

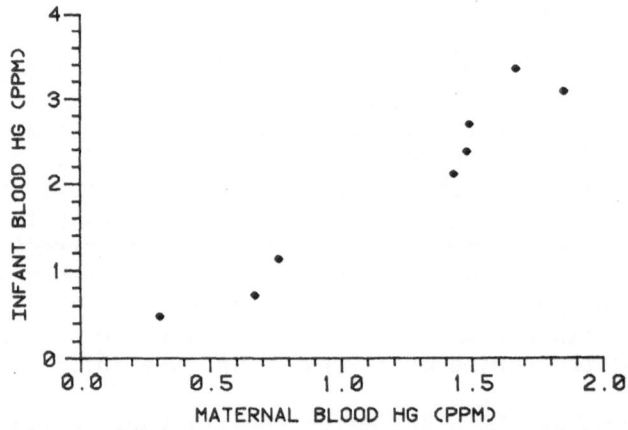

Figure 14   Total mercury blood levels at birth for infants as a
function of mother's equilibrium blood mercury level.

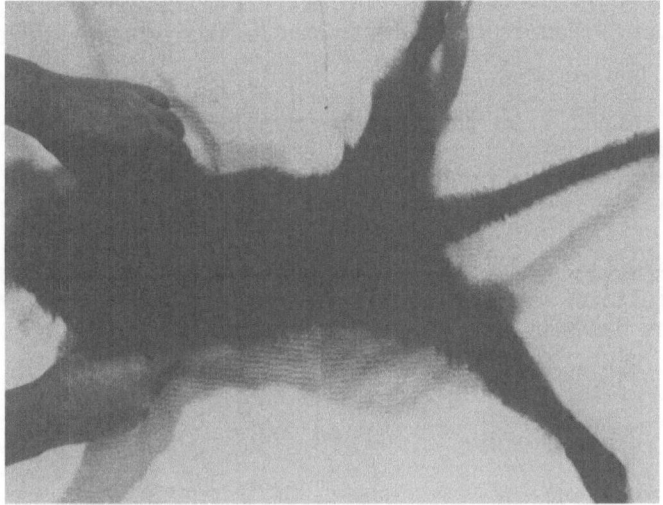

Figure 15   Monkey 110, from the 50 µg/kg/day mercury dose groups, at
            approximately three years of age. This monkey suffered
            neurological impairment; skeleton was normal.

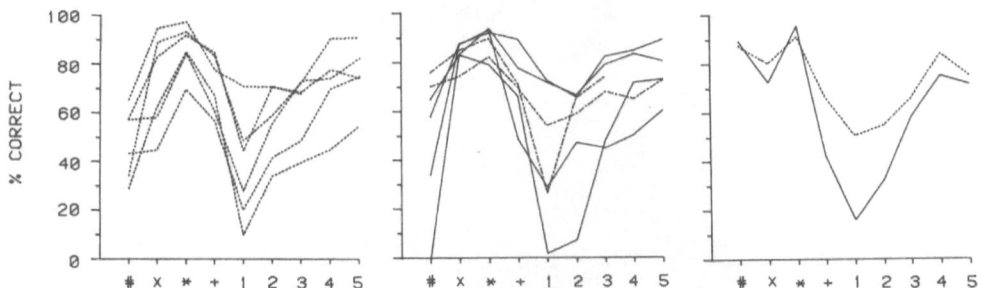

Figure 16   Percent correct for the first session for each change in
            schedule for infants on a discrimination task and series
            of reversals.   = red-dark discrimination. x = red-
            green. * = red cross-green triangle. + = cross-triangle.
            Numbers represent reversals of cross-triangle
            discrimination. Left graph represents performance of the
            six control monkeys tested at 4-8 months of age. Center
            graph represent four monkeys at the high dose (solid
            lines) and two at the middle dose (dashed lines). Right
            graph represents high dose monkeys (monkey 110) (solid
            line) and control (dashed line) tested at 9 months of age.

monkey did not perform as well initially on the form task, or during the first several reversals. Performance improved by reversal 4, however.

Another infant from this group (monkey 99) developed slight motor signs in the hind limbs and nystagmus, as well as a generalized debilitated condition, beginning at about one year of age (Figure 17).

At three years of age all of these monkeys were tested on a form discrimination and series of reversals similar to the task they had learned as infants. All but monkey 110 performed as well as

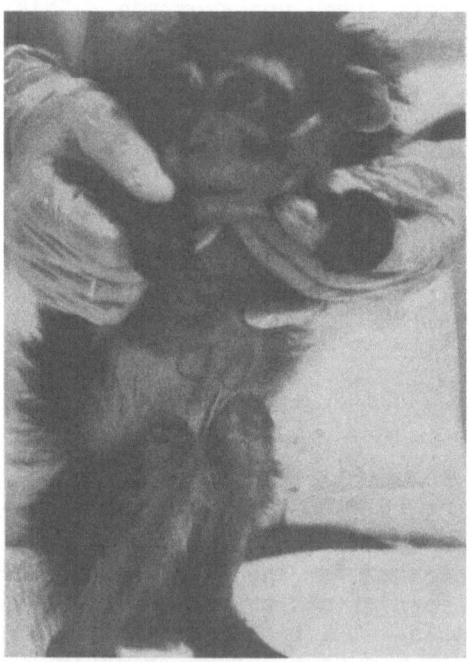

Figure 17   Monkey 99, from the mercury high dose group, at
            approximately 3 years of age. This monkey appeared
            normal until one year old, then developed slight
            neurological signs and a progressive general debilitation.
            Performance on a series of discrimination reversals was
            normal when the monkey was in this condition.

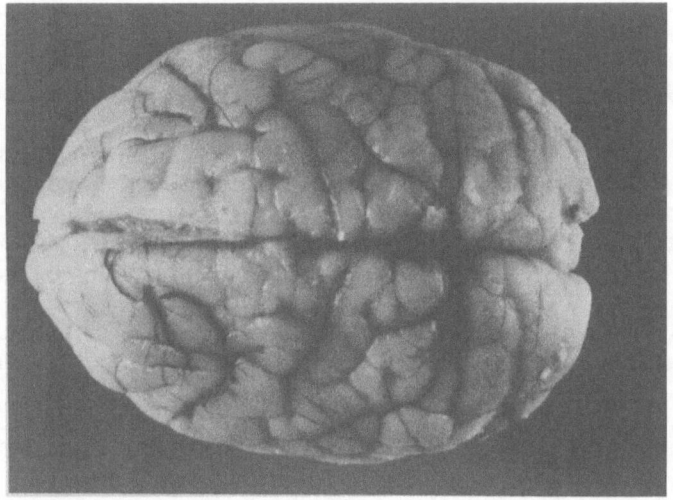

Figure 18   Brain of monkey 110, from the mercury high dose group, is
            superficially normal.

controls, although two monkeys from the high dose group (99 and 102)
refused to respond with their hands and were allowed to respond by
touching their mouths to the appropriate feeder. Monkey 110 had
severe nystagmus at this age, and although it was able to learn a
light-dark discrimination, further training was unsuccessful. Both
110 and 99 have been sacrificed. Although a detailed examination has
not yet been performed, the brains are superficially normal (Figure
18).

It appears that fetal methylmercury poisoning in the
cynomologus monkey produces neurological signs similar to those
observed in humans, but not the severe intellectual impairment that
one might expect in humans with such obvious neurological signs. We
will pursue our examination of sensory systems in these monkeys,
including both the visual and auditory systems.

In conclusion, we have found the primate an extremely useful
model with which to explore the effects of heavy metals in the young
organism. This is true for biochemical, physiological, and kinetic
studies as well as for determination of central nervous system
effects. The use of relatively sophisticated behavioral testing,
including determination of sensory system function, has allowed
detection of deficits produced by chronic exposure to low levels of
toxicants, even with small groups of monkeys.

REFERENCES

Amin-Zaki, L., Elhassani, S., Majeed, M., Clarkson, T.W., Doherty, R. and Greenwood, M.R., 1974, Studies of infants postnatally exposed to methylmercury, J. Pediatr. 85:(1)81-84.

Beattie, A., Moore, M., Goldberg, A., Finlayson, M., Graham, J., Mackie, E., Main, J., McLaren, D., Murdoch, R. and Stewart, G., 1975, Role of chronic low-level lead exposure in the aetiology of mental retardation, Lancet 3:589-592.

Chang, L.W., 1977, Neurotoxic effects of mercury - A review, Environ. Res. 14:329-373.

Clarke, P., 1981, Chance, repetition, and error in the development of normal nervous systems, Persp. in Biology and Medicine 25:2-19.

Cory-Slechta, D.A., 1982, The behavioral toxicity of lead: problems and perspectives, in: "Adv. Behav. Pharmacol. IV.", T. Thompson and P.B. Dews, eds., in press.

de la Burde, B. and Choate, M., 1975, Early asymptomatic lead exposure and development at school age, J. Pediat. 87:638-642.

de Valois, R., Morgan, H. and Snodderly, D., 1974, Psychophysical studies in monkey vision - III. Spatial luminance contrast sensitivity tests of macaque and human observers, Vision Res. 14:75-81.

Good, P., 1979, Detection of a treatment effect when not all experimental subjects will respond to treatment, Biometrics 35:483-489.

Harlow, H.F., Harlow, M.K., Schiltz, K.A. and Mohr, D.J., 1971, The effect of early adverse and enriched environments on the learning ability of rhesus monkeys, in: "Cognitive Processes of Nonhuman Primates", L.E. Jarrard, ed., pp. 121-147, Academic Press, New York.

Landrigan, P., Whitworth, R., Baloh, R., Stachling, N., Barthel, W. and Rosenblum, B., 1975, Neuropsychological dysfunction in children with chronic low-level lead absorption, Lancet 1:708-712.

Needleman, H., Gunnoe, C., Leviton, A., Reed, R., Peresie, H., Maher, C. and Barrett, P., 1979, Deficits in psychologic and classroom performance of children with elevated lead levels, N. Engl. J. Med. 300:689-695.

Rice, D.C., Gilbert, S.G. and Willes, R.F., 1979, Neonatal low-level lead exposure in monkeys: locomotor activity, schedule, controlled behavior, and the effects of amphetamine, Toxicol. Appl. Pharmacol. 51: 503-513.

Rice, D.C. and Willes, R.F., 1979, Neonatal low-level lead exposure in monkeys (Macaca fascicularis): effects of two-choice non-spatial form discrimination, J. Environ. Path. Toxicol. 2:1195-1203.

Rice, D. and Gilbert, S., 1982, Early chronic low-level methylmercury poisoning in monkeys impairs spatial vision, Science 216:759-761.

Rustam, H. and Hamdi, T., 1974, Methylmercury poisoning in Iraq - A
    neurological study, Brain 77:499.
Sabelaish, S. and Hilmi, G., 1976, Ocular manifestations of mercury
    poisoning, Bull WHO: supp. 83-86.
Willes, R., Kressler, P., and Truelove, J., 1977, Nursery rearing of
    infant monkeys (Macaca fascicularis) for toxicity studies, Lab.
    Animal Sci. 27:90-98.
Winneke, G., Brochhaus, A., Kramer, V., Ewen, U., Kujanek, G.,
    Lechner, H. and Janke, W., 1981, Neuropsychological comparison
    of children with different tooth lead levels. Preliminary
    Report. In Proceedings of International Conference, Heavy
    Metals in the Environment, pp. 553-556, WHO, Amsterdam. CEP
    Consultants: Edinburgh.
Yule, W., Landsdown, R., Miller, I., and Irbanowicz, M., 1981, The
    relationship between blood lead concentrations, intelligence
    and attainment in a school population: a pilot study, Develop.
    Med. Child Neurol. 23:567-576.

DEVELOPMENTAL TOXICITY OF METALS: IMPLICATIONS FOR PUBLIC HEALTH

J. Julian Chisolm, Jr.[1] and David J. Thomas[2]

[1]Department of Pediatrics
 Johns Hopkins School of Medicine
[2]Department of Environmental Health Sciences
 Johns Hopkins School of Hygiene and Public Health
 Baltimore, Maryland

ABSTRACT

The second National Health and Nutrition Examination Survey (NHANES II) conducted between 1976 and 1980 has provided the most comprehensive epidemiological assessment of lead absorption in the general population ever made in the United States. The data indicate that an estimated 4.0 percent, or approximately 675,000 children, aged six months to five years, have blood lead concentrations greater than the upper limit of the currently accepted "normal" range, namely $\geq$ 30 µg Pb/dl whole blood. The influence of family income and residence is striking. Increased lead absorption (PbB $\geq$ 30 µg, PbB = µg Pb/dl whole blood) is the highest among low income urban black children (18.6 percent) and the lowest among rural white children (1.2 percent). The NHANES II data suggest that average PbB for the entire population decreased from 15.8 µg to 10 µg Pb/dl whole blood between 1976 and 1980. This decrease may reflect decreases in both the lead content of food and in the use of lead additives in gasoline. If this trend is confirmed, it is likely that only old deteriorated lead-painted housing will remain as the primary environmental source of lead for young children in the United States. The prevalence of increased lead absorption in United States children, as estimated from NHANES II data, appears higher than that based upon reports from other industrialized countries.

Data in experimental animals suggest that modest increases in lead absorption during very early life do lead to subtle, but lasting impediments in neurodevelopment and cognitive function. Despite the many retrospective and cross-sectional studies on this

issue in children, the risks associated with various levels of lead
absorption remain poorly defined, particularly in regard to low
level increased lead absorption as reflected by PbBs maintained
throughout early childhood in the range of 25 to 40 µg. Hopefully,
long-term prospective studies now in progress will help to resolve
this controversial but important public health problem.

Overexposure of infants and young children to arsenic has been
limited largely to outbreaks of poisoning due to contamination of
food and drinking water. While small outbreaks may not be totally
avoidable in the practical sense, it does appear that large
epidemics such as those that have occurred in Japan, Taiwan and
Chile, could be avoided through appropriate monitoring of public
drinking water supplies and quality control in food production.
Although human data are scanty, they do suggest that neurobehavioral
and neurotoxicological assessment should be included in any future
studies and that such studies should be prospective in design.

The toxicity of methylmercury may be modified by age at
exposure. The fetus appears to be especially sensitive. Some human
studies suggest that effects on subsequent growth and development
may be produced by exposure in utero to methylmercury at levels
which produce no signs of methylmercury intoxication in pregnant
women. The consumption of methylmercury contaminated fish is the
primary source of human exposure to methylmercury. Reductions of
methylmercury intake could be achieved by reducing acceptable limits
for methylmercury in fish and/or by reducing consumption of
methylmercury-containing fish.

INTRODUCTION

The past decade has seen a great increase in the number of both
human and experimental studies on the toxicity of such metals as
lead, arsenic and methylmercury. Most of these studies have
appeared since the publication of "Effects and Dose-Response
Relationships of Toxic Metals"(Nordberg, 1976), which was based upon
proceedings of an international meeting organized by the
Subcommittee on the Toxicology of Metals of the Permanent Commission
and International Association of Occupational Health held in Tokyo
in November, 1974. In most cases these recent studies have dealt
with combined pre- and postnatal exposures. During the past decade
substantial progress has been made in the design of human studies
and in refinement of methodologies for assessing neurodevelopment
during infancy and early childhood. Even so, "no detected effect
levels" remain to be determined; although, prospective studies now
in progress on pre- and postnatal lead exposure may well narrow the
area of uncertainty concerning lead exposure and its effects on
early neurodevelopment.

LEAD

During the past century lead has been widely disseminated into the human environment, especially into the urban areas of industrialized countries. The nature and extent of the risk of adverse effects on the developing nervous system associated with such exposure remain an important, but unresolved, public health issue. Here we provide: 1) a synopsis of recent epidemiological data for the United States; 2) an overview of recent clinical studies; and 3) comments on six prospective studies now in progress on human pre- and postnatal low level lead exposure.

Epidemiological Data

The second National Health and Nutrition Examination Survey (NHANES II) conducted between 1976 and 1980 has provided the most comprehensive epidemiological assessment of lead absorption in the general population ever made in the United States (Annest et al., 1982; Mahaffey et al., 1982). Blood lead data are based entirely on venous samples, inasmuch as pilot data showed that contamination of capillary samples was unavoidable. The data indicate that an estimated 4.0 percent, or approximately 675,000 children, aged six months to five years, have blood lead concentrations $\geq$ 30 μg/dl whole blood (PbB $\geq$ 30 μg). Owing to the higher prevalence among black children, an estimated 315,000 of these 675,000 children are black. A PbB $\geq$ 30 μg is the action level proposed in the United States Center for Disease Control guidelines for the prevention of lead poisoning in children (Center for Disease Control, 1978). This action level is based upon the use of the "free" erythrocyte protoporphyrin (FEP) test as a biochemical indicator of early metabolic effect of lead. A dose-related increase in FEP occurs as PbB increases above approximately 25-30 μg in children. Table 1 shows the distribution of PbB according to race and sex in this age group. The influence of family income and residence on PbB is striking (Table 2). Increased lead absorption (PbB $\geq$ 30 μg) is highest among low income black children (18.6 percent) and lowest among rural white children (1.2 percent). Further analysis of the NHANES II data indicate that average PbB for the entire United States population decreased from 15.8 μg to 10 μg Pb/dl whole blood between 1976 and 1980 (Center for Disease Control, 1982). The decrease may reflect decreases in both the lead content of food (Schaffner, 1981) and the use of lead additives in gasoline (Center for Disease Control, 1982). This trend suggests that only old, deteriorated lead-painted housing is likely to remain as the primary environmental source of lead for young children in the United States.

In 1979 selective screening of 39 groups of children thought to be at high risk for increased lead absorption was conducted in the United Kingdom (Department of Health and Social Security, 1980).

Table 1   Distribution of PbB Levels by Race and Sex in Children Aged 6 Months – 5 Years: United States, 1976-1980*

	Estimated Population in Thousands	Mean	PbB level (μg/dl)[a]						
			<10	10-19	20-29	30-39	40-49	50-59	60-69
			Percent of Distribution[c]						
All Races[b]									
Male	8,621	16.3	11.0	63.5	21.2	4.0	0.3	0.0	0.0
Female	8,241	15.8	13.5	63.2	19.8	3.0	0.3	0.2	--
White									
Male	6,910	15.2	13.0	67.6	17.3	2.0	0.1	--	--
Female	6,732	14.7	16.1	67.3	14.8	1.6	0.1	0.1	--
Black									
Male	1,307	20.7	2.7	48.8	35.1	11.1	1.9	0.2	0.3
Female	1,277	21.0	2.2	41.6	45.3	9.2	0.9	0.8	--

[a]At the midpoint of the survey, March 1, 1978.
[b]Includes data for races not shown separately.
[c]Numbers may not add to totals due to rounding.

*Adapted from the second National Health and Nutrition Examination Survey, National Center for Health Statistics, 1982.

Table 2   Percent of Children Aged 6 Months - 5 Years with PbB Levels of 30.0 µg/dl or More: United States, 1976-80*

Demographic Variable	All [a]	Race	
		White	Black
A. Annual family income			
Under $6,000	10.9	5.9	18.5
$6,000 - $14,999	4.2	2.2	12.1
$15,000 or more	1.2	0.7	2.8
B. Degree of urbanization			
Urban, 1,000,000 persons or more	7.2	4.0	15.2
Central city	11.6	4.5	18.6
Non-central city	3.7	3.8	3.3[b]
Urban, less than 1,000,000 persons	3.5	1.6	10.2
Rural	2.1	1.2	10.3[b]

[a]Includes data for races not shown separately.
[b]Number of sample persons in cell is less than 50.
*Adapted from the second National Health and Nutrition Examination Survey, National Center for Health Statistics, 1982.

Increased lead absorption (defined as PbB > 35 µg) was found in three groups: in Glasgow, Scotland, where the lead content of household drinking water has been a major source of overexposure; in one of several groups of children of lead workers; and in one group of children living near a lead works.

Recent Clinical Studies

Five major critical reviews of the more than 20 recent human studies on the pre- and postnatal neurobehavioral and developmental effects of lead exposure have appeared since 1976 (Bornschein et al., 1980; Department of Health and Social Security, 1980; National Academy of Sciences, 1980; Needleman, 1980; Rutter, 1980). With one exception, namely, the study of de la Burde and Choate (1975), all published studies have been cross-sectional or retrospective. Most reviewers are agreed that the human studies so far reported have methodologic deficiencies, although the deficiencies vary in type and severity from one study to another. Nevertheless, there is general agreement that PbBs which are persistently raised above 60 µg are associated with an increased risk of long-lasting behavioral handicaps and an average reduction of three to four I.Q. points even in asymptomatic children. There may also be similar but lesser increased risk of adverse sequelae associated with persistently elevated PbB in the range of 40 to 60 µg/dl but this conclusion rests upon less firm data. Of particular interest is the retrospective study of Rummo (1974), which attempted to address the issue of dose-duration-response. Although she studied the children at seven to eight years of age, she had available serial PbB data from the preschool years. She divided children with repeated PbBs > 40 µg into two groups, those with PbB > 40 µg for less than six months (short-term group) and those with two PbBs > 40 µg separated by more than six months (long-term group). For the short-term group, no difference in I.Q., measured by the general cognitive index (McCarthy Scales), was found in comparison with controls who had PbB consistently < 30 µg. However, a dose-related decrement in I.Q. was found among those children with PbB in excess of 40 µg for longer than six months.

       The extent to which cognitive development may be impaired with PbB levels in the 20 to 40 µg range remains controversial. The study of Needleman et al. (1979) is generally considered the best designed clinical study to date and the findings are highly provocative. This retrospective study is based upon differences in the lead content of shed deciduous teeth. Although systematic prior serial PbB data were not available, 23 of the high dentine lead group and 58 of the low dentine lead group had blood lead tests at three to four years of age. Mean PbB in the high dentine lead group at that time was 35.5 µg (range 18-54 µg), while mean PbB was 23.8 µg (range 12-37 µg) in the low dentine lead group. Average intelligence quotient, as measured by the Wexler Intelligence Scale for Children (WISC), was four points lower in the high dentine lead group than in the low dentine lead group. Slower reaction time and shorter attention span were found in the high dentine lead group. There was a uniform shift in I.Q. scores, which were normally distributed about their means, in both the high and low dentine lead group (Needleman et al., 1982). Thus, a child in the high dentine lead group was three times more likely to have an I.Q. < 80 than a child with a low dentine lead level. This highlights the significance, from a public health perspective, of such a seemingly small decrease in average I.Q. (Rutter, 1980). More striking was the dose-related increase in the frequency of detrimental classroom behaviors reported blindly by the children's school teachers. These included, among others, short attention span, easy distractibility and decreased ability to follow a sequence of instructions. These findings have been independently confirmed by Winneke et al. (1981). Although not nearly as severe, these findings are reminiscent of the study of Byers and Lord (1943), who reported qualitatively similar but more severe neurobehavioral handicaps 40 years ago in a small group of children, many of whom had recurrent and severe symptomatic plumbism during the preschool years.

Recently, reviewers and investigators have concentrated their attention on the deficiencies of earlier studies in the hope of facilitating better designed future studies. The major deficiencies of past studies include: 1) inadequate estimation of dose; 2) inadequate control of confounding variables; 3) bias in sample selection; and 4) the overuse of global measures of intelligence and inadequate use of more sensitive neurobehavioral and neurophysiological test batteries (Needleman, 1980). A serious limitation in most of the retrospective and cross-sectional studies has been inadequate estimation of dose. Most investigators have used PbB to classify the level of lead absorption in exposed and control groups. In some follow-up studies, PbB data from the remote past were used but PbBs were not repeated at the time of neurobehavioral evaluation made during the early school years. Lead has a half-life in blood of approximately 20 days (Rabinowitz et al., 1976). Furthermore, PbB is strongly influenced by recent and current exposure and so does not provide a useful marker of past absorption in retrospective studies. On the other hand, serial PbB measurements made at three month intervals could provide a useful and practical marker for dose in long-term prospective studies. The same comments can be applied to the use of the FEP test and other biochemical indicators of lead's acute effect on heme synthesis as these are relatively short-term, reversible responses. The calcium disodium ethylenediaminetetraacetic acid mobilization test for lead is significantly correlated with PbB but does not provide evidence of excessive lead absorption in the remote past (Chisolm et al., 1976). Needleman et al. (1979) used the dentine lead content of shed deciduous teeth in their retrospective study. This marker reflects the total accumulation of lead in the tooth throughout its life span. While this approach permits an estimate of total dose in the absence of serial PbB data, it does not provide a precise estimate of the age or length of time that overexposure occurred. The combination of serial PbB data and the dentine lead content of shed deciduous teeth could in future studies provide an adequate estimate of dose.

The major concern about prenatal and early postnatal lead exposure is the relative risk that various levels of lead absorption may pose for mental retardation, learning deficits, visual-motor impairment and non-adaptive classroom behavior. A number of other factors have been shown to influence behavioral and cognitive development. These serve as confounding variables in the assessment of lead's contribution to these unwanted outcomes. Such factors include genetic endowment (parental I.Q.), socioeconomic status, inadequate prenatal care and nutrition, perinatal disease, anemia, intercurrent disease affecting the central nervous system during early life, undernutrition, parental rearing attitudes, home environment, family size, birth order, age and pica (Cowan and Leviton, 1980). The three major factors, which have not been uniformly controlled in past studies, are 1) socioeconomic class, 2) maternal intelligence and 3) the caregiving environment in the home (Bornschein et al., 1980; Rutter, 1980; Schroeder et al., 1981). The other factors, while difficult to control in retrospective studies, may be incorporated readily into the design of prospective studies. Control for socioeconomic status alone, as in many past studies, is not sufficient, as it does not fully compensate for variations in maternal I.Q. and the variable influence of caregiving in the home environment. The caregiving environment in the home may also influence the amount of nonfood lead that a young child ingests. In their assessment of factors tending to intensify pica, Lourie et al. (1963) identified "absence of mothering" as a major factor contributing to pica. Lourie et al. (1963) also viewed pica as a major response of young children to maternal stress. Heber (1970) found concordance between maternal and child intelligence. The quality of the caregiving environment in children has been assessed with the Home Observation for Measurement of the Environment (HOME) Inventory developed by Caldwell et al. (1966). Subsequently, Bradley and Caldwell (1976a,b) used the HOME Inventory to identify factors in the child's environment during the first two years of life which were related to psychometric test scores at 36 and 54 months of age. Two of the subscales on the HOME Inventory that were strongly related to later intellectual development were emotional and verbal responsivity of the mother and maternal involvement with the child. These two subscales were identified by Milar et al. (1980) as showing significant deficiencies in the environment of children with increased lead burden. The results of Milar et al. (1980) suggest the possibility that intellectual deficits found in children exposed to lead may be a direct result of deficiencies in the caregiving environment and may not be related to lead at all. However, these workers could not rule out the possibility that deficiencies in the caregiving environment during the early years were responsible for the increased lead burden and that the deficiencies seen later were due to lead. Nor could they rule out a third hypothesis, namely, that the caregiving environment and lead combined to impair subsequent intellectual development. In any event, it would appear that deficiencies in the caregiving environment in the home during the first two years of life can increase the risk of increased lead absorption if that child is overexposed to environmental lead. How potentially confounding variables are dealt with will depend on the

number of confounding variables, resources available for study and
the available sample size. If the sample size is small, subtle
deficits, if present, are not likely to be reliably identified
(Cowan and Leviton, 1980).

There is need for sensitive measures of neurobehavioral outcome
if subtle effects are to be detected (Needleman et al., 1979). In
the past, heavy reliance has been placed upon global measures of
cognitive development. Most such tests are standardized only for
children older than three to five years of age. Thus, the
assessment of neurotoxicity in very young children poses serious
problems, particularly when one considers that infants and toddlers
represent the segment of the population that is uniquely susceptible
to injury due to the immaturity of the nervous system. The design
of a battery of electrophysiological tests that is free of
linguistic, cultural and motor constraints is essential for reliable
neurotoxicological evaluation in very young children (Otto, 1981).
Otto has proposed that electrophysiological neurotoxicity tests
should meet the selection criteria required of psychometric tests.
Each test should be standardized, valid, reliable, sensitive and
objective. Preferably, such tests should also be culture-free,
non-threatening, non-invasive and as age-independent as possible.
He has classified the available electrophysiological tests suitable
for use in young children, according to these and other criteria
(Table 3).

Among these, the brainstem auditory evoked potential (BAEP) and
the pattern-reversal visual evoked potential (PREP) are, perhaps,
the best standardized and come closest to meeting the criteria. The
BAEP is not affected by changes in arousal level, and adult
latencies are reached by the age of 18 months. The visual pathway
may be particularly sensitive to the effect of lead so that
intensive work is needed to find ways to obtain the required
cooperation and visual fixation of very young children in order to
use the PREP test. In a pilot study, Otto et al. (1981) used
event-related slow visual potentials and found a positive linear
dose-related decrement over a PbB range of six to 59 µg. This test
is thought to be related to information processing, cognition and
memory; however, the study requires replication in a larger group of
children as well as further experience to evaluate its functional
significance.

Prospective Studies

Most investigators and reviewers are agreed that prospective
studies initiated as soon after conception as possible provide the
best means of evaluating the risks associated with prenatal and
early postnatal lead exposure. A conference was held in Cincinnati,
Ohio, USA, September, 1981 (Bornschein, 1981) to bring together the

Table 3 Selection Criteria for Pediatric Neurotoxicity Tests

	IQ*	BAEP*	PREP*	SEP*	SW*	CNV*
Non-verbal	-	+	+	+	+	-
Non-motoric	-	+	+	+	+	-
Non-invasive	+	+	+	+	+	+
Non-threatening	+	+	-	-	+	+
Age-independent	-	+	+	+	-	-
Culture-free	-	+	+	+	+	μ
Standardized	+	+	+	+	-	-
Valid	+	+	+	+	μ	μ
Reliable	+	+	+	+	μ	μ
Sensitive	+	+	+	+	+	μ
Objective	+	+,	+	+	+	+
Rapid	-	+	+	+	-	+
Simple	-	+	+	-	+	+
Inexpensive	+	-	-	-	-	-

*IQ-Intelligence Quotient
 BAEP-Brainstem Auditory Evoked Potential
 PREP-Pattern Reversal Visual Evoked Potential
 SEP-Somatosensory Evoked Potential
 SW-Event-related Slow Potential (visual)
 CNV-Contingent Negative Variation

Adapted from Otto (1981)

six groups of investigators who have recently initiated prospective human studies. It was hoped that some features common to all could be incorporated in each design to facilitate cross-comparisons (Table 4). Most agreed to incorporate the Bayley and McCarthy Scales in their neurobehavioral test battery and the Caldwell HOME Inventory to assess parental caregiving. Each group will employ additional but differing techniques to evaluate attentional deficits, reaction time and the processing of visual stimuli. Other important independent variables, including socioeconomic status, maternal I.Q., perinatal factors, will be controlled primarily through stratification in the statistical analyses. PbBs will be measured at least annually, although some groups will measure dentine lead at six to eight years of age in shed deciduous teeth. Another important problem is the issue of blood lead proficiency testing programs and the current lack of availability of a certified blood lead reference sample. Whether this last difficulty can be overcome remains uncertain. Proficiency in dentine lead analysis will also require close scrutiny.

Preliminary data suggest that two of the groups may be dealing with significant prenatal overexposure to lead. The Scottish group has already reported retrospective data (Moore et al., 1977), suggesting that the very high lead content of drinking water in parts of Scotland may increase the risk of mental retardation when overexposure occurs prenatally and during the first year of postnatal life. This group anticipates PbBs ranging up to 40 µg in mothers and their newly born infants. A second prospective study in Port Pirie, South Australia, where a large lead smelter is located, was initiated because the age-standardized stillbirth rate in Port Pirie was approximately 50 percent higher than the rate for the rest of South Australia during 1968-76. It is anticipated that the PbB concentrations may range up to 50 µg. These two studies may offer the best opportunity of assessing the impact of the combined effects of pre- and postnatal overexposure to lead. A third study with heavy emphasis on prenatal and early postnatal exposure and neurobehavioral assessment is being carried out in the greater metropolitan area of Sydney, Australia, where mean PbB may fall between 10 and 15 µg and few values are expected to exceed 30 µg in pregnant women. This study is intended to evaluate the impact of ambient air lead levels in this city. These three studies deal entirely with Caucasian populations.

Two prospective studies now in progress in the United States are those based in Boston, MA, and Cincinnati, OH. Both will deal with mixed populations, although the one in Boston is predominantly white, while the one in Cincinnati is predominantly black. Elevated paired maternal and infant cord blood lead values are not anticipated, so that these studies are likely to be dealing with predominantly postnatal exposure. Indeed, the Boston group has recently reported finding a mean cord PbB in 11,837 newborns of 6.56 µg (+ 3.19 µg standard deviation, Rabinowitz and Needleman, 1982). In the Cincinnati study, PbB will be determined at three month intervals prenatally and postnatally until 60 months of age. This group anticipates encountering peak PbBs in a range 10-50 µg during early childhood.

The sixth study in North Carolina is focused on follow-up of children 12 to 60 months of age, whose mothers worked in a battery factory and contaminated their homes by bringing lead-bearing dust into the home on their work clothing. The principal issues to be

Table 4 Areas of Comparability in Prospective Studies[a]

	Boston MA	Cincinnati OH	Glasgow Scotland	Wake County NC	Port Pirie Australia	Sydney Australia
No. of Subjects	249	320	151	200	800	200
Bayley Scales						
6 mo.	x	x				x
12 mo.	x	x	x			x
24 mo.	x	x	x	x	x	x
McCarthy Scales						
36 mo.		x				x
48 mo.	x	x	x		x	x
60 mo.		x				x
H.O.M.E. Scales						
6 mo.	x	x				x
12 mo.		x				x
24 mo.	x	x		x		
36 mo.		x				x
Goodman Lock Box	x			x		
Blood Lead at Yearly Intervals	x	x	x	x	x	x
Dentine Lead (Shed deciduous teeth)	x		x	x	x	

[a]Adapted from the Proceedings of the First International Lead Conference, September, 1981, Cincinnati, Ohio, U.S.A. (Bornschein, 1981)

addressed in this study are the interaction between parental care giving and lead exposure and the question of reversibility of certain effects already observed in this population. In this study heavy emphasis will be placed on electrophysiological assessment of neurotoxicity in children.· A number of substances, including lead, have been found to be toxic to the visual system in humans. A major goal of this group is evaluation of the electrophysiological neurotoxicity test battery (Table 3), using lead as a model.

ARSENIC

Arsenical polyneuropathy is well documented in adults; however, the neurodevelopmental aspects of arsenic toxicity during infancy and childhood have received scant attention (Nordberg et al., 1979; National Academy of Sciences, 1977a,b). Rather, emphasis has been focused on the question of arsenic's carcinogenic potential and its dermatological and vascular effects. Three large scale studies of children overexposed to arsenic in drinking water have been reported. Arsenic in drinking water is generally assumed to be pentavalent arsenic (Pershagen, 1979). The United States Public Health drinking water standard is $\leq$ 50 µg As/liter. Among chronically exposed villagers in southwestern Taiwan, the frequency of hyperpigmentation, keratosis, skin cancer and "Blackfoot" disease increased in a dose-dependent manner with increasing arsenic content of well-water. Wells in these villages had been in use for at least 45 years and, at the time of testing, arsenic content ranged between 17 and 1,097 µg/liter with most samples falling between 400 and 600 µg As/liter (Tseng et al., 1968). In Antofagasta, Chile, findings among children exposed for about two years to a drinking water supply containing 800 µg As/liter included recurrent bronchopneumonia and bronchiectasis, hyperpigmentation, keratosis, and peripheral vascular disease including Raynaud's Syndrome (National Academy of Sciences, 1977a). In neither of these studies were children or adults examined for clinical or subclinical neurobehavioral effects. A much smaller population of children in the western United States exposed to 108-220 µg As/liter in drinking water were compared with controls whose water contained 20 µg As/liter (Southwick et al., 1982). A slightly increased proportion of the 145 "exposed" persons showed sub-clinical slowing of nerve conduction, but none showed any dermatological changes.

Bencko and Symon (1970) reported significant hearing loss (both air and bone conduction) in 50 ten year old Czechoslovak children, who lived near a power plant, burning coal of high arsenic content. In a small group of children in the western United States exposed to airborne arsenic, no impairment of hearing was found (Milham, 1977).

A follow-up study of the Morinaga arsenic-tainted powdered milk epidemic in western Japan has provided the only evidence that

overexposure to arsenic during infancy may have long-lasting
deterimental effects on neurodevelopment (Japanese Pediatric
Society, 1973). During the summer of 1955 an estimated 12,159
babies were exposed for periods of one to three months to powdered
milk formula contaminated with arsenic trioxide (Yamashita, et al.,
1972). Sodium biphosphate of inferior grade from industrial waste,
containing arsenic and vanadium, had been used as a stabilizer in
this powdered infant milk formula. The estimated average intake of
arsenic trioxide was 1-7 mg/day. Most of the infants involved were
less than one year of age and those who became ill had consumed this
formula for at least 10 days. Several thousand infants became ill
and 131 died (Satake, 1955). Arsenic was identified in the tissues
of fatal cases, whereupon over 500,000 cans from the contaminated
lot of Morinaga powdered milk were recalled, terminating the
epidemic. Acute symptoms of poisoning included cough, rhinorrhea,
conjunctivitis, vomiting, diarrhea, melanosis, fever, abdominal
swelling secondary to hepatomegaly, anemia, granulocytopenia and
abnormal electrocardiograms. The increased density at the
metaphyseal ends of the long bones similar to the familiar
"lead-line" was striking. A small group of children was followed
for somewhat more than six months. Follow-up examinations were
concentrated upon electrocardiographic abnormalities, hepatic and
renal function tests. No mention was made of neurobehavioral
assessment; however, the few electroencephalograms that were done
were normal. Except for some retardation of growth in the ulnar
bone, all other features of the syndrome disappeared (Nagai et al.,
1956). Although there was some discussion of long-term follow-up at
the time, it appears that the issue was dropped in 1957.

It was not until some 16 years after the original episode that
groups of affected children were re-evaluated -- some by
questionnaire and some by complete clinical examinations. Among 554
affected children in Kyoto prefecture, complete examinations,
including psychometric testing, were carried out in 241 (Yamashita
et al., 1972). Of these, 73 percent had been exposed when they were
less than one year of age and an additional 22 percent were affected
between 12 and 23 months of age. Findings in the affected group at
16 years of age were compared with age-specific norms for the entire
Kyoto prefecture and with a small control group. Results were as
follows: 1) dermatological abnormalities were found in
approximately 65 percent of the affected adolescents, including
areas of both increased and decreased pigmentation; 2) average
height was reduced but weight was not; 3) four percent showed
abnormal electroencephalographic findings, six percent had seizure
disorders, and 12 percent were mentally retarded; 4) average
intelligence quotient in all school children in Kyoto was 120 while
it was 99 in 241 affected individuals; 5) the percentage of affected
individuals with an I.Q. of 85 or less (21.6 percent) was

substantially higher than that found in the general population (2 percent); 6) significant hearing loss was found in 18 percent; 7) a variety of behavioral deviations were also highly prevalent in the afflicted group. Follow-up studies in other prefectures gave similar results (Japanese Pediatrics Society, 1973; Masahiko and Hideyasu, 1973). Despite the long intervals between the original episode and the follow-up studies and other limitations inherent in such retrospective studies, the follow-up data strongly suggest that arsenic trioxide in amounts sufficient to produce acute clinical illness in infancy may cause the subsequent appearance of permanent neurobehavioral deficits.

METHYLMERCURY

The toxicity of mercury-containing compounds is largely dependent on their physical and chemical properties which determine their absorption, distribution, metabolism and clearance (MacGregor and Clarkson, 1974). For example, mercury vapor, as an uncharged species, readily crosses cell membranes and can accumulate in the central nervous system. In contrast, divalent mercury is largely excluded from this organ but rapidly accumulates in the kidney. Among alkyl and aryl mercury compounds, only methylmercury (MeHg) is relatively resistant to rapid cleavage of the carbon-mercury bond. Consequently, methylmercury has a unique pattern of distribution, binding, metabolism and clearance.

Primary emphasis in the following paragraphs will be placed on recent studies of the effects of exposure to methylmercury in utero or in early life. For general references on the toxicity of methylmercury and other mercurials, the reader is referred to MacGregor and Clarkson (1974) as well as to articles contained in a conference proceeding edited by Miller and Clarkson (1973), an article on dose-response relationships by Clarkson and Marsh (1976), and a monograph edited by Nriagu (1979). As a note of historical interest, however, mention can be made of the reported effects of inorganic mercury compounds, particularly calomel (mercurous chloride), in infants (Bilderback and Anderson, 1975). Calomel was widely used in powders which were applied to the gingiva of teething infants. Following application of these powders, some infants developed acrodynia, a condition characterized by flushing, excessive sweating, photophobia and hypotonia. Since the cessation of the use of these teething powders, acrodynia has become rare (Warkany, 1966). Taken together, these reports suggest that mercurials other than methylmercury have the potential of producing toxic effects in neonates and infants. Continuing attention to this possible hazard is needed.

In Utero Exposure to Methylmercury

The toxicity of methylmercury to the human fetus and newborn
was first recognized at Minamata Bay in Japan during the early
1950s. In some cases, pregnant women who consumed methylmercury-
containing seafood remained symptom-free but delivered infants with
so-called fetal or congenital Minamata Disease (Takizawa, 1979).
Murakami (1972) summarized the clinical and pathological findings in
26 cases of fetal Minamata Disease. Common morphological findings
included skull deformities (11 of 26), strabismus (13 of 26),
nystagmus (4 of 26), malocclusion (14 of 26) and irregular tooth
size (5 of 26). Less common features included torticollis, defects
of the chorioretinal membrane, atresia of the auditory canal,
umbilical hernia and auricular deformity. The brains of two fetal
Minimata Disease cases, which were examined by Takeuchi (1966),
showed developmental arrest and atrophy, hypoplasia and dysplasia of
neurons with poor myelination, decreased neuronal density in the
cerebrum and loss of cerebellar granule cells.

A well documented case of exposure in utero to methylmercury
occurred in the United States in 1969 (Snyder, 1971). A woman
consumed methylmercury-contaminated pork from the third to sixth
month of pregnancy. Although urinary mercury output was high, the
woman manifested no signs or symptoms of methylmercury intoxication.
At term a male infant was delivered who developed intermittent gross
tremors within one minute of birth. The EEG was normal at three
days of age, but, by three months of age, it was abnormal. At six
months of age, myoclonic jerks were present and the EEG remained
abnormal. Nystagmoid eye movement was seen at eight months of age
and evidence of visual fixation was lacking. At 16 months of age,
the child was severely impaired with development arrested at the
three-month-old level. An epileptiform EEG, myoclonic jerks,
hypotonia and lack of response to visual stimuli were found at this
time (Snyder, 1972). This carefully studied case demonstrates the
developmental hazards of exposure in utero to methylmercury.
Notably, the mother of this child manifested no signs or symptoms of
methylmercury poisoning during pregnancy despite the ingestion of
methylmercury-contaminated food. In this regard, this case resembled
fetal Minamata disease. However, the U.S. case did not exhibit some
of the severe morphological changes reported in the Japanese cases
of exposure in utero to methylmercury.

The effects of exposure in utero to methylmercury were also
examined in the Iraqi episode of 1971-1972. The original report on
this large population exposure to methylmercury (Bakir et al., 1973)
confirmed placental transfer of methylmercury by measurement of
organic mercury in the blood of the newborn and demonstrated a rough
dose-effect relationship between the concentration of organic mercury
in the blood of the neonate and the mother. Morphological studies
of the brains of two Iraqi infants exposed in utero to methylmercury

who died within one month of birth have been reported (Choi et al., 1978). Grossly, these brains exhibited shortening of the frontal lobe and simplification of the gyri. Cerebellum and brainstem appeared grossly normal. Microscopically, large numbers of heterotopic neurons were found in the white matter of cerebrum and cerebellum. Neuronal alignment and organization were disordered in the cerebral cortex. Thus, abnormal neuronal migration and consequent deranged cortical organization appeared to be a major effect of exposure in utero to methylmercury.

Follow-up studies of these infants exposed in utero to methylmercury have been conducted in order to elucidate the long-term effects of exposure. Among 15 mother-infant pairs exposed to methylmercury during pregnancy, six mothers and six infants were found to have signs and symptoms of methylmercury poisoning (Amin-Zaki et al., 1974a). Notably, children in this study were nursed by their mothers so that continuing exposure to methylmercury via milk is a confounding factor in determining the effects of exposure in utero to methylmercury. Among the six affected infants examined one to eleven months after the end of exposure to methylmercury, common findings included head circumference below the third percentile (3 of 6), fretfulness, irritability and excessive crying (6 of 6), complete blindness (4 of 6), mystagmus (1 of 6), strabismus (2 of 6), severe hearing impairment (4 of 6), increased muscle tone (3 of 6), decreased muscle tone (2 of 6), severe generalized paralysis (4 of 6), and hyperactive tendon reflexes (5 of 6). No congenital malformations were noted in any of the infants. Mercury concentrations in the blood of infants and mothers were also determined. In mothers, the lowest concentration of mercury in blood associated with the signs and symptoms of methylmercury poisoning was 300 ppb. All mothers with blood mercury concentrations > 400 ppb had signs and symptoms of methylmercury poisoning. In infants, the lowest blood mercury concentration associated with signs and symptoms of methylmercury poisoning was 546 ppb. All infants with blood mercury concentrations > 3000 ppb were severely affected. In simultaneously obtained blood samples, the mercury concentrations tended to be higher in infants than in mothers.

In another report (Amin-Zaki et al., 1976), the relationships between blood mercury concentration in mother and infant and signs of methylmercury toxicity have been examined. An infant exposed in utero to methylmercury for the first six months of gestation was normal at birth with no signs of congenital or neurological abnormalities. However, at one week of age, fever, vomiting and diarrhea developed. Following treatment with antibiotics, symptoms abated and the child remained well until 33 days of age when she was found dead in her cot. Mercury concentration in simultaneous blood samples was about two and one-half times higher in this infant than in her mother. The calculated half-time for clearance of mercury from blood was about 58 days in both mother and infant.

A later study of the developmental consequences of exposure in utero to methylmercury used the concentration of mercury in maternal hair to recapitulate the pattern of mercury exposure during fetal life (Marsh et al., 1977). Twenty-nine infants exposed in utero to methylmercury were examined between three and one-half years of age and again between four and one-half and five years of age. Children were classified on the basis of peak mercury concentration in maternal hair. Neurological abnormalities, short stature, small head circumference, mental retardation, delayed speech and convulsive disorders were all more common in children born of mothers with peak hair mercury concentrations > 100 ppm than among the offspring of women with peak hair mercury concentrations < 25 ppm. Further studies on Iraqi mother-infant pairs have indicated that the critical maternal peak hair mercury concentration for the production of developmental delay in offspring was < 67.7 ppm (Marsh et al., 1979). Based on a hair-to-blood concentration factor of about 300, this would correspond to a peak maternal blood mercury concentration of about 230 ppb. This suggests that exposure in utero to relatively small amounts of methylmercury may produce significant developmental delay. Further developmental studies of Iraqi children exposed in utero to methylmercury will undoubtedly contribute greatly to our understanding of the dose-response relationship for this toxic agent.

Postnatal Exposure to Methylmercury

Cases of exposure to methylmercury occurring exclusively in postnatal life have been reported. Amin-Zaki et al. (1974b) reported on Iraqi infants exposed by consumption of milk produced by their mothers who ate methylmercury-contaminated bread or by personal consumption of methylmercury-contaminated bread. During intake of mercury-contaminated milk and food, the blood mercury concentrations in the blood of these infants rose to exceed those found in their lactating mothers. Infants exposed postnatally to methylmercury had blood mercury concentrations exceeding 200 ppb; however, they remained free of signs or symptoms of methylmercury poisoning. This finding was notable in that a blood mercury level of 200 ppb had previously been considered the minimum concentration needed to produce signs and symptoms of methylmercury poisoning in adults (Berglund et al., 1971). These results may indicate that infants are less susceptible to methylmercury poisoning than are adults or that the evaluation of signs of methylmercury poisoning normally used in diagnosis in adults are insensitive in the infant. As suggested by Amin-Zaki and associates, long term follow-up studies are needed to assess the possible delayed effects of exposure to methylmercury in infancy.

Reproductive Status and Methylmercury Kinetics

An interesting observation made during the Iraqi episode of methylmercury poisoning involved the apparently higher susceptibility of pregnant women to the lethal effects of this agent. Bakir et al. (1973) reported case-fatality rates for pregnant women 20 to 29 years of age to be 70.5 percent and for pregnant women 30 to 39 years of age to be 16 percent. Corresponding case-fatality rates for nonpregnant women 20 to 29 years of age and 30 to 39 years of age were 8.3 percent and 5.2 percent, respectively. At present, it is uncertain whether this difference in mortality reflected a biological effect of pregnancy on the sensitivity to methylmercury intoxication, increased intake of methylmercury-contaminated food or was due to bias in hospital admissions so that deaths occurring among pregnant women exposed to methylmercury were more likely to be detected. In a related area, Greenwood et al. (1978) have shown that following ingestion of methylmercury the average half-life for clearance of mercury from the blood was faster in lactating women (42.2 days) than in nonlactating women or men (75.7 days). These differences were not accounted for by loss of mercury via milk production. Supporting studies in methylmercury-exposed mice (Greenwood et al., 1978) and rats (Magos et al., 1980) indicated that lactation does reduce the half-life of mercury in the whole body and may protect against the signs and symptoms of methylmercury poisoning. The physiological basis of these lactation-dependent differences in mercury clearance awaits further study.

Future Research Needs

Based on the current understanding of the hazards of methylmercury to developing organisms, several areas of importance for future research may be identified.

First, continuing studies of child development in methylmercury-exposed populations are required. The studies of Iraqi children in which maternal hair has been used to recapitulate the pattern of methylmercury exposure during in utero life are especially useful. Identification of new populations with relatively high methylmercury intake would also be useful for comparative studies of the dose-response relationship.

Second, further emphasis should be placed on identification of critical periods in development during which methylmercury may exert specific toxic effects. Careful definition of the duration and magnitude of exposure in utero to methylmercury or during postnatal life is needed.

Third, the role of reproductive and lactational status in the distribution and clearance of methylmercury by women requires

further study. Data from Iraq suggest that pregnancy may increase
the toxicity of methylmercury and that lactation may increase the
rate of mercury clearance from the blood. Such observations need to
be confirmed and the physiological basis understood. The
identification of pregnant or lactating women as groups at special
risk to methylmercury toxicity would be an important contribution to
evaluation of the hazards of methylmercury exposure.

     Fourth, evidence from current animal studies of the
distribution, metabolism and clearance of methylmercury during
development should be evaluated as to their application to the
assessment of the hazards of methylmercury exposure in the developing
human. Studies performed at appropriate methylmercury exposure
levels in experimental animals may be useful in identification of
critical periods in development. This information could contribute
to the design of better epidemiological studies of the hazards of
methylmercury exposure in developing humans.

SUMMARY AND IMPLICATIONS FOR PUBLIC HEALTH

     Evaluation of recently published studies indicates that lead in
food is associated with an average PbB of 8 µg while current ambient
air lead ($\leq$ 1 µg/m^3) and drinking water lead ($\leq$ 50 µg/liter)
account for an additional 2 µg, or a total of approximately 10 µg
Pb/dl whole blood on the average (Nutrition Foundation, Inc.,
1982). There is accumulating evidence, that, in children, PbB in
excess of this baseline value can be accounted for largely by lead
in dust which is transferred into the body by the hand-to-mouth
route. Mouthing, finger-sucking and other hand-to-mouth activities
are prevalent in a high percentage of children who are considered to
be healthy. Overall exposures of children through this route can be
expected to decrease in view of the downward trend during the past
five to six years in the use of lead additives in petrol as well as
the downward trend in the lead content of food. In the United
States and, perhaps, in some other areas of the western world, a
substantial stock of old housing, which still contains lead-based
paints on surfaces accessible to children, remains in use. In the
United States it is likely that several decades will elapse before
this old housing stock is either replaced or adequately renovated.
Experience with lead in gasoline and paint suggests that future
non-recycled uses of this metal must be approached with great
caution. In view of the studies of populations residing in close
proximity to large smelting operations, it would be appropriate to
locate future plants of this sort at a distance from large
population centers. The drinking water issue highlights the fact
that drinking water is contaminated with lead following purification
during its transit through older distribution systems in which water
is conveyed in lead pipes. This problem is remediable in the
short-term by measures to reduce the plumbosolvency of acidic waters

and in the long-term by minimizing exposure to drinking water to lead in the distribution system. Suppression of lead in dust is considerably more difficult. Nevertheless, the data from NHANES II in the United States, which indicate that four percent of all young children have PbB $\geq$ 30 μg, together with currently available experimental data, suggest that substantial numbers of young children in the United States remain at risk for subtle impairment in neurobehavioral development (Tables 1 and 2). The problem is particularly serious among poor, urban, black children. Data in experimental animals suggest that modest increases in lead absorption during very early life do lead to subtle, but lasting impediments in neurodevelopment and cognitive function. Despite the substantial number of epidemiological studies in children, the risks associated with various levels of lead absorption remain ill defined, particularly in regard to low level increased lead absorption as reflected by PbBs maintained throughout early childhood in the range of 25 to 40 μg. Of particular interest are two current prospective studies in which maternal PbB values during pregnancy may fall in the range of 25 to 40 μg. Data obtained in these studies may be valuable in assessing the question of exposure of women of reproductive age to increased amounts of lead in a work place.

Overexposure of young children to arsenic has been limited largely to outbreaks of poisoning due to contamination of food and drinking water but has led in some cases to fatalities. While such epidemics may not be totally avoidable in the practical sense, it does appear that large epidemics such as those occurring in Japan, Taiwan and Chile, could be avoided through appropriate monitoring of public drinking water supplies and quality control in food production. Although some have raised the concern that the increased dissemination of arsenic into the air may occur if there is a substantial increase in the burning of coal for energy, no dose-effect data are available with which to assess whether such an event would pose a significant hazard. Past experience with epidemics of arsenic poisoning do, however, suggest strongly, that neurobehavioral and neurotoxicological assessment should be included in any future prospective studies involving young children.

The toxicity of methylmercury may be modified by age at exposure. As described above, the fetus appears especially sensitive to the neurotoxic effects of this agent. In particular, some human studies suggest that effects on subsequent growth and development may be produced by exposure in utero to methylmercury at levels which produce no signs of methylmercury intoxication in the pregnant women. The production of such long-term effects in the absence of maternal poisoning suggests that the methylmercury exposure status of pregnant women should be monitored closely to insure that the hazard of injury in utero is minimized. The longitudinal studies undertaken in Iraqi infants with varying methylmercury exposure status should be especially useful in this regard. Minimization of hazard to the general population clearly depends on the careful evaluation of these highly exposed populations.

As discussed in a 1980 World Health Organization report (1980), consumption of methylmercury contaminated fish is the primary source of human methylmercury exposure. While the need to continue studies of methylmercury-exposed populations was reiterated in this report, the authors also suggested that the health hazard to individuals might be reduced by reduction of the input of methylmercury into the aquatic environment and limitation of intake of methylmercury. Reductions of methylmercury intake could be achieved by reducing acceptable limits for methylmercury in fish and/or by reducing consumption of methylmercury-containing fish.

REFERENCES

Amin-Zaki, L., Elhassani, S., Majeed, M.A., Clarkson, T.W., Doherty, R.A. and Greenwood, M.R., 1974a, Intra-uterine methylmercury poisoning in Iraq, Pediatrics 54:587-595.

Amin-Zaki, L., Elhassani, S., Majeed, M.A., Clarkson, T.W., Doherty, R.A. and Greenwood, M.R., 1974b, Studies of infants postnatally exposed to methylmercury, J. Ped. 85:81-84.

Amin-Zaki, L., Elhassani, S., Majeed, M.A., Clarkson, T.W., Doherty, R.A., Greenwood, M.R. and Giovanoli-Jakubeczak, T., 1976, Perinatal methylmercury poisoning in Iraq, Am. J. Dis. Child 130:1070-1076.

Annest, J.L., Mahaffey, K.R., Cox, D.H. and Roberts, J., 1982, Blood lead levels for persons 6 months-74 years of age: United States, 1976-80. Advanced data from vital and health statistics of the National Center for Health Statistics, number 79, pp. 1-23, May 12.

Bakir, F., Damluji, S.F., Amin-Zaki, L., Murtadha, M., Khalidi, A., Al-Rawi, N.Y., Tikriti, S., Dhahir, H.I., Clarkson, T.W., Smith, J.C. and Doherty, R.A., 1973, Methylmercury poisoning in Iraq: An interuniversity report, Science, 181:230-241.

Bencko, V. and Symon, K., 1970, The cumulation dynamics in some tissue of hairless mice inhaling arsenic, Atmos. Environ. 4:157-161.

Berglund, F., Berlin, M. Birke, G., Cederlof, R., von Euler, U., Finberg, L., Holmstedt, B., Johsson, B., Luning, K.G., Ramel, C., Skerfving, S., Swensson, A. and Jejning, S., 1971, Methylmercury in fish: Report of an expert group, Nord. Hyg. Tidskn. Suppl. 4.

Bilderback, J.B. and Anderson, J.A., 1975, Acrodynia, in: "Textbook of Pediatrics 10th Edition", V.C. Vaughan, III and R.J. McKay, eds., pp. 1682-1684, Saunders, Philadelphia.

Bornschein, R.L., ed., 1981, "Proceedings of the International
    Conference on Prospective Studies of Lead Exposure in
    Children", pp. 1-127, Department of Environmental Health,
    University of Cincinnati, Cincinnati, OH.
Bornschein, R., Pearson, D. and Reiter, L., 1980, Behavioral effects
    of moderate lead exposure in children and animal models: Part
    I - clinical studies; Part 2 - animal studies, CRC Crit. Rev.
    Toxicol. 43-99.
Bradley, R. and Caldwell, B., 1976a, Early home environment and
    changes in mental test performance in children from six to
    thirty-six months, Developmental Psychology 12:93-97.
Bradley, R. and Caldwell, B., 1976b, The relation of infants' home
    environments to mental test performance at fifty-four months:
    A follow-up study, Child Development 47:1172-1174.
Byers, R.K. and Lord, E.E., 1943, Late effects of lead poisoning on
    mental development, Am. J. Dis. Child 66:471.
Caldwell, B., Heider, J. and Kaplan, B., 1966, The inventory of home
    stimulation. Paper presented at the meeting of the American
    Psychological Association.
Center for Disease Control Statement, 1978, "Preventing Lead
    Poisoning in Young Children", Dept. of Health, Education and
    Welfare, U.S. Gov't. Printing Office, Washington.
Center for Disease Control, 1982, Morbidity and Mortality Weekly
    Report, Blood-lead levels in U.S. population, 31/10:132-134
    (March 19), Dept. of Health, Education and Welfare, Atlanta, GA.
Chisolm, J.J., Jr., Mellits, E.D. and Barrett, M.B., 1976,
    Interrelationships among blood lead concentration, quantitative
    daily ALAU and urinary lead output following calcium EDTA, in:
    "Effects and Dose-Response Relationships of Toxic Metals", G.F.
    Nordberg, ed., pp. 416-433, Elsevier, Amsterdam.
Choi, B.H., Lapham, L.W., Amin-Zaki, L. and Saleem, T., 1978,
    Abnormal neuronal migration, deranged cerebral cortical
    organizaton and diffuse white matter astrocytosis of human
    fetal brain: A major effect of methylmercury poisoning in
    utero, J. Neuropathol. Exp. Neurol. 37:719-733.
Clarkson, T.W. and Marsh, D.O., 1976, The toxicity of methylmercury
    in man: Dose-response relationships in adult populations, in:
    "Effects and Dose-Response Relationships of Toxic Metals", G.F.
    Nordberg, ed., pp. 246-261, Elsevier, Amsterdam.
Cowan, L. and Leviton, A., 1980, Epidemiologic considerations in the
    study of sequelae of low level exposure, in: "Low Level Lead
    Exposure - The Clinical Implications of Current Research", H.L.
    Needleman, ed., pp. 91-119, Raven Press, New York.
de la Burde, B. and Choate, M.S., 1975, Early asymptomatic lead
    exposure and development at school age, J. Pediat. 87:638-642.
Department of Health and Social Security, 1980, Lead and Health,
    Report of a Department of Health and Social Security working
    party on lead in the environment, Department of Health and
    Social Security, Her Majesty's Stationery Office, London.

Greenwood, M.R., Clarkson, T.W., Doherty, R.A., Gates, A.H.,
Amin-Zaki, L., Elhassani, S. and Majeed, M.A., 1978, Blood
clearance half-time in lactating and non-lactating members of a
population exposed to methylmercury, Environ. Research 16:48-54.
Heber, R., 1970, "Epidemiology of Mental Retardation", C.C. Thomas,
Springfield, Illinois.
Japanese Pediatric Society, 1973, Morinaga arsenic-tainted powdered
milk poisoning investigation special committee. Summary of
report of activities of the Morinaga arsenic-tainted powdered
milk poisoning investigation (In Japanese, translated by U.S.
EPA) (May 26, 1973).
Lourie, R.S., Layman, E.M. and Millican, F.K., 1963, Why children
eat things that are not food, Children 10:143-146.
MacGregor, J.T. and Clarkson, T.W., 1974, Distribution,
tissue-binding and toxicity of mercurials, in: "Protein-Metal
Interactions", M. Friedman, ed., pp. 463-503, Plenum Press, New
York.
Magos, L., Peristianis, G.C., Clarkson, T.W. and Snowden, R.T.,
1980, The effect of lactation on methylmercury intoxication,
Arch. Toxicol. 45:143-148.
Mahaffey, K.R., Annest, J.L., Roberts, J. and Murphy, R.S., 1982,
Blood lead levels for persons 6 months-74 years of age: United
States, 1976-80, New Engl. J. Med. 307:573-579.
Marsh, D.O., Myers, G.J., Clarkson, T.W., Amin-Zaki, L. and Tikriti,
S., 1977, Fetal methylmercury poisoning: New data on clinical
and toxicological aspects, Trans. Am. Neurol. Assoc. 102:1-3.
Marsh, D.O., Myers, G.J., Clarkson, T.W., Amin-Zaki, L., Tikriti,
S., Majeed, M. and Dabbagh, A.R., 1979, Dose-response
relationship for human fetal exposure to methylmercury,
Abstract. International Congress of Neurotoxicology, Varese,
Italy, September 27-30.
Masahiko, O. and Hideyasu, A., 1973, Epidemiological studies on the
Morinaga powdered milk poisoning incident: Final report of the
joint project team from Hiroshima and Okayama Universities for
survey of the Seno area, Jpn. J. Hyg. (Nigo Eiseigaku Zasshi),
27:500-531 (In Japanese, translated by U.S. EPA).
Milar, C.R., Schroder, S.R., Mushak, P., Dolcourt, J.L. and Grabt,
L.D., 1980, Contributions of the caregiving environment to
increased lead burden in children, Am. J. Mental Deficiency
84:339-344.
Milham, S., Jr., 1977, Studies of morbidity near a copper smelter,
Environ. Hlth. Persp. 19:131-132.
Miller, M.W. and Clarkson, T.W., eds., 1973, "Mercury, Mercurials
and Mercaptans", C.C. Thomas, Springfield, IL.
Moore, M.R., Meredith, P.A. and Goldberg, A., 1977, A retrospective
analysis of blood-lead in mentally retarded children, Lancet
1(2):717.
Murakami, U., 1972, The effect of organic mercury on intrauterine
life, in: "Drugs and Fetal Development", M.A. Klingberg, A.
Abramovici and J. Chemke, eds., pp. 309-336, Plenum, New York.

Nagai, H., Okuda, R., Nagami, H., Yati, A., Mori, C. and Wada, H.,
    1956, Subacute-chronic "arsenic" poisoning in infants --
    subsequent clinical observations, Ann. Pediatr. (Shonika Kiyo),
    2:124-132 (in Japanese, translated by U.S. EPA).
National Academy of Sciences, 1977a, Arsenic, Washington, DC.
National Academy of Sciences, 1977b, Drinking Water and Health,
    Washington, DC.
National Academy of Sciences, 1980, Lead in the Human Environment,
    Washington, DC.
National Center for Health Statistics, 1982, Second National Health
    and Nutrition Examination Survey. National Center for Health
    Statistics, Washington, DC.
Needleman, H.L., 1980, "Low Level Lead Exposure -- The Clinical
    Implications of Current Research", Raven Press, New York.
Needleman, H.L., Gunnoe, C., Leviton, A., Reed, R., Peresie, H.,
    Maher, C. and Barrett, B.S., 1979, Deficits in psychologic and
    classroom performance of children with elevated dentine levels,
    New Engl. J. Med. 13:689-695.
Needleman, H.L., Leviton, A. and Bellinger, D., 1982, Lead
    associated intellectual deficit, N. Engl. J. Med. 306:367.
Nordberg, G.F., 1976, "Effects and Dose-Response Relationships of
    Toxic Metals", Elsevier, Amsterdam.
Nordberg, G.F., Pershagen, G. and Lauwerys, R., 1979, Report to the
    Commission of European Communities, Inorganic Arsenic --
    Toxicological and Epidemiological Aspects, 1-113 (June).
Nriagu, J., ed., 1979, "The Biogeochemistry of Mercury in the
    Environment", Elsevier/North Holland, Amsterdam.
Nutrition Foundation, Inc., 1982, Assessment of the safety of lead
    and lead salts in food -- A report of the Nutrition
    Foundation's Expert Advisory Committee, (June).
Otto, D.A., 1981, Electrophysiological assessment of neurotoxicity
    in children, in: "Proceedings of the First International Lead
    Conference", R.L. Bornschein, ed., pp. 75-95, Department of
    Environmental Health, University of Cincinnati, Cincinnati, OH.
Otto, D.A. Benignus, V., Muller, K. and Barton, C., 1981, Effects of
    age and body lead burden on CNS function on young children. I.
    Slow cortical portentials, Electroenceph. Clin. Neurophysiol.
    52:229-239.
Pershagen, G., 1979, Exposure to arsenic, in "Trace Metals --
    Exposure and Health Effects", E. DiFerrante, ed., pp. 98-106,
    Pergamon Press, Oxford.
Rabinowitz, M.B. and Needleman, H.L., 1982, Temporal trends in the
    lead concentrations of umbilical cord blood, Science
    216:1429-1431.
Rabinowitz, M.B., Wetherell, G.W. and Kopple, J.D., 1976, Kinetic
    analysis of lead metabolism in healthy humans, J. Clin. Invest.
    58:260-270.
Rummo, J.H., 1974, Intellectual and behavioral effects of lead
    poisoning in children, University of North Carolina at Chapel
    Hill, Ph.D. Thesis.

Rutter, M., 1980, Raised lead levels and impaired cognitive/
    behavioral functioning: A review of the evidence, Dev. Med.
    Child. Neurol. 22:1-26.
Satake, S., 1955, Concerning the cases of arsenic poisoning caused
    by prepared powdered milk, Jpn. J. Public Health (Nihon Koshu
    Eisei Shu), 2:22-24 (In Japanese, translated by U.S. EPA).
Schaffner, R., 1981, Lead in canned foods, Food Technology
    (Chicago), 35:60.
Schroeder, S.R., Kanoy, R.C., Milar, C.R., Mushak, P. and Otto,
    D.A., 1981, Child-caregiver interactions with lead exposures,
    in: "Proceedings of the First International Lead Conference",
    R.L. Borschein, ed., pp. 61-74, Department of Environmental
    Health, University of Cincinnati, Cincinnati, OH.
Snyder, R.D., 1971, Congenital mercury poisoning, New Engl. J. Med.
    284:1014-1016.
Snyder, R.D., 1972, The involuntary movements of chronic mercury
    poisoning, Arch. Neurol. 26:379-381.
Southwick, J.W., Western, A.E., Beck, M.M., Whitley, J., Isaacs, R.,
    Petajan, J. and Hanson, C.D., 1982, Community Health Associated
    with Arsenic in Drinking Water in Millard County, Utah. U.S.
    EPA-600/S1-81-064, February.
Takeuchi, T., 1966, Pathology of Minamata disease, in: "Minamata
    Disease", M. Katsuma, ed., pp. 141-252, Study Group of Minamata
    Disease, Kumamoto University, Japan.
Takizawa, Y., 1979, Epidemiology of mercury poisoning, in: "The
    Biogeochemistry of Mercury in the Environment", J. Nriagu, ed.,
    pp. 325-365, Elsevier/North Holland, Amsterdam.
Tseng, W.P., Chu, H.M., How, S.W., Fong, J.M., Lin, C.S. and Yeh,
    Shu, 1968, Prevalence of skin cancer in an endemic area of
    chronic arsenicism in Taiwan, J. Natl. Cancer Inst. 40:453-463.
Warkany, J., 1966, Acrodynia - postmortem of a disease, Am. J. Dis.
    Child 112:147-155.
Winneke, G., Brockhaus, A., Kramer, U., Ewers, U., Kujanek, G.,
    Lechner, H. and Janke, W., 1981, Neuropsychological comparison
    of children with different tooth lead levels: A preliminary
    report, in: "Proceedings of the International Conference on
    Heavy Metals in the Environment", pp. 553-556, WHO, Geneva.
World Health Organization, 1980, Consultation to Re-examine the
    World Health Organization Environmental Health Criteria for
    Mercury, EHE/EHC/80.22, April 21-25, p. 18, Geneva.
Yamashita, N., Doi, M. Nishio, M., Hojo, H. and Tanaka, M., 1972,
    Current state of Kyoto children poisoned by arsenic tainted
    Morinaga dry milk, Jpn. J. Hyg. (Nihon Eiseigaku Zasshi),
    27:364-399 (In Japanese, translated by U.S. EPA).

SESSION 5. PRENATAL ASPECTS OF THE METABOLISM OF METALS

Chairpersons: *Richard K. Miller and Zahir A. Shaikh*

THE PLACENTA: RELEVANCE TO TOXICOLOGY

Richard K. Miller,[1,2] Wendy W. Ng,[1,2] and
Arthur A. Levin[3]

Departments of Obstetrics/Gynecology[1] and
Pharmacology/Toxicology[2],
University of Rochester, Rochester, New York
Department of Toxicology and Pathology[3]
Hoffmann-LaRoche, Inc., Nutley, New Jersey

ABSTRACT

The placenta and its extraembryonic membranes are central to
the survival of the developing mammal in utero. These membranes are
the interfaces between the maternal and embryonic environments. As
such, the trophoblast regulates the movement of molecules and
controls both the maternal and fetal physiology by the production
and release of hormones. Alterations of placental functions can
compromise the developing organism. These placental alterations may
range from decreased nutrient transfer to placental necrosis. The
responses of the placenta may reflect a direct action of the toxin
on the placenta or an indirect effect, e.g., a decrease in
utero-placental blood flow. Trophoblastic neoplasia can also be
induced in mothers exposed to chemicals only during pregnancy.
Thus, the responses of the placenta to toxic insults must be
considered when evaluating the effects on the embryo and fetus.

INTRODUCTION

The placenta and its extraembryonic membranes are tissues with
diverse structures and functions. Even though the early development
of most embryos is similar, substantial species differences are
present for the placenta and the extraembryonic membranes.
Throughout gestation, modifications of both structure and function
in these membranes are occurring. Any discussion of developmental
toxicology must contend with a placenta that not only differs among

569

species but changes throughout gestation. This tissue of embryonic origin - the trophoblast, is both a conduit for embryonic and fetal nutrition, and a controller of the maternal and fetal environments.

Among the functions the trophoblast performs are the regulation of transfer for nutrients, waste products and xenobiotics between mother and conceptus, the synthesis and release of steroid and protein hormones, and the biotransformation and retention of a wide variety of chemicals. An additional function of the placenta is the modulation of the maternal immunological system to ensure the survival of the conceptus as an allograft (McIntyre et al., 1981; McIntyre and Faulk, 1982, 1983; Billington and Bell, 1982; Levine, 1983). The subject of placental immunology will not be addressed in this chapter. The reader is referred to excellent reviews by Faulk (1981), Beer and Sio (1982), and Klopper (1982).

This chapter will review: a. the comparative morphology, b. endocrinology, metabolism and receptors, c. transport physiology and d. toxicology of the placenta.

MORPHOLOGY

Placental structures are quite different from species to species and even changes during the course of gestation. However, all placentae are similar in that one surface of the placenta is exposed to the maternal circulation/environment, and through the trophoblastic tissue run fetal capillaries which carry nutrients back to the fetus. There are considerable interspecies variations in the: 1) arrangement of the fetal blood vessels, 2) shape of the placenta, 3) type of attachment to the mother, 4) relationship to the maternal circulation, 5) placental cell type, and 6) number of cell layers. The placenta comprises not only the chorioallantoic placenta but also the extraembryonic membranes, which include the amnion and the yolk sac. In many species, the chorioallantoic placenta and the yolk sac placenta perform complementary functions even though their structures are substantially different.

The basic functional unit of the placenta is the cotyledon. Each cotyledon consists of the trophoblast and the fetal vessels associated with it. In the distal portion of the cotyledon run fetal capillaries, and each cotyledon is bathed with maternal blood from specific arteries. In the human and primate, the cotyledons are grouped together into one or two placental discs. A duplex placenta for the rhesus monkey is noted in Figure 1. The human placenta also may have this conformation. Other species such as the sheep and cow have a multicotyledonary implantation (Figure 1). Each cotyledon is independent, and they are distributed over the entire surface of the decidua. Regardless of the grouping of the implanted cotyledons, the form of the whole placenta may vary.

For the dog, cat and ferret, the implantation of the chorioallantoic placenta is zonary or ring-shaped (Figure 1).

The placenta is perfused by two separate blood supplies (fetal-umbilical circulation; maternal-uterine/decidual circulation). The maternal circulatory patterns is species- specific, e.g., channels (labyrinths) for rodents, pools (lacunae) for primates (Ramsey, 1982). Power (1972) has demonstrated that the perfusion overlap for the maternal and fetal circulations can vary within and between cotyledons. Yet when taken in toto, the reserve capacity of the chorioallantoic placenta usually allows for adequate function to sustain the conceptus.

While the cotyledon is the major anatomical unit, the essential functional interface between the maternal and fetal circulations is the trophoblast. Species differences are also present for the number of trophoblastic layers present: two for primates; three for rodents (Figure 2). In the early human placenta, there are two distinct trophoblast cell layers: the syncytiotrophoblast and the cytotrophoblast. During fetal development, the cytotrophoblast cells become less numerous, and the distance between the maternal

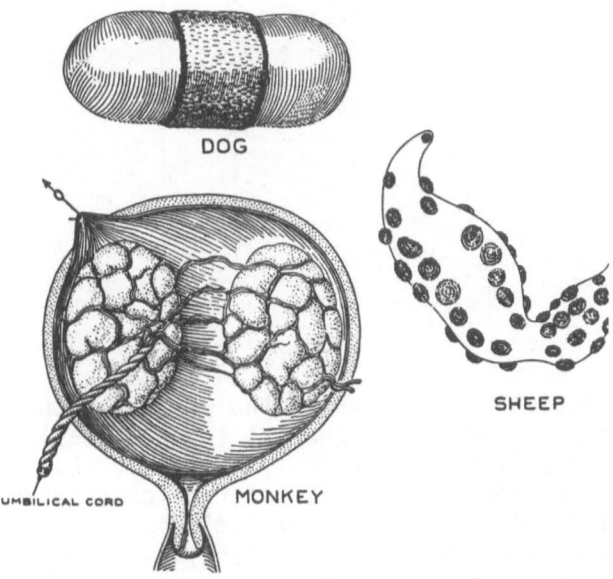

Figure 1   Morphological differences in placentae from the dog, monkey and sheep. From Faulk (1981), published with permission of the University of Rochester.

and fetal blood decreases from 25 microns during the first trimester
to 8-10 microns at term. The syncytiotrophoblast is covered by
microvilli (Figure 3). These microvilli substantially increase the
surface area of the trophoblast and are present before implantation
and throughout gestation (Figure 3).

Besides the trophoblast, which is of embryonic origin, there
may be a number of other embryonic as well as maternal cell layers
separating the blood supplies. In Figure 2, there are three examples
of the number of layers separating the circulations. Even with six
cell layers separating the maternal and fetal blood, adequate
movement of nutrients, e.g., oxygen and sodium, are maintained
(Flexner et al., 1948).

Another major interspecies difference is the presence of a
functional yolk sac and vitelline circulation. In the rodent
(Figure 4), the yolk sac consists of columnar epithelium which is
supplied by the vitelline circulation in the conceptus. Early in

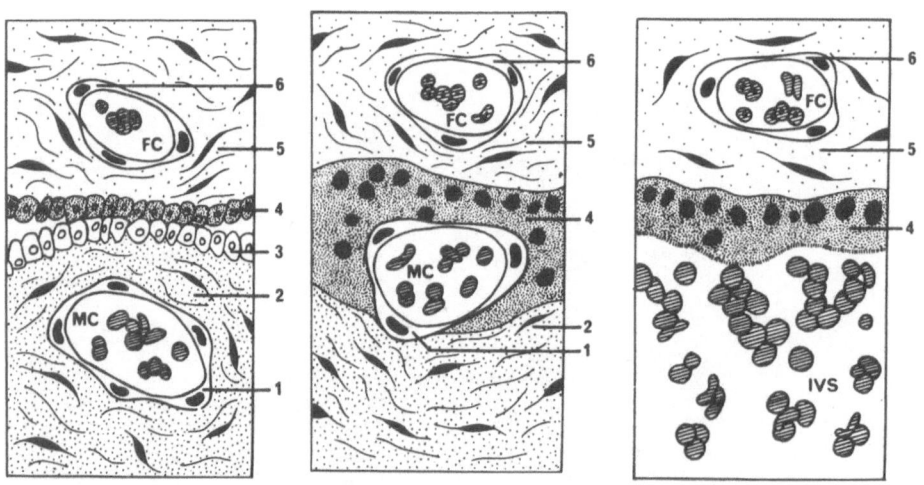

Figure 2   Histological evaluation of the epithelio chorial (horse
            and pig), endothelial chorial (dog and cat) and
            haemochorial (human, rodent, primate). 1. maternal
            capillary endothelium, 2. maternal connective tissue, 3.
            uterine epithelium (endometrium), 4. trophoblast, 5.
            fetal connective tissue, 6. fetal capillary endothelium.
            FC. fetal capillary lumen - note nucleated fetal
            erythrocytes; MC. maternal capillary lumen; IVS.
            intervillous space with maternal erythrocytes. From
            Panigel (1981), with permission from the University of
            Rochester.

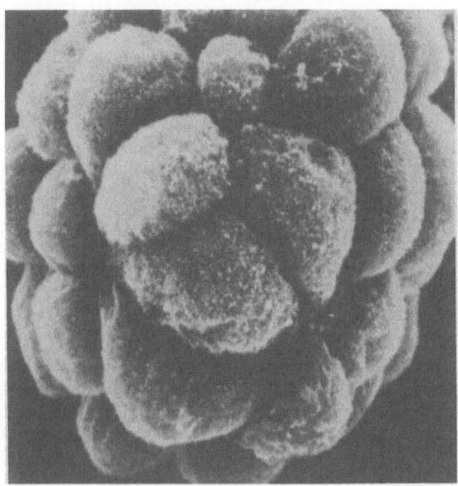

Figure 3   Preimplantation embryo from a baboon at the morula stage
            with the zona pellucida removed. This scanning electron
            microscopic view demonstrates the microvilli and cyto-
            plasmic projections. The inner cell mass cannot be seen.
            However, even at this stage the pictured cells are tropho-
            blast. From Panigel (1981), with permission from the
            University of Rochester.

development, this yolk sac supplies the primary nutritional needs of
the embryo; however, as the embryo develops, it rapidly exceeds the
nutritional capacity of the yolk. As this occurs, the yolk sac
eventually collapses and inverts with the absorptive surface now
being exposed to the uterine environment (Figure 4). As gestation
progresses (about day 17 of gestation in the rat), the parietal yolk
sac and Reichert's membrane rupture, which is the result of altered
cellular synthesis, e.g., collagen (Clark et al., 1975). At this
time, the yolk sac is in direct contact with the maternal uterine
fluids. In the rodent, yolk sac function persists throughout
gestation; however in the human, the yolk sac does not appear to
function beyond the first trimester.

     Thus, distinct interspecies developmental differences in
morphology and function can be identified for the trophoblast. The
role of these morphological differences in the placenta and the
extraembryonic membranes must be taken into consideration in
developmental toxicity evaluations.

     The comparative anatomy of the placenta has been recently
reviewed in a volume by Ramsey (1982). In addition, ultrastructural
reviews of various species are available (Björkman, 1976; Kaufmann ·
and Davidoff, 1977).

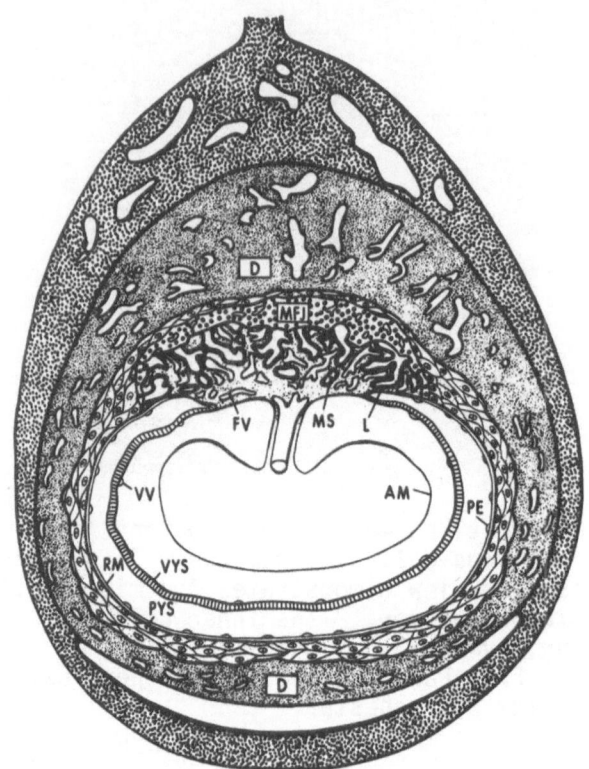

Figure 4   Schematic representation of a cross section of the
            feto-placental unit of the rat on day 11 of gestation.
            The embyro is not depicted, but the umbilical vessels are
            shown and are connected to the chorioallantoic placenta
            which consists of the labyrinth (L) and the maternal-
            fetal junction (MFJ). The labyrinth or the region for
            maternal-fetal exchange has both the fetal vessels (FV)
            and the maternal blood space (MS). The other
            extraembryonic membranes that surround the conceptus are
            the amnion (AM), the visceral yolk sac (VYS), Reichert's
            membrane (RM) and the parietal yolk sac (PYS).
            Surrounding these extraembryonic membranes are the
            maternal decidual tissues (D). The visceral yolk sac
            connects with the conceptus via the vitelline vessels
            (VV), and is the alternative circulation for nourishing
            the conceptus. On the fetal side of the Reichert's
            membrane are the parietal endodermal cells (PE) which
            maintain the Reichert's membrane until day 17-18 of
            gestation, when both the Reichert's membrane and the
            parietal yolk sac rupture and retract to the periphery of
            the chorioallantoic placenta. From Miller et al. (1976),
            with permission from Elsevier Press.

ENDOCRINOLOGY, METABOLISM AND RECEPTORS

Endocrine Function

The placenta is the controller of the maternal was well as the fetal environment. This control is accomplished via the hormones released by the trophoblast. Even prior to implantation, the trophectoderm secretes hormones. Among the ones most readily detected is chorionic gonadotropin (CG), which is used for the diagnosis of pregnancy. As pregnancy progresses, the trophoblast increases its production of chorionic gonadotropin, which mimics luteinizing hormone (LH) and stimulates ovarian secretion of steroids. These steroids are essential to the maintenance of the endometrium and the quiescence of the uterus, conditions which are necessary for the maintenance of the pregnancy.

In the rat, both the ovary and placenta supply the appropriate steroid hormones for maintaining the pregnancy. However in the human, the production of steroid hormones occurs primarily in the trophoblast by the end of the first trimester. This increase in placental steroid production consolidates the control of the placenta over both the mother and the conceptus.

These synthetic pathways for hormones can be investigated for an evaluation of toxic responses. Clinically, the metabolism of estrogens during pregnancy is routinely used to assess feto-placental compromise. The metabolism of estrogen precursors to estriol requires a functional fetal liver, adrenal, pituitary and placenta.

In the human, pregnancy-related proteins are also produced by the placenta (Table 1). Besides CG, the detection of placental protein hormones such as chorionic thyrotropin (cTSH), chorionic ACTH (cACTH), and chorionic follicle stimulating hormone (cFSH), implicates specific trophoblastic protein hormones for controlling both maternal and fetal physiology (Villee, 1977). Human chorionic gonadotropin and human placental lactogen (PL) are still the two primary protein hormones that have been associated with altered maternal physiology during pregnancy (Klopper, 1982, 1983). The PAPP A,B,C, and D as well as the SP proteins are not conclusively associated with any physiological functions at this time (Klopper, 1982,1983; Table 1).

Nutrient Metabolism

The placenta is the site of absorption, transfer and metabolism for all fetal nutrients, and serves also to modulate the maternal metabolism, e.g., glucose metabolism. In the sheep and cow, the trophoblast converts glucose to fructose. A glucose load given to

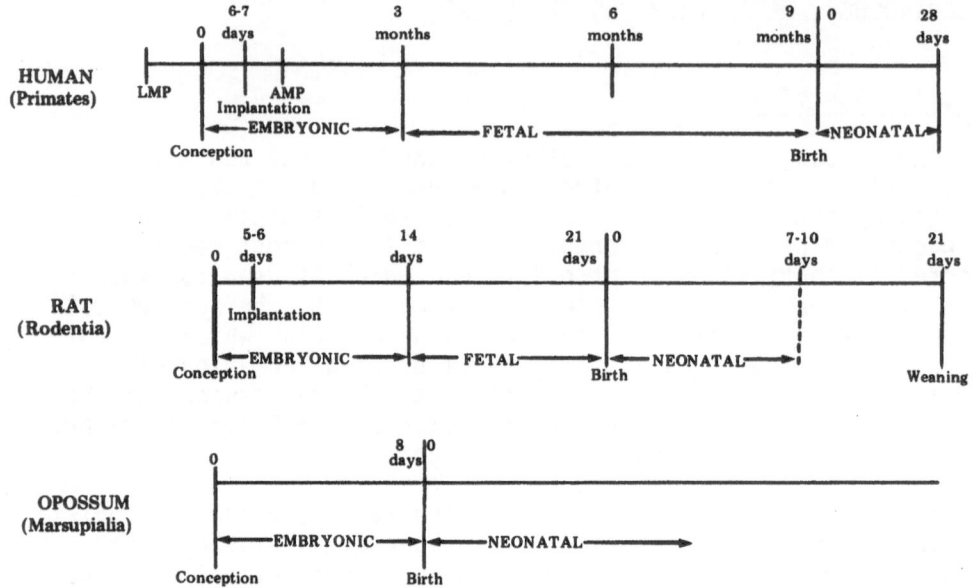

Figure 5   Comparative perinatal development in the human, rat and
            opossum. The periods of development are defined for each
            species. LMP, last menstrual period; AMP, anticipated
            menstrual period. The menstrual cycle in the average
            human female is 28 days with ovulation occurring about
            day 14. As noted for the rat, since in utero development
            is abbreviated compared to the human (21-22 days vs 9
            months), the maturation of the rat newborn is
            substantially different than in the human. It has been
            proposed that the 7-10 day old neonate may be more
            comparable to the human at birth. The opossum presents
            an entirely different pattern: 1. there is no
            chorioallantoic placenta, and 2. the neonate is still in
            an embryonic form. Even with these differences, the
            effects of environmental agents in all three species can
            be established; however, the timing of the exposure, route
            of administration, and developmental stage must be
            considered when comparing effects among species. From
            Miller (1983), with permission from A.R. Liss, Inc.

the mother does not result in increasing levels of glucose in the
fetus. Instead, fructose levels in the fetus rise substantially
(Battaglia, 1981). The placenta also contains glycogen as an energy
store for metabolic processes, e.g., amino acid transport (Longo et
al., 1972). Furthermore, the placenta alters the maternal
metabolism to ensure an adequate nutrient source for fetal growth

Table 1   Protein and Steroid Hormones and Other Proteins Produced
             by the Human Placenta

Chorionic ACTH

Chorionic Gonadotropin, CG

Placental Lactogen, PL

Corticotropin, CT

Thyrotropin, TT

Estrone, E_1

Estradiol, E_2

Estriol, E_3

Progesterone

Pregnancy - Associated Plasma Proteins
                      PAPP A
                      PAPP B
                      PAPP C
                      PAPP D

Placental Protein 5, PP5

Pregnancy Zone Protein, PZP

Pregnancy Specific Protein, SP-1

---

and development. In the human, placental lactogen induces an
increase in fatty acid metabolism as a source of energy, thus,
sparing glucose for fetal use.

     In addition to carbohydrates, lipids and low density
lipoprotein appear to play a role in placental metabolism. The
precursor for steroid synthesis is often cholesterol which is
transported into the placenta via low density lipoproteins.
Cholesterol has been found in primary human trophoblastic tissue
culture studies to be derived from low density lipoproteins (Winkel
et al., 1981). Acetate incorporation into cholesterol was inhibited
by increasing concentrations of low density lipoproteins (Winkel et
al., 1981). Thomas and associates (1983) have demonstrated in the

perfused guinea pig placenta that free fatty acids will cross the placenta but certainly not to the same extent as fatty acids when triglycerides are given to the mother. The trophoblast rapidly converts the triglycerides to fatty acids and appears to store the fatty acids besides releasing them into the fetal circulation. In these experiments, triglycerides were not detectable in the fetal perfusate.

Xenobiotic Metabolism

The metabolism of xenobiotics by the trophoblast has been observed in most species. Such metabolism reflects the presence of numerous enzymes, e.g., Cytochrome P_{450} monoxygenases, reductases, epoxide hydrases, sulfatases, glucuronidases, sulfotransferases, and glucuronyltransferases (Pelkonen, 1980; Juchau, 1980,1982). Some enzymes of the placenta are induced by exposures to chemicals in the environment, e.g., 3 methyl-cholanthrene and benzo(α)pyrene, phenobarbital, dioxin. The fact that placentae from cigarette smokers have increased levels of mixed function oxidases (Welch et al., 1969) also reflects induction of enzymes by xenobiotics. One such enzyme, arylhydrocarbon hydroxylase, in the human placental is often induced 8-10 fold in cigarette smokers. However, not all placentae from smoking mothers are induced.

The difference in placental enzyme inducibility may be directly related to the genome of the embryo (Shum et al., 1979). Heterogeneity in embryonic responses as noted in the placenta may partially account for the teratogenic responsiveness of certain embryos compared with others. The formation of reactive intermediates from polycyclic hydrocarbons has been documented in human placental enzyme preparations. This fact was confirmed for benzo(α)pyrene by covalent binding to DNA (Berry et al., 1977) and by positive mutagenic responses in the Ames test (Jones et al., 1977; Juchau et al., 1978). The presence of xenobiotic metabolism in the placenta indicates that the placenta may participate in the activation and deactivation of environmental chemicals.

For in depth discussions of xenobiotic metabolism by the placenta, the reader is referred to reviews by Juchau (1980, 1982) and Pelkonen (1980).

Receptors

Many functions of the placenta may be mediated by surface membrane or cytosolic receptors (Table 2). A number of the cell surface receptors on the trophoblast appear to be related to the selective ingestion of nutrients and molecules important to the development of the conceptus. Among the compounds having specific

Table 2   Receptors in the Human Trophoblast

Beta-Adrenergic, β_1 and β_2

Epidermal Growth Factor (EGF)

Glucocorticoid

Immunoglobulin - IgG-F_c

Insulin

Low Density Lipoprotein (LDL)

Opiate

Somatomedin

Testosterone

Transcobalamin II-Vitamin B_{12} (TC II)

Transferrin

---

placental binding sites are low density lipoprotein (Winkel et al., 1981), Immunoglobulin-G (Brambell, 1970; Faulk, 1981; Wild, 1981), transferrin (Seligman et al., 1979; Wada et al., 1979; Galbraith et al., 1980, 1981; Enns and Sussman, 1981) and transcobalamin II-vitamin-B12 (Friedman et al., 1977; Seligman and Allen, 1978; Nexø and Hollenberg, 1980; Ng et al., 1981).

Modulation of placental functions by neurochemicals is suggested by the presence of adrenergic and opiate receptors. In the placental non-brush border villus membrane there are both beta-1 and beta-2 adrenergic receptors, which are present in approximately equal proportions in the human placenta (Shocken et al., 1980; Moore and Whitsett, 1981). These receptors appear in the same membrane fraction as the placental adenylate cyclase, which is responsive to catecholamines (Whitsett et al., 1978, 1980). The placenta also contains opiate receptors (Valette et al., 1980; Ahmed et al., 1981) which are presumed to mediate the opiate reduction of human term placental amino acid accumulation (Barnwell and Sastry, 1983).

The search for placental receptors for neurochemicals has been stimulated partially by the discovery of neurochemicals in the placenta even though it is not innervated. The neurochemicals found in the placenta are: acetylcholine and its synthetic enzymes (Sastry et al., 1976, 1977, 1983; Welsch et al., 1981), methionine enkephaline (Sastry et al., 1981), substance P (Sastry et al., 1981), beta-lipotrophin and beta-endorphin (Nakai et al., 1978; Odagiri et al., 1979).

Placental receptors may also mediate or regulate placental hormone actions. Such hormones include insulin (Posner and Montreal, 1974; Marshall et al., 1974; Galbraith and Faulk, 1979), human chorionic gonadotropin (Benveniste and Scommegna, 1981), glucocorticoids (Coulam and Spelsberg, 1983), testosterone (Coulam and Spelsberg, 1983) and somatomedin (Marshall et al., 1974).

The secretion of human chorionic gonadotropin is stimulated by epidermal growth factor in the trophoblast (Benveniste and Scommegna, 1981). The receptor for epidermal growth factor is present in the placenta at least by the tenth week of gestation, and epidermal growth factor is not displaced by insulin, growth hormone, prolactin, follicle stimulating hormone, human chorionic gonadotropin, or luteinizing hormone (Benveniste et al., 1980).

In the placenta, glucocorticoids have been associated with production of CG (Wilson and Jaward, 1982) and heat-stable alkaline phosphatase (Speeg and Harrison, 1979). Coulam and Spelsberg (1983) have identified a glucocorticoid receptor in the human placenta. Thus, such alterations of placental function by glucocorticoids appear to be based upon specific binding. Similar relationships have been observed for androgen activity in the human placenta (Barile et al., 1979; McCormick et al., 1981; Coulam and Spelsberg, 1983).

Substantial controversy has developed concerning the actual presence of both estrogen and progesterone receptors in the human placenta. Since estrogens and progesterones are produced by the trophoblast in substantial amounts, many have hypothesized that receptors for these steroids must be present. The most recent exhaustive experiments by Coulam and Spelsberg (1983) have not demonstrated these steroid receptors in the cytosol or nucleus of the trophoblast. Unfortunately, it is extremely difficult to be positive that there are no specific high affinity receptors in a tissue producing large amounts of the steroids.

Thus, the placenta does respond to many exogenous and endogenous substances, e.g., certain chemicals, hormones, and proteins, as a result of substrate binding to specific trophoblastic receptors.

TRANSPORT PHYSIOLOGY

The placenta is the organ of transport for nutrients, waste products and xenobiotics, and the mechanisms of placental transport have been investigated using a variety of in vitro and in vivo technics. Proper interpretation of these in vivo and in vitro studies is important. Often the methods utilized especially for in vivo studies are dependent upon the species selected. Many of the gas-exchange studies have utilized the sheep, while many of the drug and toxin distribution studies have utilized rodents. Unfortunately, limited pharmacokinetic studies for drugs and/or toxins are available in the human. Specific methods for analyzing placental transfer processes will not be discussed in detail. The reader is referred to reviews on microvesicles (Bissonette, 1982), trophoblast cultures (Stromberg, 1980), in vitro slices, in vitro and in situ perfusions, and in vivo evaluations (Longo, 1972; Miller et al., 1976; Smith, 1981; Wallenburg et al., 1981; Young et al., 1981). Specific discussions for the transport of metals is available in Chapter 25, Miller and Shaikh (1983). Discussions of metal transport are also found in Chapters 26, 28 and 30 by Dencker et al., 1983; Levin et al., 1983 and Suzuki et al., 1983.

There are at least four major processes involved in the transport of molecules across placental membranes (Table 3). In many instances, a compound may utilize more than one process depending upon the concentration gradients established in the maternal blood, trophoblast, and fetal blood. For example, the bidirectional movement of an amino acid in the human placenta is dependent upon both a diffusional and an active transport from mother to fetus, while diffusion appears to be the primary process from fetus to mother (Wier et al., 1983a). Such examples are common, since the actual concentration gradients can determine the capacity of the carrier-mediated processes to transport compounds (Miller et al., 1976, 1977).

Simple diffusion: The diffusion of a compound is dependent upon its molecular weight (<1000 daltons), lipid solubility, ionic charge and degree of protein binding. A difficult problem is the assessment of the toxicity of a compound on the transplacental kinetics for other molecules, e.g., amino acids, which are both actively and passively transfered. The kinetics for simple diffusion must be separated from that for active processes. If one wishes to maximize for diffusion, amounts in excess of the carrier capacity of the molecule in question can be utilized or direct comparison to substances that are transferred by simple diffusion can be used. A number of investigators have examined the kinetics of substances known to be only passively transferred, e.g., antipyrine, urea, creatinine, H_2O, L-glucose (Schneider et al., 1972; Miller et al., 1976; Moll, 1981; Faber and Thornberg, 1981).

Table 3   Selected Substances Transferred by the Placenta

Mechanism	Compounds
Simple Diffusion:	Antipyrine L-Glucose Gases (Oxygen, carbon dioxide nitrous oxide) Creatinine Urea
Carrier-mediated Transport:	
Facilitated Diffusion:	D-Glucose
Active Transport:	Sodium/Potassium Calcium Creatine Amino acids Vitamin C

Receptor-Mediated Endocytosis:	Immunoglobulins
	   (IgG)
	Vitamin B_{12}
	   -transcobalamin II
	Iron-transferrin

In some instances, investigators may attribute changes in placental transfer of a substance to a direct effect on the trophoblast. However, in many instances, the decreased transfer results from alterations in blood flow (Longo, 1981; Power and Dale, 1981). Diffusion across the placenta is flow-limited. Thus, one must be careful in the interpretation of decreased placental transport of a substance and evaluate alterations in utero-placental flow as a possible mechanism.

Carrier-Mediated Transport: Many ions are transported across the placenta against a gradient, e.g., sodium, potassium and calcium (Flexner, 1948; Van Dijk, 1981). Different enzymes have been involvement with the movement of these ions. A Mg^{++}-dependent, $Na^+ + K^+$-activated ATPase and a Ca^{++} ATPase have been identified in placentae (Shami and Radde, 1972; Miller and Berndt, 1973). These ATPases are associated not only with the movement of ions but also the generation of sodium gradients which are coupled with amino acid transfer (Miller and Berndt, 1974). This ion require-ment has also been noted for creatine (Miller et al., 1977, 1979).

Amino acids have been the principal compounds used to assess toxicity related to placental transfer. The evaluations of transport function have included: 1. carrier-specificity for basic, acidic, A- and L- neutral amino acids and variations in between, 2. the energy and ion requirements, 3. the development of concentrations gradients both in the tissue and between fetal and maternal circulations, and 4. the clearance from or appearance in the respective maternal and fetal circulations of the amino acid. Usually a non-metabolized neutral amino acid, α-aminoisobutyric acid, has been utilized for this transport assessment to avoid the evaluation of protein incorporation of amino acids, e.g., alanine and glycine. However, under some experimental conditions, it may be helpful to have an index of protein incorporation (Olson and Massaro, 1980).

Besides carrier specific processes for active transport, the placental transport of d-glucose is via a facilitated diffusional process (Schroder et al., 1975; Leichtweiss, 1981). No direct energy utilization is necessary for transport of d-glucose, nor is there any concentration of glucose against a gradient. However, the transfer of d-glucose is a carrier-specific process, which is inhibited specifically by phloretin, but not phlorizin.

Endocytosis: Endocytosis is another means of uptake for extracellular materials. This process of macromolecular and particle ingestion involves the formation of vesicles, intracellular transportation of the vesicles, fusion with lysosomes and exocytosis to maintain cell volume and to excrete metabolites. These cellular processes require the presence of some or all of the following: functional cell membrane, cytoskeleton, lysosomes, protein synthesis and energy production (Silverstein et al., 1977).

Endocytosis has been subdivided into phagocytosis and pinocytosis, which are distinguished by the size of their substrates and their differential sensitivity to low temperature (Silverstein et al., 1977). Pinocytosis is further divided into specific and non-specific uptake of soluble macromolecules, and is labeled as receptor-mediated endocytosis and fluid-phase pinocytosis, respectively.

In the placenta, endocytotic activities during early stages of gestation have been described by Beck (1976) as histiotrophic when the placental cells ingest surrounding decidual cells to provide for embryonic nutrition. As the chorioallantoic placenta becomes established, nutrient transfer occurs directly between the maternal plasma and trophoblast surface and is described as the hemotrophic phase of gestation.

The pinocytotic mode of placental transfer has been studied extensively in the visceral yolk sac placenta of the rodent, and is

considered the means for uptake and degradation of maternal serum
proteins, which contribute to the fetal amino acid pool (Livesey and
Williams, 1979; Ibbotson and Williams, 1979). Serum albumin,
colloidal gold, polyvinylpyrrolidine and horseradish peroxidase are
commonly used as markers of this process (Steinman and Cohn, 1972;
Brown and Segal, 1977; Agarwal and Moore, 1978; Livesey and
Williams, 1979; Sharma and Peel, 1979; Roberts et al., 1980; Huxham
and Beck, 1981; Lloyd, 1980; Duncan et al., 1981; Livesey and
Williams, 1982; Dickson et al., 1981).

Pinocytotic processes also occur in the chorioallantoic
placenta, but, due to the ease of in vitro preparation and the
endogenous rate of uptake, pinocytosis in the placenta has been
investigated more frequently in the visceral yolk sac. In vivo,
pinocytotic markers are localized in the chorioallantoic placenta
and the cells in close proximity (Sharma and Peel, 1979). The
regional differences in pinocytotic uptake of marker molecules may
be due to the physical proximity of the tissue to the maternal
source (Myagkaya et al., 1979), and cannot be demonstrated under in
vitro conditions.

Pinocytosis in the visceral yolk sac has been reported to be
eliminated by metabolic inhibitors, such as 2,4-dinitrophenol
(Duncan and Lloyd, 1978), but some investigators report that it does
not demonstrate a significant sensitivity to low temperature or
metabolic inhibition (Ockelford and Clint, 1980; Sharpey-Shafer and
Ockleford, 1978). The possibility remains that pinocytosis requires
minimal energy or alternate energy sources such as phosphocreatine
(Miller et al., 1979; Ng and Miller, 1983).

Non-specific pinocytosis is also subject to hormonal and other
influences. Pinocytosis can be stimulated by the use of glucagon
(Brown and Segal, 1977). This effect may be mediated by the cyclic
nucleotides. Other agents such as polyanions and polycations may
also stimulate the rate of pinocytosis (Duncan et al., 1979).

The detrimental effects of the inhibition of degradative
pinocytosis may be ameliorated by the ability of the placenta to
actively transport amino acids, if placental pinocytosis is a means
to provide the conceptus with amino acids. However, interruptions
of receptor-mediated endocytosis may be more deleterious because
this specific transfer of intact macromolecules is essential to
normal growth and development of the conceptus and neonate.

Receptor-mediated endocytosis was first proposed by Brambell
(1970) and elaborated by Wild (1976, 1981) to explain the transfer
of maternal immunoglobulins to the conceptus. Immunoglobulins bind
to a surface membrane receptor which is specific for the
immunoglobulins and the binding triggers the formation of a
clathrin-coated vesicle. The coated vesicles do not fuse with

lysosomes as do other pinocytotic vesicles thereby conserving the
receptor-bound proteins. The proteins are transported to the basal
membrane for exocytosis into the fetal blood stream. Alternatively,
it has been proposed that the coated vesicles fuse with lysosomes
and only the receptor-bound proteins are protected from the
enzymatic lysis. Brambell's hypothesis of protective endocytotic
transfer of immunoglobulins is supported by the finding of a
placental membrane receptor specific for immunoglobulin G (IgG) in
the human term placental tissue (McNabb et al., 1976; Van der
Meulen, 1980; Johnson and Brown, 1981). On the other hand, Williams
and Ibbotson (1980) have shown that the rodent visceral yolk sac
degrades up to 70 percent of the absorbed IgG. The accumulating
evidence indicates that both degradative and protective endocytosis
of immunoglobulins exist in the placenta.

Receptor-mediated endocytosis is also suggested as the means
for the materno-conceptal transfer of a number of other
macromolecules. For example, the vital nutrient, cobalamin (cbl,
vitamin B_{12}) which is bound to one of its plasma carriers,
transcobalamin II (TCII), may bind to surface membrane receptors in
the human placenta that are specific for TCII-cbl (Friedman et al.,
1977; Seligman and Allen, 1978; Nexø and Hollenberg, 1980). In
cells other than the placental tissues, this receptor-bound TCII-cbl
forms coated vesicles -- which fuse with lysosomes. The degradation
of TCII releases the cobalamin moiety for cellular utilization
(Finkler and Hall, 1967; Savage and Green, 1976; Ostroy and Gams,
1977; Rothenberg et al., 1978). However in the placenta, the
receptor-mediated uptake of TCII-cbl is followed by degradative as
well as protective endocytosis. The cobalamin released from
TCII-cbl supplies the metabolic requirements of the placenta and any
excess cobalamin may be bound to placental cobalamin binder for
release (Ng and Miller, 1983). The protective receptor-mediated
endocytosis supplies the conceptus with intact maternal TCII-cbl, a
process which enables the congenital human TCII-deficient conceptus
to sustain normal intrauterine growth (Hakami et al., 1971; Hitzig
et al., 1974; Hall et al., 1979). The proportion of cobalamin
entering the conceptus via protective endocytosis has not been
determined for placental IgG uptake.

Besides TCII-cbl and IgG, receptor-mediated endocytosis is also
suggested for a number of other nutrients and hormones such as low
density lipoprotein, epidermal growth factor, insulin, human
chorionic gonadotrophin, opiates, transferrin, and ferritin (see
section on receptors). Coated vesicles isolated from human term
placenta has been shown to contain ferritin, transferrin and
immunoglobulins (Pearse, 1982).

Future investigations of placental receptor-mediated
endocytosis, will provide insight into the mechanism of endocytotic
transfer of specific macromolecules, interaction of the various

receptor-bound molecules, the intracellular pathways of the coated vesicles, and the physiological importance of pinocytosis to intrauterine growth and development of the conceptus, and further understanding of the toxic actions of agents such as Trypan blue, yolk sac antisera, compounds which disrupt the cytoskeleton, e.g. methylmercury (Sager et al., 1982), colchicine and cytochalasins (Lees and Lin, 1979), or compounds that affect lysosomal action, e.g., tertiary amines (Livesey et al., 1980). Investigators may also look forward to the possibility of intrauterine therapy by specific endocytotic delivery systems (Sly, 1980).

While pinocytosis benefits the conceptus by nutrient transfer, phagocytosis may provide mixed blessings. Like the macrophage the placental tissue may ingest large cells. In the ruminants and most carvinores, the placenta engulfs and digests extravasated maternal erythrocytes and neighboring cells (Myagkaya et al., 1979). Phagocytosis may play an important role in the implantation of the conceptus in the initial stages of gestation. However, phagocytosis may be the route of transplacental transmission of parasites (Delgado and Santos-Buck, 1978) and provide the means for infection of the fetus.

Thus, the transport characteristics for any substance in the placenta can be best summarized in the following three principles originally defined for nutrients by Dancis (1981).

"1.   Ask not whether a maternal nutrient (substance) crosses the placenta. Ask rather how, how much, and how fast. Ask also as to fetal need.

2.   Beware of the treachery of generalizations for they will surely lead you into error. All humans are animals, but not all animals behave like humans.

3.   Behold what the placenta takes and behold what it delivers, for verily they may not be the same."

With these three principles firmly in mind, the placental toxicity of a substance can be evaluated.

TOXICOLOGY

Toxic effects on the placenta are not widely recognized. It has been postulated that the placenta may be directly involved in many instances of early spontaneous abortions, fetal death, and intrauterine growth retardation (Faulk, 1981; McIntyre and Faulk, 1983), and a number of substances and conditions have been associated with alterations in the functions of the trophoblast and yolk sac. However, conclusive in vivo and in vitro evidence is limited.

It is difficult to resolve the specificity of the toxic actions of various agents in vitro when multiple methods and high doses are used. In vitro tissue preparations such as microvesicles, slices, organ cultures or cell culture monolayers often does not indicate the potential for toxic responses in vivo. As reviewed by Kelman (1979) and Goodman et al. (1982), these in vitro studies routinely require doses in the micromolar to millimolar range, but the effective circulating levels of a toxic agent are quite often in the nanomolar range. The placental responses to such high doses may indicate generalized cellular toxicity instead of specific placental toxicity.

An alternative means of monitoring placental functions and fetal distress induced by exogenous chemicals is the determination of steroid metabolism. In the human, biochemical assessments of fetal and placental metabolism of estrogens, the production of estriol, and the metabolism of dihydroepiandrosterone have been used as an index of fetal well being in clinical situations (Alsat et al., 1983). It has been noted that in the human, when there is a decrease in estriol production it may reflect utero-placental blood flow alterations as well as possible placental and/or fetal effects. Similarly, in instances of intoxication, fetal distress may be the result of either decrease utero-placental blood flow or effects on the placenta or fetus directly.

The association between cigarette smoking with altered trophoblast structure and function, premature delivery and increased abortion rates is of growing concern, and the investigations of the mechanisms of the toxic actions illustrate some of the challenges in placental toxicology. Recent evidence indicates that fetal serum thiocyanate levels are significantly increased in mothers who smoke and also in mothers who are passively exposed to cigarette smoke (Bottoms et al., 1982). Thus, a mother need not be a smoker to expose the conceptus to the constituents of cigarette smoke.

The placenta may be changed structurally as well as biochemically by cigarette smoking. Reports by Assmussen (1978) and Peereboom-Stegeman and associates (1979, 1981, 1982) have indicated that in placentae from cigarette smokers there are alterations at the ultrastructural level, particularly in the basement membrane. More recently Van der Veen and Fox (1982) has indicated an increase in the incidence of necrosis and cell clumping. Placentae from smokers have increased activities of enzymes which metabolize polycyclic hydrocarbons, e.g., benzo(α)pyrene (Welch et al., 1969; Juchau, 1980). Thus, it appears that the morphology can be changed as well as the enzymes of placentae from smokers.

The constituents in cigarette smoke are associated with altered blood flow and potential direct effects on the placenta. Among the constituents of cigarette smoke are carbon monoxide, nicotine, cyanide, polycyclic hydrocarbons, and heavy metals such as cadmium. Under in vitro conditions, all of these agents have been documented to produce cellular dysfunction. Rowell (1981) also reports altered amino acid accumulation under in vitro conditions in placenta from smoking mothers. However, to produce acute toxic insult, concentrations of these agents are usually from 10 to 1000 fold higher concentrations than the circulating toxic levels in the blood. The placenta is also known to concentrate numerous substances, but especially metals (Miller and Shaikh, 1983).

Nicotine, a constituent of cigarette smoke, may be affecting the placenta either directly or perhaps indirectly by altering uterine blood flow. Nicotine can alter the growth and development of the embryo (Garrett, 1975; Rowell and Clark, 1982; Hammer and Mitchell, 1979), increase fetal mortality, decrease placental weight to a greater degree than fetal weight and depress placental iron-transferrin uptake (Garett, 1975). One complicating factor in these iron studies was substantial maternal weight loss in the nicotine group with no pair-fed controls.

The effects of nicotine may be mediated via the placental cholinergic agents, which has been postulated to modify or regulate amino acid transfer (Sastry et al., 1977; Welsch et al., 1981). Under in vitro conditions, nicotine in low doses will increase the release of acetylcholine from the human placenta, while at high doses will decrease acetylcholine release (Olubadewo and Sastry, 1978a; Sastry et al., 1977). The release of acetylcholine, the addition of the acetylcholinesterase inhibitor atropine, and the presence of acetylcholine analogs have been correlated with a depression of amino acid uptake (Sastry et al., 1977; Rowell and Sastry, 1978; Welsch et al., 1981). Nicotine at 10^{-4}M or higher did depress α-aminoisobutyric acid uptake (Olubadvewo and Sastry, 1978; Rowell and Sastry, 1978; Barnwell et al., 1983). Other agents such as morphine and cocaine and cholinergic analogs, have produced similar decreases in amino acid uptake (Barnwell et al., 1983).

However, Rowell and Clark (1982) did not demonstrate that chronic nicotine administration can alter mouse placental acetylcholine content, acetylcholinesterase, acetyltransferase or intracellular water space. Chronic oral nicotine administration during pregnancy in the mouse results in reduced fetal and placental weight, but the in vitro placental amino acid uptake was not reduced except at the highest dose (100 μg/ml drinking water). This amino acid uptake was evaluated only at 60 min under in vitro conditions. This lack of nicotine effect on the cholinergic system of the mouse placenta would indicate that nicotine may not be producing its effects in the mouse through placental cholinergic processes but rather other processes. Such effects could be directly on the placenta or indirectly through the mother.

The comparison between chronic in vivo exposure to nicotine in animals and the acute responses to nicotine under in vitro conditions in human placental preparations demonstrates that nicotine does have the potential to alter trophoblast function; however, the underlying mechanisms are not clearly established.

Other substances (mercury, polychlorinated biphenyls) have been recently suggested to alter the amino acid transfer across the rodent placenta (Gerber et al., 1978; Olson and Massaro, 1980; Kihlstrom, 1982). After chronic oral administration of polychlorinated biphenyls in the guinea pig, the placental transfer of amino acids was investigated using an in situ perfusion technic. Accumulation of α-aminoisobutyric acid in the fetal circulation was apparently decreased. This decrease in amino acid transport by the placenta was attributed to the inhibition of Mg^+ - Na^+ + K^+-activated ATPase by hexachlorobiphenyl in the placenta. This hypothesis is based upon the effects of polychlorinated biphenyls on other tissues but is not confirmed by the measurement of the perfused placental tissue ATPase activity. It is interesting to note that the commercial preparation of polychlorinated biphenyls, Clophen-A50, is not as potent in producing a decreased appearance of α-aminoisobutyric acid in the fetal perfusate but is more potent in producing fetal death and reabsorption (Brunstrom, 1982). The exact relationship between altered placenta function and polychlorinated biphenyls requires further detailed investigation.

In some instances the parameters selected for toxicological evaluations are often not the most sensitive ones, e.g., placental transport of amino acids. The placenta has the capability for both aerobic and anaerobic metabolism (Longo et al., 1972; Miller and Berndt, 1974). Therefore, the introduction of cyanide, elimination of oxygen or other toxicants which will uncouple oxidation from phosphorylation can reduce uptake of amino acids to some degree but not entirely eliminate it. This reserve capacity and large transport capacity in the placenta itself may be the limiting factors. In a number of species especially the human, the transport of amino acids is dependent upon sodium transport (Miller et al., 1976), and different kinetics may be involved in these processes. To inhibit them with various toxicants, e.g., cadmium and mercury, may require huge concentrations (Goodman et al., 1982), although in the human and rodent placentae, 10^{-8} molar concentrations of ouabain are effective in inhibiting this process. This ouabain effect indicates a specificity for toxic interaction in the trophoblast, and the interactions of these metals and other substances may be non-specific by interfering with any cellular carrier proteins or other structural proteins. Joshi et al. (1981) have reported similar changes in organ culture when measuring CG production.

There are scattered reports in the literature suggesting that certain agents have direct placental toxic interactions. Trypan blue and anti-yolk sac antisera are two examples of direct placental toxic agents which affect pregnancy outcome. Trypan blue has been shown to be teratogenic presumably due to its ability to inhibit endocytosis in the visceral yolk sac during organogenesis. Trypan blue is localized in the visceral yolk sac vesicles via adsorptive pinocytosis but it is not found in the embryo. Under in vitro tissue incubation conditions the 17.5-day visceral yolk sac concentrated Trypan blue to a concentration of 100 μg/ml, above which the rate of endocytosis began to decrease. The teratogenic effects of Trypan blue may be due to the inhibition of lysosome degradation of macromolecules or intracellular movements of vesicles (pinosomes), although formation of pinosomes is not inhibited until Trypan blue concentration reaches 100 μg/ml or higher. The precise mechanism of its interference with in utero nutrient transfer is not clear.

Similar to Trypan blue, anti-yolk sac sera can be teratogenic or an abortifacient (Brent et al., 1983). Localization of the antibodies in the rodent visceral yolk sac has been observed. Freeman and associates (1981) demonstrated that such antisera disrupt endocytosis and the subsequent protein degradation. Whether the abortigenic and teratogenic actions of the yolk sac antisera are related solely to the inhibition of endocytosis remains to be examined.

The only agent evaluated in depth as a direct placental toxic agent is cadmium. Its placental toxicity was originally noted by Parizek in 1964. A single maternal injection of cadmium will result in placental necrosis and fetal death within 24 hours. These placental alterations were not observed following direct fetal injections of cadmium (Levin and Miller, 1980). Additional studies (Levin et al., 1981, 1983) demonstrate that there are early cellular changes in the trophoblast prior to any fetal death or significant alterations in the utero-placental blood flow. These early effects are expressed as increased mitochondrial calcium levels and ultrastructural changes in the trophoblast, and have not been seen with the direct administration of metallothionein-cadmium to pregnant dams (Plautz et al., 1980). One of the interesting observations with cadmium is that it is not readily transfered to the fetus but is highly accumulated by the placenta. Similar observations have been noted for the human placenta under in vitro perfusion conditions (Wier et al., 1983b).

Webb and Samarawickrama (1981) have demonstrated that on day 12 of gestation in the rat, single in vivo doses of cadmium will inhibit the embryonic accumulation of zinc, which is essential for normal in utero development. Excess zinc administered during pregnancy will reduce some of the fetal growth retardation effects of cadmium (Ahokas et al., 1980). Since cadmium does not readily penetrate into the embryo at this stage in development, it is proposed that the placenta and the extraembryonic membranes may be regulating the toxic response to cadmium.

The common end point of placental necrosis in animals can be achieved via other interventions besides cadmium administration. These include the administration of serotonin (Robson and Sullivan, 1965), induction of vitamin E deficiency by feeding peroxidized lipids (Kaunitz et al., 1962) and the injection of endotoxin (McKay and Huang, 1962). The necrosis of the trophoblast due to serotonin administration appears to be related to alterations in utero-placental blood flow, while the cause of the histological changes induced by vitamin E deficiency or a reaction to endotoxin are currently not established. Thus, it appears that a number of agents can produce placental toxicity without substantial effects on the mother.

Placental toxicity may also be expressed by the induction of trophoblastic neoplasia in the mother. In mice and rats, ethylnitrosourea is embryotoxic, teratogenic and carcinogenic following only a single maternal exposure (Rice, 1979). In Patas monkeys treated with ethylnitrosourea during pregnancy, trophoblastic neoplasia developed (Rice et al., 1981). This appearance of trophoblastic neoplasia in the adult females treated during pregnancy with ethylnitrosourea is the first demonstration of a chemically-induced choriocarcinoma. Choriocarcinoma is the equivalent of the trophoblast growing in an extrauterine site usually the lungs and/or brain. The neoplasia has similar morphologic characteristics to trophoblastic tissue, and the neoplasia secretes numerous placental hormones including CG. Hence, it is possible to induce maternal toxicity via the placenta.

What are appropriate transport markers for the evaluation of placental toxicity Preliminary studies by Dencker (unpublished observations), indicate that the placental transport of amino acids in the mouse is unaffected following cadmium exposure, while the placental transport of vitamin B_{12} is substantially reduced. Like immunoglobulin G, vitamin B_{12} is transported across the placenta apparently via receptor-mediated endocytosis. It has been noted that intrauterine growth retarded human neonates have significantly lower levels of vitamin B_{12}, folate and pantothenate than their normal-birth weight counterparts, despite similar normal maternal levels of vitamins (Baker et al., 1977). Further studies indicate that the human placenta concentrates vitamin B_{12} in the maternofetal transfer of the vitamin (Baglan et al., 1981; Ng et al., 1981; Ng and Miller, 1983). The human placental transfer of vitamin B_{12} may also be sensitive to the effects of cadmium as the process in the rodent and merits further investigation. Since receptor-mediated endocytosis is a much more complex transfer process, it may be a more sensitive indicator of toxic response. Another possible marker of placental toxicity may be the proliferation of X-cells in placental tissue. Placental tissues from intrauterine growth retarded pregnancies, especially those accompanied by chronic ischemia, have altered morphology which includes a proliferation of X-cells (review by Altshuler, 1981).

It is essential to attempt a correlative study of in vivo and in vitro responses. The use of drugs in the in vitro perfused placenta lobules for prolonged perfusions in excess of 8 hours may be helpful in establishing the responsiveness of the human placenta to toxicants. Such evaluations of this tissue can include steroid and protein hormone metabolism, transport, membrane integrity, fetal oxygen consumption and blood flow characteristics as well as morphological criteria based upon ultrastructural analysis. Perhaps through a combination of these efforts, we can begin to understand the relationship of the placenta to toxicologic studies of development.

In summary, the placenta and its extraembryonic membranes especially the yolk sac can be involved in numerous functions, the transfer of immunoglobulins, heavy metals and other agents, the production of hormonal regulators and the survival of the tissue itself. A number of agents have been noted to alter the functions of the placenta under in vitro conditions; however, under in vivo conditions, in many instances the effects have not been well studied. Under some conditions, the alterations in placental functions appeared to reflect an effect on utero-placental blood flow or an effect directly on the placenta or yolk sac, e.g., cadmium, visceral yolk sac, antisera and trypan blue. Among the most devastating possibilities for toxicity is the potential for an agent to induce specific tissue tumors. This induction of trophoblastic neoplasia appears to be the case for ethylnitrosourea. Hopefully, this chapter and the other chapters in this volume will stimulate investigators to explore the questions of trophoblastic functions and their importance to both conceptus and mother.

ACKNOWLEDGEMENTS

The original research presented was supported in part by NIEHS 01247, 02774 and the R.W. and M.S. Goode Gift. The authors gratefully acknowledge the critical reviews by Drs. Raymond Baggs, Henry Thiede, Ellen Henry and Patrick Weir.

REFERENCES

Agarwal, P. and Moore, A.T., 1978, The pinocytosis of chemically modified albumin, in: "Protein Transmission through Living Membranes", pp. 171-183, Amsterdam: Elsevier/North Holland.

Ahmed, M.S., Byrne, W.L. and Klee, W.A., 1981, Solubilization of opiate receptors from human placenta, Placenta 3:115-121.

Ahokas, R.A., Dilts, P.V. and Lahaye, E.B., 1981, Cadmium-induced fetal grwoth retardation: protection by excess dietary zinc, Am. J. Obstet. Gynecol. 136:216-221.

Alstat, E., Bedin, M., Gisele, T., Thoumsin, H. and Cedard, L., 1983, In vivo and in vitro studies of the factors limiting the metabolism of DHA-S in different cases of impaired estrogen secretion, Trophoblast Res., in press.

Altshuler, G., 1981, "Diseases of the placenta and their effects on transport", pp. 35-43, Meade Johnson Symposium on Perinatal and Developmental Medicine 18, Meade Johnson and Co., Evansville, Indiana.

Assmussen, I., 1978, Ultrastructure of the human placenta at term - observations on placentas from newborn children of smoking and nonsmoking mothers, Acta Obst. Gynecol. Scand. 56:119-126.

Awasthi, Y.C. and Dao, D.D., 1981, Glutathione-mediated detoxification mechanisms of human placenta, Placenta 3:289-301.

Baglan, J.C., Brill, A.B., Schubert, A., Wilson, D., Larsen, K., Baker, H., Frank, O., Deangelis, B., Feingold, S. and Kaminetzky, H.A., 1981, Role of placenta in maternal-fetal vitamin transfer in humans, Amer. J. Ostet. Gyn. 141:792-796.

Baker, H., Thind, I.S., Frank, O., DeAngelis, B., Caterini, H. and Louria, D.B., 1977, Vitamin levels in low-birth-weight newborn infants and their mothers, Amer. J. Obstet. Gyn. 129:521-524.

Barile, G., Nagiani, S., Montemuro, A., Mango, D. and Scirpa, P., 1979, Evidence for a testerone binding macromolecule in human placental cytosol, J. Steroid Biochem. 11:1247-1252.

Barnwell, S.L. and Sastry, B.V.R., 1983, Depression of amino acid uptake in human placental villus by nicotine, morphine and cocaine, Trophoblast Res., in press.

Battaglia, F., 1981, Metabolism of the placenta: its physiologic applications, in: "Placental Transport", Mead Johnson Symposium on Perinatal Medicine and Developmental Medicine, No. 18. pp. 9-13, Mead Johnson and Co., Evansville, Indiana.

Beck, F., 1982, "Model Systems in Teratology Research", K. Snell, ed., pp. 11-32, Praeger, New York.

Beck, F., 1976, Comparative placental pathology and function, Environ. Hlth. Persp. 18:5-12.

Beckman, D., Jensen, M., Burman, M., Koszalka, T.R. and Brent, R.L., 1981, Rat trophoblastic cell antigenicity, Placenta 3:75-84.

Beer, A.E. and Sio, J.O., 1982, Placenta as an immunological barrier, Biol. Reprod. 26:15-27.

Benveniste, R. and Scommegna, A., 1981, Human chorionic gonadotropin and free alpha subunit secreted by cultured human choriocarcinoma (JEG-3) cells, Placenta 3:241-250.

Benveniste, R., Chase, R. and Scommegna, A., 1980, Characteristics of epidermal growth factor receptors in early, midterm and term placentas, Abstracts of the 8th Rochester Trophoblast Conference.

Berry, D.L., Zachariah, P.K., Slaga, R.J. and Juchau, M.R., 1977, Analysis of biotransformation of benzo(α)pyrene in human fetal and placental tissues with high-pressure liquid chromatography, Europ. J. Canc. 13:667-675.

Billington, W.D. and Bell, S.C., 1982, Immunoregulatory factors in pregnancy: essential or irrelevant in the maintenance of the fetal placental allograft, Placenta 4:13-23.

Bishcof, P., Geinoz, A., Herrman, W.L. and Sizonenko, P.C., 1983, Inhibition of complement activity by pregnancy-associated plasma protein A: Studies on the molecular mechanism of inhibition, in: "Fetal Nutrition, Metabolism, and Immunology: Role of the Placenta", R.K. Miller, and H.A. Thiede, eds., Plenum Press, New York, in press.

Bissonnette, J.M., 1982, Membrane vesicles from trophoblast cells as models for placental exchange studies, Placenta 3:99-106.

Bjorkman, N., 1970, "An Atlas of Placental Fine Structure", Williams and Wilkins Co., Baltimore, MD.

Bottoms, S.F., Kuhnert, B.R., Kuhnert, P.M. and Reese, A.L., 1982, Maternal passive smoking and fetal serum thiocyanate levels, Amer. J. Obstet. Gynecol. 144:787-791.

Brambell, F.W.R., 1970, "The Transmission of Passive Immunity from Mother to Young", American Elsevier, New York.

Brent, R.L., Jensen, M., Koszalka, T.R., Beckman, D.A. and Damjanov, I., 1983, Pathological findings in rat embryonic sites exposed to teragenic yolk sac, in: "Fetal Nutrition, Metabolism and Immunology: Role of the Placenta, R.K.Miller and H.A.Thiede, eds., Plenum Press, New York, in press.

Brunstrom, B., Kihlstrom, I. and Lundkvist, U., 1982, Studies of foetal death and foetal weight in guinea pig fed polychlorinated biphenyls (PCB), Acta Pharm. Tox. 50:100-103.

Buehrdel, P., Willigerodt, H., Keller, E., Theile, H. and Emmrich, P., 1974, Intrauterine dystrophy in rats due to placental insufficiency caused by hormonally induced prolonged gestation, Biol. Neonate 24:57-65.

Brown, J.A. and Segal, H.L., 1977, Effect of glucagon on pinocytosis by the yolk sac of the rat, J. Biol. Chem. 252:7151-7155, 1977.

Clark, C.C., Tomichek, E.A., Koszalka, T.R., Minor, R.R. and Kefolides, N.A., 1975, The embryonic rat parietal yolk sac. The role of the parietal endoderm in the biosynthesis of basement membrane collagen and glycoprotein in vitro, J. Biol. Chem. 250:5259-5267.

Coulam, C.V. and Spelsberg, T.C., 1983, The placenta as a target tissue for steroids, Trophoblast Res., in press.

Dancis, J., 1981, Placental transport of amino acids, fats and minerals, in: "Placental Transport," Mead Johnson Symposium on Perinatal and Developmental Medicine, Number 18, Evansville: Mead Johnson, pp. 25-32.

Dancis, J., Ghosh, N.K., Jansen, V., Schneider, H., Fallon, R.J., and Cox, R.P., 1979, Secretory proteins in the perfused human placenta, Biol. Neonate 35:188-193.

Delgado, M.A. and Santos-Buch, C.H., 1978, Transplacental
    transmission and fetal parasitosis of trypanosome cruzi in
    outbred white Swiss mice, Am. J. Trop. Med. Hyg. 27:1108-1115.
Dencker, L., Danielsson, B., Khayat, A. and Lingren, A., 1983,
    Disposition of metals in the embryo and fetus, in:
    "Reproductive and Developmental Toxicity of Metals", T.
    Clarkson, G. Norberg and P. Sager, eds., Plenum Press, New
    York, this volume.
Dickson, R.B., Willingham, M.C. and Pastan, I., 1981,
    α_2-Macroglobulin adsorbed to colloidal gold: a new probe in
    the study of receptor-mediated endocytosis, J. Cell. Biol.
    89:29-34.
Duncan, R. and Lloyd, J.B., 1978, Pinocytosis in the rat visceral
    yolk sac. Effects of temperature, metabolic inhibitors and
    some other modifiers, Biochem. Biophys Acta 544(3):647-655.
Duncan, R., Pratten, M.K., Cable, H.C., Ringsdorf, H. and Lloyd,
    J.B., 1981, Effects of molecular size of ^{125}I-labelled
    poly(vinylpyrrolidine) on its pinocytosis by rat visceral yolk
    sacs and rat peritoneal macrophages, Biochem. J. 196:49-55.
Duncan, R., Pratten, M.K. and Lloyd, J.B., 1979, Mechanism of
    polycation stimulation of pinocytsis, Biochem. Biophys. Acta
    587:463-475.
Duncan, R., Rejmanova, P. Kopecek, J. and Lloyd, J.B., 1981,
    Pinocytic uptake and intracellular degradation of N (2-
    hydropolproply)-methacrylamide copolymers. A potential drug
    delivery system, Biochem. Biophys. Acta 678:143-150.
Enns, C.A. and Sussman, H.H., 1981, Characterization of the
    transferrin-binding protein in the human trophoblast, Placenta
    3:23-32.
Faber, J.J. and Thornburg, K.L., 1981, The forces that drive inert
    solutes and water across the epitheliochorial placentae of the
    sheep and goat and the haemochorial placentae of the rabbit and
    guinea pig, Placenta 2:203-214.
Faulk, W.P., 1981, Tropohoblast and extraembryonic membranes in the
    immunobiology of the human pregnancy, in: "Placenta:
    Receptors, Pathology, and Toxicology", R.K. Miller and H.A.
    Thiede, eds., pp. 3-22, W.B. Saunders, London.
Finkler, A.E. and Hall, C., 1967, Nature of the relationship between
    vitamin B_{12} binding and cell uptake, Arch. Biochem. Biophys.
    120:79-85.
Flexner, L.B., Cowie, D.B., Hellman, L.M., Wilde, W.S. and Vosburgh,
    G.J., 1948, The permeability of the human placenta to sodium in
    normal and abnormal pregnancies and the supply of Na^+ to the
    human fetus as determined with radioactive Na^+, Am. J.
    Obstet. Gyn. 55:469-480.
Freeman, S.J., Beck, F. and Lloyd, J.B., 1981, The role of the
    visceral yolk sac in mediating protein utilization by rat
    embryos cultured in vitro, J. Embryol. Exptl. Morph. 66:223-234.

Friedman, P.A., Shia, M.A. and Wallace, J.C., 1977, A saturable
    high affinity binding site for transcobalamin II-vitamin B_{12}
    complexes in human placental membrane preparations, J. Clin.
    Invest. 59:51-58.
Galbraith, G.N.P., Galbraith, R.N., Temple, A. and Faulk, W.P.,
    1980, Demonstration of transferrin receptors on human placenta
    trophoblast, Blood 55:240-242.
Galbraith, R.N. and Faulk, W.P., 1979, Immunologic considerations of
    the materno-fetal relationship in diabetes mellitus, in: "The
    Diabetic Pregnancy", I.R. Merkatz and P.A.J. Adams, eds.,
    pp. 111-121, Grune and Stratton, London.
Galbraith, R.N., Werner, P., Kantor, R. and Galbraith, G.M.P., 1981,
    Studies of the interaction between human transferrin and
    specific receptors on the trophoblast membrane, Placenta
    3:49-60.
Garrett, R.J.B., 1975, Nicotine and placental iron transport,
    Experientia 31:486-488.
Gerber, G., Maes, J. and Deroo, J., 1978, Effect of dietary lead on
    placental blood flow and on fetal uptake of alph-amino
    iosbutyrate, Arch. Toxicol. 41:125-131.
Goodman, D.R., James, R.C. and Harbison, R.D., 1982, Placental
    toxicology, Fd. Chem. Toxicol. 20:123-128.
Hakami, N., Neiman, P.E., Canellos, G.P. and Lazerson, J., 1971,
    Neonatal megaloblastic anemia due to inherited transcobalamin
    II deficiency in two siblings, New Engl. J. Med. 285:1163-1170.
Hall, C.A., 1973, Congenital disorders of vitamin B_{12} transport
    and their contribution to concepts, Gastroenterology 65:684-686.
Hall, C.A., Hitzig, W.H., Green, P.D. and Begley, J.A., 1979,
    Transport of therapeutic cyanocobalamin in the cogenital
    deficiency of transcobalamin II (TC II), Blood 53:251-263.
Hammer, R.E. and Mitchell, J.A., 1979, Nicotine reduces embryo
    growth, delays imnplantation and retards parturition in rats,
    Proc. Soc. Exp. Biol. Med. 162:333-336.
Hitzig, W.H., Dohmann, U., Pluss, H.J. and Vischer, D., 1974,
    Hereditary transcobalamin II deficiency: clinical findings in
    a new family, J. Peds. 85:622-628.
Huxman, M. and Beck, F., 1981, Receptor-mediated coated vesicle
    transport of rat IgG agross the 11.5 day in vitro rat yolk sac
    endoderm, Cell. Biol. Int. Rep. 5:1073-1081.
Ibbotson, G.E. and Williams, K.E., 1979, Rate of pinocytic capture
    of macromolecular substrates by rat yolk sac incubated in
    serum-free culture medium, Biochem. J. 178:785-792.
Johnson, P.M. and Brown, P.J., 1981, Review article: Fc gamma
    receptors in the human placenta (review), Placenta 2:355-370.
Jones, A.H., Fantel, A.G., Kocon, R.A. and Juchau, M.R., 1977,
    Bioactivation of procarcinogens to mutagens in human fetal and
    placental tissues, Life Sci. 21:1831-1837.
Jones, C.J. and Fox, H, 1978, An ultrastructural study of the
    placenta in materno-fetal rhesus incompatibility, Virchows
    Arch. (Pathol. Anat.) 379:229-41.

Joshi, S.G., Bank, J.F. and Makarachi, A., 1980, An in vitro model
    to study anti-trophoblastic agents in women, Abstracts of the
    8th Rochester Trophoblast Conference, p. 5.
Juchau, M.R., Nornkung, M.J., Jones, A.H. and DiGiovanni, J., 1978,
    Biotransformation and bioactivation of 7,12-dimethyl-
    benz(α)anthracene in human fetal and placental tissues, Drug
    Metabol. Dispos. 6:273-281.
Juchau, M.R., 1980, Drug biotransformation in the placenta,
    Pharmacology Therapeutics 8:501-524.
Juchau, M.R., 1982, The role of the placenta in developmental
    toxicology, in: "Developmental Toxicolgy", K. Snell, ed., pp.
    187-210, Praeger, New York.
Kaunitz, H., Malins, D.C. and McKay, D.G., 1962, Studies of the
    generalized Schwartman reaction produced by diet II: feeding of
    fraction of oxidized cod liver oil, J. Expt. Med. 115:1127-1136.
Kaufmann, P. and Davidoff, M., 1977, "The Guinea-Pig Placenta",
    Springer-Verlag, Berlin.
Kelman, B.J., 1979, Effects of toxic agents on movements of material
    across the placenta, Fed. Proc. 38:2246-2250.
Kihlstrom, I., 1982, Placental transport of the non-metabolizable
    α-aminoisobutyric acid in guinea pigs given a commercial
    chlorobiphenyl preparation or a defined pure chlorobiphenyl,
    Acta Pharmacologia et Toxicologia 51:428-433.
Klopper, A., ed., 1982, "Immunology of Human Placental Proteins",
    Praeger, New York.
Klopper, A., 1983, Steroid and protein metabolism by the
    trophoblast, in: "Fetal Nutrition, Metabolism, and
    Immunology: Role of the Placenta", R.K. Miller, and H.A.
    Thiede, eds., Plenum Press, New York, in press.
Kuhnert, P.M., Kuhnert, B.R., Bottoms, S.F. and Erhard, P., 1982,
    Cadmium levels in maternal blood, fetal cord blood, and
    placental tissues of pregnant women who smoke, Amer. J. Obstet.
    Gyn. 142:1021-1025.
Lees, A. and Lin. S., 1979, 7-acetylcytochalasin B: differential
    effects on sugar transport and cell motility, J. Supramol.
    Struct. 12:185-194.
Leichtweiss, H.P., 1981, Carrier - mediated placental transfer,
    Placenta 1:115-124.
Leiser, R. and Enders, A.C., 1980a, Light- and electron-microscopic
    study of the near-term paraplacenta of the domestic cat. I.
    Polar zone and paraplacental junctional areas, Acta Anat.
    (Basel) 106:293-311.
Leiser, R. and Enders, A.C., 1980b, Light- and electron-microscopic
    study of the near-term paraplacenta of the domestic cat. II.
    Paraplacental hematoma, Acta Anat. (Basel) 106:312-326.
Levin, A.A. and Miller, R.K., 1980, Fetal toxicity of cadmium in the
    rat: maternal vs. fetal injections, Teratology 22:1-6.
Levin, A.A., Plautz, J.R., di Sant'Agnese, P.A. and Miller, R.K.,
    1981, Cadmium: placental mechanisms of fetal toxicity,
    Placenta 3:303-318.

Levin, A.A., Kilpper, R. and Miller, R.K., 1983, Organ specific kinetics of a fetal toxic injection of CdCl$_2$ in the pregnant rat, Toxicol. Appl. Pharmacol., in press.

Levin, A.A., Miller, R.K. and di Sant'Agnese, P.A., 1983, Heavy metal alterations of placental functions: A mechanism for the induction of fetal toxicity by cadmium, in: "Reproductive and Developmental Toxicity of Metals", T. Clarkson, G. Nordberg and P. Sager, eds., Plenum Press, New York, this volume.

Levine, P., 1983, Antibody-induced abortion, in: "Women in Three Different Studies", Trophoblast Res., in press.

Levy, G., 1981, Pharmacokinetics of fetal and neonatal exposure to drugs, Obstet. Gyn. 58:9S-16S.

Livesey, G. and Williams, K.F., 1979, Hydrolysis of an exogenous ^{125}I-labelled protein by rat yolk sacs. Evidence for intracellular degradation within lysomes, Biochem. J. 184:519-526.

Livesey, G. and Williams, K.E., 1981, Rates of pinocytic capture of simple proteins by rat yolk sacs incubated in vitro, Biochem. J. 198:581-586.

Livesey, G. and Williams, K.E., 1982, Heterogeneity of binding site for adsorptive pinocytosis of simple proteins by rat yolk sacs, Eur. J. Biochem. 122:147-151.

Livesey, G., Williams, K.E., Knowles, S.E. and Ballard, F.J., 1980, Effects of week bases on the degradation of endogenous and exogenous proteins by rat yolk sac, Biochem. J. 188:895-903.

Lloyd, J.B., 1980, Insights into mechanisms of intracellular protein turnover from studies on pinocytosis, in: "Protein Degradation in Health and Disease", Ciba Foundation Symposium 75:151-165.

Longo, C.D., 1972, Disorders of placenta transfer, in: "Pathophysiology of Gestation", A. Assali, ed., Volume II, pp. 1-76, Academic Press, New York.

Longo, C.D., 1981, The interrelations of maternal-fetal transfer and placental blood flow, Placenta 2:45-64.

Longo, L.D., Yuen, P. and Gusseck, D.J., 1972, Anaerobic glycogen-dependent transport of amino acids by the placenta, Nature (London) 243:531-534.

McCormick, P.D., Razel, A.J., Spelsberg, T.C. and Coulam, C.B., 1981, Absence of high-affinity binding of progesterone (R5020) in human placenta and fetal membranes, Placenta 3:123-132.

McIntyre, J.A., Faulk, W.P. and O'Sullivan, M.J., 1981, Interaction of trophoblast membranes with lymphocytes and other cells, Placenta 3:95-102.

McIntyre, J.A. and Faulk, W.P., 1982, HLA and the generation of diversity in human pregnancy, Placenta 4:1-11.

McIntyre, J.A. and Faulk, W.P., 1983, Effective cellular immunity and recurrent spontaneous abortions, Trophoblast Res., in press.

McKay, D.G. and Wong, T.C., 1962, Studies of the generalized Schwartman reaction produced by diet. I: Pathology, J. Expt. Med. 115-1117-1126.

McNabb, T., Koh, T.Y., Dorrington, K.J. and Painter, R.H., 1976, Structure and function of immunoglobulin domains. V. Binding of immunoglobulin G and fragments to placental membrane preparations, J. Immunol. 117:882-888.

Magos, L. and Webb, M., 1983, The influence of weight and other physiological changes during pregnancy and lactation on toxicities of mercury and cadmium, in: "Reproductive and Developmental Toxicity of Metals", T. Clarkson, G. Nordberg and P. Sager, eds., Plenum Press, New York, in press.

Marshall, R.N., Underwood, L.E., Voina, S.J., Founshee, D.V. and Van Wyk, J.J., 1974, Characterization of the insulin and somatomedin-C receptors in human placental cell membranes, J. Clin. Endocrinol. Metab. 39:283-292.

Miller, D.S. and Holliday, C.W., 1982, $HgCl_2$ inhibition of L-leucine transport in hamster placental slices, Environ. Res. 28:32-38.

Miller, R.K. and Shaikh, Z., 1983, Prenatal metabolism: metals and metallothionein, in: "Reproductive and Developmental Toxicity of Metals", T. Clarkson, G. Nordberg and P. Sager, eds., Plenum Press, New York, this volume.

Miller, R.K., 1983, Perinatal toxicology: its recognition and fundamentals, Amer. J. Indust. Med. 4:205-244.

Miller, R.K. and Berndt, W.O., 1973, Evidence for Mg^{++}-dependent, Na^+ and K^+-activated ATPase and Ca^{++}-ATPase in the human term placenta, Proc. Soc. Exptl. Biol. Med. 143:118-122.

Miller, R.K. and Berndt, W.O., 1974, Characterization of neutral amino acid accumulation by human placenta slices, Am. J. Physiol. 227:1236-1242.

Miller, R.K. and Thiede, H.A., eds., 1981, "Placenta: Receptors, Pathology and Toxicology", W.B. Saunders, London.

Miller, R.K. and Thiede, H.A., eds., 1983, "Fetal Nutrition, Metabolism and Immunology: Role of the Placenta", Plenum Press, New York.

Miller, R.K., Davis, B.M., Brent, R.L. and Koszalka, T.R., 1977, Placental transport of creatine in the rat, Am. J. Physiol. 233:E308-E315.

Miller, R.K., Koszalka, T.R. and Brent, R.L. 1976, Transport mechanisms for molecules across placental membranes, in: "Cell Surface Reviews", G. Poste and G. Nicolson, eds., pp. 145-332, Elsevier/North-Holland, Amsterdam.

Miller, R.K., Reich, K.A., Fox, H.E. and Koszalka, T.R., 1979, Creatine Transport and Energy Metabolism by the Human Placenta, Rochester Trophoblast Conf. 7:80-83.

Mobbs, I.G. and McMillan, D.B., 1981, Transport across endodermal cells of the chick yolk sac during early stages of development, Am. J. Anat. 160:285-308.

Moll, W., 1981, Diffusional placental transfer, Placenta 1:101-112.

Moore, J.J. and Whitsett, J.S., 1981, The beta-adrenergic receptors from human placenta: Receptor subtype analysis (B_1 and B_2) and partial characterization of the solubilized receptor, Placenta 3:103-115.

Moore, J.J., Baker, J.V. and Whitsett, J.A., 1983, Protein kinases in human placenta, Trophoblast Res., in press.

Myagkaya, G., Schellens, J.P., Vreeling-Sindelarova, H., 1979, Lysosomal breakdown of erythrocytes in the sheep placenta. An Ultrastructural study, Cell Tissue Res. 197:79-94.

Nakai, Y., Nakaok, K., Oki, S. and Imura, H., 1978, Presence of the immunoreactive beta-lipotropin and beta-endophin in human placenta, Life Sci. 23:2013-2018.

Nexø, E. and Hollenberg, M.D., 1980, Characterization of the particulate and soluble acceptor for transcobalamin II from human placenta and rabbit liver. Biochim. Biophys. Acta 628:190-200.

Ng, W.W., Catus, R. and Miller, R.K., 1981, Macromolecule transfer in the human trophoblast: Transcobalamin II-vitamin B12 uptake, Placenta 3:145-160.

Ng, W.W. and Miller, R.K., 1983, Transport of nutrients in the early human placenta: Amino acid, creatine and vitamin B12, Trophoblast Res., in press.

Ockleford, C.D. and Clint, J.M., 1980, The uptake of IgG by human placental chiorionic villi: A correlated autoradiographic and wide aperture counting study, Placenta 1:91-111.

Odagiri, E., Sherrell, D.J., Mount, C.D., Nicholson, W.E. and Orth, D.N., 1979, Placental immunoreactive corticotropin, lipotropin, and beta-endophin: evidence for a common precursor, Proc. Natl. Acad. Sci. USA 77:2027-2031.

Olson, F.C. and Massaro, E.J., 1980, Developmental pattern of cAMP, adenyl cyclase, and cAMP phosphodiesterase in the palate, lung and liver of the fetal mouse: alterations resulting from exposure to methylmercury at levels inhibiting palate closure, Teratol. 22:155-166.

Olubadewo, J.O. and Sastry, B.V.R., 1978, Human placental cholinergic system: stimulation-secretion coupling for release of acetylcholine from isolated placental villus, J. Pharm. Expt. Therap. 204:433-445.

Ostroy, F. and Gams, R.A., 1977, Cellular fluxes of vitamin B12, Blood 50:877-887.

Panigel, M., 1981, Placental function: toxicology and pathology, in: "Placenta: Receptors, Pathology and Toxicology", R.K. Miller, and H.A. Thiede, eds., pp. 275-288, W.B. Saunders, London.

Parizek, J., 1964, Vascular changes at sites of estrogen biosynthesis produced by injection of camdium: a destruction of the placenta by cadmium, J. Reprod. Fertil. 7:263-264.

Parizek, J., 1964, The peculiar toxicity of cadmium during pregnancy: an experimental toxemia of pregnancy induced by cadmium, J. Reprod. Fertil. 9:111-112.

Pearse, B.M., 1982, Coated vesicles from human placenta carry ferritin, transferrin and immunoglobulin G, Proc. Natl. Acad. Sci. USA 79:451-455.

Peereboom, J.W. Copius, de Voogt, P., van Hattum, B., van de Velde, W. and Peereboom-Stegeman, J.H.J., 1979, The use of the human placenta as a biological indicator for cadmium exposure, Int. Conf.: Management and Control of Heavy Metals in the Environment.

Peereboom, J.W. Copius, and Peereboom, J.H.J. Copius, 1981, Exposure and health effects of cadmium, Part 2. Toxic effects of cadmium to animals and man, Tox. Environ. Chem. Rev. 4:67-178.

Peereboom-Stegeman, J.H.J., Jongstra-Spaapen, E., Letschert, J. and Dessing, H., 1981, Effects of cadmium exposure on female reproductive organs, Int. Conf.: Heavy Metals in the Environment.

Peereboom-Stegeman, J.H.J. Copius, van der Velde, W.J. and Dessing, J.W.M., 1982, Influence of cadmium on placental structure, Ecotox. Environ. Safety, in press.

Pelkonen, O., 1980, Environmental influences on human fetal and placental xenobiotic metabolism, Eur. J. Clin. Pharmacol. 18:17-24.

Penfold, P., Drury, L., Simmonds, R. and Hytten, F.E., Studies of a single placental cotyledon in vitro: I. The preparation and its viability, Placenta 2:149-154.

Penfold, P. and Illsley, N.P., 1983, Placental amino acid transfer and metabolism in oxygenated conditions using the human placenta perfused in vitro, in: "Fetal Nutrition, Metabolism and Immunology: Role of the Placenta", R.K. Miller, and H.A. Thiede, eds., Plenum Press, New York, in press.

Plautz, J.R., Levin, A.A. and Miller, R.K., 1980, Fetal and maternal toxicity of cadmium metallothionein and its distribution in the pregnant Wistar rat, Teratology 21:61a.

Posner, B.I. and Montreal, M.D., 1974, Insulin receptors in human and animal placental tissue, Diabetes 23:209-217.

Pratten, M.K., Duncan, R., Cable, H.C., Schnea, R., Ringsdorf, H. and Lloyd, J.B., 1981, Pinocytic uptake of divinyl ethyaleic anhydride (pyran copolymer) and its failure to stimulate pinocytosis, Chem. Biol. Interact. 35:319-330.

Power, G.G., 1972, The Placental Sluice: Maternal Effects on the Fetal Circulation in Respiratory Gas Exchange and Blood Flow in the Placenta, L.D. Longo and H. Bartels, eds., pp. 191-201, DHEW Publication No. NIH73-361.

Power, G.G. and Dale, P.S., 1981, Placental water transfer with uneven blood flow, Placenta 2:215-228.

Ramsey, E.M., 1982, "The Placenta. Human and Animal", Praeger, New York.

Rice, J.M., eds., 1979, Perinatal Carcinogenesis, Bethesda, MD: NCI Monograph 57, DHEW Publication No. 79-1633.

Rice, J.M., Williams, G.M., Palmer, A.E., London, W.T. and Sly, D.L., 1981, Pathology of gestational choriocarcinoma induced in Patas monkeys by ethylnitrosourea given during pregnancy, in: "Placenta: Receptors, Pathology, and Toxicology", R.K. Miller and H.A. Thiede, eds., pp. 223-230, W.B. Saunders, London.

Roberts, G., Williams, K.E. and Lloyd, J.B., 1980, Mechanism of stimulation of pinocytosis by trypan blue, Chem. Biol. Interact. 32:305-310.

Robson, J.M. and Sullivan, F.M., 1966, analysis of actions of 5-hydroxytryphamine in pregnancy, J. Physiol. (London) 184:717-732.

Rothenberg, S.P., Weiss, J.P. and Cotter, R., 1978, Formation of transcobalamin II-vitamin B_{12} complex by guinea-pig ileal nucosa in organ culture after in vivo incubation with intrinsic factor-vitamin B_{12}, Brit. J. Haematol. 40:401-414.

Rowell, P.P., 1981, The effect of maternal cigarette smoking on the ability of human placental villae to concentrate alpha-aminoisobutyric acid in vitro, Res. Comm. Subst. Abuse 2:253-266.

Rowell, P.P. and Clark, M.J., 1982, The effect of chronic oral nicotine administration on fetal weight and placental amino acid accumulation in mice, Tox. Appl. Pharmacol. 66:30-38.

Rowell, P.P. and Sastry, B.V.R., 1978, The influence of cholinergic blockade on the uptake of α-aminoisobutyric acid by isolated human placental villi, Tox. Appl. Pharmacol. 45:79-93.

Rowell, P.P. and Sastry, B.V.R., 1981, Human placental cholinergic system: Depression of the uptake of α-aminoisobutyric acid in isolated human placental villi by choline acetyltransferase inhibitors, J. Pharmacol. Exp. Ther. 216:232-238.

Sager, P.R., Doherty, R.A. and Rodier, P.M., 1982, Effects of methylmercury on developing mouse cerebellar cortex, Exp. Neurol., 77:179-193.

Sastry, B.V.R., Barnwell, S.L., Tayeb, O.S., Janson, B.E. and Owens, L.K., 1980, Occurrence of methionine enkephalin in human placental villus, Biochem. Pharmacol. 29:475-478.

Sastry, B.V.R., Olubadewo, J., Harbison, R.D. and Schmidt, D.E., 1976, Human placental cholinergic system: occurrence, distribution and variation with gestational age of acetylcholine in human placenta, Biochem. Pharmacol. 25:425-431.

Sastry, B.V.R., Olubadewo, J.O. and Boehm, F.H., 1977, Effects of nicotine and cocaine on the release of acetylcholine from isolated human placental villi, Arch. Internat. Pharm. 229:23-36.

Sastry, B.V.R., Tayeb, O.S., Barnwell, S.L., Janson, B.E. and Owens, L.K., 1981, Peptides from human placenta: methionine enkephalin and substance P, in: "Placenta: Receptors, Pathology and Toxicology", R.K. Miller and H.A. Thiede, eds., pp. 327-337, Saunders Ltd., London.

Sastry, B.V.R., Moore, R.D., Barnwell, S.L. and Rowell, P.P., 1983, Factors affecting the uptake of alpha-amino acid by human placental villus: acetylcholine, phospholipid, methylation, calcium and cytoskeletal organization, Trophoblast Res., in press.

Savage, C.R., Jr. and Green, P.D., 1976, Biosynthesis of transcobolamin II by adult rat liver parenchymal cells in culture, Arch. Biochem. Biophys. 173:691-702.

Schneider, H., Panigel, M. and Dancis, J., 1972, Transfer across the
    perfused human placenta of antipyrine, soidum, and luecine,
    Amer. J. Obstet. Gyn. 114:822-829.
Schocken, D., Caron, M. and Lefkowitz, R., 1980, The human placenta
    - a rich source of β-adrenergic receptors: characterization of
    the receptors in particulate and solubilized preparation, J.
    Clin. Endocr. Metabol. 50:1082-1087.
Schroder, H., Leichtweiss, H.P. and Madee, W., 1975, The transport
    of D-glucose, L-glucose, and D-mannose across the isolated
    guinea pig placenta, Pflugers Arch. Europ. J. Physiol.
    356:267-275.
Seligman, P.A. and Allen, R.H., 1978, Characterization of the
    receptor for TC II isolated from human placenta, J. Biol. Chem.
    253:1766-1772.
Seligman, D.A., Scheichter, R.B. and Allen, R.H., 1979, Isolation
    and characterization of the transferrin receptor from human
    placenta, J. Biol. Chem. 254:9943-9946.
Shami, Y. and Radde, I.C., 1972, The effect of the Ca^{++}/Mg^{++}
    concentration ratio on placental (Ca^{++}-Mg^{++}) ATPase
    activity, Biochim. Biophys. Acta 255:675-679.
Sharma, R. and Peel, S., 1979, Uptake of marker proteins by
    glycoprotein-containing cells of the pregnant rat uterus and
    placenta, J. Anat. 129:707-718.
Sharpey-Shafer, J.M. and Ockleford, C.O., 1978, Uptake of protein by
    cultured human trophoblast cells, Cell Biol. Int. Rep.
    2:579-589.
Shum, S., Jensen, N.M. and Nebert, D.M., 1979, The murine ah locus:
    in utero toxicity in teratogenesis associated with genetic
    differences in benzyo(α)pyrene metabolism, Teratology
    20:365-376.
Silverstein, S.C., Steinman, R.M. and Cohn, Z.A., 1977, Endocytosis,
    Ann. Rev. Biochem. 46:669-722.
Sly, W.S., 1980, Multiple recognition forms of human beta-
    glucuronidase and their pinocytosis receptors: implications
    for enzyme therapy, Birth Defects 16:115-128.
Smith, C.H., 1981, Incubation techniques and investigation of
    placental transport mechanisms in vitro, Placenta 2:163-172.
Speeg, K.P., Jr. and Harrison, R.W., 1979, The ontogeny of the human
    placental glucocorticoid receptor and inducibility of heat
    stable alkaline phosphatase, Endocrinology 104:1364-1368.
Steinman, R.M., Silver, J.M. and Cohn, Z.A., 1974, Pinocytosis in
    fibroblasts. Quantitative studies in vitro, J. Cell. Biol.
    63:949-969.
Steinman, R.M. and Cohn, Z.A., 1972, The interaction of soluble
    horseradish peroxidase with mouse peritoneal macrophages in
    vitro, J. Cell Biol. 55:186-204.
Stromberg, K., 1980, The human placenta in cell and organ culture,
    Methods in Cell Biology 21B:227-252.

Suzuki, T., 1983, Methylmercury metabolism in pregnant mice: its modification by selenium with particular reference to prenatal toxicity of these compounds, in: "Reproductive and Developmental Toxicity of Metals," T. Clarkson, G. Nordberg, and P. Sager, eds., Plenum Press, New York, this volume.

Thomas, C.R., Lowy, C., St. Hillaire, R.J. and Brunzell, J., 1983, The clearance and placental transfer of free fatty acids and triglycerides in the pregnant guinea pig, in: "Fetal Nutrition, Metabolism and Immunology: Role of the Placenta", R.K. Miller, and H.A. Thiede, eds., Plenum Press, New York, in press.

Valette, A., Reme, J.M., Pontonnier, G. and Cros, J., 1980, Specific binding for opiate-like drugs in the placenta, Biochem. Pharmacol. 29:2657-2661.

Van Der Meulen, J.A., McNabb, T.C., Haeffner-Cavaillon, N., Klein, M. and Dorrington, K.J., 1980, The Fc$_\alpha$ receptor on human placental plasma membrane. I. Studies on the binding of homologous and heterologous immunoglobulin G, J. Immunol. 124:500-507.

Van der Veen, F. and Fox, H., 1982, The effects of cigarette smoking on the human placenta: A light and electron microscopic study, Placenta 3:243-256.

Van Dijk, H.P., 1981, Active transfer of the plasma-bond compounds calcium and iron across the placenta, Placenta 1:139-164.

Villee, C., 1977, Synthesis of proteins in the placenta, J. Gynecol. Invest. 8:145-161.

Villee, C.A., 1983, Enzymes, receptors, metabolism and placental function, in: "Fetal Nutrition, Metabolism and Immunology: Role of the Placenta", R.K. Miller, and H.A. Thiede, eds., Plenum Press, New York, in press.

Wada, H.G., Hass, P.E. and Sussman, H.H., 1979, Transferrin receptor in human placental brush-borders, J. Biol. Chem. 254:12629-12635.

Wallenburg, H.C.S., Van Kreel, B.K. and Van Dijk, J.P., eds., 1981, "Transfer Across the Primate and Non-Primate Placenta", W.B. Saunders, London.

Waddell, W.J. and Marlowe, C., 1981, Transfer of drugs across the placenta, Pharmac. Therap. 14:375-390.

Webb, M. and Samarawickrama, G.P., 1981, Placental transport and embryonic utilization of essential metabolites in the rat at the teratogenic doses of cadmium, J. Appl. Toxicol. 1:270-278.

Welch, R.M., Harrison, J.E., Commi, B.W., Poppers, P.I., Finster, M. and Convey, A.H., 1969, Stimulatory effect of cigarette smoking and the hydroxylation of benzo(α)pyrene by enzymes in human placenta, Clin. Pharmacol. Therap. 10:100-110.

Welsch, F., 1979, Release of human chorionic somatomammotrophin from isolated perfused lobules and superfused fragments of term placenta: spontaneous liberation and the effects of cholinergic drugs, dibutyrylcyclic adenosine monophosphate and calcium, Res. Comm. Chem. Pathol. Pharm. 24:211-222.

Welsch, F., Wenger, W.C. and Stedman, D.B., 1981, Acetylcholine in the term placenta: tissue levels and intact fragments after inhibition in vitro both choline and acetyltransferase in relationship to ^{14}C alpha-amino isobutyric acid uptake, in: "Placenta: Receptors, Pathology and Toxicology", R.K. Miller and H.A. Thiede, eds., pp. 223-230, W.B. Saunders, London.

Whitsett, J., Johnson, C., Hawkins, K., 1978, Differences in the localization of adenylate cyclase and insulin receptors of the human placenta, Am. J. Obstet. Gyn. 133:479.

Whitsett, J., Johnson, C., Noguchi, A., Darovec-Buckerman, C. and Costello, M., 1980, Beta-adrenergic receptors and catecholamine-sensitive adenylate cyclase on the human placenta, J. Clin. Endocrinol. Metab. 50:27-32.

Wier, P., Miller, R.K. and Maulik, D., 1983a, The bidirectional transport of alpha-aminoisobutyric acid by the human perfused placental lobule, Trophoblast Res.. 1: in press.

Wier, P., Miller, R.K. and Maulik, D., 1983b, Transfer and accumulation of cadmium by the perfused human placental lobule, Teratology, in press.

Wild, A.E., 1976, Mechanism of protein transport across the rabbit yolk-sac endoderm, in: "Maternofoetal Transmission of Immunoglobulins", W.A. Hemmings, ed., pp. 155-165, Cambridge: Cambridge University Press.

Wild, A.E., 1981, Endocytic mechanisms of protein transfer across the placenta, Placenta 1:165-186.

Williams, K.E., 1982, Biochemical mechanisms of teratogenesis, in: "Developmental Toxicology", K. Snell, ed., pp. 93-129, Praeger, New York.

Williams, K.E. and Ibbotson, G.E., 1979, In vitro studies of the fate of ^{125}I-labelled IgG within rat visceral yolk sac, in: "Protein Transmission through Living Membranes", W.A. Hemmings, ed., pp. 185-195.

Wilson, E.A. and Jaward, M.J., 1982, Stimulation of human chorionic gonadotropin secretion by glucocorticoids, Am. J. Obstet. Gyn. 42:344-349.

Winkel, C.A., MacDonald, P. and Simpson, E.R., 1981, The role of receptor-mediated low-density lipoprotein uptake and degrdation in the regulation of progesterone biosynthesis and cholesterol metabolism by human trophoblasts, in: "Pathology and Toxicology", R.K. Miller and H.A. Thiede, eds., pp. 133-144, W.B. Saunders, London.

Young, M., Boyd, R.D.H., Longo, L.D. and Telegdy, G., 1981, in: "Placental Transfer: Methods and Interpretations", W.B. Saunders, London.

DISPOSITION OF METALS IN THE EMBRYO AND FETUS

Lennart Dencker, Bengt Danielsson, Amir Khayat and
Arne Lindgren

Department of Toxicology
Uppsala University
Uppsala, Sweden

ABSTRACT

The distribution of a number of metals of significance in the
work environment has been studied in pregnant experimental animals.
Particular interest has been paid to cadmium, inorganic and metallic
mercury, lead, chromium and arsenic in different forms. The degree
of uptake in the conceptus and the embryonic and fetal distribution
patterns vary considerably between different metals and with the
stage of development. Cadmium and inorganic mercury showed high
placental but low fetal concentrations, except for the early
organogenetic period. Metallic mercury was more easily transferred
to the fetus than inorganic mercury and was retained in several
fetal organs after oxidation to inorganic mercury. Lead was slowly
transferred to the fetus; lead levels increased during gestation, a
pattern observed with other foreign compounds. Highest levels of
lead were seen in fetal blood, liver and skeleton. Arsenite and
arsenate both passed relatively freely to the fetus throughout
gestation and accumulated preferentially in squamous epithelia.
Chromium VI reached higher fetal levels than chromium III and was
also more toxic to embryonic cells in vitro, which explains its
higher fetotoxicity as compared to chromium III. A number of fetal
organs and parental reproductive organs are also listed according to
their tendency to accumulate toxic metals.

INTRODUCTION

There are a number of reports where the adverse effects of
metals on the human fetus have been described. Methylmercury has
probably been the most disastrous one with the episodes in Japan

and Iraq where ingestion of contaminated fish or treated grain respectively has caused cerebral palsy and mental retardation (Matsumoto et al., 1965; Murakami, 1972; Amin-Zaki et al., 1974). Lead has been reported to increase the incidence of abortion and stillbirth (Angle and McIntire, 1964; Cantarow and Trumper, 1944) and is suspected of causing mental retardation (Beattie et al., 1975; Moore et al., 1977). Heavy ingestion of inorganic arsenic has caused neonatal death (Lugo et al., 1969). There is a case report on the transplacental carcinogenesis of arsenic. A 32-year-old man, whose mother was treated with Fowler's solution during pregnancy, developed multiple basaliomas (Aldick and Fabry, 1973), which is the typical form of skin cancer induced by arsenic. For most of the metals discussed in the toxicological literature, a number of reports on teratogenic effects in experimental animals have appeared.

It is striking how little we still know about mechanisms of teratogenic action of foreign chemicals. To restrict the present discussion to metals, one can propose three principally different modes of the adverse effects. Some metals cross the placenta and may directly influence developmental processes in the embryo. Others accumulate in the placenta and may disturb transport mechanisms, thus impairing fetal nutrition. Still another possibility is that the metal is so toxic to the maternal organism that this may secondarily disturb fetal development or even interrupt gestation.

The aim of this paper is to describe the pattern of placental and fetal distribution of a number of metals that we have lately been particularly interested in. Most of them also belong to the group of metals that have been most often discussed in the toxicological literature. First, we will review some general aspects of placental transfer of foreign compounds. Then each individual metal will be described separately and discussed in relation to what is known about its fetotoxicity. After that, a number of fetal organs and parental reproductive organs will be listed and their tendency to accumulate metals discussed. Most of our results are derived from experiments in mice or golden hamsters and occasionally in monkeys.

GENERAL ASPECTS OF PLACENTAL TRANSFER OF FOREIGN COMPOUNDS

When effects of foreign chemicals on the progress of gestation and fetal development are considered, it is essential to keep in mind the particular period of gestation. Roughly, one should distinguish between the early, organogenetic period when malformations may be induced, and later stages when one can expect more adult-type organ toxicity or functional disturbances. The same distinction should be made when one discusses embryonic and fetal uptake and distribution of chemicals.

Technically, it is difficult to measure concentrations of chemicals in early embryos, especially if they are low; contamination of excised embryos with maternal tissues or fluids may give unreliable results. It is even more crucial to determine concentrations in single embryonic organs. In a series of studies we have therefore used autoradiography to follow the placental passage and fetal accumulation of a number of organic compounds as well as metals. In this technique, thin sections (attached to tape) are cut through whole frozen animals and the dried sections are subsequently used for autoradiography (Ullberg, 1954, 1977).

In early gestation, the whole reproductive apparatus (ovaries, oviducts, uterus and cervix) is removed and frozen in a horizontal plane so that it is possible to section through all embryos at the same time (Dencker, 1976, 1979). In this way most single organs can be surveyed. One can keep the reference to maternal tissues by sectioning, e.g. the maternal liver and kidney together with the uterus. One has to keep in mind that it is radioactivity which is registered, and most often it is not possible to distinguish between the parent compound and possible metabolites. Embryonic tissues are usually not available in quantities large enough to allow the use of separation methods.

Results from autoradiographic studies on a variety of potential teratogens have been reviewed earlier (Ullberg, 1973; Waddell and Marlowe, 1976; Dencker, 1979; Ullberg et al., 1981; Dencker, 1982). The technique has provided new and interesting information related to the pattern of distribution in the conceptus. It has especially generated new information on how this pattern changes with the developmental stage of the embryo and fetus, and has also shown that one particular drug may be blocked by the placenta in one (most often early) stage but transferred in another (late) stage. The main reason for these differences appears to be that in rodents there are two placental structures, namely the yolk sac placenta, operating mainly in early gestation, and the chorioallantoic placenta, starting to function around day 11 in the mouse. They apparently show differences in their discrimination of foreign chemicals (Dencker, 1979, 1982).

Another reason for the often observed increase in fetal uptake of foreign compounds in the latter part of gestation may be changes that occur in the fetus. Such parameters include binding to fetal plasma proteins, cellular or extracellular proteins (e.g. arsenic to keratin), or calcified areas of the skeleton (several elements like lead, chromium, barium). Also, the capacity of fetal organs to transform foreign compounds metabolically increases with age. This tends to increase their retention in the fetal tissues, either as a result of the relatively higher polarity of the metabolites, or their firmer binding to tissue components. This is of importance especially for organic compounds, but also for some metals such as metallic mercury (see below).

METALS

Zinc - Cadmium

It seems pertinent to begin this survey of metals in the fetus
with a comparison of zinc and cadmium. These two metals, being in
the same group in the periodic system, often accompany each other in
minerals and organic matter. Cadmium interferes in a number of the
physiological functions of zinc. This is evidenced by the fact that
zinc often counteracts the toxicity of cadmium, including the
teratogenic effects, and the two metals to some extent bind to the
same sites on proteins.

The kinetics of the two related compounds in the conceptus are
very different. Zinc is readily taken up in embryonic and fetal
structures, apparently in a pattern that mirrors its role as a
co-factor in cellular processes related to replication and growth.
It can thus be recovered in the neuroepithelium and in the
developing endodermal structures, such as gut and liver, and the
somites (Dencker, 1976) (Figure 1). Cadmium, on the other hand, is
almost totally prevented from reaching the fetus and at the same
time is accumulated by the placental structures (Berlin and Ullberg,
1963b; Dencker, 1975) (Figure 2); cadmium may cause placental
necrosis and fetal wastage in the latter part of gestation (Parizek,
1964). Gale and Ferm (1973) observed malformation in the hamster
when cadmium was given during a restricted period of the early
organogenetic period; they also reported that when radioactive
cadmium was administered to the dams, very low levels could be
recovered in embryonic tissues (Ferm et al., 1969). A more detailed
localization of radioactive cadmium in the embryo showed that it was
restricted mainly to the primitive gut wall and vitelline duct
(Dencker, 1975) (Figure 3). When the pattern of embryonic uptake of
cadmium was followed with time, it was found to stop abruptly at the
time when the communication between the yolk sac and the primitive
gut through the vitelline duct was closed (around day 9 in the
hamster, day 9.5 in the mouse). This largely coincided with the
period of teratogenic sensitivity in the hamster and mouse as
reported by Gale and Ferm (1973) and Schluter (1970), respectively.

As mentioned before, accumulation of cadmium occurs, throughout
gestation, in the yolk sac placenta and chorioallantoic placenta.
It is not well established what influence on interference in
placental function may have on fetal development, in terms of
malformations. We think it is reasonable to assume that the early
accumulation of cadmium in the endoderm of the primitive gut may
influence the development of the endoderm derivatives and
neighbouring structures developing in close association with the
endoderm. Cadmium causes severe facial malformations, and these
develop in close contact to and with the direct participation of the
foregut endoderm. In parallel with this direct influence within the

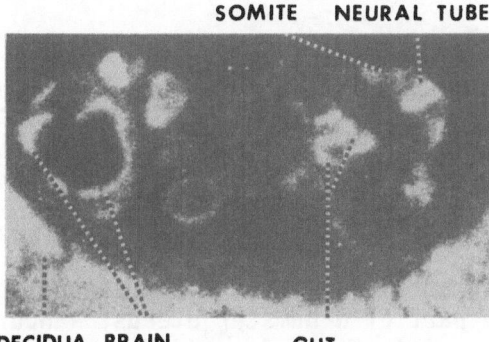

SOMITE   NEURAL TUBE

DECIDUA BRAIN   GUT

Figure 1   Autoradiogram of a hamster embryo, 24 hours after
           intravenous injection of $^{65}ZnCl_2$ into the mother on
           day 8 of gestation. High concentrations (white areas) can
           be seen in rapidly growing structures in a pattern similar
           to that of thymidine. The highest levels are found in
           epithelial structures such as the neuroepithelium of the
           developing brain and neural tube, and in the endoderm of
           the gut. (Dencker, 1976, courtesy of Acta Pharmacology
           and Toxicology)

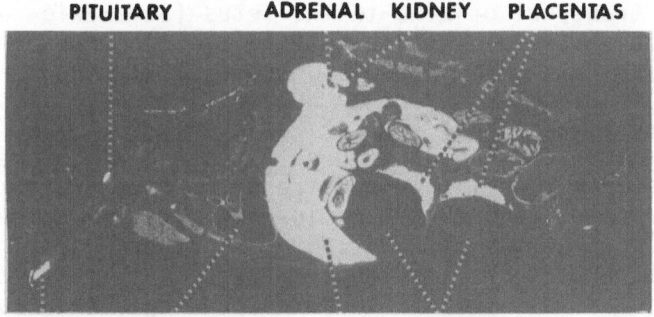

PITUITARY   ADRENAL KIDNEY   PLACENTAS

TOOTH   BLOOD OF HEART   LIVER   FETUSES

Figure 2   Whole-body autoradiogram of a mouse, 4 hours after
           intravenous injection of $^{109}CdCl_2$ on day 16 of
           gestation. There is a marked accumulation of cadmium in
           the chorioallantoic placentas and in the liver and kidney
           of the mother. However, no radioactivity can be seen in
           any fetal structure. (Dencker, 1975, courtesy of Journal
           of Reproduction and Fertility)

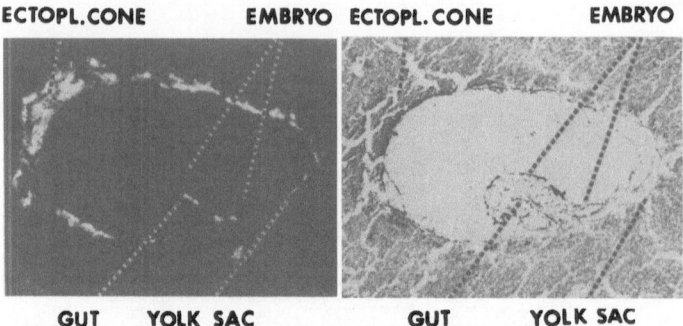

Figure 3   Autoradiogram (left) and the corresponding section (right)
            showing a part of a hamster uterus, 4 hours after
            intravenous injection of $^{109}CdCl_2$ on day 8 of
            gestation. High concentrations can be seen in the
            ectoplacental cone, the visceral yolk sac and the gut of
            the embryo. At this stage of development the communication
            between the mother and the embryonic gut is still open
            through the vitelline duct. One day later this duct
            closes and after that period no intraembryonic
            accumulation occurs.

embryo, cadmium apparently disturbs fetal nutrition by its
accumulation in the placenta. It has been shown that cadmium
decreases the transport of zinc to the fetus (Samarawickrama and
Webb, 1979), which is interesting in view of the common interactions
between zinc and cadmium. There is, however, evidence that cadmium
decreases the fetal uptake of other nutrients as well, such as
vitamin B_{12} and amino acids, even at relatively low doses of
cadmium (Danielsson and Dencker, to be published). The reduction in
nutrient transfer may explain the decrease in fetal weight gain
after subtoxic doses of cadmium to mice and rats as was reported by
Webster (1979) and Ahokas et al. (1980). Further support for a
placental mechanism is the finding that cadmium injected directly
into the fetus was less toxic than corresponding concentrations
after administration to the mother (Levin and Miller, 1980).

Mercury

        The disposition of inorganic mercury (Hg^{2+}) in the conceptus
is similar to that of cadmium. A heavy accumulation is observed in
the placenta, and only small amounts are recovered in the fetus,
although more than the amount found for cadmium. Like cadmium,
Hg^{2+} also is accumulated in the primitive gut of the early embryo
(Dencker, 1976).

Lately, we have compared Hg^{2+} to metallic mercury (Hg^0), after inhalation by the mother, during both early and late gestation (Khayat and Dencker, 1982). Figure 4 shows that considerably more Hg^0 is transferred to the fetus than Hg^{2+}, especially in the latter part of gestation. Similar results were reported earlier by Clarkson et al. (1972). In early gestation, however, only traces of mercury (after Hg^0 inhalation) could be found in the embryonic tissues (as seen by autoradiography). It should be said that what is registered in the body after Hg^0 inhalation most likely represents exclusively Hg^{2+}, oxidized from Hg^0 in the tissues by the catalase-hydrogen peroxide complex (Clarkson et al., 1961; Nielsen-Kudsk, 1969). One reason for the increase in fetal accumulation of Hg^0 with advancing fetal development is that the fetal organs increase their capacity to oxidize Hg^0. This could be seen in organs such as the liver, myocardium and brain (Figure 5A).

Further evidence that Hg^0 is oxidized in the fetal tissues and not transferred to the fetus in the form of Hg^{2+} after oxidation in the mother is the change in fetal distribution that can be induced by ethanol. Ethanol has been shown to inhibit the oxidation of Hg^0 in most adult organs except in the liver since it partly utilizes catalase for its metabolic degradation. The resulting increase in the liver/carcass ratio that is seen in adult mice was found also in the fetuses (Khayat and Dencker, 1982). Furthermore, ethanol caused a redistribution of mercury in the fetal as well as in the maternal liver (Figure 5B).

Somewhat unexpectedly, ethanol increased the total accumulation of Hg^0 in the fetal carcass by about 4-fold, while at the same time the concentration in the maternal carcass decreased. The only apparent explanation for this is that the maternal serum concentration of Hg^0 was increased by the ethanol, allowing an increase in the net transfer to the fetus. Methylmercury is accumulated considerably more in fetal tissues than is inorganic mercury (Berlin and Ullberg, 1963a; Satoh and Suzuki, 1979). The fetal brain showed a high concentration.

Lead

Inorganic lead is transferred to the fetus in substantial amounts after maternal exposure (McClain and Becker, 1975; Singh et al., 1976; Kelman and Walter, 1980). Carpenter et al. (1973) showed embryonic concentrations in early gestation in the hamster, but found most of the lead to be restricted to the yolk sac placenta.

In our preliminary studies on inorganic lead (administered intravenously as lead acetate), this metal was found in embryonic and fetal tissues at all stages of gestation, although more in late than in early stages (Table 1). This probably depends in part on

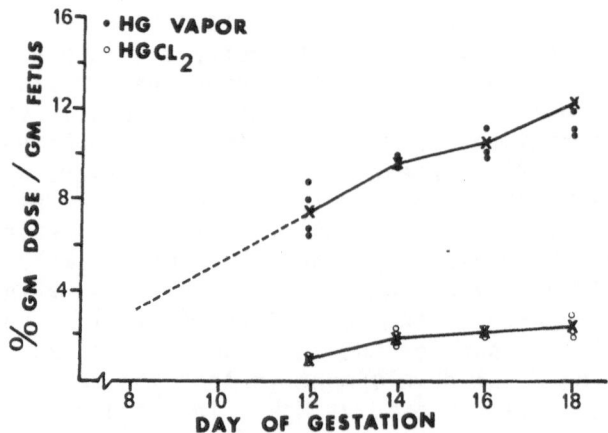

Figure 4   Fetal concentration of radioactivity, 60 minutes after a
           1-hour period of ^{203}Hg vapor inhalation or 90 minutes
           after intravenous injection of ^{203}HgCl$_2$ in pregnant
           mice on different days (12-18) of gestation. The dotted
           line indicates the approximate embryonic concentrations
           earlier in gestation as judged from concomitant
           autoradiographic studies. More Hg vapor (in percent of
           the given dose) accumulated in the fetus as compared to
           Hg^{2+}, especially in the latter part of gestation. This
           may be due to the increasing capacity of fetal organs to
           oxidize Hg vapor to Hg^{2+}, which was then retained.
           (Khayat and Dencker, 1982, courtesy of Biological Research
           in Pregnancy)

the marked accumulation in the fetal skeleton, which was observed
from day 13 to 14 and onwards. The transfer to the fetus appeared
to be rather slow as the fetal concentration was regularly higher at
24 hours as compared to 4 hours after maternal injection (Table 1).

     Except for the skeleton, the highest fetal concentrations of
lead were seen in the blood and in the liver (Figure 6). Due to the
high energy of the ^{203}Pb radiation, the autoradiographic resolution
was decreased. It was, however, possible to identify an accumulation
of lead in the embryonic blood on day 8 to 9 and later, and in the
embryonic liver as early as day 12 and then increasing later in
gestation. These sites of lead accumulation - the blood, liver and
skeleton - were found in the adult as well. The fetal kidney,
however, did not show any specific accumulation of lead.

     It is interesting to speculate why lead in the soft tissues is
restricted to the blood and liver more in the fetus than in the
adult. Lead is known to inhibit several enzymes in the production

BRAIN   SPINAL CORD   KIDNEY

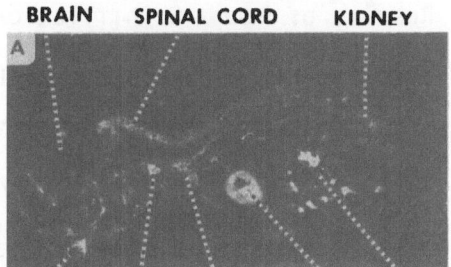

EYE   THYROID   THYMUS   MYOCARD   LIVER

BRAIN   SPINAL CORD

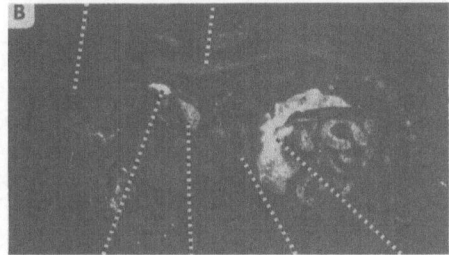

THYROID   THYMUS   MYOCARD   LIVER

Figure 5   Autoradiograms of mouse fetuses at day 18 of gestation after the dams had inhaled ^{203}Hg vapor as described in Figure 4. In (B) the dam was pretreated with ethanol (2 g/kg) 30 minutes before inhalation of the Hg vapor. The fetus in (A) shows a high concentration especially in the myocardium and a spotty pattern of accumulation in the liver, presumably due to high catalase activity in these tissues. Ethanol, which inhibits catalase, caused a redistribution of the radioactivity within the fetus and an increase in the liver concentration compared to most other organs. (Khayat and Dencker, 1982, courtesy of Biological Research in Pregnancy)

of heme. In adults, the lead in blood is known to be gradually concentrated in the red blood cell, where it is bound mainly to the globin moiety of hemoglobin. Ong and Lee (1980) have shown that hemoglobin of fetal origin (HbF) has a much greater affinity for lead than adult hemoglobin (HbA). This may explain why lead in the fetus tends to accumulate in blood rather than being distributed in the extracellular space.

As reported here and by Carpenter et al. (1973), lead accumulates in the yolk sac placenta. The embryonic red blood cells are formed exclusively in the visceral yolk sac placenta during the first part of gestation. It seems possible that the yolk sac

Table 1   Preliminary Results of Gamma Scintillation Experiments at
          Various Days of Gestation and Different Time Intervals
          after Administration of ^{203}Pb-Acetate to Pregnant Mice

CONCENTRATIONS (dpm/g)

Day of gestation	Interval (hr) between injection and autopsy	Maternal Liver X 10^6	Kidney X 10^6	Placenta X 10^3	Fetus X 10^3
13	4	14	19	750	83
	24	2.5	12	420	121
15	4	22	42	853	187
	24	3.5	16	494	245
16	4	11	33	784	215
	24	2.4	18	537	272
18	4	11	63	1065	248

Note that while placental and maternal organ concentrations
decrease with time after injection, fetal concentrations
increase in spite of a "diluting" effect of fetal growth.
This indicates that there is a continuous transfer to the
fetus at least up to 24 hours after administration of
lead. There is also an increasing fetal concentration from
day 13 to day 18 of gestation. Dose: 8.8 X 10^6 dpm/g
body weight. Values are means from two animals.

placenta at this period restricts lead from reaching embryonic
tissues, but that lead is incorporated into the globin of red blood
cells formed in the yolk sac, and can then be traced in the embryonic
blood. In the latter part of gestation (from around day 12), fetal
erythropoiesis takes place in the liver. The accumulation of lead
in the fetal liver from day 12 and later may be a reflection of
hemoglobin production and a subsequent binding of lead to the newly
formed globin.

     Brain hemorrhages have been reported both in chick (Ridgway and
Karnofsky, 1952) and rat (McClain and Becker, 1975), and Carpenter
and Ferm (1977) suggested that edematous blebs and hemorrhages
preceded the caudal defects in tail and sacral skeleton. It is
tempting to speculate that this edema and bleeding might be secondary
to fetal anemia or other defects in the blood caused by lead.

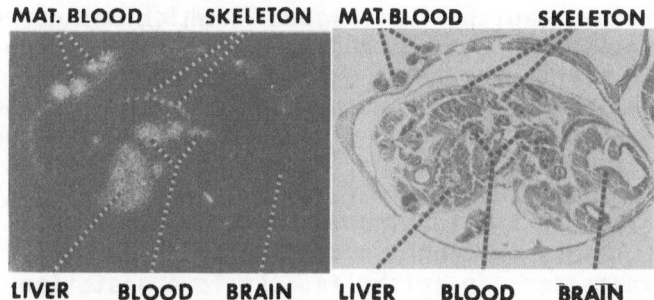

MAT. BLOOD   SKELETON   MAT.BLOOD   SKELETON

LIVER   BLOOD   BRAIN   LIVER   BLOOD   BRAIN

Figure 6   Autoradiogram (left) and the corresponding tissue section
            (right) showing a fetus 24 hours after intravenous
            injection of ^{203}Pb-acetate to the mother on day 13 of
            gestation. Note the high concentration of lead in the
            fetal blood, liver and skeleton. The fetal blood
            concentration is only slightly lower than the maternal.
            (Lindgren, Danielsson and Dencker, personal communication)

Arsenic

We have studied the distribution of inorganic arenic (As) in
the forms of As III (NaAsO$_2$, arsenite) and As V (Na$_2$ HAsO$_4$, arsenate)
in mice and hamsters (Lindgren et al., 1982), and it may be pertinent
to mention here the more significant differences in the distribution
pattern of the two forms in adult tissues. The whole body retention
is longer for As III than for As V (about three times more at 72
hours). As III is accumulated by the liver and excreted via the bile
more than As V, which is eliminated more via the urine.

Both forms accumulate in skin and hair, and in the squamous
epithelia of the oral cavity, esophagus and esophageal part of the
stomach (Figure 11) which correlates well with the presence of
keratin in these epithelia. Further, they accumulate slowly but
selectively in the colloid of the thyroid gland, in distinct parts
of the eipdidymis and, finally, in the ocular lens where they are
retained up to 30 days after administration. In addition to these
sites, As V, but not As III, accumulates rapidly in the calcified
areas of the skeleton, most likely due to the similarities between
(AsO$_4$)$^{3-}$ and (PO$_4$)$^{3-}$ ions.

The fetal uptake and distribution of the two forms do not
differ greatly, except for the accumulation of As V in the fetal
skeleton in late gestation. They both pass freely to the fetus in
all stages of gestation. Hanlon and Ferm (1977) reported a
placental permeability of arsenate in early embryogenesis in the
hamster. In the organogenetic period, accumulation could be

observed in the neuroepithelium (Figure 7) which may correlate with severe malformations in the CNS and eyes such as exencephaly, anophthalmy and microphthalmy reported by Beaudoin (1974) and Hood and Bishop (1972). After the organogenetic period (around days 12-14), a more even distribution was observed. During the last days of gestation, from day 15 onwards, accumulation was found in the skin and upper gastrointestinal tract, as seen in the adults. As arsenic has been reported to bind to keratin (Webb, 1966), this accumulation probably reflects an increasing differentiation, and thus keratin formation, in epithelia. In late gestation, arsenic accumulated in the lens, and As V accumulated in the fetal skeleton. In contrast to adults, no thyroid radioactivity could be detected in the fetuses.

Inorganic arsenic is partly transformed to dimethylarsenic in several species, including the rodent. Dimethylarsenic (labeled with ^{74}As) differed from inorganic arsenic in its distribution. For example, no specific uptake was seen in the skin and squamous epithelia or in the skeleton. There was a transfer of dimethylarsenic to the fetuses and an accumulation in the fetal lens (Vahter, Lindgren and Dencker, personal communication).

In the Marmoset monkey, As III reached high fetal levels, and the distribution was similar to that observed in the mother. An accumulation was observed in the skin, oral mucosa and esophagus, and the liver. There was a marked blood-brain barrier to the As III (Lindgren and Dencker, personal communication) (Figure 8).

Multiple basalioma of the skin are a recognized side effect of medication with arsenicals, and there is one case report of the transplacental induction of such skin cancer (see INTRODUCTION). The prominent accumulation of arsenic in skin and oral mucosa, presumably in the keratin, observed both in the mouse and in the monkey is consistent with the hypothesis that a transplacental induction of such a cancer might occur. Keratin belongs to a group of intermediate filaments in the cytoplasm of epithelial cells, which have been proposed to be essential for cell-shape changes that occur during locomotion and cell division (Sun et al., 1979; Lazarides, 1980).

As III has been reported to be more toxic than As V (Byron et al., 1967). We have used an in vitro spot culture system (based on chick embryonic fibroblasts differentiating into chondrocytes) to show that cartilage formation is inhibited by As III at a concentration of 5-10 µM (ED_{50}). As V was not inhibitory at the highest concentration tested (200 µM). These results fit well with the higher teratogenicity reported for As III compared to As V (Hood, 1972; Hood and Bishop, 1972).

FETUSES

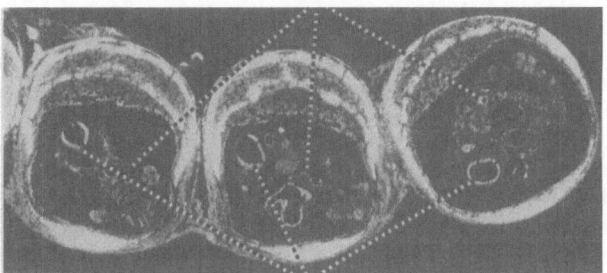

NEUROEPITHELIUM

Figure 7   Autoradiogram of a uterus, 4 hours after intravenous injection of [74]As-arsenate (As V) to a dam on day 10 of gestation. High concentrations of radioactivity are seen in the fetal tissues and especially in the neuroepithelium. (Lindgren and Dencker, personal communication)

BRAIN   SKIN   LUNG

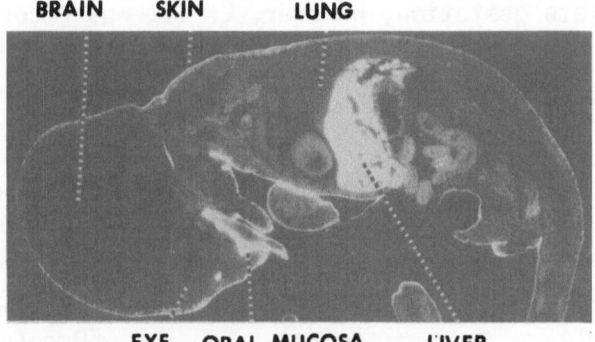

EYE   ORAL MUCOSA   LIVER

Figure 8   Autoradiogram of a Marmoset monkey fetus in late gestation, 8 hours after an injection of [74]As-arsenite (As III) to the mother. There is marked accumulation of arsenic in the skin and the squamous epithelium of the tongue and oral cavity, presumably due to binding to keratin in these epithelia. Also note the high concentration in the liver. Little arsenic crossed the blood-brain barrier. (Lindgren and Dencker, personal communication)

     To conclude the results on arsenic, it appears that the differences in teratogenicity between As III and As V most likely depend on differences in the direct toxicity of the two forms on the embryonic cells rather than on the pharmacokinetics in the placenta, embryo or fetus. The accumulation in skin in late gestation may be noted as a potential risk for transplacental carcinogenesis.

Chromium

For chromium (Cr), we have also studied two of the forms commonly present in the work environment, Cr III (CrCl$_3$) and Cr VI (Nc$_2$Cr$_2$O$_7$) (Danielsson et al., 1982). The distribution patterns of these two forms differ from each other in many respects. In the blood, the concentration of which is critical for the transfer to the fetus, Cr VI is accumulated in red blood cells, with a low concentration in the serum. Cr III on the other hand is bound mostly to plasma proteins.

Despite the lower serum concentration of Cr VI compared to Cr III (Table 2), Cr VI is more readily transferred to the embryo and fetus. During the organogenetic period, no Cr III could be detected autoradiographically in embryonic tissues, and, as measured by impulse counting, the concentration was still very low on day 13 (Table 2). In late gestation, however, Cr III was recovered in the fetus where the radioactivity was almost exclusively confined to the calcified areas of the skeleton.

Table 2   Comparison of Concentrations in Maternal Serum and Whole Fetuses and the Toxicity In Vitro of Cr III and Cr VI

	Concentrations in vivo		Toxicity in vitro
	Maternal serum (µg/ml)	Whole fetus (µg/g)	ED$_{50}$ (µg/ml)
Cr III	8.3 ± 0.9	0.03 ± 0.003	>15
Cr VI	2.6 ± 0.2	0.3 ± 0.01	~0.03

Cr III (^{51}CrCl$_3$) and Cr VI (Na$_2$ ^{51}Cr$_2$O$_7$) were injected i.v. to mice on day 13 of gestation in doses of 10 µg Cr/g body weight. This dose of Cr VI has been reported to be teratogenic in the hamster (Gale, 1978). The animals were sacrificed after one hour. In the in vitro studies, the two forms of Cr were added (for 1-4 days) to chick limb bud fibroblasts differentiating into chondrocytes. The production of sulfated proteoglycans was measured by alcian blue staining and incorporation of ^{35}SO$_4$ $^{2-}$. As can be seen, the fetal concentrations of Cr VI (but not Cr III) are considerably higher than those required for causing toxic effects in vitro.

Cr VI was transported to the embryo and fetus throughout gestation (Figure 9), although the concentration was always lower than the maternal. Activity was seen in most tissues at 1 and 4 hours after administration to the mother. In late gestation, Cr VI concentrated more in the calcified areas of the skeleton (as did Cr III), and this increased with time after injection.

Although little is known about the teratogenicity of chromium in experimental animals, there are indications that Cr VI is more teratogenic than Cr III (Gale, 1978; Matsumoto et al., 1976). This could be due to the higher embryonic concentrations of Cr VI and/or that Cr VI is more toxic to the embryonic cells. To test the toxicity per se, $CrCl_3$ (Cr III) and $K_2Cr_2O_7$ (Cr VI) were added to spot cultures of chick embryonic fibroblasts (see Arsenic). This system records effects on cartilage formation, which is pertinent in this case, as skeletal malformations (Gale, 1978) and achondroplasia (Ridgway and Karnofsky, 1952) have been reported after chromium was administered to pregnant hamsters or injected directly into eggs.

For Cr VI, the dose which inhibited cartilage formation by 50 percent (ED_{50}) was 0.03 µg/ml medium. For Cr III, we did not register any inhibition at the highest dose tested, 15 µg/ml. Table 2 gives concentrations of Cr III or Cr VI, respectively, in maternal serum and fetal tissues, on day 13, after a dose of chromium to the mother which is reported teratogenic for Cr VI, compared to the toxicity of the two forms on the embryonic cells in vitro. These experiments thus indicate that Cr III may be less teratogenic because: 1) it is less directly toxic to the embryonic cells; and 2) it is not transferred to the embryo to a significant degree as compared to Cr VI.

Interference with the embryotrophic nutrition (exemplified by trypan blue) may be a mechanism of early teratogenic effects. It is possible that Cr III in particular, which binds strongly to proteins, inhibits the intracellular digestion of proteins in the yolk sac epithelium, thus depriving the embryo of essential nutrients (see below, Placenta).

FETAL ORGANS

Placenta

As has been mentioned in the preceding section, some metals accumulate in the different placental structures (yolk sac and chorioallantoic placentas). Cadmium, inorganic mercury, lead and chromium (both Cr III and Cr VI) (Figure 9) all accumulate in the yolk sac placenta during early gestation. Cadmium and mercury accumulate in the chorioallantoic placenta as well (Figure 2).

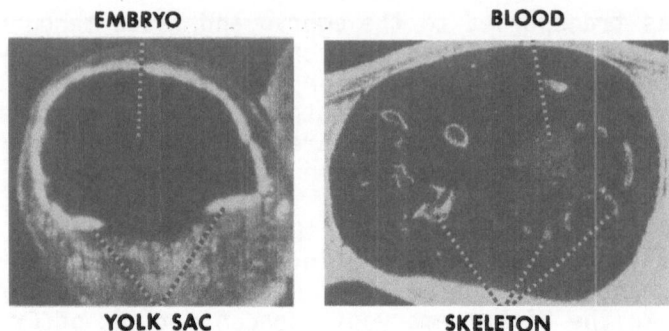

Figure 9   (Left) Autoradiogram showing part of a uterus of a mouse
           (on day 11 of gestation), 1 hour after intravenous
           injection of chromium (^{51}Cr III). There is a strong
           accumulation in the yolk sac placenta but no radioactivity
           can be detected in the embryonic tissues. (Right) One
           hour after intravenous injection of chromium (^{51}Cr VI)
           on day 16 of gestation. Cr VI passes more freely to the
           fetus than does Cr III. The highest concentration can be
           seen in the calcified areas of the skeleton and in the
           blood. (Danielsson, Hassoun and Dencker, 1982, courtesy
           of Archives of Toxicology)

     The yolk sac placenta appears to be more discriminatory with
regard to the transfer of foreign compounds than is the
chorioallantoic placenta. Possibly as a consequence of this, many
metals have a marked tendency to accumulate in the yolk sac. For
the metals that are not further transferred to the embryo, such as
cadmium, mercury and Cr III, the yolk sac placenta may be considered
a dead end.

     An important question is whether accumulation in the placenta
per se can be considered a risk for the embryonic development. The
yolk sac placenta is the only structure which mediates the transfer
of nutrients to the embryo from the time just after implantation to
around day 11 in the mouse. As has been suggested for trypan blue
(Beck et al., 1967), that interference with early embryonic
nutrition, via the yolk sac, may lead to severe malformations. It
is likely that the metals discussed here are bound to serum proteins,
which are transported to the yolk sac. These proteins are intended
to be degraded and serve as nutrients for the embryo. Metals bound
to these proteins may interfere with the proteolysis (e.g. chromium
binds strongly to proteins), or they may be released upon degradation
of the proteins and then rebind to functional groups in the yolk sac.
It is noteworthy that the pattern of malformations caused by Cr III
and the period of teratogenic sensitivity in the mouse (Matsumoto et

al., 1976) are very similar to what has been reported for trypan blue (Schluter, 1970).

As has been discussed above (see Zinc - Cadmium; Figure 2), cadmium is accumulated in the chorioallantoic placenta, which may lead to interference with nutrition followed by growth inhibition or fetal death in the latter part of gestation. It is possible that other metals such as mercury may also interfere in the function of this placenta. This is a field where further research is essential. Placental mechanisms may be of clinical significance, for example, as a basis for the frequent reports on low birth weights under various exposure conditions.

Fetal Skeleton

Skeletal defects are among the most frequent malformations recorded in experimental teratology. These defects may be induced early in gestation by interference with somite or limb bud formation and chondrogenesis through an interaction with differentiation processes. As described above, metals such as chromium VI and arsenic III may interfere in cartilage formation in vitro. Nickel (Olsen and Jonsen, 1979) and cobalt (Flodh, 1968) are known to accumulate specifically in adult and fetal cartilage.

Another way a chemical may disturb skeletal formation is to interact in the calcification process. A great number of elements are known to be specifically accumulated in bone tissues, e.g. strontium and barium (due to their resemblance to calcium), nickel, chromium, arsenic (As V), lead, cobalt, and the essential metals, iron and zinc. In addition, a number of less common elements such as the lanthanoides and the actinoides accumulate in calcified tissues. All these elements can be recovered in the fetal skeleton as well, provided they are transferred through the placenta. In many cases, such as with Cr III, strontium and barium, the fetal radioactivity, after injection of these radioactive elements to the mother, is almost exclusively restricted to the skeleton. Most elements mentioned here are probably incorporated into the apatite crystal as cations substituting for calcium. Arsenic, in the form of arsenate and chromium (Cr VI), however, are most likely incorporated as anions.

It is not likely that elements incorporated into bone cause direct toxic effects on the permanent bone. At the high concentrations attained in these areas, they may, however, disturb enzyme systems involved in the calcification process. Bone may also serve as a storage organ and that toxic influence may be exerted in other organs upon release of the elements.

Fetal Liver

While the adult liver often stores metals in high
concentrations, this is most often not the case in the fetus. Some
metals, such as zinc and selenium are, however, specifically
accumulated in the fetal liver, which may serve as a physiological
storage.

Metallic mercury is oxidized in the liver, and a specific
accumulation of what is most probably inorganic mercury (after
oxidation of metallic mercury) occurs in the peripheral cells of the
liver lobuli (Figure 5A). Accumulation of mercury, as well as lead,
could be seen by day 12 to 13 of development. For lead, it is
possible that this accumulation is due to an uptake in the
hematopoietic cells that appears in the liver around day 12, after
which the liver is the main blood-forming organ.

Fetal Kidney

Many of the metals discussed in this review, such as cadmium,
mercury, lead and chromium (Cr VI), accumulate in the renal tubuli
of adult animals and may cause nephropathy. It is noteworthy that
there is usually no renal accumulation of these metals in the fetuses
even in late gestation, although metallic mercury and lead accumulate
in the fetal liver, even in midgestation. Although the murine fetal
kidneys are partially mature in late gestation, as they produce
urine, the lack of accumulation of these metals probably reflects
some biochemical immaturity.

Fetal Brain

The focus on damage to the developing brain has been first on
the early organogenetic period when severe morphological
malformations can be induced, and second on the perinatal period
when several chemicals have been shown to cause behavioural
disturbances. When the distribution pattern of foreign chemicals in
fetal tissues is followed during development, interesting changes
can be recorded. In many cases the neuroepithelium of the early
brain accumulates chemicals; this is more evident for organic
chemicals but was observed also for arsenic (Figure 7). In late
gestation, development of the blood-brain barrier reduces
accumulation (Figure 8). Its presence, however, does not prevent
uptake of some metals, such as methylmercury (Berlin and Ullberg,
1963a) and metallic mercury (Khayat and Dencker, 1982) (Figure 5A)
which can be observed in the fetal brain.

Lead has been suspected of causing behavioural disturbances
transplacentally in man (Beattie et al., 1975; Moore et al., 1977),

which could not be confirmed in experimental animals (Minsker et al., 1979). Such effects are, however, well known in children after ingestion of lead-containing paints. The concentration of inorganic lead in the fetal brain was very low in our studies (Figure 6).

Other Fetal Organs

Metallic mercury accumulates in organs such as the thyroid and myocardium after apparent oxidation to inorganic mercury (Figure 5). Dimethylmercury and arsenic are specifically concentrated in the lens of the fetal eye. Arsenic binds to the squamous epithelia of the skin and upper gastrointestinal tract (Figure 8).

PARENTAL REPRODUCTIVE ORGANS

Ovary

Some metals like cadmium and mercury accumulate selectively in ovarian tissues, although in different patterns. For mercury (Figure 10), the inorganic form, Hg^{2+}, is concentrated in the granulosa cells of the graafian follicles (Dencker, 1976). Metallic mercury, on the other hand, accumulates in the corpora lutea (Khayat and Dencker, 1982), indicating a high capacity of oxidation in the luteal cells; cadmium also accumulates mainly in the corpora lutea. To our knowledge, high resolution autoradiography or other methods have not been used to localize metals in the oocyte.

Testis and Epididymis

Most metals seem to be restricted from entering the spermatogenetic epithelium but at the same time are concentrated in the interstitial tissues. This is true for cadmium, which is specific in producing testicular necrosis, for mercury (Hg^0 and Hg^{2+}), and for chromium.

For arsenic, there did not appear to be a blood-testis barrier. In the Marmoset monkey, arsenite injection resulted in an accumulation in the seminiferous tubules (Vahter et al., 1982). Arsenic (As III and As V) given to mice, hamsters or monkeys was also concentrated in the lumen of the duct, especially in the body, of the epididymis (Figure 11). High concentrations of radioactivity were observed in the seminal duct as long as 8 days after [74]As administration. This suggests that the semen will be exposed to arsenic for long periods of time. This ought to be remembered in connection with the reports of reproductive disturbances in families around a smelter in northern Sweden, where both parents or fathers only were employed (Beckman, 1978).

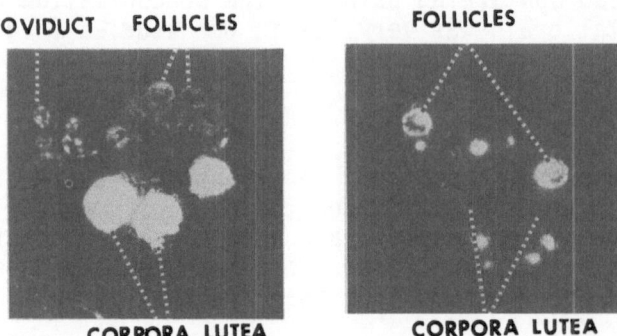

Figure 10   Autoradiograms of ovaries after ^{203}Hg vapor inhalation (left) and ^{203}HgCl$_2$ injection (right). Hg vapor accumulated preferentially in the corpora lutea, most likely after oxidation to Hg^{2+} in the luteal cells. Hg^{2+}, on the other hand, concentrated in the follicular granulosa cells.

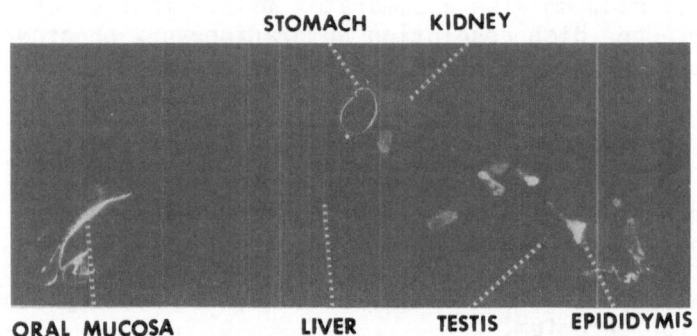

Figure 11   Autoradiogram of male syrian hamster, 24 hours after intravenous injection of ^{74}As-Arsenate (As V). The distribution pattern is characterized by an accumulation in the skin and gastric mucosa, and in the body of the epididymis and the ampullae of the vas deferens. This radioactivity appears to be contained in the lumen of the ducts, which means that the semen will probably be exposed to the arsenic for long periods of time. (Lindgren, et al., 1982, courtesy of Acta Pharmacology and Toxicology)

CONCLUSIONS

In conclusion, it can be said that the degree of embryonic and fetal uptake of metals varies widely. Methylmercury and arsenic reach fetal concentrations close to that found in maternal tissues. Lead, metallic mercury and chromium VI fall in an intermediate group where moderate embryonic and fetal concentrations are recovered. Cadmium, inorganic mercury and chromium III show undetectable levels or traces only in embryonic and fetal tissues. One exception is the high concentration of cadmium, and to some extent inorganic mercury, in the gut endoderm before the placental barrier is fully developed in the first stages of organogenesis. Especially those metals which are inhibited from reaching the fetus tend to accumulate in the placental structures.

The distribution within the fetus also varies greatly between metals. The skeleton is a common target organ for lead, chromium, arsenic V, strontium, and barium. Lead is also found in the blood and in the liver. Arsenic accumulates in the neuroepithelium in early gestation and in the skin and other squamous epithelia in late gestation. Metallic mercury is oxidized and retained in brain, myocardium, liver and thyroid.

The patterns of distribution that have been recorded are sometimes in accordance with known effects of the respective metals on fetal development. In other cases, these patterns may, for certain organ indicate risks that have not hitherto been considered.

ACKNOWLEDGEMENTS

This study was supported by grants from the Swedish Work Environment Fund and the Swedish Medical Research Council.

REFERENCES

Ahokas, A., Dilts Jr., P.V., and LaHaye, E.B., 1980, Cadmium-induced fetal growth retardation: Protective effect of excess dietary zinc, Am. J. Obstet. Gynecol. 136:219-222.

Aldick, H.J. and Fabry, H., 1973, Multiple Basaliome durch Arseneinwirkung in der Fetalperiode, Der Hautarzt 24:496.

Amin-Zaki, L., Elhassani, S., Majeed, M.A., Clarkson, T.W., Doherty, R.A. and Greenwood, M.R., 1974, Intra-uterine methylmercury poisoning in Iraq, Pediat. 54:587-595.

Angle, C.R. and McIntire, M.S., 1964, Lead poisoning during pregnancy: fetal tolerance of calcium disodium edetate, Amer. J. Dis. Child. 108:436-439.

Beattie, A.D., Moore, M.R., Goldberg, A., Finlayson, M.J.W.,
    Mackie, E.M., Graham, J.F., Main, J.C., McLaren, D.A., Murdock,
    R.M. and Stewart, G.T., 1975, Role of chronic low-level lead
    exposure in the aetiology of mental retardation, Lancet
    1:589-592.
Beaudoin, A.R., 1974, Teratogenicity of sodium arsenate in rats,
    Teratology 10:153-158.
Beck, F., Lloyd, I.B. and Griffiths, A., 1967, Lysosomal enzyme
    inhibition by trypan blue; a theory of teratogenesis, Science
    157:1180-1182.
Beckman, L., 1978, The Ronnskar smelter - occupational and
    environmental effects in and around a polluting industry in
    northern Sweden, Ambio 7:226-236.
Berlin, M. and Ullberg, S., 1963a, Accumulation and retention of
    mercury in the mouse. III. An autoradiographic comparison of
    methylmercuric dicyandiamide with inorganic mercury, Arch.
    Environ. Health 6:610-616.
Berlin, M. and Ullberg, S., 1963b, The fate of Cd^{109} in the
    mouse. An autoradiographic study after a single intravenous
    injection of Cd^{109}Cl$_2$, Arch. Environ. Health 7:686-693.
Byron, W.R., Bierbower, G.W, Brouwer, J.B. and Hansen, W.H., 1967,
    Pathological changes in rats and dogs from two-year feeding of
    sodium arsenite or sodium arsenate, Toxicol. Appl. Pharmacol.
    10:132-147.
Cantarow, A. and Trumper, M., 1944, "Lead Poisoning", Williams
    and Wilkins, Baltimore.
Carpenter, S.J. and Ferm, V.H., 1977, Embryopathic effects of lead
    in the hamster: a morphological analysis, Lab. Invest.
    37:369-385.
Carpenter, S.J., Ferm, V.H., and Gale, T.F., 1973, Permeability of
    the golden hamster placenta to inorganic lead:
    radioautographic evidence, Experienta 29:311-313.
Clarkson, T.W., Gatzy, J. and Dalton, C., 1961, Studies on the
    equilibration of mercury vapor with blood, University of
    Rochester, AEP Report No. 582.
Clarkson, T.W., Magos, L. and Greenwood, M.R., 1972, The transport
    of elemental mercury into fetal tissues, Biol. Neonate
    21:239-244.
Danielsson, B., Hassoun, E., and Dencker, L., 1982, Embryotoxicity
    of chromium: distribution in pregnant mice and effects on
    embryonic cells in vitro, Arch. Toxicol. (in press).
Dencker, L., 1975, Possible mechanisms of cadmium fetotoxicity in
    golden hamsters and mice: Uptake by the embryo, placenta and
    ovary, J. Reprod. Fertil. 44:461-471.
Dencker, L., 1976, Tissue localization of some teratogens at early
    and late gestation related to fetal effects, Acta Pharmacol.
    Toxicol. 39:1-113.
Dencker, L., 1979, Embryonic-fetal localization of drugs and
    nutrients, in: "Advances in the Study of Birth Defects, Vol.
    I: Teratogenic Mechanisms", T.V.N. Persaud, ed., pp. 1-18, MTP
    Press Ltd., Lancaster, England.

Dencker, L., 1982, Disposition of chemicals in the developing embryo and fetus, Biol. Res. Pregn. 3:144-121.

Ferm, V.H., Hanlon, D.P. and Urban, J., 1969, The permeability of the hamster placenta to radioactive cadmium, J. Embryol. Exp. Morph. 22:107-113.

Flodh, H., 1968, Autoradiographic studies on distribution of radiocobalt chloride in pregnant mice, Acta Radiol.(Ther.) 7:121-126.

Gale, T.F., 1978, Embryotoxic effects of chromium trioxide in hamsters, Environ. Res. 16:101-109.

Gale, T.F. and Ferm, V.H., 1973, Skeletal malformations resulting from cadmium treatment in the hamster, Biol. Neonat.(Basel) 23:149-160.

Hanlon, D.P. and Ferm, V.H., 1977, Placental permeability of arsenate ion during early embryogenesis in the hamster, Experientia 33:1221-1222.

Hood, R.D., 1972, Effects of sodium arsenite on fetal development, Bull. Environ. Contam. Toxicol. 7:216-222.

Hood, R.D. and Bishop, S.L., 1972, Teratogenic effects of sodium arsenate in mice, Arch. Environ. Health. 24:62-65.

Kelman, B.J. and Walter, B.K., 1980, Transplacental movements of inorganic lead from mother to fetus, Proc. Soc. Exp. Biol. Med. 163:278-282.

Khayat, A. and Dencker, L., 1982, Fetal uptake and distribution of metallic mercury vapor in the mouse: influence of ethanol and aminotriazole, Biol. Res. Pregn. 3:38-46.

Lazarides, E., 1980, Intermediate filaments as mechanical integrators of cellular space, Nature 283:249-256.

Levin, A.A. and Miller, R.K., 1980, Fetal toxicity of cadmium in the rat: Maternal vs fetal injections, Teratology 22:1-5.

Lindgren, A., Vahter, M. and Dencker, L., 1982, Autoradiographic studies on the distribution of arsenic in mice and hamsters administered [74]As-arsenite and -arsenate, Acta Pharmacol. Toxicol. 51(3):253-265.

Lugo, G., Cassady, G. and Palmisano, P., 1969, Acute maternal arsenic intoxication with neonatal death, Amer. J. Dis. Child. 117:328-330.

Matsumoto, H., Koya, G. and Takeuchi, T., 1965, Fetal Minamata disease: A neuropathological study of two cases of intrauterine intoxication by a methyl mercury compound, J. Neuropathol. Exp. Neurol. 24:563-574.

Matsumoto, N., Jijima, S. and Katsunuma, H., 1976, Placental transfer of chromic chloride and its teratogenic potential in embryonic mice, J. Toxicol. Sci. 2:1-13.

McClain, R.M. and Becker, B.A., 1975, Teratogenicity, fetal toxicity and placental transfer of lead nitrate in rats, Toxicol. Appl. Pharmacol. 31:72-82.

Minsker, D.H., Moskalski, N., Peter, C.P., Robertson, R.T. and Bokelman, D.L., 1979, Effects of lead exposure in utero or postpartum on brain histomorphology and behaviour in rat offspring, Teratology 19:40A.

Moore, M.R., Meredith, P.A. and Goldberg, A., 1977, A retrospective analysis of blood-lead in mentally retarded children, Lancet 1:717-719.

Murakami, U., 1972, Organic mercury problem affecting intrauterine life, in: "Proc. of the Int. Symp. on the Effects of Prolonged Drug Usage on Fetal Development, Adv. Exp. Med. Biol.", M.A. Klingberg, ed., pp. 301-336, Plenum Press, New York.

Nielsen-Kudsk, F., 1969, Uptake of mercury vapour in blood in vivo and in vitro from Hg-containing air, Acta Pharmacol. Toxicol. 27:149-160.

Olsen, I. and Jonsen, J., 1979, Whole body autoradiography of ^{63}Ni in mice throughout gestation, Teratology 12:165-172.

Ong, C.N. and Lee, W.R., 1980, High affinity of lead for fetal haemoglobin, Brit. J. Ind. Med. 37:292-298.

Parizek, J., 1964, Vascular changes at sites of oestrogen biosynthesis produced by parenteral injection of cadmium salts: the destruction of placenta by cadmium salts, J. Reprod. Fertil. 7:263-265.

Ridgway, L.P. and Karnofsky, D.A., 1952, The effects of metals on the chick embryo: Toxicity and production of abnormalities in development, Ann. N.Y. Acad. Sci. 55:203-215.

Samarawickrama, G.P. and Webb, M., 1979, Acute effects of cadmium on the pregnant rat and embryo-fetal development, Environ. Health Perspect. 28:245-249.

Satoh, H. and Suzuki, T., 1979, Effects of sodium selinite and methylmercury distribution in mice of late gestational period, Arch. Toxicol. 42:275-279.

Schluter, G., 1970, Embryotoxische Wirkungen von Trypanblau bei Mausern in Abhangigkeit vom Behandlungszeitpunkt, Naunyn Schmiedeberg's Arch. Pharmacol. 267:20-30.

Singh, N.P., Thind, I.S., Vitate, L.F. and Pawlow, M., 1976, Lead content of tissues of baby rats born of, and nourished by lead-poisoned mothers, J. Lab. Clin. Med. 87:273-280.

Sun, T.T., Shih, C. and Green, H., 1979, Keratin cytoskeletons in epithelial cells of internal organs, Proc. Natl. Acad. Sci.(USA) 76:2813-2817.

Ullberg, S., 1954, Studies on the distribution and fate of S^{35}-labelled benzylpenicillin in the body, Acta Radiol. (Stockh.) 118:1-110.

Ullberg, S., 1973, Autoradiography in fetal pharmacology, in: "Fetal Pharmacology", L.O. Boreus, ed., pp. 55-73, Raven Press, New York.

Ullberg, S., 1977, The technique of whole body autoradiography. Cryosectioning of large specimens, Science Tools, the LKB Instrument Journal, Special Issue on Whole-Body Autoradiography, Bromma, Sweden.

Ullberg, S., Dencker, L. and Danielsson, B., 1981, The distribution of drugs and other agents in the fetus, in: "Developmental Toxicology", K. Snell, ed., pp. 123-163, Croom Helm Ltd. Publishers, London.

Vahter, M., Marafante, E., Lindgren, A. and Dencker, L., 1982, Tissue distribution and subcellular binding of arsenic in Marmoset monkeys after injection of ^{74}As-arsenite, <u>Arch. Toxicol.</u> (in press).

Waddell, W.J. and Marlowe, G.C., 1976, Disposition of drugs in the fetus, <u>in</u>: "Perinatal Pharmacology and Therapeutics", B.L. Mirkin, ed., pp. 119-268, Academic Press, New York.

Webb, J.L., 1966, "Enzyme and Metabolic Inhibitors", Vol. 3, Academic Press, New York.

Webster, W.S., 1979, Cadmium-induced fetal growth retardation in mice and the effects of dietary supplements of zinc, copper and selenium, <u>J. Nutr.</u> 109:1646-1651.

HEAVY METAL ALTERATIONS OF PLACENTAL FUNCTION: A MECHANISM FOR THE INDUCTION OF FETAL TOXICITY IN CADMIUM

Arthur A. Levin[1,2,3], Richard K. Miller[2,3],
P. Anthony di Sant'Agnese[4]

[1]Department of Toxicology and Pathology,
 Hoffman-LaRoche, Nutley, New Jersey
[2]Department of Obstetrics and Gynecology; [3]Department
 of Pharmacology/Toxicology; [4]Department of Pathology,
 University of Rochester, Rochester, New York

ABSTRACT

Cadmium induces fetal death and placental necrosis in the rat following exposure late in gestation. Fetal death is produced despite limited fetal accumulation of cadmium. Using direct fetal injections of cadmium, it was demonstrated that cadmium concentrations 8-fold higher than those associated with fetal toxic maternal injection could be tolerated by fetuses. Thus, fetal death was not the result of direct effects of cadmium on the fetus. The placentae of dams treated with 40 µmoles Cd/kg (subcutaneously) demonstrated trophoblastic necrosis, hemorrhage and congestion of the maternal vascular spaces. These changes were indicative of local circulatory alterations. Blood flow to the placentae of dams treated with 40 µmoles Cd/kg was reduced within 12-16 and 18-24 hours following injections of $CdCl_2$, prior to the occurrence of fetal death.

The placenta rapidly accumulated cadmium following either subcutaneous or intravenous injection. The rapid and extensive accumulation of cadmium may alter placental structure and function. Cell death in the trophoblast was observed biochemically as early as eight hours after acute exposure to cadmium. The biochemical alteration was accompanied by alterations in placental ultrastructure especially of trophoblast layer II. Webb and Samarawickrama (1981) have demonstrated that acute exposure of rats to cadmium also reduced placental transport of zinc. Thus, acute exposure to cadmium alters placental viability, structure, and function. In conclusion, acute studies in rodents have established that the placenta is a target organ for cadmium. Chronic exposure regimens and human placental preparations will aid in determining the effects of environmental exposures of humans to cadmium.

INTRODUCTION

The placenta is a multifunctional, dynamic organ for homeostatic regulation of the fetus. In the past, the placenta was thought to be a barrier between mother and fetus. Although it serves as a barrier between maternal and fetal circulations, it is actually an organ of transport for many substances including many xenobiotics. The placenta mediates a broad range of functions including oxygen and carbon dioxide exchange, transfer of metabolic waste products, hormonal regulation, absorption of nutrients, as well as glycogen storage and biotransformation of xenobiotics. Thus, the placenta is an in utero equivalent of the lung, kidney, ovary, pituitary, gastrointestinal tract and liver. It is not surprising then, that alteration of placental function through disease processes or through physical or chemical means has a profound impact on the well being of the embryo or fetus.

Most previous investigations in teratology have focused on the description of the direct effects of toxicants on fetal structure or function with little emphasis on the role of placental or maternal factors in the etiology of toxic effects. However, reports on the effects of cadmium in late pregnancy have, from the outset (Parizek, 1964) suggested a placental mechanism of toxicity. Recent investigations have demonstrated this hypothesis to be correct.

The multiplicity of functions performed by the placenta makes it vulnerable to numerous different toxic effects. For example, compounds which inhibit steroid metabolism could seriously affect the endocrine function of the placenta while inhibitors of transport processes can alter the nutrient-waste exchange function of the placenta. Similarly, the placental gas exchange function will be affected by agents which alter fetal or maternal blood flow to the placenta. Thus, with toxicants like cadmium it can be envisioned that a number of different placental target sites could be affected.

This chapter will discuss the effects of cadmium in late gestation and will emphasize recent results which demonstrate placental sensitivity to cadmium, as well as fetal resistance to direct exposure to cadmium. In addition, a discussion of the permeability of the placenta to cadmium and the effects of cadmium on uteroplacental blood flow and placental transport function will be used to demonstrate that in the rodent, acute exposure to cadmium induces fetal distress by altering placental viability. The possible effects of cadmium on human fetal development and the accumulation of cadmium in the placentae of pregnant women who smoke cigarettes will also be discussed.

EFFECTS OF CADMIUM IN PREGNANCY

In early gestation in rodents, exposure to cadmium produces teratogenic effects. The specific nature of the teratogenic effects depends on species, strain and time of exposure. The teratogenic effects include limb malformations, exencephaly, renal agenesis, and embryo death and resorption (Chernoff, 1973; Ferm, 1971; Gale and Ferm, 1973; Barr, 1973).

Exposure of laboratory rodents to a single injection of cadmium salts late in gestation induces fetal death, placental necrosis and maternal distress (Parizek, 1964; Chiquoine, 1965). Parizek (1964) reported that subcutaneous injections of 20-40 μmoles Cd/kg caused 100 percent fetal death and placental necrosis in Wistar Porton rats. The fetal toxic doses of cadmium salts were also lethal to a large percentage (70 percent) of the dams. In late gestation there is an apparent decrease in the LD_{50} of rats from 1.77 mg Cd/kg in virgin females to 1.05 mg Cd/kg injected intravenously on day 20 of pregnancy (Samarawickrama and Webb, 1979). However, this apparent sensitivity of pregnant rats may be due to the increase in weight in late gestation (Samarawickrama and Webb, 1981). The maternal toxicity was characterized by lethargy, hematuria and occasionally, convulsions. Microscopic examination of maternal tissues revealed generalized venous congestion, with intense pulmonary congestion and hemorrhagic edema. The kidneys were swollen and hyperemic (Parizek, 1965; Samarawickrama and Webb, 1979). The combination of renal and placental toxicity, generalized hemorrhage, and the observation of convulsions prior to maternal death were suggestive of a cadmium-induced toxemia of pregnancy (eclampsia).

Placental Permeability and Fetal Accumulations of Cadmium

The rodent placenta is relatively impermeable to cadmium. The fetus or embryo accumulates very small amounts of cadmium from injection, oral administration or inhalation of cadmium during pregnancy. Intravenous injection of ^{109}Cd on day 18 did not result in autoradiographically detectable fetal accumulations of cadmium in the mouse (Berlin and Ullberg, 1963). While exposure of rodents to cadmium earlier in gestation also produced very low embryonic accumulations (Ferm et al., 1969), Dencker (1975) localized these embryonic accumulations to the primitive gut. Radiochemical analysis of fetal accumulations following intravenous injection in late gestation (day 20) revealed that at fetal toxic doses, 0.015 percent of the dose was accumulated per gram fetal tissue (Sonawane et al., 1975). In rats, subcutaneous injections of

40 μg/kg CdCl$_2$ on day 18 of gestation resulted in fetal body burden of 8.6 + 4.4 nmoles or concentration of 5 nmoles/g fetal weight. These body burdens were associated with a fetal mortality of 76 percent (Levin and Miller, 1980). Ahokas and Dilts (1979) demonstrated that less than 1.4 x 10^{-5} percent of a 1000 μg CdCl$_2$ oral dose was accumulated by the day 17 fetus. Inhalation exposure to 0.4 mg/m^3 throughout gestation resulted in fetal growth retardation, yet fetal liver concentration was only 0.4 nmoles/gram, which is less than 2 percent of the maternal liver concentration (Prigge, 1978). Thus, the fetal toxicity and the teratogenicity of cadium are associated with very low accumulation of cadmium in the fetus or embryo.

Fetal Sensitivity to Cadmium

The low fetal concentrations of cadmium and the high fetal lethality suggested that fetuses were either extremely sensitive to cadmium or that cadmium was toxic through placental or maternal sites of action. To test the sensitivity of fetuses to cadmium, fetuses were directly exposed in utero (Levin and Miller, 1980). Dams were laparotomized and the uterine horns were exposed on day 18 of gestation. Individual fetuses were injected intraperitoneally with 3 μl of saline or CdCl$_2$ using a 10 μl Hamilton syringe. The uterine horns were then replaced and the dams were allowed to recover. Fetal viability was determined on day 21 of gestation following caesarian delivery. Fetuses were injected with doses of cadmium which ranged from 0.4 nmoles to 120 nmoles. The highest dose was 60 μmoles/kg fetal weight, one and one-half times greater than with the dose given the dams to induce fetal death. The body burdens of the directly-injected fetuses at the highest dose were eight times greater than those from the dose given the dams to induce fetal death. The body burdens of the directly injected fetuses at the highest dose were eight times greater than the body burdens associated with fetal toxic maternal injections, yet mortality was only 12 percent. Fetal mortality from maternal injections was 75 percent (Table 1).

Differences in distribution of cadmium within the fetus did not explain the apparent insensitivity of the fetuses to direct injections, since organ concentrations of cadmium were higher for all organs measured following fetal exposure than in fetuses of exposed dams. Thus, cadmium-induced fetal toxicity was not the result of a direct effect on the fetus. However, the placentae of the fetuses from exposed dams had higher accumulations of cadmium than the placentae following fetal injection (Table 2). The observations, of fetal insensitivity to cadmium injected directly and the apparent correlation of fetal death and placental cadmium concentration, support the hypothesis that placental effects of the toxicant induce fetal death.

Table 1   Comparison of Percent Fetal Death and Fetal Body Burden
After Maternal or Fetal Injection of $CdCl_2$

Injection	Fetal Body Burden	Percent Fetal Death
Maternal	8.6 ± 4.4 (38,12)	75.0 (38,12)
Fetal	74.6 ± 34.8 (25,7)	11.5 (52,11)

[a]Maternal injection was 40 μmoles/kg and fetal
injection was 60 μmoles/kg fetal weight (120 nmoles/
fetus). Values for fetal body burden are means ± S.D.
Number of fetuses and number of litters are given in
parentheses. (Levin and Miller, 1980, courtesy of
Teratology)

Effect of Cadmium on Uteroplacental Blood Flow

The cadmium-induced placental lesion which accompanied fetal
death was characterized by necrotic changes in the pars fetalis,
generalized edema, as well as congestion and hemorrhage of the
maternal vascular spaces (Parizek, 1964; Levin and Miller, 1981).
The presence of edema, congestion, and hemorrhage in the placentae
of cadmium-exposed rats is indicative of local circulatory
derangement. Since cadmium is known to induce circulatory change in
the testis, the effects of cadmium on uteroplacental blood flow were
investigated as a cause of fetal death and placental pathologic
changes.

A single subcutaenous injection of 40 μmoles $CdCl_2$/kg on day
18 of pregnancy to Wistar rats resulted in decreased uteroplacental
blood flow within 12 hours (Levin and Miller, 1981). Blood flow to
maternal organs and placentae was determined using 15 μm Co^{57}
microspheres. At 12-16 hours and 18-24 hours, uteroplacental blood
flow was decreased 40 percent and 73 percent from the control value
(2.1 ± 0.3 ml/min/gram fetal placenta). Uteroplacental blood flow
was depressed in the absence of significant decrease in maternal
cardiac output or change in blood flow to any maternal organ with
one exception; blood flow to the adrenals was decreased 35 percent
and 45 percent from control values at 12-16 and 18-24 hours. No
blood flow changes were observed prior to 12 hours. The depression
or uteroplacental blood flow occurred concurrently with the
incidence of fetal death (Figure 1). However, further examination
of the data revealed that the uteroplacental blood flow associated
with live fetuses in compromised litters was also reduced, compared

Table 2 Concentrations of Cadmium in Fetuses and Fetal Tissues
Following Maternal or Direct Fetal Injection of $CdCl_2$

Tissue	Cadmium Concentration (nmol/g)	
	Maternal subcutaneous injection	Fetal intraperitoneal injection
Liver	28.4 ± 14.6[a] (14,4)	75.5 ± 38.4[b] (20,7)
Kidney	3.3 ± 2.2 (14,4)	19.6 ± 10.8 (20,7)
Gastrointestinal tract	5.0 ± 2.6 (14,4)	25.9 ± 16.1 (20,7)
Heart and lungs	2.1 ± 1.4 (12,2)	28.2 ± 13.0 (20,7)
Fetus (whole)	3.1 ± 1.3 (38,12)	21.0 ± 9.3 (16,5)
Chorioallantoic placenta	113.1 ± 34.4 (38,12)	9.5 ± 8.0 (25,7)
Visceral yolk sac	16.5 ± 6.5 (38,12)	38.5 ± 18.6 (25,7)

[a]Maternal injection was 40 μmol/kg and fetal injection
was 60 μmol/kg (120 μmol/fetus). Values are mean ± S.D.
Number of fetuses and number of litters are given in
parentheses.
[b]Levin and Miller, 1980, courtesy of Teratology.

to controls. Thus, blood flow was depressed to live fetuses, and
therefore blood flow change may in fact precede and be the cause of
fetal death.

A 40-70 percent reduction in uteroplacental blood flow would
result in fetal hypoxia or undernutrition and finally fetal death.
The alteration of uteroplacental blood flow and the morphologic
changes in the placenta may also be related. Greater than 95
percent of all dead fetuses showed microscopic evidence of placental
changes. In addition, placental necrosis was observed prior to
fetal death, but the exact cause and effect relationship between
blood flow change and the onset of placental necrosis could not be
determined.

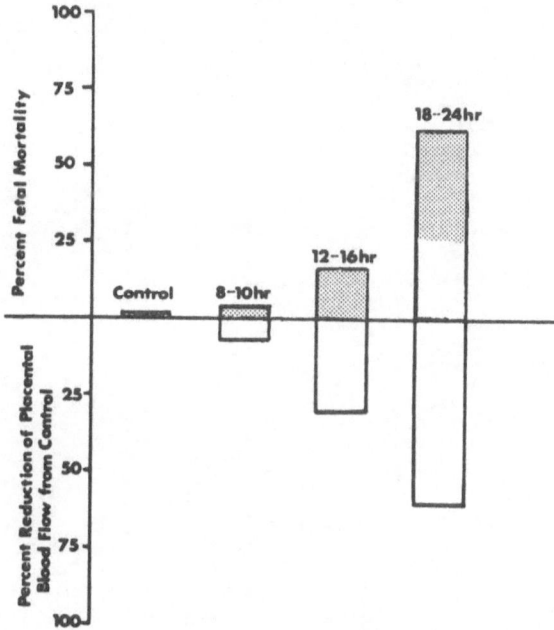

Figure 1   Percent fetal mortality and percent reduction of placental
           blood flow after injection of CdCl₂. Percent fetal
           mortality at 8-10 hour (n = 9), 12-16 hour (n = 14), and
           18-24 hour (n = 13) is shown with percentage decrease in
           placental blood flow vs controls (1.24 ml/min/g; n = 13)
           for the same periods. Mortality increased concurrently
           with decrease in uteroplacental blood flow. (Levin and
           Miller, 1981, courtesy of Toxicology and Applied
           Pharmacology)

     Morphologic changes in the placenta 12-16 hours following
CdCl₂ administration, as reported by Levin and Miller (1981), were
less severe than those changes observed by Parizek (1964). These
morphologic changes may precede the alterations previously
described. The early changes were characterized by a loss of
cytoplasm from the trophoblast, resulting in a thinning of the
trophoblast. The trophoblast also showed nuclear changes such as
karyorrhexis, karyolysis and loss of nucleolar definition. In the
maternal vascular spaces, infiltration of polymorphonuclear
leukocytes was observed (Figures 2 and 3). Samarawickrama and Webb
(1979; 1982) also described early changes in the maternal fetal
junctional zone of the rat placenta, but neither light microscopic
(Levin and Miller, 1981) nor electron microscopic examination of
placentae (di Sant'Agnese et al., 1983; Levin et al., 1981) in rats
injected subcutaneously could differentiate degenerative changes

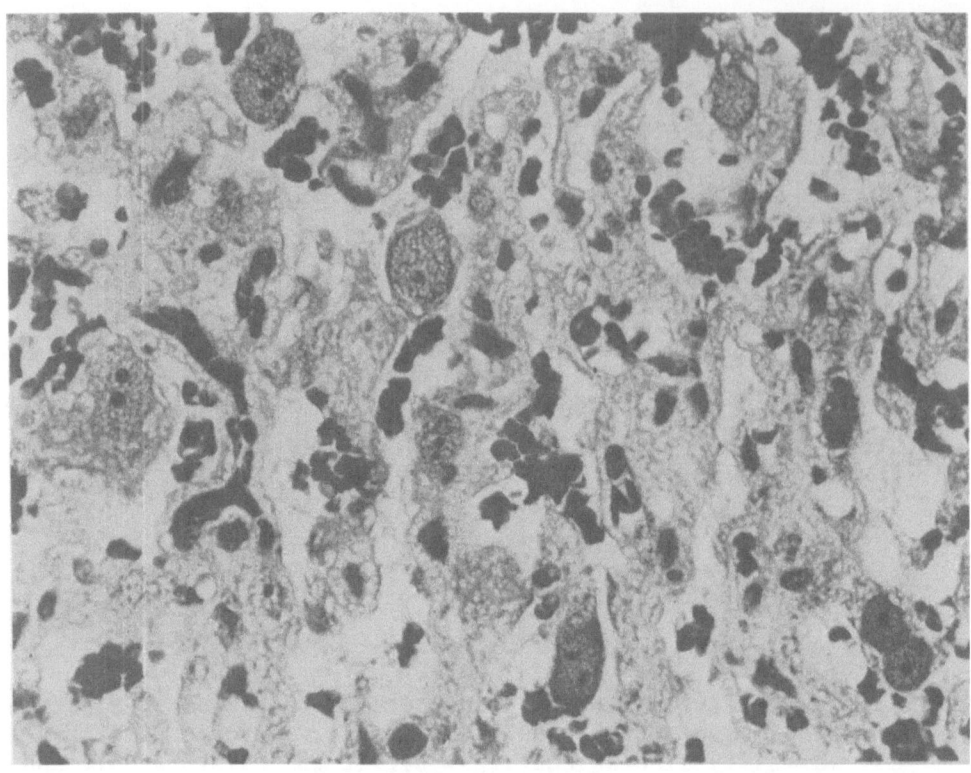

Figure 2   High-power photomicrograph of a placenta from a control
            rat on day 19 of gestation. Trophoblastic tissue with
            normal cytoplasm and nuclei are shown. Hematocxylin and
            eosin, x 500. (Levin and Miller, 1981, courtesy of
            Toxicology and Applied Pharmacology)

that normally occur in this region in late gestation from cadmium-
induced changes.

    Alterations in uteroplacental blood flow may play a role in the
induction of placental necrosis. Previous reports have described
similarly swollen, congested and hemorrhagic placentae following
treatment of rats late in pregnancy with agents that alter
uteroplacental blood flow (Robson and Sullivan, 1966). However, the
earlier changes observed in the trophoblast may represent direct
effects of cadmium on the placenta.

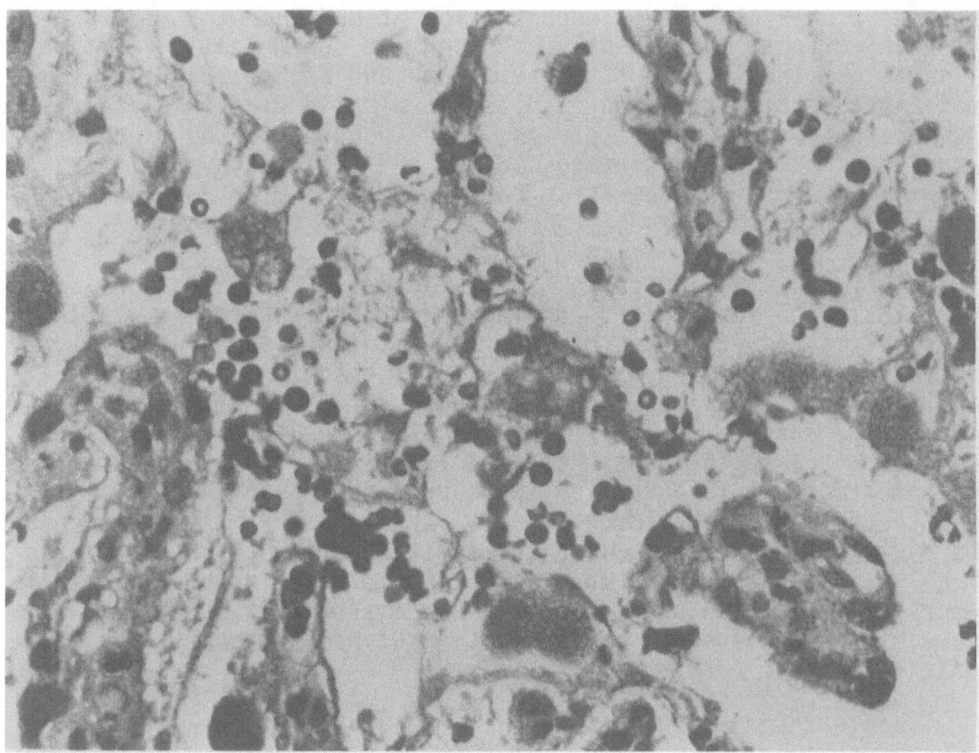

Figure 3 High-power photomicrograph of a placenta from a treated
          rat on day 19 of gestation, 18-24 hours after cadmium
          injection. Necrotic trophoblastic tissue with cytoplasmic
          thinning, pyknosis, karyorrhexis, and disruption of
          placental organization are evident. Leukocytic
          infiltration is also apparent. Hematoxylin and eosin, x
          500. (Levin and Miller, 1981, courtesy of Toxicology and
          Applied Pharmacology)

The Distribution and Toxicokinetics of Cadmium in Pregnancy

Following exposure in late gestation, the rat placenta
accumulated cadmium to a greater degree than did any maternal organ
except the liver (Samarawickrama and Webb, 1981; Levin et al.,
1983). The accumulation of cadmium in the placenta even exceeded
the renal concentration despite the fact that the kidney is often
the target organ for cadmium toxicity. Both subcutaneous (40
μmoles/kg) and intravenous (14 μmoles/kg) injections of fetal toxic
doses produced rapidly decreasing blood concentration following an
early peak; the exponential decay phases were followed by a
relatively constant blood level. Intravenous administration

produced a peak placental concentration of cadmium at 5 minutes after injection. Subsequently, the cadmium concentration in the placenta declined slowly (Samarawickrama and Webb, 1981). Subcutaneous administration resulted in a rapid rise in placental and maternal organ concentrations, corresponding to the exponential decay phase of the circulating cadmium and followed by a linear increase in organ concentration corresponding to the constant blood concentration phase.

The placenta and adrenals had peak cadmium concentrations at 12 hours following subcutaneous dosing. Note that subsequent to 12 hours, blood flow to these organs was diminished and hence delivery of cadmium to the organ was impaired. Although analog computer modeling of the data provides satisfactory fits to all maternal organs, the model did not predict the placental and adrenal concentrations at 18 hours. The model, in fact, overshoots the data concentrations at 18 hours for these organs, supporting the hypothesis that blood flow alteration, beginning at 12 hours, changes the distribution of cadmium to the affected organ (Figure 4; Levin et al., 1983). Note that the toxicokinetic model used a mathematic description of the blood concentration data which was obtained by curve stripping, assuming a constant input beginning at t = o. The equation was

$$\text{Blood [Cd]} = 22.1e^{-6.65t} + 1.78e^{-0.95t} + 1.16 \text{ nmol/ml.}$$

This empirically determined function was used as a forcing function with each organ analog receiving cadmium from that mathematically described blood curve analog. Each organ was modeled assuming there were two fractions of the cadmium, one that was freely exchangeable with the blood and one that was non-exchangeable, or irreversibly bound. Without the non-exchangeable compartment, satisfactory fits to the data were not obtained (Figure 5). The necessity of including a non-exchangeable compartment suggested that cadmium was rapidly bound with high affinity in many organs, including the placenta. The high affinity of cadmium for free sulfhydryl groups may explain this irreversibly-bound component.

The intravenous injection of 14 μmoles Cd/kg (Samarawickrama and Webb, 1981) and the subcutaneous injection of 40 μmoles Cd/kg (Levin et al., 1981) resulted in fetal toxicity and placental necrosis. These doses also produced similar peak cadmium concentrations in the chorioallantoic placenta 60 of nmoles/gram and 70 nmoles/gram. The similarity of the concentrations in the placenta suggest the existence of a critical concentration of cadmium for the induction of necrosis. Not only was the extent of accumulation significant, but the rapidity of the accumulation was also remarkable. Although it is not surprising that intravenous injection of cadmium resulted in rapid accumulation of cadmium in the placenta, the speed of placental accumulation following subcutaneous injection was notable.

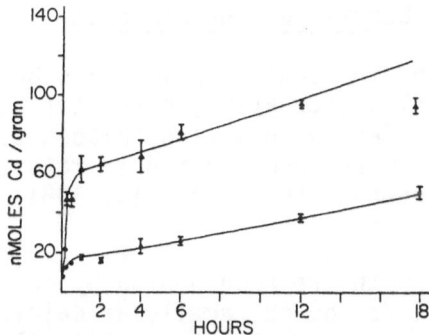

Figure 4   The cadmium concentration data of placenta and maternal
           kidney. The solid lines are computer simulations of the
           data. Placental uptake of cadmium was rapid and the
           placental level of cadmium at 1 hour exceeded renal
           cadmium levels through 18 hours. Note that the model for
           the placenta does not predict the 18-hour time point (see
           text). O = kidney; Δ = placenta. (Mean ± S.E.; n = 3-5).

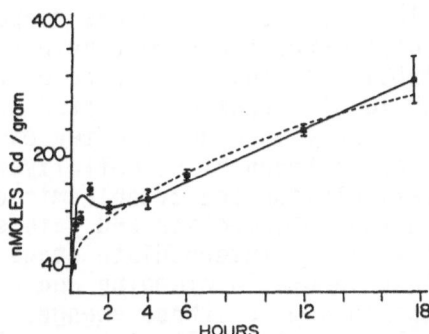

Figure 5   Computer-generated curves for the cadmium concentration
           data of maternal liver with (———) and without (- - -) a
           non-exchangeable tissue compartment.

Greater than 75 percent of the total accumulation in the placenta
occurred within the first hour after injection (Figure 4). The rapid
accumulation of cadmium in the placenta should be investigated at
earlier times than those in the previous studies on the alteration
of uteroplacental blood flow. Early cadmium accumulation and early
insult of the placenta were consistent with the appearance of
placental lesions at 12-16 hours, since light microscopic changes
often take 8-12 hours to develop following insult.

The Direct Effects of Cadmium on the Placenta

To investigate the temporal relationships between fetal death, uteroplacental blood flow alteration, placental accumulation of cadmium, and placental lesion formation, placental ultrastructure and cellular viability were investigated in rats exposed to 40 μmole Cd/kg on day 18 of pregnancy (Levin et al., 1981; di Sant'Agnese et al., 1983).

Cell injury and death are accompanied by cell water and ion balance changes. Influxes of extracellular calcium have been associated with irreversible cell injury and cell death (Schanne et al., 1979). Mitochondria actively take up calcium for intracellular calcium regulation (Lehninger, 1970). Thus, fluxes of calcium into cells will be reflected in mitochondrial calcium levels. Measurements of calcium in mitochondria isolated from placentae of treated dams showed increased calcium concentrations with time beginning as early as 6 hours following cadmium administration (Figure 6). The changes in placental mitochondrial calcium were not accompanied by consistent changes in maternal liver or kidney mitochondrial calcium. Thus, cadmium was altering cellular viability in the placenta as early as 6 or 8 hours after injection.

The biochemical index of cell death was supported by the observations of placental ultrastructure (Levin et al., 1981; di Sant'Agnese et al., 1983). A single exposure of rats to cadmium (40 μmoles/kg s.c.) on day 18 of pregnancy resulted in alterations in placental morphology as early as 6 hours after exposure. The earliest change appeared in trophoblast cell layer II and consisted mainly of lysosomal vesiculation and cytoplasmic edema. These changes intensified in the intermediate and late stages of toxicity (Figures 7 and 8). Additional intermediate stage alterations included unusual nuclear chromatin clumping and nucleolar disorganization. Although some of these changes were observed in the other trophoblast layers, layer II was predominately affected. In the late stages of cadmium placental toxicity, trophoblast cell layer II underwent necrosis with extensive calcification (in the form of crystalline apatite) of the mitochondria in this cell layer (Figures 9 and 10). Trophoblast layer II was the first to undergo necrosis, although the other layers soon followed. The fetal endothelium was remarkably unaffected even when the trophoblast layers were sloughed off, leaving denuded fetal capillaries. The sparing of the fetal capillaries may be related to the failure of the cadmium to transit the placenta in significant quantities. Thus, cadmium may not reach the fetal endothelial tissue of the placental vasculature.

It should also be noted that no pathologic changes were observed in the maternal uterine vasculature after cadmium exposure. Therefore, injury to the uterine vessels is not the

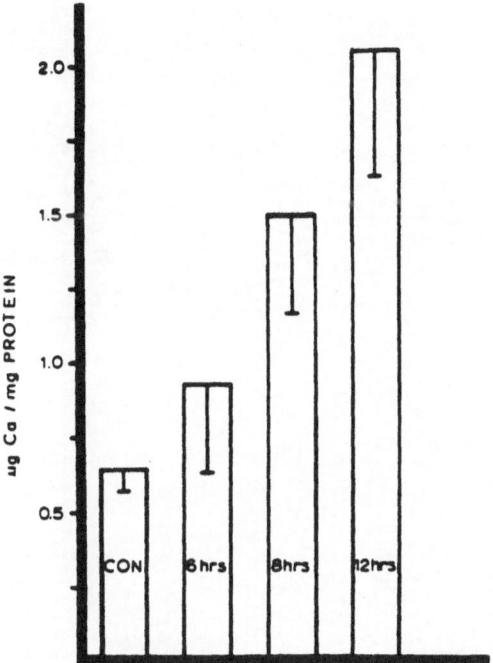

Figure 6   The calcium levels in placental mitochondria isolated from
            rats, 6, 8, and 12 hours after cadmium treatment (CdCl$_2$,
            40 μmol/kg) and control rats. The data are expressed as
            means + S.D. The results represent the placentae from 3
            dams at 6 and 12 hours, 5 dams at 8 hours and 6 control
            dams. Calcium levels at 8 and 12 hours after treatment
            differed significantly from controls (p<0.05). (Levin et
            al., 1981, courtesy of Placenta)

stimulus for the depression of uteroplacental blood flow that was
observed. Thus, the biochemical and ultrastructural studies
indicate that cadmium has a direct effect on the placenta leading to
changes in placental structure and function.

The Effects of Cadmium on Placental Transport

The inhibition of placental transport function after a single
exposure of cadmium was described by Webb and Samarawickrama
(1981). Transport of $^{65}Zn^{2+}$ was inhibited in a dose-dependent
fashion on day 12 of gestation (Figure 11). The inhibitory doses
correlated well with the teratogenic doses of cadmium. Although at
this stage of gestation, the chorioallantoic placenta is not fully
functional. These data are suggestive of effects on placental

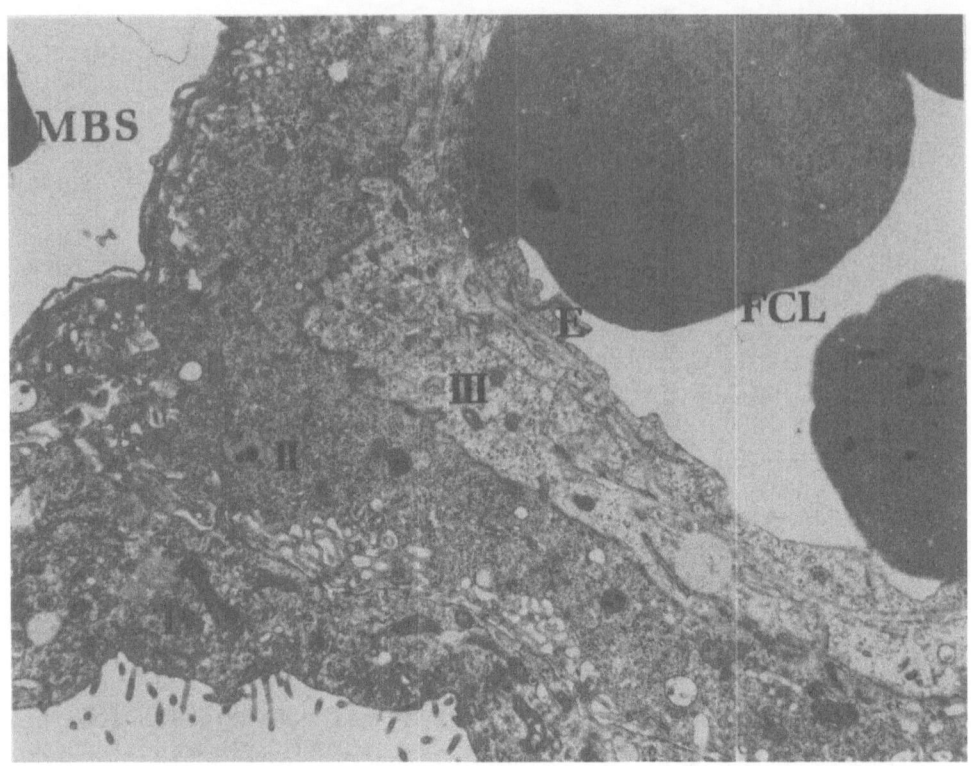

Figure 7   Control placenta demonstrating three trophoblast layers
(I,II,III) and fetal endothelium (E). Maternal blood
space (MBS) and fetal capillary (FCL) are also shown, x
7,300.

function. The inhibition of transport was in the absence of
necrotic effects. The inhibition of zinc transport might be an
alteration of yolk sac function since at this stage of gestation the
yolk sac is the principal site of nutrient absorption. However,
previous investigations (Dencker, 1975) have demonstrated high
accumulations of cadmium in the ectoplacental cone around this
period of gestation, thus suggesting that the inhibition of
$^{65}Zn^{2+}$ transfer might be the result of an effect on the early
placenta.

      Other heavy metals inhibit placental transport function. Olson
and Massaro (1978) demonstrated that placental amino acid uptake was
inhibited by methylmercury. This inhibition of placental transport
may play a role in the depressed protein synthesis and growth
retardation associated with prenatal exposure to the toxicant. The

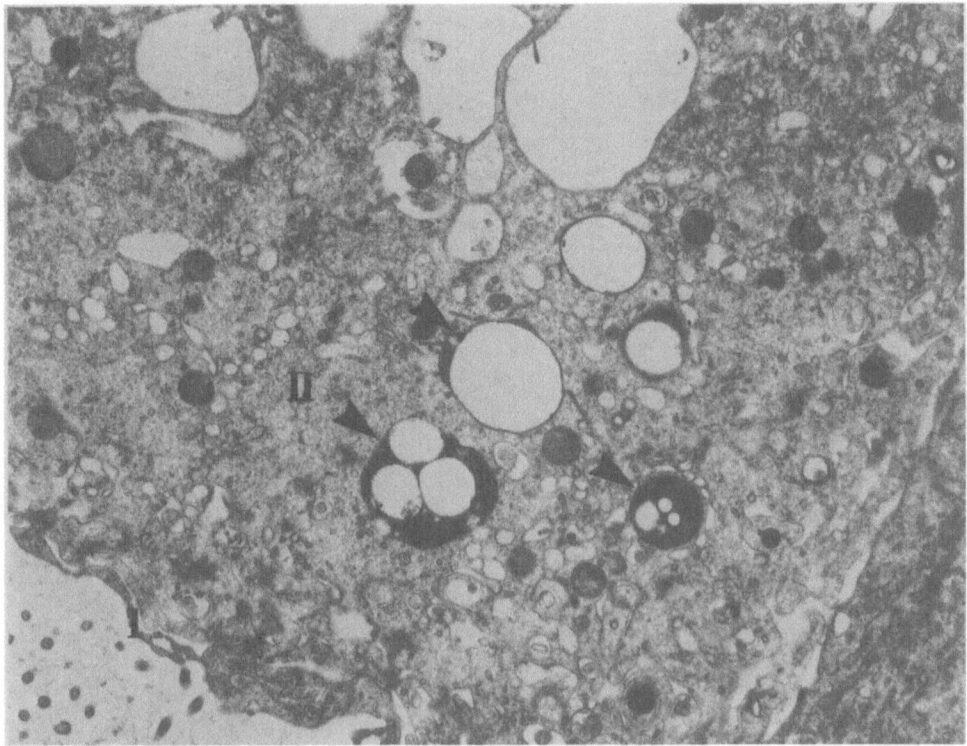

Figure 8   Marked lysosomal vesiculation (arrowheads) and diffuse
           cytoplasmic edema is seen in trophoblast layer II
           demonstrating an intermediate stage of toxicity, x 10,500.

reduction of fetal growth associated with methylmercury-inhibited
placental transport and the inhibition of zinc transport by cadmium
serve as examples of subacute toxicities affecting placental
function.

     The use of high-dose single exposures has helped identify the
placenta as a target organ for cadmium. Low-dose exposure of rats
to cadmium over two generations resulted in decreased fertility
(Schroeder and Mitchener, 1971). Using a drinking water exposure
regimen, Webster (1978) demonstrated that cadmium induced growth
retardation and fetal anemia which were reversible following
parenteral iron supplement. However, the data are not conclusive as
to whether the effect of cadmium is inhibition of maternal iron
uptake from the gut or of placental iron transport. Martin et al.
(1977) have demonstrated that iron-stressed dams were more
susceptible to cadmium-induced fetal death. Again, it is not clear
if this sensitivity was the result of cadmium inhibition of iron
transport to the already stressed fetus.

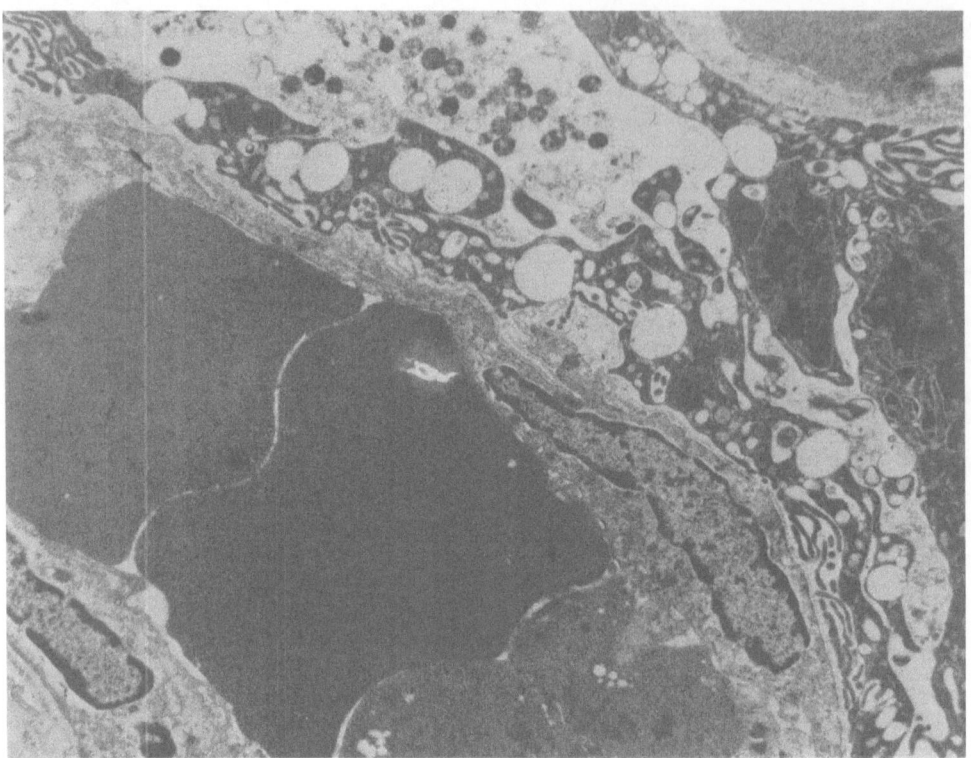

Figure 9   Late stage cadmium toxicity. Note the congestion in the
           fetal capillary and the intact endothelium, even in the
           presence of necrotic trophoblast (at lower left).
           Remnants of layer II show calcified mitochondria (bottom),
           x 9,400.

        Chronic exposure studies in pregnancy are necessary to further
evaluate the risks of environmental exposure to cadmium during human
gestation. The chronic exposure protocols will necessitate the use
of other animal models with longer gestation periods. However, the
placenta is unique in the availability of human tissue. Evaluation
of human risk to the effects of cadmium on the placenta can be
estimated through studies of human placental preparations in vitro.

The Effects of Cadmium on Human Placental Preparations

        In vitro data supporting the hypothesis of direct effects of
cadmium on the placenta have been obtained using human placental
preparations. In two abstracts, Goodman et al. (1978,1979), using

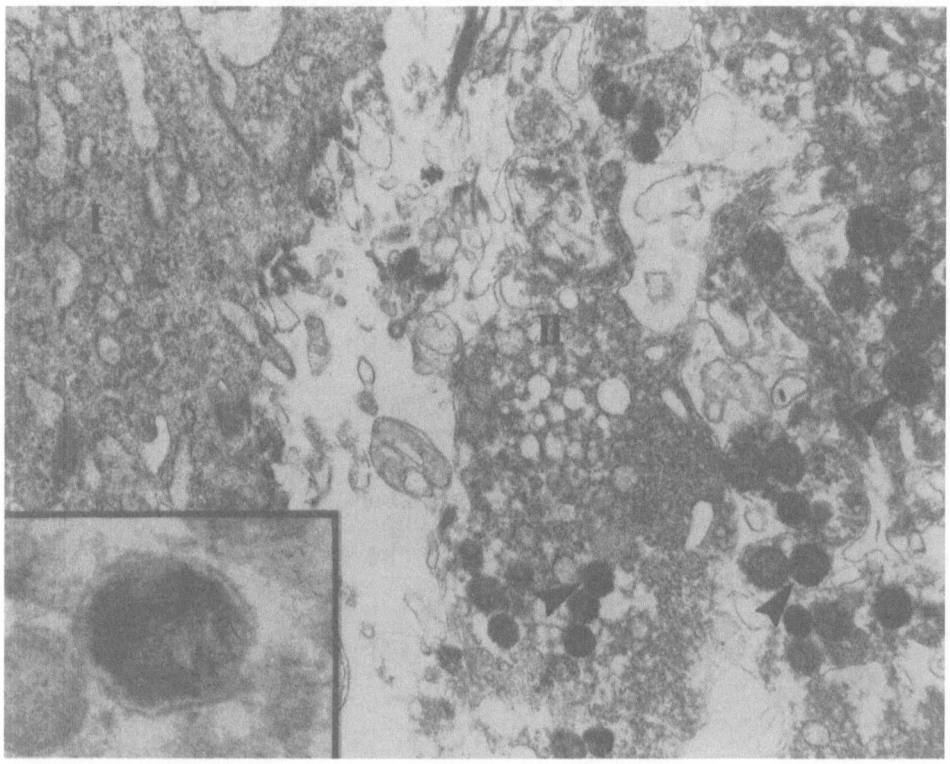

Figure 10 Late stage toxicity with necrosis of layer II and numerous
          mitochondria with electron dense crystalline apatite
          (arrowheads and inset). Note layer I is intact with only
          slight dilatation of the rough endoplasmic reticulum, x
          13,650. Inset x 81,000.

placental membrane vesicles, have demonstrated that mercury and
cadmium altered the uptake and equilibration of a non-metabolizable
amino acid, α-aminoisobutyric acid (AIB). The concentrations of
mercury and cadmium required to inhibit AIB transport were 100 μM to
800 μM. AIB uptake by human placental slices was inhibited by 100
μM $CdCl_2$ but not by 10 μM $CdCl_2$. The high concentrations
required to produce the effects on placental slices and membrane
preparations may indicate that these inhibitory effects are
nonspecific in nature (Levin and Miller, unpublished data). Studies
are needed to correlate the in vitro inhibition observed with human
placental preparations and the in vivo effects of cadmium and other
heavy metals.

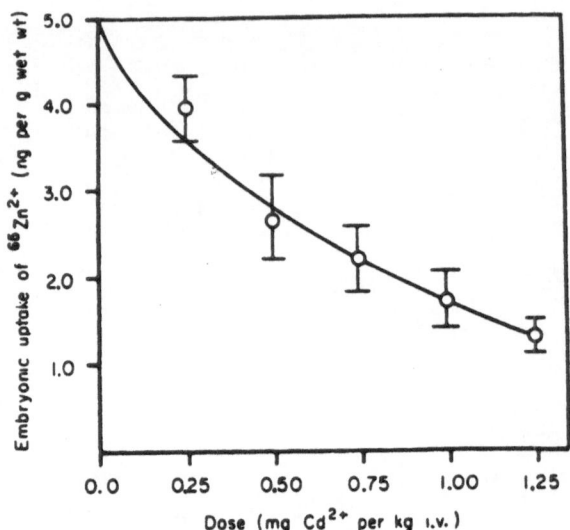

Figure 11   Uptake of $^{65}Zn^{2+}$ by embryos at 4 hours after
            intravenous injection of various doses of Cd^{2+} into
            12-day pregnant rats (mean $\pm$ S.D.). (Webb and
            Samarawickrama, 1981, courtesy of Journal of Applied
            Toxicology)

        Weir et al. (1983) have used human, isolated, perfused human
placental lobules to determine the permeability of human placenta to
cadmium. Although it is reported that human fetuses are born with
less than 1 μg cadmium (Friberg et al., 1974), there was no direct
evidence on the placental permeability in humans. Preliminary
results (Weir et al., 1983) indicate that ratios of greater than 1
to 10 exist between the placental cadmium concentration and the
maternal perfusate concentration. Negligible concentration of
cadmium was detected in the fetal perfusate when initial maternal
perfusate concentration was 10 nmoles/ml. The négligible fetal
level indicates that human placental permeability to cadmium is very
limited and similar to the rodent placenta. This is in contrast to
the guinea pig placenta which is thought to be relatively permeable
to cadmium (Kelman and Walter, 1977; Kelman, 1979).

        The role of cadmium in the prenatal effects of cigarette
smoking is a question that needs to be investigated further.
Smoking during pregnancy is associated with low birth-weight
babies. Roels et al. (1978) and Miller and Gardner (1981) have
reported that the placentae from mothers who smoke during pregnancy
have 30-fold higher cadmium concentrations than do the placentae
from non-smokers. In addition, cigarette smoking is associated with
alterations in placental morphology (Asmussen, 1979) and function
(Rowell, 1981). Rowell has reported that the placental slices from

smokers have decreased ability to take up AIB. Although other
factors associated with smoking, such as carboxyhemoglobin and
cyanide levels, increased aryl hydrocarbon hydroxylase activity and
nicotinic effects may play a role in altered prenatal development
and alterations of placental morphology, it is clear that the
effects of cadmium on the human placenta must also be considered.
The substantial differences in cadmium concentrations between
smokers and non-smokers may be a useful tool for evaluation of the
chronic effects of cadmium on the placenta.

CONCLUSION

The acute effects of cadmium, which induce fetal death, may
result from rapid and extensive accumulations of cadmium in the
placenta. The direct effects of the high cadmium concentrations on
the placenta may result in the alterations of morphology and
cellular viability in the placenta observed biochemically and by
electron microscopy. The presence of injured placental tissue may
induce local circulatory alterations leading to decreased
uteroplacental blood flow. The decrease in blood flow can lead to
fetal death through anoxia, or decreased nutrient flow due to blood
flow alterations and altered placental function. Thus, in late
gestation the rodent placenta is a target organ for cadmium, and
fetal death is the result of the placental effects of the toxicant.

The chronic effects of cadmium on placental function need
further investigation to allow for extrapolation to humans.
Certainly the role of cadmium in the lowered birth-weight babies of
cigarette smoking mothers needs to be explored. Because of the
short gestation of laboratory rodents and the very short functional
period of the mouse and rat placenta, it is necessary for future
studies to employ animal models which will facilitate long-term
chronic exposure of cadmium to placentae. This type of study will
allow us to differentiate the high-dose acute effects of cadmium on
placental morphology and function from low-dose chronic
alterations. The use of human placental preparations has already
demonstrated conclusively that the human placenta is relatively
impermeable to cadmium. It is hoped that future investigation will
allow us to establish threshold levels of cadmium below which
functional deficits are absent. Thus, although studies on placental
toxicity are hampered by species and gestational differences in
structure and function, the ability to obtain human tissue may allow
for direct determination of human placental sensitivity to cadmium.

ACKNOWLEDGEMENTS

The expert technical assistance of Karen Jensen-Demesy in
performing the electron microscopy is acknowledged. We would also

like to acknowledge the assistance of Joanne Quate and Linda Smith in the preparation of this manuscript. This work was supported in part by The Richard W. and Mae Stone Good Gift and National Research Service Award ES-07026.

REFERENCES

Ahokas, R.A. and Dilts, P.V., 1979, Cadmium uptake by the rat embryo as a function of gestational age, Am. J. Obstet. Gynecol. 135:219-222.

Asmussen, I., 1979, Effects of maternal smoking on the fetal cardiovascular system, Cardiovasc. Med. 4:777-790.

Barr, M., 1973, Teratogenicity of cadmium chloride in two stocks of Wistar rats, Teratology 7:237-242.

Berlin, M. and Ullberg, S., 1963, The fate of Cd^{109} in the mouse: an autoradiographic study after a single intravenous injection of $Cd^{109}Cl_2$, Arch. Environ. Health 7:686-693.

Chernoff, N., 1973, Teratogenic effects of cadmium in the rat, Teratology 8:29.

Chiquone, A.D, 1965, Effect of cadmium chloride on the pregnant albino mouse, J. Reprod. Fertil. 10:263-265.

Dencker, L., 1975, Possible mechanisms of cadmium fetotoxicity in golden hamsters and mice: uptake by the embryo, placenta, and ovary, J. Reprod. Fertil. 44:461-471.

di Sant'Agnese, P.A., DeMesy-Jensen, K., Levin, A.A. and Miller, R.K., 1983, Placental toxicity of cadmium in the rat: an ultrastructural study, Placenta (in press).

Ferm, V.H., Hanlon, D.P. and Urban, J., 1969, The permeability of the hamster placenta to radioactive cadmium, J. Embryol. Exp. Morphol. 22:107-113.

Ferm, V.H., 1971, Developmental malformations induced by cadmium, Biol. Neonate 19:101-107.

Friberg, L., Piscator, M., Nordberg, G.F. and Kyellstrom, T., 1974, "Cadmium in the Environment", 2nd Edition, CRC Press, Cleveland, Ohio.

Gale, T.F. and Ferm, V.H., 1973, Skeletal malformations resulting from cadmium treatment in the hamster, Biol. Neonate 23:149-160.

Goodman, D.R., Fant, M.E. and Harbison, R.D., 1978, Placental toxicity of mercury and cadmium: evidence for direct effects on placental plasma membranes, The Pharmacologist 20:262.

Goodman, D.R., Fant, M.E. and Harbison, R.D., 1979, Direct effect of the heavy metals mercury and cadmium on alpha-amino-isobutyric acid transport across human placental membranes, Fed. Proc. 38:535.

Kelman, B.J., 1979, Effects of toxic agents on movements of materials across the placenta, Fed. Proc. 38:2246-2250.

Kelman, B.J. and Walter, B.K., 1977, Passage of cadmium across the perfused guinea pig placenta, Proc. Soc. Exp. Biol. Med. 156:68-71.

Lehninger, A.L., 1970, Mitochondria and calcium ion transport, Biochem. J. 119:129-138.

Levin, A.A. and Miller, R.K., 1980, Fetal toxicity of cadmium in the rat: maternal vs. fetal injections, Teratology 22:1-6.

Levin, A.A. and Miller, R.K., 1981, Fetal toxicity of cadmium in the rat: decreased uteroplacental blood flow, Toxicol. Appl. Pharmacol. 58:297-306.

Levin, A.A., Plautz, J.R., di Sant'Agnese, P.A. and Miller, R.K., 1981, Cadmium: placental mechanisms of fetal toxicity, Placenta Suppl 3:303-318.

Levin, A.A., Kilpper, R.W. and Miller, R.K. 1983, Organ specific kinetics of a fetal toxic injection of $CdCl_2$ in the pregnant rat, Toxicol. Appl. Pharmacol. (in press).

Miller, R.K. and Gardner, K.A., 1981, Cadmium in the human placenta: relationship to smoking, Teratology 23:51A.

Martin, P.G., Hitchock, B.B. and King, J.F., 1977, Interactions of Cd, Zn, Cu and Fe in the anemic rat, in: "Trace Substances in Environmental Health", XI, D.D. Hemphill, ed., pp. 201-210, Univ. of Missouri Press, Columbia, MO.

Olson, F.C. and Massaro, E.J., 1978, Effect of methylmercury on murine fetal amino acid uptake, protein synthesis and palate closure, Teratology 16:187-194.

Parizek, J., 1964, Vascular changes at sites of oestrogen biosynthesis produced by parenteral injection of cadmium salts: the destruction of the placenta by cadmium salts, J. Reprod. Fertil. 7:263-264.

Parizek, J., 1965, The peculiar toxicity of cadmium during pregnancy: an experimental toxemia of pregnancy induced by cadmium salts, J. Reprod. Fertil. 9:111-112.

Prigge, E, 1978, Inhalative cadmium effects in pregnant and fetal rats, Toxicology 10:297-309.

Robson, J.M. and Sullivan, F.M., 1966, Analysis of actions of 5-hydroxytryptamine in pregnancy, J. Physiol. 184:717-732.

Roels, H., Hubermont, G., Buchet, J.P. and Lauwerys, R.R., 1978, Placental transfer of lead, mercury, cadmium and carbon monoxide III, Environ. Res. 16:236-247.

Rowell, P.P., 1981, The effect of maternal cigarette smoking on the ability of human placental villi to concentrate α-amino-isobutryic acid in vitro, Res. Comm. Subst. Abuse 2:253-266.

Samarawickrama, G.P. and Webb, M., 1979, Acute effects of cadmium during pregnancy and embryo-fetal development in the rat, Environ. Health Perspect. 28:345-349.

Samarawickrama, G.P. and Webb, M., 1981, The acute toxicity and teratogenicity of cadmium in the pregnant rat, J. Appl. Toxicol. 1:264-269.

Schanne, F.A.X., Kane, A.B., Young, E.E. and Farber, J.L., 1979, Calcium dependence of toxic cell death: a final common pathway, Science 206:700-702.

Schroeder, H.A. and Mitchener, M., 1971, Toxic effects of trace elements of mice and rats, Arch. Environ. Health 23:102-109.

Sonawane, B.R., Nordberg, M., Nordberg, G.F. and Lucier, G.W., 1975, Placental transfer of cadmium in rats: influence of dose and gestational age, Environ. Health Perspect. 28:248-249.

Webb, M. and Samarawickrama, G.P., 1981, Placental transport and embryonic utilization of essential metabolites in the rat at the teratogenic dose of cadmium, J. Appl. Toxicol. 1:270.

Webster, W.S., 1978, Cadmium-induced fetal growth retardation in the mouse, Arch. Environ. Health 33:36-42.

Weir, P., Miller, R.K. and Manlik, D., 1983, Cadmium: placental transfer and accumulation by the perfused human placental lobule, Teratology (in press).

ENDOGENOUS METAL-BINDING PROTEINS IN THE CONTROL OF ZINC, COPPER, CADMIUM AND MERCURY METABOLISM DURING PRENATAL AND POST-NATAL DEVELOPMENT

Michael Webb

Toxicology Unit
MRC Laboratories
Carshalton, Surrey, United Kingdom

ABSTRACT

Livers of prenatal and neonatal animals contain high concentrations of metallothioneins, which appear to function in copper (Cu) and/or zinc (Zn) homeostasis. In the newborn of some species the hepatic metallothioneins contain only small amounts of copper and seem to control only the metabolism of zinc. Before intestinal closure in such species (e.g. the rat), copper absorption may be regulated by a specific copper-binding complex. Neonates of certain other species (e.g. the Syrian hamster) appear to lack this intestinal copper-complex and to regulate the metabolism of copper and zinc by the synthesis of hepatic metallothionein.

The intestinal copper-complex and hepatic metallothionein of the newborn rat provide immediately-available binding sites for cadmium (Cd) and mercury (Hg). The former limits the transport of these metals across the intestine, whilst the latter binds them by replacement of zinc.

Both cadmium and mercury inhibit the placental transport of zinc and copper and, when administered in mid-gestation are teratogenic, possibly because of their effects on these processes. Newborn rat pups, from dams dosed with cadmium in late gestation, are deficient in hepatic zinc-metallothionein and their gain in body weight is retarded.

Interference with transport processes in both the maternal intestine and placenta contribute to the susceptibility of the fetus at chronic exposure of the dam to cadmium.

ADULT MECHANISMS OF METAL ION HOMEOSTASIS

Absorption of toxic, unessential metals, such as cadmium and mercury, must take place by intestinal transport processes that operate for certain essential metals. Competitive interactions occur, therefore, between the essential and nonessential metals for common carrier sites. Although surprisingly little information seems to be available on the interactions of mercury with other metallic ions, particularly at the sites of gastrointestinal absorption, interactions between cadmium and zinc, copper, calcium and iron are well-established (e.g. Bremner, 1974, 1979). Thus, not only do these essential metals antagonize the uptake of cadmium, but the latter may induce nutritional deficiencies of the former; for example, copper deficiency in rats (Campbell and Mills, 1974), sheep (Mills and Delgarno, 1972), goats (Anke et al., 1970; Grun et al., 1979) and iron deficiency in experimental animals (Samarawickrama, 1979) and man (Lauwerys et al., 1974). As, at least in the adult animal, anaemia is severe only when cadmium is given intragastrically, interactions other than at the site of iron absorption (Hamilton and Valberg, 1974; Ragan, 1977; Hamilton, 1978) seem of minor significance. Deficiencies of calcium (Pond and Walker, 1975; Washko and Cousins, 1975,1976,1977) and zinc (Petering et al., 1971) enhance the absorption of cadmium, the former probably because the calcium transport pathway provides a mechanism for cadmium absorption and, the synthesis of the calcium-binding protein, which binds cadmium with almost equal affinity (Bredderman and Wasserman, 1974), is increased by calcium deficiency (Washko and Cousins, 1975,1976,1977).

All of the essential metallic ions, some more so than others, can be toxic if present within living cells in the wrong concentrations or ratios. Thus, the biological response of the whole animal to variations in the supply of any one of them, although less clear-cut than in unicellular organisms (e.g. Bowen, 1966) will range through the deficiency phases, both severe and mild, to the optimal and then to the toxic phases. The optimum concentration ranges for certain trace metals may be extremely narrow, and thus regulatory mechanisms, which control absorption and distribution, are needed to maintain homeostasis or metabolic equilibrium. In the adult animal, such a regulatory mechanism in the control of zinc metabolism has been ascribed to metallothionein, the synthesis of which is inducible in cells of the intestinal mucosa, liver and kidneys (e.g. Webb, 1979). According to Cousins (1979), for example, zinc metabolism is regulated by the synthesis of intestinal and hepatic metallothioneins which, respectively, control the efflux of the cation from the mucosal cells to the blood and its uptake from the blood by the liver. Similar mechanisms have been proposed for the regulation of the absorption of copper (Evans, 1979) and cadmium (Squibb et al., 1976; Cherian et al., 1978; Kotsonis and Klaassen, 1978; McGivern and Mason, 1979).

In all of these proposed models, the metal is considered to be retained in the dose-dependent metallothionein pool, until eliminated by desquamation of the mucosal cells. The presence of cadmium-metallothionein in the mucosa, however, does not interfere with the intestinal uptake and transfer of either zinc or cadmium (Kello et al., 1979; Sugawara, 1981) and is not a determinant in cadmium absorption (Kello et al., 1979). Hall et al. (1979) also find that, under normal conditions, mechanisms other than incorporation into metallothionein, regulate the absorption of copper. Furthermore, Jackson et al. (1981), in agreement with Schwartz and Kirchgessner (1977), have shown that, in normal rats, absorption of zinc occurs predominantly by a slow, carrier-mediated process, and is proportional to dietary intake whilst body retention is controlled by the rate of excretion. At low dietary levels of zinc, absorption is increased, not as a result of decreased mucosal binding, but by the activation of a second high-affinity transport mechanism. Starcher et al. (1980), however, find: 1) a direct proportionality between zinc absorption and intestinal metallothionein concentration in mice; and 2) preadministration of actinomycin-D before zinc or stress, prevents both thionein synthesis and zinc absorption. These results, which are considered to imply a significant role for metallothionein in zinc uptake, provide no evidence that the metalloprotein, itself, acts as a carrier in the transport process. It is possible, for example, that the metallothionein forms a metal-ion buffer, which increases zinc transport by a gradient effect. Thus, as discussed in more detail elsewhere (Webb and Cain, 1982), whilst there is no doubt that zinc, copper, and cadmium can induce the synthesis of metallothioneins in the intestine, the precise function of these metalloproteins in absorptive processes is far from clear.

ZINC AND COPPER METABOLISM IN THE FETUS AND NEONATE

Irrespective of the control mechanisms, however, the adult intestine seems to provide an efficient barrier to the uptake of excessive amounts of zinc and copper and normally the concentration of the hepatic metallothionein, which reflects the plasma levels of these metals, is low (e.g. Webb, 1979). In contrast, the fetuses and/or newborn of all mammalian species thus far investigated contain large amounts of metallothionein in their livers. In some species, for example, human beings (Riordan and Richards, 1980; Bakka and Webb, 1981) and sheep (Bremner et al., 1977), the concentration of the metallothionein, which contains both zinc and copper, is maximal during gestation. The relative proportions of the bound cations, however, are not constant, but alter with gestational age. Also, at least in human fetal liver, a soluble zinc-rich metallothionein coexists with an insoluble, copper-rich metallothionein (Riordan and Richards, 1980). The latter is probably identical with the particulate-bound mitochondrocuprein of

prenatal human (and bovine) liver, which yields a copper-rich,
partially disaggregated metallothionein in the presence of strong
reducing agents (Porter, 1971,1974). A previous report (Ryden and
Deutsch, 1978) that the hepatic metallothionein from the human
fetus, as well as immature laboratory animals, is predominantly a
copper-metalloprotein now seems erroneous, due to an artefact in the
isolation procedure (Riordan and Richards, 1980).

In the fetal rat, in contrast with the human or ovine fetus,
metallothionein accumulates in the soluble fraction of the liver
only after the 16th day of gestation (Bakka et al., 1981) or,
according to Kern et al. (1981), the 14th day post-fertilization.
The threshold concentration of liver zinc, above which thionein
synthesis occurs, seems to be about 20 μg/g wet weight (Bakka et
al., 1981) and this is appreciably less than that (30 μg/g wet
weight) in the adult (Bremner et al., 1973). The concentration of
this metalloprotein, which contains much more zinc than copper,
increases in parallel with the total hepatic zinc to a maximum at 2
days postpartum (Bakka et al., 1981). Thereafter, it decreases with
age to reach the low adult level at, or shortly after, weaning
(Mason et al., 1981a). According to Bell (1980), the hepatic
metallothionein of either the 7-day-old or 28-day-old rat is
undersaturated with zinc. This, however, may be due to an artefact;
partial loss of zinc is likely to occur during the isolation of the
native metalloprotein by gel filtration (e.g. Sokolowski and Weser,
1975; Webb, 1979), a procedure that can be used to measure
dissociation constants of zinc protein complexes (Dixon, 1976).

Studies on the effect of maternal cadmium exposure on the
accumulation and loss of the metallothionein during prenatal and
postnatal development in the rat (Bakka et al., 1981) and on the
change in distribution of zinc between the particulate and soluble
components of the liver with age after birth (Mason et al., 1981a)
suggest that the metalloprotein has two major functions: firstly,
to regulate the metabolism of zinc, particularly before the
development, with closure of the intestine, of the adult homeostatic
mechanisms; and secondly, to provide a source of zinc for the
maintenance of the concentration of this metal at functional sites
in the liver cytosol. Possibly, therefore, the conclusion of Mills
and Davies (1979) that "the sensitivity of the fetus or newborn to
changes in the supply of essential elements will be influenced by
the efficiency of placental and mammary transport and the capacity
of the fetus to accumulate reserves", might be extended to include
"the capacity of the newborn to maintain these reserves". The
neonatal mouse, in which the concentration of thionein-bound zinc
decreases very rapidly after 2 days of age (Bakka and Webb, 1981),
for example, is extremely susceptible to zinc deficiency (Beach et
al., 1980).

In newborn animals, mechanisms for the control of the absorption of various metals are poorly developed until the intestinal mucosa acquires the structure and function of the adult (e.g. Jugo, 1977, 1979; Walter, 1979). Before this change occurs, uptake of both essential (e.g. copper, zinc, iron) and non-essential (e.g. cadmium, mercury, lead) cations is attributed to non-specific pinocytotic absorption of metal-protein complexes (Jugo, 1979; Mills and Davies, 1979) and is much greater than in the mature animal. If intestinal homoeostasis is inadequate, it seems possible that other mechanisms exist to limit the interactions of potentially toxic cations with sensitive, functional sites. As the decrease in the hepatic concentration of thionein-bound zinc, which occurs between 2 and 21 days of age in newborn rats, can be prevented or even reversed by the oral administration of zinc (M. Webb and D. Holt, unpublished observations), it seems that, as mentioned previously, metallothionein synthesis in the liver provides one such mechanism. In this species, the hepatic concentration of copper, in contrast with that of zinc, remains low for the first five to six days after birth and then increases to a maximum at about 14 to 15 days of age (Mason et al., 1981b). Although a small increase in the copper concentration of fetal rat liver between 19 and 21 days postfertilization, possibly related to the appearance of the copper-metallothionein polymer, mitochondrocuprein, has been reported by Kern et al. (1981), the amount of soluble thionein-bound copper remains small throughout the first two or more weeks of neonatal life (Mason et al., 1981b). Most of the copper absorbed from the maternal milk during this period seems to accumulate in the intestine, not in the liver. Thus, the copper concentration in the whole intestine of the Wistar rat increases from about 17 μg/g wet weight at birth to as much as 140 μg/g wet weight at 2 days postpartum (Mason et al., 1981b). This copper is not evenly distributed but increases from the proximal to the distal end of the intestine and is maximal (over 200 μg/g wet weight) in the ileum (D. Dinsdale, D. Holt and M. Webb, unpublished observations), the predominant site of copper absorption in the newborn rat (Mistilis and Mearrick, 1969). Also, in agreement with the suggestion of Mistilis and Mearrick (1969) that ileal uptake of copper probably involves a pinocytotic mechanism, much of the absorbed copper seems to be concentrated within apical cytoplasmic vesicles (D. Dinsdale, D. Holt and M. Webb, unpublished observations).

The increase in intestinal copper concentration immediately after birth is accompanied by the appearance and accumulation of a soluble, polydisperse copper-complex in the mucosal cells (Mason et al., 1981b). Although an analogous copper-rich fraction from the intestine of the 5-day-old Long-Evans rat, which also contains zinc, has been resolved by Johnson and Evans (1980a) into two main components, the amino acid compositions of which characterize them as isometallothioneins, the crude copper-complex from the intestinal mucosa of the newborn Wistar rat contains at least ten components (Figure 1) and, as none of them incorporates labelled cysteine (administered via the maternal milk), even the tentative assumption that some of them are polymeric copper-metallothioneins is unjustified. Between the 13th and 15th days after birth, the concentration of the intestinal copper-complex decreases rapidly and, at 21 days, only small amounts of copper remain in association with two clearly defined fractions, the second of which also contains zinc and has the properties of a metallothionein (Mason et al., 1981b). The development of this pattern of distribution, which is similar to that in the intestine of the adult, thus occurs at about the time of intestinal closure. In the rat, for example, the columnar absorptive cells lose the capacity to ingest proteins and colloids when the ultrastructure of the intestinal epithelial cells changes from the primitive pattern of multiple membrane invaginations and apical cytoplasmic vesiculation to the microtubular cytoplasmic network, characteristic of the adult, at 18 days (Clark, 1959), 20 days (Walter, 1979) or three weeks (Hagihira, 1965) of age. It has been suggested, therefore, that before these changes occur, copper

Figure 1   Resolution of the crude copper-complex, isolated from the intestine of the 6-day-old rat by gradient polyacrylamide gel electrophoresis (K. Cain, unpublished observations).

absorption is regulated by the copper-complex (Mason et al., 1981b), or by the intestinal metallothionein in the Long-Evans rat (Johnson and Evans, 1980b), whilst the metabolism of zinc is controlled by the hepatic metallothionein (Mason et al., 1981b).

This hypothesis, if true for the neonatal rat, cannot be of general application. As in the human fetus and newborn infant, the hepatic metallothioneins of fetal and newborn rabbits, Syrian and Chinese hamsters and mice vary greatly in metal content and composition according to age, as well as species (Bakka and Webb, 1981). Thus, in either the rabbit or Chinese hamster, the metallothionein is a zinc-metalloprotein, which contains only small amounts of copper, whereas that of the Syrian hamster contains much more copper than zinc. This last species, however, does not accumulate copper in its intestine, either as a polydisperse copper-complex, or in any other form (D. Holt and M. Webb, unpublished observations). It seems possible, therefore, that in the Syrian hamster, as in the guinea pig (Sasser and Jarboe, 1980), intestinal closure occurs at or before birth and, in consequence, the hepatic metallothionein functions in the regulation of the metabolism of copper as well as zinc.

UPTAKE, DISTRIBUTION AND TOXICITY OF CADMIUM AND MERCURY IN THE NEWBORN

At least in newborn rats, excessive absorption and intestinal retention is a characteristic feature of the uptake of certain essential (copper, iron) and unessential (cadmium, cerium, (^{95}Zr) zirconium, (^{95}Nb) niobium, mercury, strontium, lead) metals (Matsusaka et al., 1972; Inaba and Lengemann, 1972; Shiraishi and Ichikawa, 1972; Forbes and Reina, 1972; Kello and Kostial, 1977a,b; Sasser and Jarboe, 1977; Kostial et al., 1974,1979). Enhanced absorption of heavy metals in the sucking animal until weaning is attributed to the combination of a milk diet and the nonselective permeability of the undeveloped intestine (Jugo, 1977). The effect of a milk diet on the absorption of various metals (lead, cadmium, mercury), but not the reason for it, is well established (Kostial et al., 1971; Kello and Kostial, 1973,1977b; Jugo, 1976,1977; Engstrom and Nordberg, 1978). Nonselective permeability usually is ascribed to nonspecific pinocytosis although, according to Sasser and Jarboe (1980), species differences in cadmium absorption do not seem to correlate well with species differences in the absorption of macromolecules. Comparative studies with 1-day-old pigs, rats and guinea pigs, for example, show that the pig, which probably has the greatest capacity for protein absorption at this age, absorbs much less cadmium than the guinea pig although the latter has the more mature gastrointestinal system at birth. Nevertheless, intestinal retention of cadmium does appear to correlate inversely with intestinal maturity (Sasser and Jarboe, 1980).

Both the intestinal copper-complex and the hepatic metallothionein of the newborn rat provide additional, immediately available high-affinity binding sites for foreign cations, such as cadmium and mercury. Binding of cadmium to the copper-complex, for example, probably explains the observation of Sasser and Jarboe (1977,1980) that this metal persists in the gastrointestinal tract of the neonatal rat as a metallothionein-like protein until excreted by extrusion of the mucosal cell into the intestinal lumen. Also, the accumulation of the copper-complex from an undetectable level at birth to a maximum at 2 days of age (Mason et al., 1981b) offers an explanation for the six-fold greater systemic absorption of cadmium in 2-hour-old rat pups than in 24-hour-old pups, observed by Sasser and Jarboe (1977). The greater retention of cadmium in the gastrointestinal tract of the sucking rat also is relevant to the apparent differences in toxicity of this cation in newborn and adult animals. Although the observations of Bell (1980) suggest that the LD_{50} of subcutaneously administered cadmium may be lower in 7-day-old than in 28-day-old rats, the results of Kostial et al. (1979) show no increased susceptibiltiy of sucking animals to intraperitoneally-administered cadmium. In contrast, however, the data of Kostial et al. (1979) indicate high toxicity of orally-administered cadmium in sucking animals (Table 1). Nevertheless, if the LD_{50} values (Table 1) are corrected for differences in intestinal retention and transport, it seems that, in terms of systemic uptake, the toxicity of cadmium is similar in neonatal and mature animals. Thus, at oral LD_{50} values of 18.4 and 202 mg Cd/kg in 1-week-old and 18-week-old animals, the calculated systemic absorption of cadmium is 1.45 and 1.15 mg Cd/kg, respectively. Jugo (1977) also concludes that the toxicity of heavy metals is lower for young animals than for adults but is overwhelmed by a much higher absorption rate, lower excretion and unfavourable distribution.

Retention of orally-administered mercury (790 µg Hg/kg body weight) in the intestine also is much greater in the 5-day-old sucking rat than in the 21-day-old weanling and, at 18 hours after dosing, accounts for most of the body burden (Webb and Holt, 1982). At this dose, binding of mercury to the copper-complex, which is present in the intestine of the suckling, but not of the weanling or adult, accounts for an appreciable fraction of the retained cation in the neonate. At low-dose levels (e.g. 100 µg/kg body weight), however, most of the mercury in the soluble fraction of the suckling intestine is associated with the high molecular weight proteins, not with the copper-complex. The pattern of distribution is somewhat different after administration of cadmium. Binding of this metal to the high molecular weight proteins increases disproportionately with the dose and, at low dose levels, a greater percentage of the total is bound to the copper-complex (M. Webb and D. Holt, unpublished observations). These differences in binding of cadmium and mercury to the copper-complex seem relevant to the observation of Kostial et al. (1980) that supplementation of cow's milk with iron, zinc,

Table 1   Acute Toxicities of Parenterally- and Orally-Administered CdCl$_2$ in Rats in Relation to Age and Sex[a]

	LD$_{50}$ values (mg Cd/kg body weight) and, in brackets, 95 confidence limits at 8 days after			
Age (weeks)	Intraperitoneal Administration		Oral Administration	
	Males	Females	Males	Females
2	10.7(10.0-11.4) 7.6(6.8- 8.5)		47.0(43.0-51.0)[b] 18.4(15.2-22.0) 12.7(10.5-15.3)	
3	14.5(12.2-17.3)	11.8(9.4-14.8)	227(162-317)	240(198-291)[b]
6	7.6(5.2-11.2)	8.5(6.9-10.5)	260(207-328)	211(182-252)[b]
18	11.0(6.9-17.6)	9.6(7.0-13.1)	202(136-299) 166(144-197)	170(140-206)[b] 168(137-207)
52	2.0(1.7- 2.4)	1.8(1.4- 2.2)	145(116-180) 131(106-162)	109(86-136)[b] 128(106-154)

[a]Kostial et al., 1979.
[b]Kostial et al., 1978 (courtesy of Environmental Health Perspectives).

manganese and copper significantly increases the whole body retention of cadmium in sucking rats, but has no effect on the retention of mercury. From the data of these authors, it can be calculated that the dose of cadmium (about 20 µg Cd/animal) was about ten times that of mercury (approximately 2 µg Hg/animal) on a weight basis, or about 18 times greater on a molar basis. The results of Webb and Holt (1982) suggest that, at this low dose mercury would bind predominantly to the cytosolic high molecular weight proteins and thus intestinal retention would not be influenced greatly by changes in the concentration of the copper-complex. At the higher dose of cadmium, however, binding of this metal to the complex not only would be appreciable, but also probably would be influenced by the increased intestinal concentration of the latter, caused by the presence of copper in the trace metal supplement.

The foregoing observations on the intestinal binding of cadmium and mercury suggest that the copper-complex is not the primary

acceptor of these metals in the gut of the newborn but, at least for
mercury, becomes increasingly important in retention with increasing
dose. Whilst such interactions might be expected if the complex
functions as a regulator, not as a carrier in cation transport, it
is also possible that, as the dose of either metal increases, so too
does absorption in the ileum, which contains the highest
concentration of the complex. After oral administration of a tracer
dose of ^{115m}Cd, for example, the metal is retained initially in
the upper and midsections of the intestine and an appreciable
percentage of the dose is present in the lower section only after
15-17 days (Sasser and Jarboe, 1977). In contrast with cadmium or
mercury, lead does not bind to the copper-complex (M. Webb and D.
Holt, unpublished observations). The latter, therefore, would not
be expected to regulate the absorption of lead at any dose level.
Significantly, the greater whole body retention of
orally-administered lead in sucking rats, in comparison with adults,
is known to be due to increased absorption without increased
retention in the gut (Kostial et al. 1971).

The copper-complex limits but does not prevent the transfer of
cadmium and mercury from the intestine to the blood and thus to
other organs of the body. In the sucking animal, the inter- and
intraorgan distributions of these metals are known to differ from
those in the weanling and adult (Jugo, 1979; Wong and Klaassen,
1980). After administration of mercury, for example, the ratio of
the renal:hepatic content of mercury increases with age (Jugo, 1979;
Webb and Holt, 1982). Most of the relatively large amount of
mercury retained in the liver of the suckling is bound to the
endogenous metallothionein by displacement of zinc whereas, in the
adult, less than 5 percent of the total hepatic content is in this
form (Webb and Holt, 1982). Induction of zinc-metallothionein in
the adult by pretreatment with zinc, however, does not alter the
uptake of mercury by the liver (Webb and Holt, 1982). The excessive
accumulation of mercury in the liver of the newborn, therefore,
cannot be due to the presence of the endogenous metallothionein.
Mason (1982) also finds no relationship between the concentration of
the endogenous metallothionein and the uptake of cadmium by the
liver and emphasizes that, after an intraperitoneal dose of cadmium
(1 mg Cd/kg), liver uptake is less in the 2-day-old rat, which
contains the higher content of the metalloprotein, than in the
12-day-old animal. This difference, however, is not unexpected
since, in the newborn animal, the gut is known to be a major site of
selective cadmium accumulation (Kostial et al., 1979).

Age-related differences in toxic metal distribution, therefore,
may reflect the age-related differences in the contents, or binding
affinities of carrier proteins in the blood and in the development
of various organs, particularly the kidneys. Changes in the protein

composition of serum or plasma during neonatal development can be shown easily by electrophoretic techniques (e.g. Wise et al., 1963), whilst newborn rats, when treated with an acute parenteral dose of mercury, show no evidence of renal damage before 14 days postpartum and only exhibit the adult pattern of extensive tubular necrosis when the kidney attains structural maturity at three weeks of age (Wachstein and Robinson, 1965). The significance of these differences in blood protein composition, renal structure and function, and the development of the blood-brain barrier (e.g. Dobbing, 1961) in relation to the neonatal toxicity of heavy metals and in particular, to the increased uptake of these metals in the brain of the newborn, has yet to be investigated in detail. Whereas the uptake of lead into various brain regions (cerebellum, cerebral cortex, brainstem and hippocampus) of the rat is known to be greater if the dose is given during the first 10 days after birth (Klein and Koch, 1981), and the effects on learning are known to persist in the eight- to ten-week-old adult, even though the blood lead concentration has returned to control values (Brown, 1975), the behavioral toxicology of cadmium and mercury seems a much neglected field. The observation that indirect exposure of the fetal rat to cadmium, injected into the maternal animal, appears to have no effect on the development of the central nervous system (Rohrer et al., 1979) probably is of little significance in relation to postnatal exposure, since the placenta discriminates very effectively against cadmium transport to the fetus, unless the challenge is substantial and acute (Mills and Davies, 1979).

Other areas that remain to be investigated are: 1) the differences in intestinal metal transport in the newborn of different species (e.g. Sasser and Jarboe, 1980) in relation to the differences in time of intestinal closure and to the presence or absence of an intestinal copper-complex; and 2) the effects of the interactions of foreign cations (e.g. mercury and cadmium) with both this complex and the hepatic metallothionein on the metabolism of the essential copper and zinc ions. According to Mason (1982), parenteral administration of cadmium (1 mg Cd/kg) is unlikely to influence zinc metabolism in the 2-day-old rat since, in relation to the contents of endogenous cations, the amount of cadmium incorporated into the hepatic metallothionein, apparently and unexpectedly (e.g. Irons and Smith, 1976) by displacement of copper, not zinc, is small. Thus, the metallothionein remains a zinc-rich protein with an approximate zinc:copper:cadmium ratio of 16:3:1. Similar treatment of the 12-day-old animal, however, results in a metallothionein that contains more cadmium than zinc. Mason (1982) suggests that this appreciable incorporation of cadmium may affect the rate of turnover of the metalloprotein (Cain and Holt, 1979) and thus alter the hepatic metabolism and tissue distribution of zinc and copper.

PRENATAL INTERACTIONS OF CADMIUM AND MERCURY WITH ZINC AND COPPER

Interactions of cadmium and mercury with essential metals, of course, are not confined to life after birth, but can begin in utero. Cadmium causes a dose-dependent inhibition of the placental transport of zinc (Samarawickrama and Webb, 1979; Webb and Samarawickrama, 1981), and thus rat pups, from dams that have been treated with a high dose of cadmium (1 mg Cd/kg, intravenous) on the 18th day of gestation, are deficient in hepatic zinc-metallothionein. As, however, birth eliminates the transport block, the hepatic concentrations of total and thionein-bound zinc in these pups then increase rapidly to reach maxima similar to, but about five days later than, those in the newborn of normal dams. Although pups recover from one effect of cadmium exposure during gestation, their body weights and liver weights remain below normal for at least the first 20 days after birth (Bakka et al., 1981). When administered earlier in gestation, i.e. during the critical period of organogenesis, a single acute but sublethal dose of cadmium is teratogenic. The teratogenic response, as well as the teratogenic dose, varies between and within species (e.g. Gale, 1973; Parzyck et al., 1978; Samarawickrama and Webb, 1981) but, at least in the rat, seems to be determined by the accumulation of the metallic ion in the placenta, not in the embryo. At four hours after a single intravenous injection of cadmium (1.25 mg Cd/kg) into the pregnant rat on the 12th day of gestation, for example, the concentration of cadmium in the embryo is extremely small (12-16 ng Cd/g wet weight), approximately 0.8 percent of that in the placenta (Webb and Samarawickrama, 1981). The presence of this relatively high concentration of cadmium in the latter organ at this time is sufficient to inhibit the transport of zinc and copper to the embryo. In particular, the inhibition of zinc transport is severe and leads to decreased embryonic thymidine kinase activity and incorporation of thymidine into DNA. Simultaneous administration of zinc with cadmium, which prevents the teratogenic effects of cadmium (Ferm and Carpenter, 1967), overcomes the inhibition of thymidine kinase and restores DNA synthesis to the normal level (Webb and Samarawickrama, 1981). It seems, therefore, that there may be a relationship between teratogenesis and the temporary block in the zinc supply to the embryo. Nevertheless, the teratogenic dose range for cadmium is narrow and, in particular, the difference in the inhibition of (^{65}Zn)zinc transport at the highest no-effect dose and the teratogenic dose levels is small, only about 8 percent (Webb and Samarawickrama, 1981). Also, in the Wistar rat, mercury is a less effective teratogen than cadmium, but its effects on the placental transport of zinc and other metals (copper, iron), although delayed, ultimately are greater (D. Holt and M. Webb, unpublished observations).

Maternal exposure to either cadmium or mercury increases the placental content of metallothionein. This metalloprotein also binds zinc and copper. As after cadmium treatment, metallothionein accumulation is relatively slow, whereas the inhibition of zinc transport is rapid; it is perhaps unlikely that the latter process is related to the former. In this respect, the placenta is analogous to the maternal intestine; both accumulate metallothionein in response to cadmium, but the effects of this accumulation on zinc and copper transport are conjectural. Obviously, this is an important area for further study in relation to the effects of acute and chronic exposure to cadmium and, perhaps, mercury during pregnancy. Doses of cadmium above the teratogenic range, if not lethal for the maternal rat are embryo- or fetotoxic. Although, after development of the functional placenta on the 10th or 11th day of gestation (Ahokas and Dilts, 1979), transport of cadmium to the fetus increases with dose and gestational age (Sonawane et al., 1975), the fetal concentration of cadmium invariably remains low in comparison with that in the placenta (Webb and Samarawickrama, 1981). Furthermore, comparison of the effects of cadmium when injected into the maternal animal, or directly into the fetuses, shows a lower incidence of fetal deaths under the latter conditions (Levin and Miller, 1980). Also, dietary zinc deficiency from the 4th to the 12th day of gestation which, alone, does not cause fetal reabsorptions in Holtzman rats, increases the reabsorption rate due to a single acute dose of cadmium on the 12th or 14th day (Parzyck et al., 1978). After acute maternal exposure, therefore, fetotoxicity probably results from severe and prolonged inhibition of placental transport processes and/or decreased uteroplacental blood flow, which is appreciable at 12-16 hours (Levin and Miller, 1981).

Deficiencies of copper, iron and zinc are common in both the fetus and newborn animals that are exposed to cadmium in food or drinking water before and/or during pregnancy (Anke et al., 1970; Schroeder and Mitchener, 1971; Mills and Dalgarno, 1972; Grun et al., 1979; Choudhury et al., 1978; Rohrer et al., 1978; Petering et al., 1979; Webster 1979a; Ahokas et al., 1980) and probably result mainly from interactions of the toxic metal with maternal intestinal and placental transport processes. These deficiencies, which lead to a wide range of metabolic disorders; for example, defects in DNA, RNA and protein synthesis and catabolism and in the cross linking of peptide chains in the formation of collagen, decreased reproductive performance, abnormalities in preimplantation embryos, increased infant mortality and, in the fetus, impaired development of the skeleton and central nervous system, arterial fragility, haemorrhage and umbilical hernia, are described or reviewed in detail by Hurley (1977), Oster and Salgo (1977), White and Holland (1977), Williams (1977) and Mills and Davies (1979). Inhibition by cadmium of the transport of zinc, copper and iron in the adult intestine is well established (e.g. Bremner, 1974,1979) and is likely to be of greater significance in late gestation if, as with zinc (Davies and Williams, 1977), the increased demand normally is met by increased

absorption. The additional restraint on placental transport in the
pregnant animal thus may result in fetal death or growth retardation,
the latter being attributed to limitation of the oxygen supply to the
fetus in consequence of the fetal anaemia (Webster, 1979b) or to
decreased maternal food consumption and metabolism coupled with
reduced placental zinc transport (Ahokas et al., 1980).

REFERENCES

Ahokas, R.A. and Dilts, P.V., 1979, Cadmium uptake by the rat embryo
    as a function of gestational age, Am. J. Obstet. Gynecol.
    135:219-220.
Ahokas, R.A., Dilts, P.V. and LaHaye, E.B., 1980, Cadmium-induced
    fetal growth retardation: protective effect of excess dietary
    zinc, Am. J. Obstet. Gynecol. 136:216-221.
Anke, M., Henning, A., Schneider, H-J., Ludke, H., von Gagern, W.
    and Schlegel, H., 1970, The inter-relationships between
    cadmium, zinc, copper and iron in the metabolism of hens,
    ruminants and man, in: "Trace Element Metabolism in Animals",
    C.F. Mills, ed., pp. 317-320, Livingstone, Edinburgh.
Bakka, A. and Webb, M., 1981, Metabolism of zinc and copper in the
    neonate: changes in the concentrations and contents of
    thionein-bound Zn and Cu with age in the livers of the newborn
    of various mammalian species, Biochem. Pharmacol. 30:721-725.
Bakka, A., Samarawickrama, G.P. and Webb, M., 1981, Metabolism of
    zinc and copper in the neonate: effect of cadmium
    administration during late gestation in the rat on the zinc and
    copper metabolism of the newborn, Chem.-Biol. Interact.
    34:161-171.
Beach, R.S., Gershwin, M.E. and Hurley, L.S., 1980, Growth and
    development in zinc-deprived mice, J. Nutr. 110:201-211.
Bell, J.U., 1980, Induction of hepatic metallothionein in the
    immature rat following administration of cadmium, Toxicol.
    Appl. Pharmacol. 54:148-155.
Bowen, H.M.J., 1966, "Trace Elements in Biochemistry", p. 103,
    Academic Press, London.
Bredderman, P.J. and Wasserman, R.H., 1974, Chemical composition,
    affinity for calcium and some related properties of Vitamin
    D-dependent calcium-binding protein, Biochemistry 13:1687-1694.
Bremner, I., 1974, Heavy metal toxicities, Quart. Rev. Biophys.
    7:75-124.
Bremner, I., 1979, Mammalian absorption, transport and excretion of
    cadmium, in: "The Chemistry, Biochemistry and Biology of
    Cadmium", M. Webb, ed., pp. 175-193, Elsevier/North Holland,
    Amsterdam.
Bremner, I., Davies, N.T. and Mills, C.F., 1973, The effect of zinc
    deficiency and food restriction on hepatic zinc proteins in
    rats, Biochem. Soc. Trans. 1:982-985.

Bremner, I., Williams, R.B. and Young, B.W., 1977, Distribution of copper and zinc in the liver of the developing sheep foetus, Br. J. Nutr. 38:87-92.

Brown, D.R., 1975, Neonatal lead exposure in the rat: decreased learning as a function of age and blood lead concentration, Toxicol. Appl Pharmacol. 32:628-637.

Cain, K. and Holt, D.E., 1979, Metallothionein degradation: metal composition as a controlling factor, Chem. Biol. Interact. 28:91-106.

Campbell, J.K. and Mills, C.F., 1974, Effects of dietary cadmium and zinc on rats maintained on diets low in copper, Proc. Nutr. Soc. 33:15A-17A.

Cherian, M.G., Goyer, R.A. and Valberg, L.S., 1978, Gastrointestinal absorption and organ distribution of oral cadmium chloride and cadmium metallothionein in mice, J. Toxicol. Environ. Health, 4:861-868.

Choudhury, H., Hastings, L., Merden, E., Brockman, D., Cooper, G.P. and Petering, H.G., 1978, Effect of low level prenatal cadmium exposure on trace metal body burden and behavior in Sprague-Dawley rats, in: "Trace Element Metabolism in Animals and Man-3", M. Kirchgessner, ed., pp. 549-552, Freising-Weihenstephan, Institut fur Ernahrungsphysiologie, Technische Universitat Munchen.

Clark, S.L., 1959, The ingestion of proteins and colloidal materials by columnar absorptive cells of the small intestine in suckling rats and mice, J. Biophys. Biochem. Cytol. 5:41-50.

Cousins, R.J., 1979, Regulatory aspects of zinc metabolism in liver and intestine, Nutr. Rev. 37:97-103.

Davies, N.T. and Williams, R.B., 1977, Effects of pregnancy and lactation on the absorption of zinc and lysine by the rat duodenum in situ, Br. J. Nutr. 38:417-423.

Dixon, H.B.F., 1976, Removal of bound ligands from a macromolecule by gel filtration, Biochem. J. 159:161-162.

Dobbing, J., 1961, The blood brain barrier, Physiol. Rev. 41:130-187.

Engstrom, B. and Nordberg, G.F., 1978, Effects of milk diet on gastro-intestinal absorption of cadmium in adult mice, Toxicol. 9:195-203.

Evans, G.W., 1979, Metallothionein in intestinal copper metabolism, Experientia Suppl. 34(metallothionein):321-329.

Ferm, V.H. and Carpenter, S.J., 1967, Teratogenic effect of cadmium and its inhibition by zinc, Nature (Lond.) 216:1123.

Forbes, G.B. and Reina, J.C., 1972, Effect of age on gastrointestinal absorption (Fe, Sr, Pb) in the rat, J. Nutr. 102:647-652.

Gale, T.F., 1973, The interactions of mercury with cadmium and zinc in mammalian embryonic development, Environ. Res. 6:95-105.

Grun, M., Anke, M. and Partschefeld, M., 1979, The Cd exposure of cattle and sheep in the GDR, Kadmium Symposium, pp. 253-258, Friedrich Schiller Universitat, Jena, GDR.

Hagihira, H., 1965, cited by Shiraishi, Y. and Ichikawa, R., 1972,
    Hall, A.C., Young, B.W. and Bremner, I., 1979, Intestinal
    metallothionein and the mutual antagonism between copper and
    zinc in the rat, J. Inorgan. Biochem. 11:57-66.
Hamilton, D.L., 1978, Interrelationships of lead and iron retention
    in iron-deficient mice, Toxicol. Appl. Pharmacol. 46:651-661.
Hamilton, D.L. and Valberg, L.S., 1974, Relationship between cadmium
    and iron absorption, Am. J. Physiol. 227:1033-1037.
Hurley, L.S., 1977, Zinc deficiency in prenatal and neonatal
    development, in: "Zinc Metabolism: Current Aspects in Health
    and Disease", G. Brewer and A.S. Prasad, eds., pp. 47-48, A.R.
    Liss, New York.
Inaba, J. and Lengemann, F.W., 1972, Intestinal uptake and whole
    body retention of ^{141}Ce in suckling rats, Health Phys.
    22:169-175.
Irons, R.D. and Smith, J.C., 1976, Prevention by copper of cadmium
    sequestration by metallothionein in liver, Chem.-Biol.
    Interact. 15:289-294.
Jackson, M.J., Jones, D.A. and Edwards, R.H.T., 1981, Zinc
    absorption in the rat, Br. J. Nutr. 46:15-27.
Johnson, W.T. and Evans, G.W., 1980a, Isolation of a (copper,
    zinc)-thionein from the small intestine of normal rats,
    Biochem. Biophys. Res. Commun. 96:10-17.
Johnson, W.T. and Evans, G.W., 1980b, Age dependent variation of
    copper in tissue and proteins of neonatal rat small intestine,
    Proc. Soc. Exp. Biol. Med. 165:496-501.
Jugo, S., 1976, Retention and distribution of ^{203}HgCl$_2$ in
    suckling and adult rats, Health Phys. 30:240-241.
Jugo, S., 1977, Metabolism of toxic heavy metals in growing
    organisms: a review, Environ. Res. 13:36-46.
Jugo, S., 1979, Metabolism and toxicity of mercury in relation to
    age, in: "The Biogeochemistry of Mercury in the Environment",
    J.O. Nriagu, ed., pp. 481-502, Elsevier/North Holland,
    Amsterdam.
Kello, D. and Kostial, K., 1973, The effect of milk diet on lead
    metabolism in rats, Environ. Res. 6:355-360.
Kello, D. and Kostial, K., 1977a, Influence of age on whole body
    retention and distribution of ^{115m}Cd in the rat, Environ.
    Res. 14:92-98.
Kello, D. and Kostial, K., 1977b, Influence of age and milk diet on
    cadmium absorption from the gut, Toxicol. Appl. Pharmacol.
    40:277-282.
Kello, D., Sugawara, N., Voner, C. and Foulkes, E.C., 1979, On the
    role of metallothionein in cadmium absorption by rat jejunum in
    situ, Toxicology 14:199-208.
Kern, S.R., Smith, H.A., Fontaine, D. and Bryan, S.E., 1981,
    Partitioning of zinc and copper in fetal liver subfractions:
    appearance of metallothionein-like proteins during development,
    Toxicol. Appl. Pharmacol. 59:346-354.

Klein, A.W. and Koch, T.R., 1981, Lead accumulation in brain, blood and liver after low dosing of neonatal rats, Arch. Toxicol. 47:257-262.

Kostial, K., Simonovic, I. and Pisonic, M., 1971, Lead absorption from the intestine in newborn rats, Nature (Lond.) 233:564.

Kostial, K., Maljkovic, T. and Jugo, S. 1974, Lead acetate toxicity in relation to age and sex, Arch. Toxicol. 31:265-269.

Kostial, K., Kello, D., Jugo, S., Rabar, I. and Maljkovic, T., 1978, The influence of age on metal metabolism and toxicity, Environ. Health Perspect. 25:81-86.

Kostial, K., Kello, D., Blanusa, M., Maljkovic, T. and Rabar, I., 1979, Influence of some factors on cadmium pharmacokinetics and toxicity, Environ. Health Perspect. 28:89-95.

Kostial, K., Rabar, I., Blanusa, M. and Ciganovic, M., 1980, Influence of trace elements on cadmium and mercury absorption in sucklings, Bull. Environ. Contam. Toxicol. 25:436-440.

Kotsonis, F.N. and Klaassen, C.D., 1978, The relationship of metallothionein to the toxicity of cadmium after prolonged oral administration to rats, Toxicol. Appl. Pharmacol. 46:39-54.

Lauwerys, R., Buchet, J.P., Roels, H., Brouwers, J. and Stanescu, D., 1974, Epidemiological survey of workers exposed to cadmium, Arch. Environ. Health, 28:145-148.

Levin, A.A. and Miller, R.K., 1980, Fetal toxicity of cadmium in the rat: maternal vs. fetal injections, Teratol. 22:1-5.

Levin, A.A. and Miller, R.K., 1981, Fetal toxicity of cadmium in the rat: decreased uteroplacental blood flow, Toxicol. Appl. Pharmacol. 58:297-306.

Mason, R., 1982, Metabolism of cadmium in the neonate: effect of hepatic zinc, copper and metallothionein concentrations on the uptake of cadmium in the rat liver, Biochem. Pharmacol. 31:1761-1764.

Mason, R., Bakka, A., Samarawickrama, G.P. and Webb, M., 1981a, Metabolism of zinc and copper in the neonate: accumulation and function of (Zn,Cu)-metallothionein in the liver of the newborn rat, Br. J. Nutr. 45:375-389.

Mason, R., Brady, F.O. and Webb, M., 1981b, Metabolism of zinc and copper in the neonate: accumulation of Cu in the gastrointestinal tract of the newborn rat, Br. J. Nutr. 45:391-399.

Matsusaka, N., Tanaka, M., Nishimura, Y., Yuyama, A. and Kobayashi, H., 1972, Whole body retention and intestinal absorption of $^{115m}CdCl_2$ in young and adult mice, Med. Biol. Japan 85:275-279.

McGivern, J. and Mason, J., 1979, The effect of chelation on the fate of intravenously administered cadmium in rats, J. Comp. Pathol. 89:1-9.

Mills, C.F. and Dalgarno, A.C., 1972, Copper and zinc status of ewes and lambs receiving increased dietary concentrations of cadmium, Nature (Lond.) 239:171-173.

Mills, C.F. and Davies, N.T., 1979, Perinatal changes in the absorption of trace elements, in: "Development of Mammalian Absorptive Processes", Ciba Foundation Symposium 70, Exerpta Med., pp. 247-266, Amsterdam.

Mistilis, S.P. and Mearrick, P.T., 1969, The absorption of ionic biliary and plasma radio-copper in neonatal rats, Scan. J. Gastroenterol. 4:691-696.

Oster, G. and Salgo, M.P., 1977, Copper in mammalian reproduction, Adv. Pharmacol. Chemotherap. 14:357-409.

Parzyck, D.C., Shaw, S.M., Kessler, W.V., Vetter, R.J., Van Sickle, D.C. and Mayer, R.A., 1978, Fetal effects of cadmium in pregnant rats on normal and zinc deficient diets, Bull. Environ. Contam. Toxicol. 19:206-214.

Petering, H.G., Johnson, M.A. and Stemmer, K.L., 1971, Studies on zinc metabolism in the rat. I. Dose response effects of cadmium, Arch. Environ. Health 23:93-101.

Petering, H.G., Choudhury, H. and Stemmer, K.L., 1979, Some effects of oral ingestion of cadmium on zinc, copper and iron metabolism, Environ. Health Perspect. 28:97-106.

Pond, W.G. and Walker, E.F., 1975, Effect of dietary Ca and Cd level of pregnant rats on reproduction and on dam and progeny tissue mineral concentrations, Proc. Soc. Exp. Biol. Med. 48:665-668.

Porter, H., 1971, Neonatal hepatic mitochondrocuprein. IV. Sulfitolysis of the cystine-rich crude copper protein and isolation of a peptide containing more than 35 percent half-cystine, Biochim. Biophys. Acta 229:143-154.

Porter, H., 1974, The particulate half-cystine rich copper protein of newborn liver. Relationship to metallothionein and subcellular localization in non-mitochondrial particles, possibly representing heavy lysosomes, Biochem. Biophys. Res. Commun. 56:661-668.

Ragan, H.A., 1977, Effect of iron deficiency on the absorption and distribution of lead and cadmium in rats, J. Lab. Clin. Med. 90:700-706.

Riordan, J.R. and Richards, V., 1980, Human fetal liver contains both zinc- and copper-rich forms of metallothionein, J. Biol. Chem. 255:5380-5383.

Rohrer, S.R., Shaw, S.M., Born, G.S. and Vetter, R.J., 1978, The maternal distribution and placental transfer of cadmium in zinc-deficient rats, Bull. Environ. Contam. Toxicol. 19:556-563.

Rohrer, S.R., Shaw, S.M. and Lamar, C.H., 1979, Cadmium fetotoxicity in rats following prenatal exposure, Bull. Environ. Contam. Toxicol. 23:25-29.

Ryden, L. and Deutsch, H.F., 1978, Preparation and properties of the major copper-binding component in human fetal liver, Biol. Chem. 253:519-524.

Samarawickrama, G.P., 1979, Biological effects of cadmium in mammals, in: "The Chemistry, Biochemistry and Biology of Cadmium", M. Webb, ed., pp. 341-421, Elsevier/North Holland, Amsterdam.

Samarawickrama, G.P. and Webb, M., 1979, Acute effects of cadmium during pregnancy and embryo-fetal development, Environ. Health Perspec. 28:245-249.

Samarawickrama, G.P. and Webb, M., 1981, The acute toxicity and teratogenicity of cadmium in the pregnant rat, J. Appl. Toxicol. 1:254-269.

Sasser, L.B. and Jarboe, G.E., 1977, Intestinal absorption and retention of cadmium in neonatal rats, Toxicol. Appl. Pharmacol. 41:423-431.

Sasser, L.B. and Jarboe, G.E., 1980, Intestinal absorption and retention of cadmium in neonatal pigs compared to rats and guinea pigs, J. Nutr. 110:1641-1647.

Schroeder, H.A. and Mitchener, M., 1971, Toxic effects of trace elements on the reproduction of mice and rats, Arch. Environ. Health 23:102-106.

Schwartz, F.J. and Kirchgessner, M., 1977, Studies on the regulation of the intestinal absorption of zinc, in: "Trace Element Metabolism in Man and Animals", M. Kirchgessner, ed., pp. 110-115, Freising-Weinhenstephan, Technische Universitat Munchen.

Shiraishi, Y. and Ichikawa, R., 1972, Absorption and retention of ^{144}Ce and ^{95}Zr-^{95}Nb in newborn, juvenile and adult rats, Health Phys. 22:373-378.

Sokolowski, G. and Weser, U., 1975, Circular dichromism and X-ray photoelectron spectroscopy of hepatic Zn-thionein, Hoppe-Seyler's Zeit. Physiol. Chem. 356:1715-1726.

Sonawane, B.R., Nordberg, M., Nordberg, G.F. and Lucier, G.W., 1975, Placental transfer of cadmium in rats: influence of dose and gestational age, Environ. Health Perspect. 12:97-102.

Squibb, K.S., Cousins, R.J., Silbon, B.L. and Levin, S., 1976, Liver and intestinal metallothionein: function in acute cadmium toxicity, Exp. Mol. Pathol. 25:163-171.

Starcher, B.C., Glauber, J.C. and Madaras, J.G., 1980, Zinc absorption and its relationship to intestinal metallothionein, J. Nutr. 110:1391-1397.

Sugawara, N., 1981, Role of metallothionein in zinc uptake from rat jejunum, Proc. U.S.-Japan Workshop on Metallothionein, March 1981, Cincinnati, OH.

Wachstein, M. and Robinson, M., 1965, Neonatal resistance to nephrotoxic renal tubular necrosis in the rat, Fed. Proc. 24:619.

Walter, W.A., 1979, Intestinal host defence: importance of gut closure in control of macromolecular transport, in: "Development of Mammalian Absorptive Processes", Ciba Foundation Symposium 70, Excerpta Med., pp. 201-207, Amsterdam.

Washko, P.W. and Cousins, R.J., 1975, Effect of low dietary calcium on chronic cadmium toxicity in rats, Nutr. Rep. Internat. 2:113-127.

Washko, P.W. and Cousins, R.J., 1976, Metabolism of [109]Cd in rats fed normal and low-calcium diets, J. Toxicol. Environ. Health 1:1055-1066.

Washko, P.W. and Cousins, R.J., 1977, Role of dietary calcium and calcium-binding protein in cadmium toxicity in rats, J. Nutr. 107:920-928.

Webb, M., 1979, The metallothioneins, in: "The Chemistry, Biochemistry and Biology of Cadmium", M. Webb, ed., pp. 195-266, Elsevier/North Holland, Amsterdam.

Webb, M. and Samarawickrama, G.P., 1981, Placental transport and embryonic utilization of essential metabolites in the rat at the teratogenic dose of cadmium, J. Appl. Toxicol. 1:270-277.

Webb, M. and Cain, K., 1982, Functions of metallothionein, Biochem. Pharmacol. 31:137-142.

Webb, M. and Holt, D., 1982, Endogenous metal binding proteins in relation to the differences in absorption and distribution of mercury in newborn and adult rats, Arch. Toxicol. 49:237-245.

Webster, W.S., 1979a, Iron deficiency and its role in cadmium-induced fetal growth retardation, J. Nutr. 109:1640-1645.

Webster, W.S., 1979b, Cadmium-induced fetal growth retardation in mice and the effect of dietary supplements of zinc, copper, iron and selenium, J. Nutr. 109:1646-1651.

White, I.G. and Holland, M.K., 1977, Aspects of the involvement of heavy metals in reproduction and fertility control, Inorgan. Perspect. Biol. Med. 1:137-172.

Williams, R.B., 1977, Trace elements and congenital abnormalities, Proc. Nutr. Soc. 36:25-32.

Wise, R.W., Ballard, F.J. and Ezekiel, E., 1963, Developmental changes in the plasma protein pattern of the rat, Comp. Biochem. Physiol. 9:23-30.

Wong, K-L. and Klaassen, C.D. 1980, Tissue distribution and retention of cadmium during postnatal development: minimal role of metallothionein, Toxicol. Appl. Pharmacol. 53:343-353.

THE CELLULAR ACCUMULATION AND SUBCELLULAR LOCALIZATION OF

METALLOTHIONEIN IN RAT LIVER DURING POSTNATAL DEVELOPMENT

M. George Cherian, M. Panemangalore and D. Banerjee

Department of Pathology, Health Sciences Centre
University of Western Ontario
London, Ontario, Canada

ABSTRACT

Metallothionein (MT), a low molecular weight, cysteine rich protein has been detected in high concentrations in livers of foetal and newborn mammals. This intracellular metalloprotein occurs bound mainly to zinc and copper in livers of newborn rats. In our study, the concentrations of both hepatic zinc and metallothionein remained high for the first 14 days after birth and then decreased rapidly to adult levels by 24 days of age in newborn rats. The ratio of metallothionein to zinc in liver also decreased with age, suggesting a rapid degradation of metallothionein during postnatal development.

The localization of metallothionein in rat liver during postnatal development was achieved by immunohistochemical technique of peroxidase-antiperoxidase using a specific anti-rat liver metallothionein serum. The results showed intense intranuclear staining for metallothionein in foetal and newborn rats which persisted until the 11th day after birth. The nuclear staining for metallothionein decreased with age; at 14 days, metallothionein was mainly localized in the cytoplasm and was similar to that observed in adult rat liver. The intranuclear localization of metallothionein in liver of foetal and newborn rats could be considered a typical foetal-neonatal morphological pattern and its subsequent presence in the cytoplasm, an adult pattern. Although metallothionein was localized exclusively in the cytoplasm in adult rat liver, the induction of metallothionein synthesis by injection of $ZnSO_4$ or $CdCl_2$ resulted in its movement into the nucleus of the hepatocytes. The presence of metallothionein in the nucleus of the cell could be indicative of active synthesis of metallothionein.

Despite the high basal levels of hepatic zinc and
metallothionein in 5-day-old rats, injection of ZnSO₄ (20 mg Zn/kg)
further induced the synthesis of metallothionein and increased the
accumulation of hepatic zinc and metallothionein, a response similar
to that in the adult rat. However, similar treatment with CdCl₂
(1 mg Cd/kg) resulted in displacement of zinc from metallothionein
and binding of cadmium to the pre-existing metallothionein wihout
any change in metallothionein synthesis. These results, along with
previous studies, suggest that metallothionein can serve as an
effective zinc storage protein during growth and development in
neonates and also after excessive exposure to zinc in newborn and
adult rats. Thus, metallothionein may function in zinc metabolism
in a manner similar to ferritin in iron metabolism. The immunohistochemical localization studies also support the view that
metallothionein is mainly an intracellular protein in normal cells
and it may have only a limited role in the transport of metals. The
synthesis of metallothionein may be directly influenced by the
cytoplasmic level of free thionein which could act as a repressor in
the induced synthesis of metallothionein.

INTRODUCTION

The biological role of metallothionein and its induced synthesis
in various tissues have attracted much attention in recent years
(Kagi and Nordberg, 1979; Foulkes, 1982a). Metallothionein is an
intracellular metalloprotein which binds various divalent metals,
both essential (Zn^{2+} and Cu^{2+}) and non-essential (Cd^{2+} and
Hg^{2+}). The presence of bound Zn^{2+} is a characteristic property
of this protein whether naturally occurring or induced by exposure
to other metals. Recent structural studies of metallothionein using
[113]Cd nuclear magnetic resonance spectroscopy (Briggs and Armitage,
1982) have identified two distinct metal clusters in metallothionein,
one of which may be a specific Zn^{2+} binding cluster. The high
concentration of Zn^{2+} and Cu^{2+} associated with metallothionein
in livers of term foetuses and newborn mammals has been reported
from various laboratories (Bremner et al., 1977; Bell, 1979; Wong
and Klaassen, 1979; Riordan and Richards, 1980; Mason et al., 1980).
Since all RNA and DNA polymerases and a number of other enzymes
contain tightly bound Zn^{2+}, the requirement for Zn^{2+} may well be
universal during postnatal development for catalysis of metabolic
processes, nucleic acid metabolism and protein biosynthesis. The
elevated levels of hepatic metallothionein in neonates may serve as
a storage protein for zinc and copper (Webb and Cain, 1982). The
rapid degradation of metallothionein in neonatal rats during
development also suggests the release of these metals for rapid
growth.

In this report, we will describe some of the recent work from
our laboratory on the changes in metallothionein levels and

subcellular localization of metallothionein in newborn rat liver. In addition, we will discuss the significance of these results in relation to the biosynthesis of metallothionein in adult rats and excessive exposure to metals in neonates.

HEPATIC LEVELS OF ZINC AND METALLOTHIONEIN IN POSTNATAL DEVELOPMENT

Elevated levels of zinc and copper have been reported in foetal and neonatal mammalian livers (Bergel et al., 1957; Porter, 1974; Kaszper et al., 1976; Terao and Owen, 1977). Recent studies showed that more than 50 percent of zinc in foetal liver was bound to metallothionein (Bremner et al., 1977; Hartmann and Weser, 1977; Bell, 1979; Wong and Klaassen, 1979; Riordan and Richards, 1980; Mason et al., 1980). A copper-binding metallothionein was also isolated from human foetal liver in the presence of reducing agents. Wong and Klaassen (1979) have demonstrated that the newborn rat liver metallothionein was similar to zinc-induced metallothionein in adult rat liver. Two types of metal clusters in calf liver metallothionein (a three-metal or a four-metal binding site), with marked specificity for Cu^{2+} and Zn^{2+} ion binding, have been identified recently by ^{113}Cd nuclear magnetic resonance spectroscopy (Briggs and Armitage, 1982). These were similar to the metal clusters in metallothionein, isolated from adult animals (Otvos and Armitage, 1980; Winge and Miklossy, 1982).

The changes in metallothionein levels during postnatal development in rat liver (Wong and Klaassen, 1979; Bell, 1979; Mason et al., 1980) and other mammalian species (Bakka and Webb, 1981) have also been reported recently. However, in most of these studies, metallothionein levels were reported as a zinc-bound fraction and not as concentration of the protein. Only in a few studies was the actual quantitation of metallothionein attempted (Wong and Klaassen, 1979; Bell, 1979). We have recently measured concentration of metallothionein (μg/g) in 11 different tissues in adult rat (Onosaka and Cherian, 1981) by a simple method (Cd-hem method) which is based on the saturation of metallothionein with Cd^{2+} and the removal of the excess free Cd^{2+} and other cadmium-binding proteins with rat hemoglobin and heat treatment (Onosaka et al., 1978). The testis of adult rat contained the highest basal metallothionein level of all the tissues studied. There was also a good correlation between metallothionein measurements by Cd-hem method and polarographic analysis (Onosaka and Cherian, 1982b) in rat liver and kidney. This method has enabled us to measure and compare the induction pattern of metallothionein synthesis in various organs of the adult rat after exposure to Cd^{2+} and Zn^{2+} salts. In a recent study (Panemangalore et al., personal communication), the concentration of metallothionein in rat liver and kidney during postnatal development was measured by the Cd-hem method and compared to the hepatic zinc concentration. The results are shown in Table 1.

Newborn rats were sacrificed on day 1, 2, 5, 9, 14, 19, 25 or 31 after birth and livers were removed for analysis of zinc and metallothionein.

The highest concentrations of metallothionein (1150 µg/g) and zinc (98 µg/g) were observed in rat liver within 24 hours after birth and remained almost constant for the first five days. After this initial period, the concentration of both zinc and metallothionein decreased slowly until the 14th day and then declined more rapidly to reach near adult level by 25 days. The data showed that the total hepatic zinc content increased gradually with age, while the total metallothionein content in liver was unaltered until the 14th day and then decreased rapidly. These results confirm the studies of Mason et al. (1980) which showed that the decrease in hepatic zinc concentration in newborn rats was essentially due to an increase in liver weight until the 16th day. It is also interesting to note for our results that, although the ratio of metallothionein to zinc concentration declined with age, a high ratio was maintained up to 14 days of age. After this period, the ratio decreased rapidly to day 25 when metallothionein concentration reached the adult level.

Further comparison of zinc and metallothionein concentrations in the livers of developing neonatal rats by multiple regression analysis indicated a direct linear relationship (Figure 1). The

Table 1   Concentrations of Zinc and Metallothionein in Rat Livers During Postnatal Development[a]

Age (days)	Number Rats	Zinc µg/g[c]	Metallothionein[b] µg/g[c]	Metallothionein: Zinc Ratio
1	(9)	98.8 + 5.3	1159.0 + 86.3	11.8 + 0.5
2	(9)	73.0 ∓ 3.7	906.4 ∓ 67.3	12.3 ∓ 0.5
5	(7)	103.0 ∓ 2.9	902.1 ∓ 49.1	8.9 ∓ 0.5
9	(6)	72.8 ∓ 3.1	728.0 ∓ 70.2	9.9 ∓ 0.7
14	(5)	54.2 ∓ 2.1	497.2 ∓ 14.8	9.2 ∓ 0.3
19	(6)	33.9 ∓ 2.9	162.4 ∓ 35.5	4.6 ∓ 0.8
25	(6)	39.8 ∓ 0.9	33.5 ∓ 4.1	1.1 ∓ 0.1
31	(6)	28.8 ∓ 1.8	27.3 ∓ 1.2	0.9 ∓ 0.1

[a]Data from Panemangalore et al. (personal communication).
[b]Measured by Cd-hem method described in Onosaka and Cherian (1981).
[c]Values are mean ± S.E.

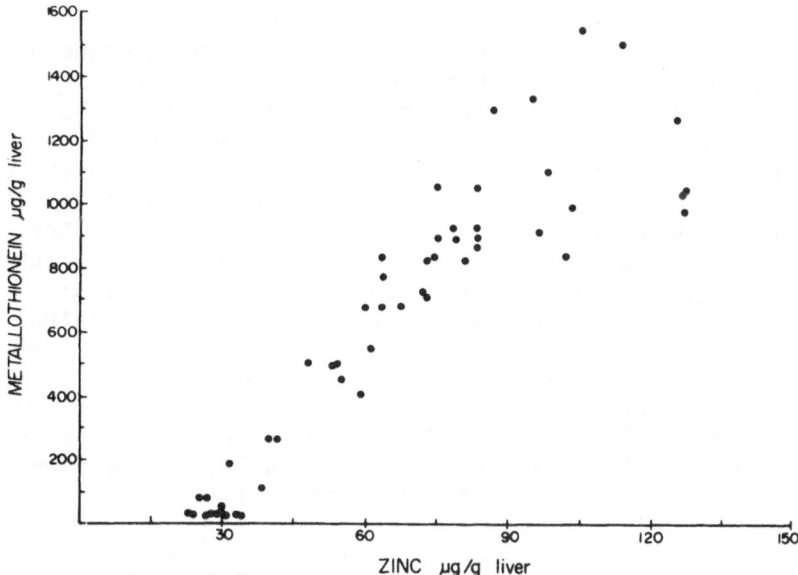

Figure 1   Relationship between hepatic concentrations of zinc and
metallothionein in newborn rats (from Panemangalore et al.,
personal communication). Rats were sacrificed on 1, 2, 5,
9, 14, 19, 25 or 31 days after birth and concentrations of
zinc and metallothionein in liver were measured (see Table
1). A positive linear relationship was obtained between
hepatic zinc and metallothionein levels. The regression
equations showed metallothionein = 13.6 (Zn)-286. The
correlation coefficient of the regression line was 0.85
and was statistically significant (p<0.001).

slope of the regression line was 13.58. We reported a similar type
of relationship (slope 14.6) in adult rat liver after injection of
increasing doses of $ZnSO_4$ (Onosaka and Cherian, 1982a).
Therefore, both in adult rat after excessive exposure to zinc salts
and in newborn rat with naturally-occurring high levels of zinc, the
concentration of hepatic metallothionein was directly related to the
zinc content of the liver. However, a certain threshold tissue zinc
level was required for induction and deposition of metallothionein.
This was about 25 to 30 µg/g in liver as shown in Figure 1.

These results suggest that metallothionein can act as a
temporary reservoir for hepatic zinc or serve as an effective
storage protein for zinc during growth and development in neonates.
The biological role of metallothionein thus seems analogous to that
of ferritin in iron metabolism. It should be mentioned that
ferritin was also found in high concentration in livers of foetal

and newborn mammals (Linder et al., 1972; Linder and Munro, 1972). In addition, both ferritin (Redman, 1969) and metallothionein (Shapiro and Cousins, 1980; Cherian et al., 1981) were preferentially synthesized on the free polysomes rather than on membrane-bound polysomes in rat liver. Thus, the site of metallothionein biosynthesis in rat liver was also indicative of a non-secretory, intracellular nature of this protein with little role in transport of metals. It is not clearly understood whether metallothionein has any direct role in the homeostasis of zinc or copper. Although such a role has been postulated for metallothionein to act as a resistor in the movement of zinc across intestinal epithelium and in the control of zinc absorption (Richards and Cousins, 1975), it is unlikely that metallothionein can directly influence the transport of metals across the cellular membrane (Foulkes, 1982b; Jackson et al., 1981). However, the presence of metallothionein in the cell could markedly influence the form of metals after they were transported into the cell.

LOCALIZATION OF HEPATIC METALLOTHIONEIN IN NEWBORN RATS

The intracellular distribution of metallothionein by biochemical techniques suggests that it is mainly a cytoplasmic protein (Kägi and Nordberg, 1979). The immunochemical localization of this protein has been difficult because of its poor antigenicity. A previous report (Kojima and Hamashima, 1978), using immuno-fluorescent techniques, also suggests that it may be localized in the cytoplasm in tissues from adult mammals. Thus, the localization of metallothionein by both these methods is identical in adult mammals. We have recently localized metallothionein in livers and kidneys of rats by an immunoperoxidase-antiperoxidase method (Banerjee et al., 1982).

The immunohistochemical technique of peroxidase-antiperoxidase is about 1000 times more sensitive than the immunofluorescent method (Sternberger, 1979) and can be described as follows. Tissues are first fixed in 10 percent buffered formalin and embedded in paraffin. Five-micron sections are deparaffinized and used for metallothionein localization. They are first incubated with normal swine serum to reduce nonspecific staining and then incubated with normal rabbit serum or rabbit anti-rat-metallothionein serum diluted 1:100 in phosphate buffered saline. These sections are further incubated in sequence with swine anti-rabbit IgG (Immunoglobulin G), peroxidase-rabbit antiperoxidase antibody complex and DAB(3,3'-diaminobenzidine) in the presence of hydrogen peroxide. The immunohistochemical reaction using rabbit anti-metallothionein serum showed specific staining for metallothionein since none of the negative control procedures gave any staining. The absorption of rabbit anti-metallothionein with added rat liver metallothionein abolished all staining and the use of normal rabbit serum in place of antiserum did not produce any staining. Also, no staining was observed when the primary antiserum (anti-metallothionein) was omitted from the procedure. Thus, this immunohistochemical technique provided a sensitive method to localize metallothionein specifically in tissue sections.

In a recent study, (Banerjee et al., 1982), using this unlabelled peroxidase-antiperoxidase immunohistochemical technique (Sternberger, 1979) with a rabbit antibody specific to rat liver metallothionein, we were able to identify the intracellular localization of metallothionein in the livers of control and cadmium chloride-injected adult rats. This has provided new information concerning the distribution of metallothionein within liver and kidney cells. In control rats, metallothionein was mainly localized in the cytoplasm of hepatocytes, renal collecting duct epithelium and distal convoluted tubular epithelium. In rats injected with cadmium chloride, metallothionein was initially present in the nuclei which were largely negative in control rats. However, metallothionein was subsequently localized both in nuclei and cytoplasm in renal and hepatic cells of rats repeatedly injected with cadmium chloride.

The significance of the presence of metallothionein in the cytoplasm in control rats and its localization in both the nucleus and cytoplasm following induced synthesis of metallothionein by injection of metal salts is not yet clear. Since the newborn rats contained a high concentration of metallothionein in liver and as it was rapidly degraded during postnatal development, this model provided us with an interesting system to study the localization of metallothionein and its cellular developmental changes. Recent reports by Mason et al. (1980) suggested that the zinc concentration of the particulate fraction of newborn rat liver decreased with age and was consistent with a decrease in hepatic zinc concentration. However, no estimation of zinc bound to metallothionein in the particulate fraction was reported. Since metallothionein is a low molecular weight protein, it may be difficult to prevent its leakage from cell organelles to the cytoplasm during biochemical isolation. Therefore, immunohistochemical localization of metallothionein may be more reliable than biochemical subcellular fractionation.

The localization of metallothionein in livers of rats during postnatal development by immunohistochemical technique showed intense staining for metallothionein in the nuclei of hepatocytes in newborn rats, two to five days of age (Panemangalore et al., personal communication). There was little cytoplasmic staining in the livers of newborn rats. The nuclear staining for metallothionein decreased with age (Figures 2 A-D) and on the 9th day after birth, metallothionein was localized both in nucleus and cytoplasm. The pattern of staining for metallothionein changed rapidly thereafter, and by day 14, localization of metallothionein was mainly in the cytoplasm. A similar cytoplasmic staining of less intensity was also observed in rat liver on the 25th day of age (Figure 3). Further studies showed that the cytoplasmic staining for metallothionein with little nuclear staining persisted in rat liver during later growth. Thus, the presence of metallothionein in the cytoplasm of hepatocytes was an adult distribution pattern for metallothionein while its nuclear localization could be considered a typical foetal-neonatal distribution pattern. The biological significance of the presence of metallothionein in the nucleus of hepatocytes in foetal and newborn rats and its subsequent redistribution to the cytoplasm with age is intriguing and requires further investigation.

The biological and toxicological implications of nuclear cytoplasmic interactions of metals are poorly understood and have been reviewed (Bryan, 1981). In our previous study (Banerjee et al., 1982), the induction of metallothionein synthesis in adult rats resulted in the nuclear localization of metallothionein in liver, a distribution pattern similar to that in foetal-neonatal rat liver. Thus, the presence of metallothionein in the nucleus of the cell seems to indicate an increased synthesis of metallothionein.

INDUCED SYNTHESIS OF METALLOTHIONEIN IN ADULT RAT

Although the recent findings using cDNA probe and genomic clones have clearly shown specific inducible mRNA for metallothionein, the exact role of metals in the induced synthesis of metallothionein is unclear (Ohi et al., 1981). In addition to metals, metallothionein synthesis can also be induced in rat liver by starvation and various other stress conditions (Oh et al., 1978). However, Klaassen (1981) has shown that the injection of adrenocortical steroids and other stress conditions can increase the concentration of metallothionein in hamster liver by only 50 to 80 percent while injection of Zn^{2+} or Cd^{2+} can increase the metallothionein level by 700 to 2,000 percent. Thus, there is a definite difference in the magnitude of induction of metallothionein synthesis by metals and stressful conditions.

The induction of hepatic metallothionein synthesis has been reported in a number of species on exposure to high amounts of zinc salts (Webb, 1972; Bremner and Marshall, 1974). However, the data

Figure 2 A, B Localization of metallothionein in newborn rat liver by unlabelled peroxidase-antiperoxidase (PAP) method. Intense intranuclear staining for metallothionein in both liver sections 400 x. 2A 3-day-old; 2B 5-day-old.

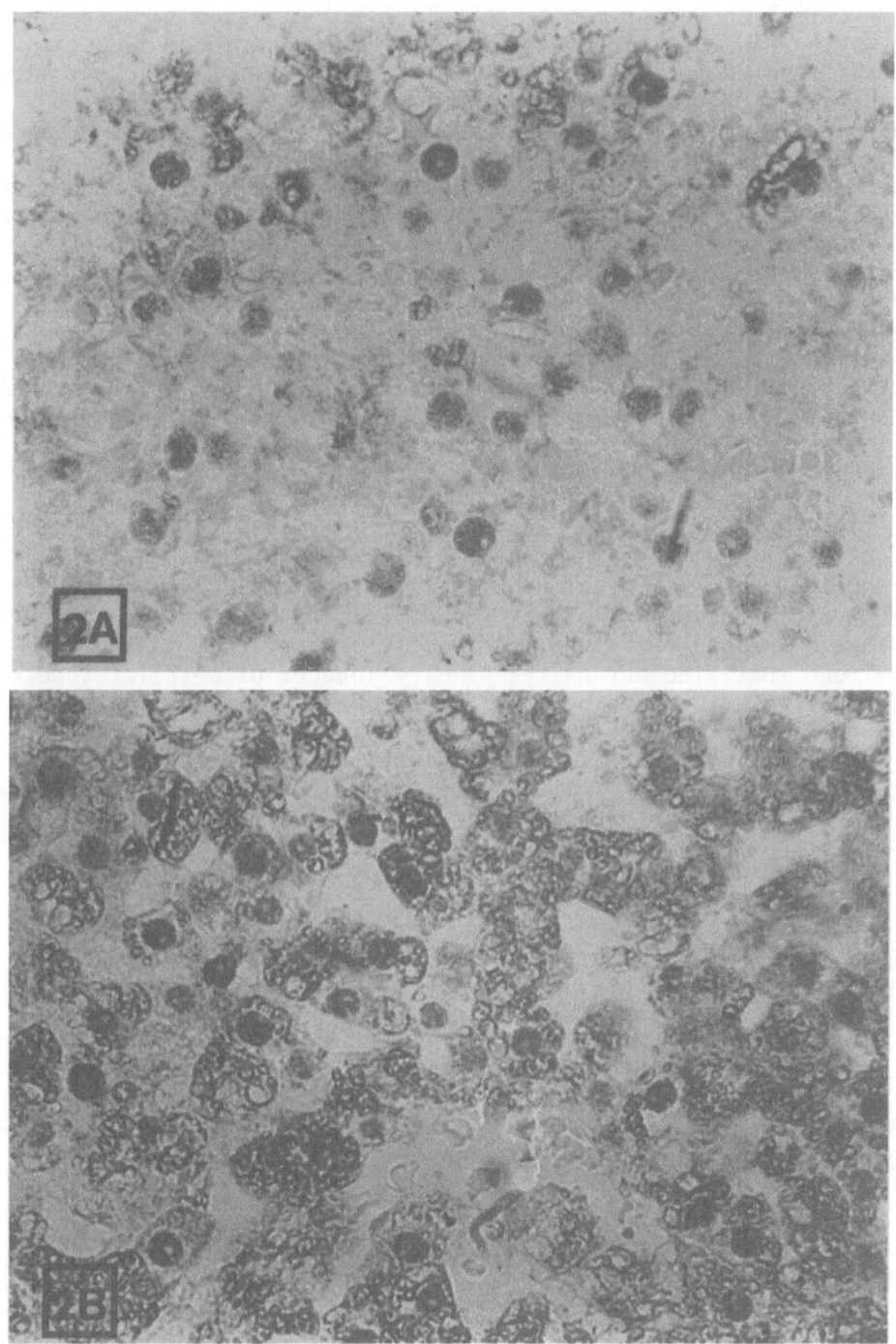

on the quantitation of metallothionein levels in various tissues
from control and experimental animals after exposure to metals are
limited. This information is essential to compare the induction and
deposition of metallothionein in various organs. In a recent study
(Onosaka and Cherian, 1982a), we measured metallothionein
concentrations in 11 tissues of rats injected with various doses of
$ZnSO_4$ and demonstrated an increase in metallothionein levels in
pancreas, liver, small intestine and kidney with similar induction
capacity in all four organs. A direct positive correlation between
the deposition of zinc and metallothionein in each tissue was
observed, even though the tissue metallothionein levels were
different. The slope of the regression equation between hepatic
zinc and metallothionein concentrations could provide the apparent
capacity of liver to induce metallothionein synthesis in response to
zinc deposition. These values were very similar for liver in adult
rats injected with $ZnSO_4$ (Onosaka and Cherian, 1982a) and during
postnatal development in newborn rats (Panemangalore et al.,
personal communication).

They can be expressed as follows: metallothionein (μg/g liver)
= a(Zn μg/g)+b. Thus, in adult rat metallothionein = 14.6(Zn) - 363
and during postnatal development metallothionein = 13.6(Zn) - 282.
These results demonstrate that the deposition of metallothionein in
adult and newborn rat liver is directly proportional to the zinc
level and that zinc may be the primary inducer of metallothionein.
The re-utilization of zinc from injected zinc-metallothionein has
also been shown in vivo in rats (Cherian, 1977). Moreover, the zinc
in zinc-metallothionein was metabolically as active as zinc salts
after administration to rats. Thus, metallothionein can effectively
function as a zinc storage protein in the liver after excessive
exposure to zinc salts in adult rats and in neonates with high
hepatic zinc content.

A new model has been proposed for the induced synthesis of
metallothionein by metals, based on recent results from our
laboratory on the localization of metallothionein under various
experimental conditions (see above).

Preliminary studies (Banerjee et al., 1982) on the localization
of metallothionein in tissue sections by immunohistochemical methods
provided, for the first time, evidence that metallothionein may be
present in cell nuclei and not just within the cytoplasm. The

Figure 2 C, D Localization of metallothionein in newborn rat liver
               by PAP method 400 x. 2C 11-day-old - both nuclear
               and cytoplasmic staining for metallothionein; 2D
               14-day-old - mainly cytoplasmic staining with little
               metallothionein in the nucleus.

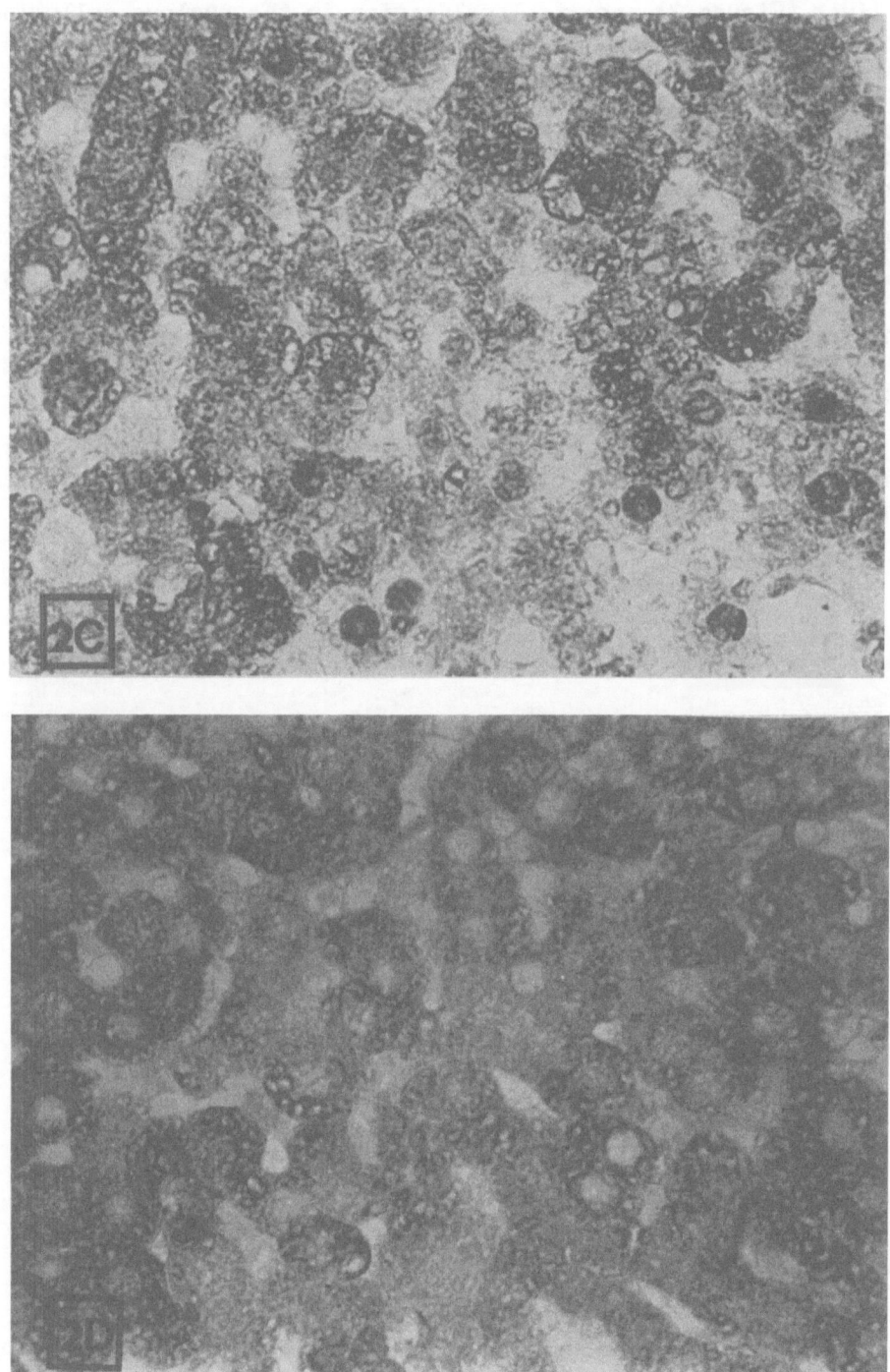

presence of metallothionein exclusively in the cytoplasm in control
rat liver (Figure 3) and its localization in the nucleus following
injection of metals and also in foetal-newborn tissue (Figures 2A -
C) are indications of a unique regulation where the protein
(thionein) in the cytoplasm could exert a post-transcriptional
control on the inhibition or destabilization of its own mRNA. We
postulate that the small amount of metal-free thionein in cytoplasm
of adult rat hepatocytes could inhibit thionein mRNA translation and
thus prevent further synthesis of thionein. On exposure to metals
(Zn^{2+} or Cd^{2+}), the free thionein in the cytoplasm would bind to
metals and enter the nucleus to bind to nuclear components. This
could then result in increased synthesis of thionein mRNA and
thionein. Thus, transcriptional control may be the main factor
during induced synthesis of metallothionein by metals (Richards and
Cousins, 1975; Ohi et al., 1981). With repeated exposure to Zn^{2+}
or Cd^{2+}, the newly synthesized thionein could bind to metals and
accumulate in the cytoplasm and nucleus as metallothionein. As long
as excess metal was available for binding to thionein, there could
be no accumulation of free thionein, and therefore no inhibition of

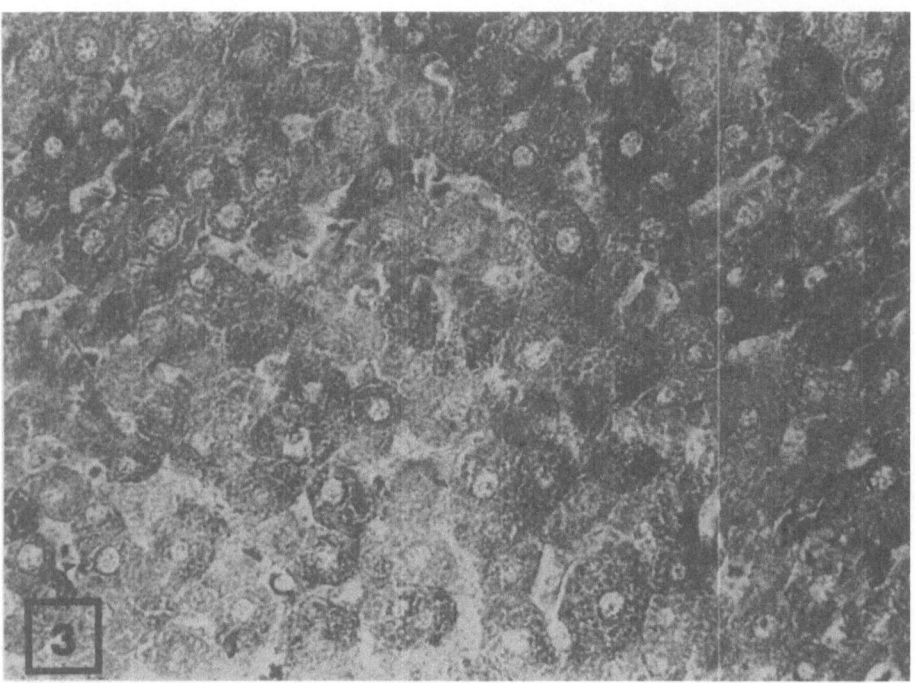

Figure 3   Localization of metallothionein in adult rat liver by PAP
           method.   Cytoplasmic staining for metallothionein and no
           nuclear staining.   400 x

thionein mRNA was possible. This may be a unique regulation where the level of free thionein in the cytoplasm can act as a repressor for its own synthesis. In this model, the cells could actively synthesize thionein until an excess of free thionein accumulated, resulting in inhibition of thionein mRNA and metallothionein synthesis. Experiments are under way to explore this hypothesis. Although this is an attractive model for the control of metallothionein synthesis, no free thionein has been isolated from the cell so far.

INDUCTION OF METALLOTHIONEIN SYNTHESIS IN NEONATES

The administration of large doses of cadmium salts to pregnant animals can cause lethal toxic effects in foetuses because of placental damage rather than by direct effect on the foetus (Parizek, 1964; Levin and Miller, 1980). However, even at low doses, a portion of cadmium injected to the pregnant rat was incorporated to the foetal liver metallothionein (Kelman et al., 1979). Different effects on foetal metallothionein were observed in pregnant rats and rabbits when they were exposed to cadmium salts. The maternal cadmium administration resulted in a decrease of foetal hepatic metallothionein level in rats (Waalkes and Bell, 1980; Sasser, et al., 1981) while an increase of foetal hepatic metallothionein level was observed in rabbits (Waalkes et al., 1982). Bakka et al. (1981) also reported reduced hepatic metallothionein levels in neonates when pregnant rats were injected with cadmium chloride. The toxicological implications of the alterations in maternal-placental functions and changes in foetal metallothionein level on maternal exposure to nonessential metals such as cadmium during gestational period are not yet understood.

The discussions in the preceding sections of this article support the hypothesis that one of the major biological roles of metallothionein may be to function as a hepatic storage protein for Zn^{2+} and Cu^{2+} during growth and development in mammalian neonates. However, little is known on the detoxification of toxic metals (Cd^{2+} or Hg^{2+}) by metallothionein in neonates, although the role of metallothionein in the metabolism of cadmium in adult animals is more defined (Webb, 1972; Sabbioni and Marafante, 1975; Cherian and Goyer, 1978; Panemangalore and Brady, 1978). The recent reports from Klaassen's laboratory (Klaassen and Wong, 1982) suggested that the high hepatic concentration of metallothionein in neonates neither decreased the toxicity of cadmium nor markedly increased the hepatic distribution of cadmium. Chronic cadmium administration in newborn rats produced tissue damage similar to that in adult rats (Wong et al., 1980). The hepatic metallothionein levels in 5-day-old rats were altered only after injection of high doses of cadmium (6 mg Cd/kg). At lower doses, the injected cadmium could bind with preexisting metallothionein by displacing zinc in a dose-dependent manner (Bell, 1979). However, the dose of cadmium (6 mg Cd/kg) required for induction of metallothionein synthesis in newborns in this study was more than the LD_{50} value.

We have recently studied the metabolism of parenterally-administered zinc and cadmium in newborn rats (Panemangalore and Cherian, 1982). A single subcutaneous injection of Zn^{2+} (20 mg Zn/kg) along with either $^{65}ZnSO_4$ or ^{35}S-cysteine increased the liver zinc concentration of 5-day-old rats within 24 hours. This increase in hepatic zinc level was accompanied by a concomitant elevation of metallothionein concentration (Table 2). The de novo synthesis of metallothionein was indicated by a significant increase in ^{35}S-cysteine incorporation into the protein as compared to ^{35}S-cysteine incorporated into metallothionein of the saline-injected controls. Also, more than 50 percent of the cytosolic zinc was associated with metallothionein in livers of 5-day-old rats. The single injection of zinc also increased the incorporation of zinc into metallothionein by 146 percent to that of the control.

Table 2   Hepatic Zinc and Metallothionein in Livers of 5-Day-Old Rats After Injection with $CdCl_2$ and $ZnSO_4$[a]

Treatment[b]	Zinc µg/g[c]	Metallothionein µg/g[c]
Saline (control)	106.18 + 10.39	804.1 + 108.4
Saline + ^{35}S-cys	104.56 ∓ 3.65	798.6 ∓ 76.7
Zn + ^{65}Zn	196.38 ∓ 8.77[d]	1579.9 ∓ 72.7[d]
Zn + ^{35}S-cys	165.61 ∓ 8.06[d]	1437.2 ∓ 36.5[d]
Cd + ^{109}Cd	125.03 ∓ 3.74	739.1 ∓ 35.7
Cd + ^{35}S-cys	105.51 ∓ 6.37	795.6 ∓ 61.3

[a]Adapted from Panemangalore and Cherian (1982).
[b]Rats were injected subcutaneously with: 0.1 ml of saline (control); Zn: 20 mg/kg as $AnSO_4$ or $^{65}ZnSO_4$ (2.5 µCi); Cd: 1 mg/kg as $CdCl_2$ or $^{109}CdCl_2$ (2.5 µCi) with or without ^{35}S-cysteine (5 µCi). Rats were sacrificed 24 hours later and metallothionein was estimated by the method of Onosaka et al. (1978).
[c]Values are mean ± S.E.
[d]Significantly different from others in the same column (p < 0.001).

In contrast, a single subcutaneous injection of Cd^{2+} (1 mg Cd/kg) did not produce any of the dramatic changes in the liver which were observed after zinc administration; however, the dose of zinc was 34 times that of cadmium, on a molar basis. In addition, more importantly, we found that all the cadmium in the liver cytosol was bound to pre-existing metallothionein by displacement of zinc. Cadmium was essentially distributed between the nuclei and the cytosol in the liver, about 20 percent and 80 percent, respectively. No changes in hepatic zinc and metallothionein concentration were observed.

The distribution of copper in the cytosol, metallothionein and particulate fractions remained unaltered by either zinc or cadmium administration. This may be due to the higher affinity of copper than cadmium or zinc to metallothionein. We also found that the renal zinc, copper and metallothionein were unaffected by either zinc or cadmium treatment in neonate rats.

In conclusion, our findings indicate that livers of newborn rats respond to zinc administration by induction and synthesis of metallothionein despite the high concentration of preexisting metallothionein; that the synthesis and deposition of zinc in metallothionein are directly related to the concentration of zinc in the liver, thus reaffirming the role of metallothionein in zinc storage during growth and development. It is not clear whether metallothionein could be involved in detoxification of cadmium or other nonessential metals in neonates, even though administered cadmium was sequestered exclusively by hepatic metallothionein.

REFERENCES

Bakka, A. and Webb, M., 1981, Metabolism of zinc and copper in the neonate: changes in the concentrations and contents of thionein bound zinc and copper with age in the livers of newborn of various mammalian species, Biochem. Pharm. 30:721-275.

Bakka, A., Samarawickrama, G.P. and Webb, M., 1981, Metabolism of zinc and copper in the neonate, Chem-Biol. Interact. 34:161-171.

Banerjee, D., Onosaka, S. and Cherian, M.G., 1982, Immunohistochemical localization of metallothionein in cell nucleus and cytoplasm of rat liver and kidney, Toxicology 24(2):95-105.

Bell, J.U., 1979, Native metallothionein levels in rat hepatic cytosol during perinatal development, Toxicol. Appl. Pharm. 50:101-107.

Bell, J.U. and Waalkes, M.P., 1982, Role of hepatic metallothionein during perinatal development in the rat, in: "Biological Roles of Metallothionein", E.C. Foulkes, ed., p. 99, Elsevier/North Holland, Amsterdam.

Bergel, F., Everett, A.J.L., Martin, J.B. and Webb, J.S., 1957, Cellular constitutents, major and minor metals in normal and abnormal tissues, J. Pharm. 9:522-531.

Bremner, I. and Marshall, R.B., 1974, Hepatic copper and zinc binding proteins in ruminants. I. Distribution of Cu and Zn among soluble proteins of liver of varying Cu and Zn content, Br. J. Nutr. 32:283-291.

Bremner, I., Williams, R.B. and Young, B.W., 1977, Distribution of copper and zinc in the liver of the developing sheep foetus, Brit. J. Nutr. 38:87-92.

Briggs, R.W. and Armitage, I.M., 1982, Evidence for site selective metal binding in calf liver metallothionein, J. Biol. Chem. 257:1259-1262.

Bryan, S.E., 1981, Heavy metals in the cells nucleus, in: "Metal Ions in Genetic Information Transfer", G.L. Eichorn and L. Marzilli, eds., p. 87-101, Elsevier/North Holland, Amsterdam.

Cherian, M.G., 1977, Studies on synthesis and metabolism of zinc-thionein in rats, J. Nutr. 107:965-972.

Cherian, M.G. and Goyer, R.A., 1978, Metallothioneins and their role in the metabolism and toxicity of metals, Life Sci. 23:1-10.

Cherian, M.G., Yu, S. and Redman, C.M., 1981, Site of synthesis of metallothionein in rat liver, Can. J. Biochem. 59:301-306.

Foulkes, E.C., 1982a, ed., "Biological Roles of Metallothionein", Elsevier/North Holland, Amsterdam.

Foulkes, E.C., 1982b, Role of metallothionein in the transport of heavy metals, in: "Biological Roles of Metallothionein", E.C. Foulkes, ed., p. 131-140, Elsevier/North Holland, Amsterdam.

Hartmann, J-J. and Weser, U., 1977, Copper-thionein from fetal bovine liver, Biochem. Biophys. Acta. 491:211-222.

Jackson, M.J., Jones, D.A. and Edwards, T.H., 1981, Zinc absorption in the rat, Br. J. Nutr. 46:15-27.

Kägi, J.H.R., and Nordberg, M., 1979, "Metallothionein", Birkhäuser Verlag, Basel.

Kaszper, B.W., Piotrowski, J.K., Marciniak, W. and Sielcznska, M., 1979, Comparative study of the level of metallothionein-like proteins, cadmium and zinc in the livers and kidneys of rats, Bromat. Chem. Toksykol. 9:315-326.

Kelman, B.J., Ozga, J.A., Walter, B.K. and Sasser, L.D., 1979, Cadmium-binding in the pregnant and fetal rat, Toxicol. Lett. 4:135.

Klaassen, C.D., 1981, Induction of metallothionein by adrenocortical steroids, Toxicology 20:275-279.

Klaassen, C.D. and Wong, K-L., 1982, Minimal role of the high concentration of hepatic metallothionein in the newborn rat in the toxicity, distribution and excretion of cadmium, in: "Biological Roles of Metallothionein", E.C., Foulkes, ed., p. 113-130, Elsevier/North Holland, Amsterdam.

Kojima, Y. and Hamashima, Y., 1978, Immunohistological study of equine renal metallothionein, Acta. Histochem. Cytochem. 11:205-211.

Levin, A.A. and Miller, R. K., 1980, Fetal toxicity of cadmium in the rat: Maternal vs. fetal injections, Teratology 22:1-6.

Linder, M.C., Moor, J.R., Scott, L.E. and Munro, H.N., 1972, Pre- and postnatal changes in content and species of ferritin in rat liver, Biochem. J. 129:455-462.

Linder, M.C. and Munro, H.N., 1972, Iron and copper metabolism in development, Enzyme 15:111-138.

Masón, R., Bakka, A., Samarawickrama, G.P. and Webb, M., 1980, Metabolism of zinc and copper in the neonate: accumulation and function of (Zn-Cu) metallothionein in the liver of newborn rat, Brit. J. Nutr. 45:375-389.

Oh, S.H., Deagen, J.T., Whanger, P.D. and Wesweig, P.H., 1978, Induction of metallothionein by various stresses, Am. J. Physiol. 234:E282-E285.

Ohi, S., Cardenosa, G., Pine, R. and Huang, P.C., 1981, Cadmium induced accumulation of metallothionein mRNA in rat liver. J. Biol. Chem. 256:2180-2184.

Onosaka, S. and Cherian, M.G., 1981, The induced synthesis of metallothionein in various tissues of rat in response to metals. I. Effect of repeated injection of cadmium salts, Toxicol. 22:91-101.

Onosaka, S. and Cherian, M.G., 1982a, The induced synthesis of metallothionein in various tissues of rat in response to metals. II. Influence of zinc status and specific effect on pancreatic metallothionein, Toxicol. 23:11-20.

Onosaka, S. and Cherian, M.G., 1982b, Comparison of metallothionein determination by polarographic and cadmium saturation methods, J. Toxicol. Appl. Pharm. 63:270-274.

Onosaka, S., Tanaka, D., Dio, M. and Okahara, K., 1978, A simplified procedure for determination of metallothionein in animal tissues, Eisei Kagaku 24:128-133.

Otvos, J.D. and Armitage, I.M., 1980, Structure of metal clusters in rabbit liver metallothionein, Proc. Natl. Acad. Sci., U.S.A. 77:7094-7098.

Panemangalore, M. and Brady, F.O., 1978, Induction and synthesis of metallothionein in isolated perfused rat livers, J. Biol. Chem. 253:7898-7904.

Panemangalore, M. and Cherian, M.G., 1982, Interaction of injected zinc and cadmium with hepatic metallothionein in newborn rats, Fed. Proc. Abstr. 41:2180.

Parizek, J., 1964, Vascular changes at sites of oestrogen biosynthesis produced by parenteral injection of cadmium salts, J. Reprod. Fertil. 7:263-265.

Porter, H., 1974, The particulate half cysteine rich copper protein of newborn liver. Relationship to metallothionein and subcellular localization in non-mitochondrial particles possibly representing heavy lysosomes, Biochem. Biophys. Res. Commun. 56:661-668.

Redman, C.M., 1969, Biosynthesis of serum proteins and ferritin by free and attached ribosomes of rat liver, J. Biol. Chem. 244:4308-4315.

Richards, M.P. and Cousins, R.J., 1975, Influence of parenteral Zn and actinomycin D on tissue Zn uptake and synthesis of a Zn binding protein, Bioinorg. Chem. 4:215-224.

Riordan, J.R. and Richards, V., 1980, Human fetal liver contains both zinc and copper rich forms of metallothionein, J. Biol. Chem. 255:5380-5383.

Sabbioni, E. and Marafante, E., 1975, Heavy metals in rat liver cadmium binding protein, Environ. Physiol. Biochem. 5:132-141.

Sasser, L.B., Charles-Shannon, V.L., Berquist, B.D. and Kelman, B.J., 1981, The effect of zinc and cadmium on hepatic metallothionein in the fetal rat, Toxicologist 1:30.

Shapiro, S.G. and Cousins, R.J., 1980, Induction of metallothionein mRNA and its distribution between free and membrane bound polyribosomes, Biochem. J. 190:755-765.

Sternberger, L.A., 1979, "Immunohistochemistry", p. 104, John Wiley and Sons, New York.

Terao, T. and Owen, C.A., 1977, Copper metabolism in pregnant and postpartum rat pups, Am. J. Physiol. 232:E170-E179.

Waalkes, M.P. and Bell, J.U., 1980, Depression of metallothionein in fetal rat liver following maternal cadmium exposure, Toxicol. 18:103-110.

Waalkes, M.P., Thomas, J.A. and Bell, J.U., 1982, Induction of hepatic metallothionein in the rabbit fetus following maternal cadmium exposure, Toxicol. Appl. Pharm. 62:211.

Webb, M., 1972, Protection by zinc against cadmium toxicity, Biochem. Pharm. 21:2767-2771.

Webb, M. and Cain, K., 1982, Functions of metallothionein, Biochem. Pharm. 31:137.

Winge, D.R. and Miklossy, K.A., 1982, Domain nature of metallothionein, J. Biol. Chem. 257:3471-3476.

Wong, K-L. and Klaassen, C.D., 1979, Isolation and characterization of metallothionein which is highly concentrated in the newborn rat liver, J. Biol. Chem. 254:12399-12403.

Wong, K-L., Cachia, R. and Klaassen, C.D., 1980, Comparison of the toxicity and tissue distribution of cadmium in newborn and adult rats after repeated administration, Toxicol. Appl. Pharm. 56:317-325.

METHYLMERCURY METABOLISM IN PREGNANT MICE: ITS MODIFICATION BY
SELENIUM WITH PARTICULAR REFERENCE TO PRENATAL TOXICITY OF THESE
COMPOUNDS

Tsuguyoshi Suzuki

Department of Human Ecology
University of Tokyo
Tokyo, Japan

ABSTRACT

Since selenium protection against methylmercury embryotoxicity
and teratogenicity is variable according to the dose-combinations of
both chemicals, modification of methylmercury metabolism by selenium
in pregnant mice has been reviewed.

The effect of selenite on the placental transfer and fetal
accumulation of methylmercury is not considered to be the
explanation for the modification of toxicity, while the fetal
accumulation of selenium is enhanced by administration of
methylmercury.

From these modifications by selenite of the dose-response
relationships for methylmercury, an additive (or synergistic)
influence by selenite on the embryo- and fetolethal effect of
methylmercury is proposed. These relationships were observed for
mercury concentrations on maternal blood and amniotic fluid versus
the total embryonic and fetal death rate, and the toxicity of
selenite itself in the fetoplacental complex.

INTRODUCTION

Embryotoxicity and teratogenicity, including behavioral
aberrations of methylmercury have been well documented in various
animal species (Ramel, 1967; Matsumoto et al., 1967; Moriyama, 1967;
Inoue et al., 1972; Casterline and Williams, 1972; Nolen et al.,
1972a,b; Harris et al., 1972; Spyker and Smithberg, 1972; Spyker et
al., 1972; Khera and Tabacova, 1973; Scharpf et al., 1973; Ware et

693

al., 1974; Mottet, 1974; Chang and Sprecher, 1976; Su and Okita, 1976a,b; Snell et al., 1977; Musch et al., 1978; Olson and Massaro, 1977, 1980; Fuyuta et al., 1978, 1979; Robins et al., 1978; Fujimoto et al., 1979; Bornhausen et al., 1980; Cortese et al., 1980). Humans exposed to methylmercury during the fetal stage were also noted to have various neurological abnormalities after birth (Engelson and Herner, 1952; Harada, 1968, 1978; Snyder, 1971; Bakir et al., 1973; Amin-Zaki et al., 1974, 1976, 1979; Choi et al., 1978; Marsh et al., 1980; Snyder and Seelinger, 1976; Brenner and Snyder, 1980). Although protective effects of selenium compounds against the toxicity of methylmercury had been extensively described before the mid-1970s in experimental animals (Ganther et al., 1972; Iwata et al., 1973; Johnson and Pond, 1974; Potter and Matrone, 1974; Stilling et al., 1974; Stoewsand et al., 1974; Ohi et al., 1975a,b, 1976), little was known regarding the effect of selenium on the embryotoxicity and teratogenicity of methylmercury. Our previous report was the first to deal with this topic (Nobunaga et al., 1979); it revealed variability in selenium protection against methylmercury toxicity, in contrast with the uniform protection noted in adult animals. The teratogenic effect of methylmercury appeared to be either augmented or reduced according to the amount of selenite added in relation to the dose of methylmercury (Figure 1). Similar observations were reported in the same year in experiments using a different strain of mice and a different route of administration (Lee et al., 1979). In both studies, selenite treatment alone caused changes in the fetal weight without being accompanied by gross malformations. These findings contradict the large body of evidence indicating that selenium uniformly reduces methylmercury toxicity (Calabrese, 1981). Therefore, our efforts have centered on resolution of this issue.

As reviewed in Table 1, the mode of embryonic nutrition differs with the period of gestation in mice; accordingly, the critical or target organ may also vary with the period. In histiotrophic nutrition, local macromolecules are mainly responsible for the maintenance of the embryo; in hemotrophic nutrition, exchange of material is constantly maintained between the maternal and the fetal circulation (Beck, 1976).

Effects of methylmercury on maternal physiology also should be considered with respect to embryotoxicity and teratogenicity. For instance, cleft palate in mice has been associated with high maternal plasma corticosterone levels (Barlow et al., 1975; Hemm et al., 1977). If methylmercury induces high levels of circulating corticosterone, the "teratogenicity" can be considered a secondary outcome of toxicity. This corticosterone theory was first postulated by Lee et al. (1979). The adrenal glands were markedly hypertrophic but the elevation of serum corticosterone was not recognized in male rats chronically poisoned with methylmercury (Burton and Meikle, 1980).

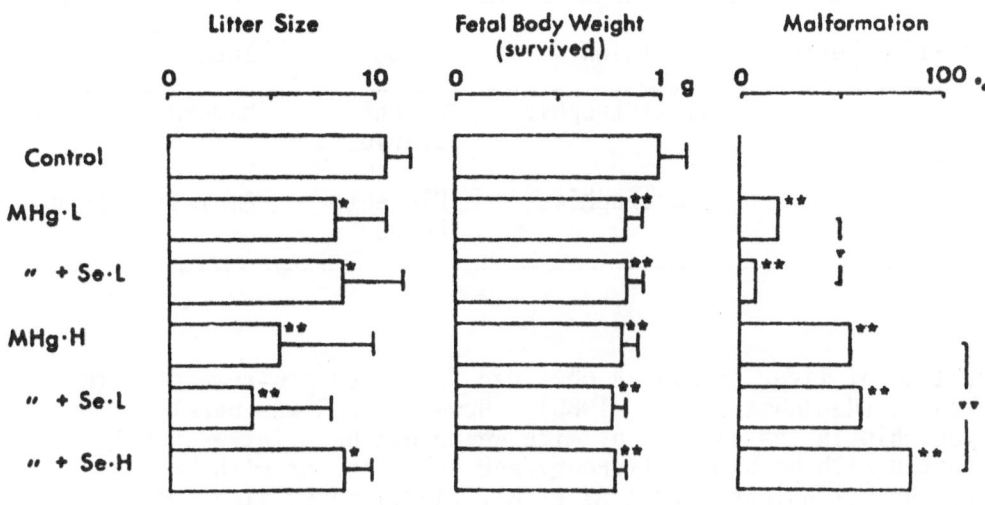

Figure 1   Modification by selenite of methylmercury toxicity on
           mouse embryos and fetuses. Methylmercury chloride (MeHg)
           was fed via drinking water to IVCS female mice from 30
           days before mating through day 18 of gestation.

METABOLISM OF METHYLMERCURY AND SELENITE IN PREGNANT MICE

Interpreting the interactions between two chemicals in pregnant
animals poses special problems since both the mother and embryo/fetus
are involved in the metabolism. We must consider the following
parameters: 1) maternal metabolism; 2) placental transfer; and 3)
embryonic or fetal metabolism.

Maternal Metabolism

Metabolism of methylmercury and selenium appears to be
different in non-pregnant and pregnant females. However, the basic
metabolic mechanism should be identical in both cases. When
methylmercury and selenite were added to rabbit blood,
bis(methylmercuric) selenide (BMS, $(CH_3Hg)_2Se$) was formed
(Naganuma and Imura, 1980). The homogenates, soluble fraction, or
insoluble fraction of mouse liver, kidney, spleen, and brain were
also capable of forming BMS from the methylmercury and selenite.
BMS was also formed when methylmercury was added to the soluble

Table 1   Different Mode of Nutrition in Embryos and Fetuses of
          Mice by Period of Gestation

Gestation Period	Nutrition	Target	Index Media
Early	Histiotrophic	Uterus Embryo	Maternal blood
Middle Late	Hemotrophic	Placenta Fetus	Amniotic fluid

fraction of liver or kidney obtained from mice pre-treated with
selenite (Naganuma et al., 1980). However, BMS was barely
detectable in the tissues of mice which had been intravenously
injected with both methylmercury and selenite, or with BMS itself.
From these findings, Naganuma et al. (1980) postulated the following
chain of events to occur in the mouse: rapid formation of BMS in
the blood and transport into tissues followed by a cycle of
degradation and resynthesis. BMS injection produced remarkable
accumulation of both mercury and selenium in the mouse brain.
Maternal blood reaching the uterus and the placenta may contain BMS,
methylmercury and selenium, or, BMS may be formed in the uterus and
placental tissue, after simultaneous administration of methylmercury
and selenite.

The next process to be considered is the cleavage of the
carbon-mercury bond of methylmercury. As already reviewed elsewhere
(Suzuki, 1977), the cleavage of the covalent bond occurs in various
animal species. The cleavage is inversely dose-dependent in guinea
pigs (Iverson and Hierlihy, 1974), rats (Syverson, 1974), and
squirrel monkeys (Berlin et al., 1975). The accumulation of
inorganic mercury in the liver and kidneys proceeds with time after
administration of methylmercury in rats (Omata et al., 1980) or
during the feeding of methylmercury in mice (Suzuki and Shishido,
1976).

Does simultaneous administration of selenium enhance the
cleavage of the covalent bond of methylmercury? Several studies in
vivo suggest that this may be true. An increase in the accumulation
of inorganic mercury in rat liver was observed after feeding of
methylmercury and selenite for 70 days (Figure 2) (Ohi et al.,
1976). As shown in Figure 3, two-week-feeding of methylmercury and
selenite produced an increase in inorganic mercury concentration in
mouse liver in a manner associated with the dose of selenium
(Yamamoto and Suzuki, 1981). Respiratory exhalation of ^{14}C was
markedly enhanced in rats when selenite was administered

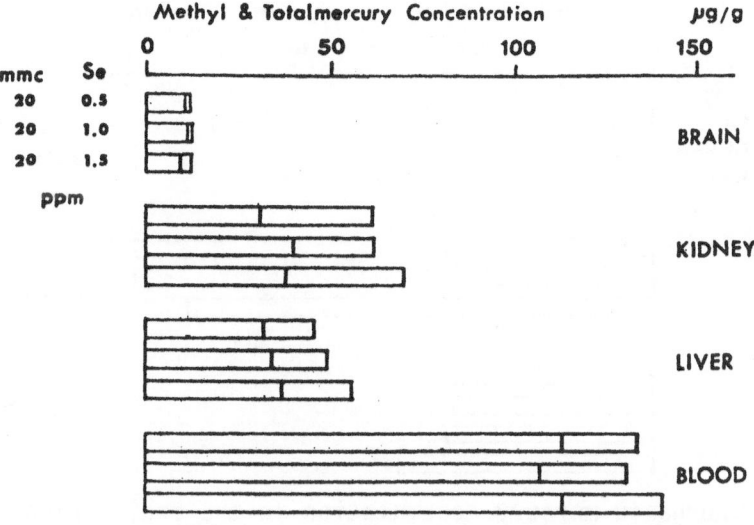

Figure 2 Inorganic mercury accumulation in organs and tissues of
          rats fed methylmercury chloride and selenite for over 70
          days. Methylmercury chloride (mmc) at 20 ppm in the feed;
          selenite (Se) at 0.5, 1.0, 1.5 ppm in the feed. Shaded
          part of column indicates methylmercury concentration;
          entire length of column represents total mercury
          concentration (Ohi et al., 1976).

simultaneously with ^{14}C-labeled methylmercury, compared with rats
dosed with ^{14}C-methylmercury alone (Yamane et al., 1977). These
results from in vivo experiments provide indirect evidence suggesting
the accelerated cleavage of the covalent bond of methylmercury in
the presence of selenite. The site of demethylation is proposed to
be in the liver. Nevertheless, no direct evidence from in vitro
experiments for this effect of selenium has been obtained (Ishihara
and Suzuki, 1976).

Placental Transfer and Maternal and Fetal Body Distribution

     Placental transfer of methylmercury and selenite was first
studied by Iijima et al. (1978). On day 15 of gestation each
chemical alone or both chemicals simultaneously were injected into
pregnant mice. Simultaneous injection of selenium and methylmercury
produced an increase in methylmercury accumulation in maternal brain
but produced a decrease in methylmercury content in the fetus
compared with administration of methylmercury alone. Simultaneous
injection of both chemicals increased selenium accumulation both in

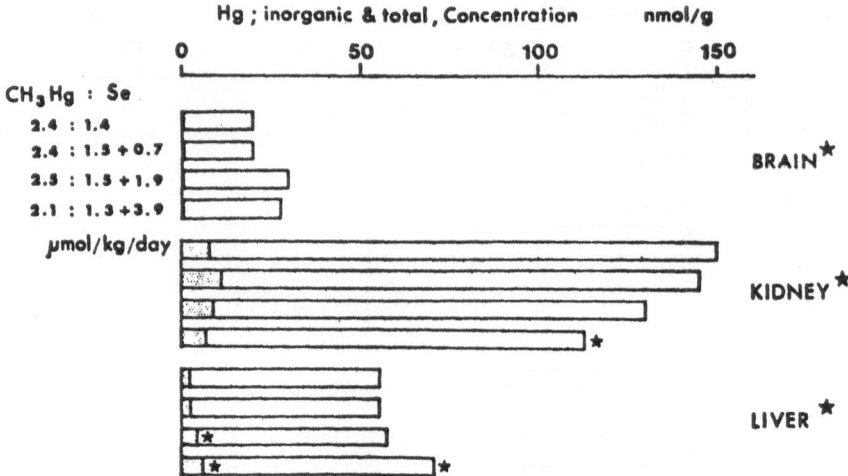

Figure 3   Inorganic mercury accumulation in the brain, kidney and
           liver of mice fed methylmercury chloride and selenium for
           two weeks. Methylmercury and selenium (chemical form
           unidentified) were fed via feed and selenite, via drinking
           water. Figures in each column show the daily intake: for
           selenium, the figure on the left shows the amount from the
           feed and on the right, from drinking water. Shaded
           portion of the bar represents inorganic mercury; entire
           length represents total mercury. Star (*) by organ name
           indicates significant differences due to the level of
           selenium (Yamamoto and Suzuki, 1981).

the maternal brain and fetus, compared with the injection of
selenium alone. A single dose level of each compound and a single
dose-combination were used and none of the fetal organs were
examined.

     Figures 4 through 10 present simplified diagrams of a pregnant
mouse; the compartments are numbered. In the following figures, an
arrow in each compartment shows either an increase (upward arrow) or
decrease (downward) in the concentration of the indicated chemical.
In each case, simultaneous administration of two chemicals or BMS
administration was compared with the administration of a single
chemical. A slanted arrow indicates a statistically non-significant
increase or decrease.

     Figures 4 through 7 show the results of our recent experiments
to determine whether BMS passes more easily through the placenta and
accumulates in the fetus, compared with administration of

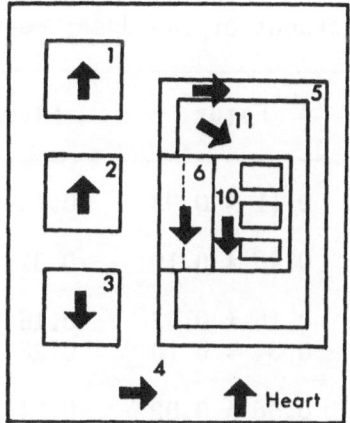

Figure 4   Total mercury contents or concentrations in organs and
tissues: comparison of simultaneous administration of
methylmercury and selenite with methylmercury alone.
Chemicals were labeled with radioactive mercury or
selenium and injected intravenously; measurements were
conducted 1 hr after injection. 1. Maternal brain;
2. Maternal liver; 3. Maternal kidney; 4. Maternal blood;
5. Uterus; 6. Placenta; 10. Fetus; 11. Amniotic fluid.
↑ increased content or concentration; ↓ decreased
content or concentration; → no change; ↘, ↗ statistically
non-significant decrease or increase.

methylmercury alone or with coadministration of methylmercury and
selenite (Yonemoto et al., 1983).   The data are also shown in Tables
2 and 3.   For single or simultaneous administration, pregnant JCR
mice were injected with [^{203}Hg]CH$_3$HgCl (1.5 μmol/kg) and/or
[^{75}Se]Na$_2$SeO$_3$ (0.75 μmol/kg) on day 16 of gestation; mice were
killed 1 hour after injection. BMS, [^{203}Hg,^{75}Se](Ch$_3$Hg)$_2$Se
(0.75 μmol/kg), was similarly administered. Figures 4 and 5
indicate the following: 1) the accumulation of mercury in the
maternal organs and tissues is in accordance with the previous
results in non-pregnant mice; as shown in Table 4, the maternal

Table 2 Selenium and Mercury Contents in Fetus, Placenta and Amniotic Membrane From Pregnant Mice 60 minutes after Injection of Sodium Selenite and/or Methylmercury, or $(CH_3Hg)_2Se$. (percent of the dose; mean ± S.D.)[a]

Treatment	No.		Fetus	Placenta	Amniotic Membrane
Na_2SeO_3	4	Se	0.11 ± 0.03	0.14 ± 0.02	0.03 ± 0.01
Ch_3HgCl	4	Hg	0.45 ± 0.19	0.31 ± 0.14	0.05 ± 0.02
Na_2SeO_3 + CH_3HgCl	4	Se	0.16 ± 0.03	0.16 ± 0.03	0.03 ± 0.01
		Hg	0.34 ± 0.10	0.26 ± 0.06	0.03 ± 0.01
$(CH_3HG)_2Se$	4	Se	0.06 ± 0.02	0.14 ± 0.03	0.03 ± 0.01
		Hg	0.33 ± 0.07	0.23 ± 0.09	0.03 ± 0.01

[a]Yonemoto et al., 1983.

Table 3 Selenium and Mercury Concentration in Blood and Amniotic Fluid of Pregnant Mice 60 minutes after Injection of Sodium Selenite and/or Methylmercury, or $(CH_3Hg)_2Se$. (nmol/ml; mean ± S.D.)[a]

Treatment	No.		Whole blood	Plasma	Erythrocyte	Amniotic Fluid
Na_2SeO_3	4	Se	0.72±0.06	1.19±0.10	0.28±0.03	0.02±0.01
CH_3HgCl	4	Hg	6.92±1.41	1.56±0.85	11.87±2.39	0.03±0.02
Na_2SeO_3 + CH_3HgCl	4	Se	0.71±0.08	1.15±0.11	0.34±0.06	0.02±0.01
		Hg	7.03±1.11	0.93±0.23	12.66±2.16	0.01±0.01
$(CH_3Hg)_2Se$	4	Se	0.98±0.37	1.72±0.70	0.29±0.07	0.02±0.01
		Hg	3.76±2.14	0.68±0.29	6.61±4.13	0.02±0.01

[a]Yonemoto et al., 1983.

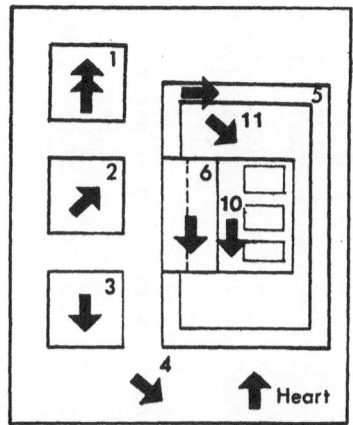

Figure 5   Total mercury contents or concentrations in organs and
            tissues: comparison of bis(methylmercuric) selenide (BMS)
            administration with simultaneous administration of
            methylmercury and selenite, and comparison of BMS with
            methylmercury alone. Measurements were made as in Figure
            4. Double arrow shows increase in BMS group, compared
            with both simultaneous administration and methylmercury
            alone groups. Single arrows show increase or decrease of
            total mercury concentration in BMS group, compared with
            methylmercury alone group. 1. Maternal brain; 2. Maternal
            liver; 3. Maternal kidney; 4. Maternal blood; 5. Uterus;
            6. Placenta; 10. Fetus; 11. Amniotic fluid.
            ↑ increased content or concentration; ↓ decreased
            content or concentration; →no change;↘,↗statistically
            non-significant decrease or increase.

Table 4   Selenium and Mercury Concentration in Maternal Tissues and Fetus 60 minutes after Injection of Sodium Selenite and/or Methylmercury, or $(CH_3Hg)_2Se$.   (nmol/g tissue; mean (S.D.)[a]

Treatment	No.		Brain	Liver	Kidney	Spleen	Heart	Muscle	Uterus	Fetus	Placenta	Amniotic Membrane
Na_2SeO_3	4	Se	0.07 (0.03)	5.49 (0.93)	3.19 (0.22)	0.63 (0.05)	0.98 (0.33)	0.18 (0.06)	0.50 (0.11)	0.06 (0.02)	0.45 (0.14)	0.22 (0.09)
CH_3HgCl	4	Hg	0.23 (0.10)	2.65 (1.05)	9.76 (2.67)	4.59 (0.76)	1.79 (0.36)	0.53 (0.21)	1.34 (0.68)	0.48 (0.17)	1.92 (0.92)	0.71 (0.37)
Na_2SeO_3	4	Se	0.21[c] (0.04)	4.40 (0.40)	3.41 (0.41)	0.63 (0.14)	1.34 (0.26)	0.22 (0.04)	0.56 (0.12)	0.08 (0.01)	0.47 (0.11)	0.26 (0.07)
+ CH_3HgCl		Hg	0.80[c] (0.29)	5.67[b] (1.29)	5.14[b] (1.17)	4.72 (1.39)	4.31[c] (0.87)	0.80 (0.30)	1.20 (0.27)	0.37 (0.07)	1.48 (0.37)	0.54 (0.22)
$(CH_3Hg)_2Se$	4	Se	0.91[b,d] (0.32)	3.72 (1.32)	2.76 (0.40)	1.13 (0.45)	2.90[c,e] (0.38)	0.38[b] (0.13)	0.43 (0.09)	0.03[b,e] (0.01)	0.42 (0.05)	0.17 (0.04)
		Hg	2.24[b,e] (0.57)	3.91[b] (0.64)	4.74[b] (1.74)	3.65 (0.45)	5.78[c,d] (0.64)	1.40[b] (0.43)	1.42 (0.40)	0.33 (0.03)	1.38 (0.03)	0.42 (0.09)

[a] Yonemoto et al., 1983.
[b] $p < 0.05$. Significantly different from the control (as for Se, Na_2Se_3 alone group; for Hg, CH_3HgCl group).
[c] $p < 0.01$.
[d] $p < 0.05$.
[e] $p < 0.01$. Significantly different from simultaneous injection of both Se and Hg.

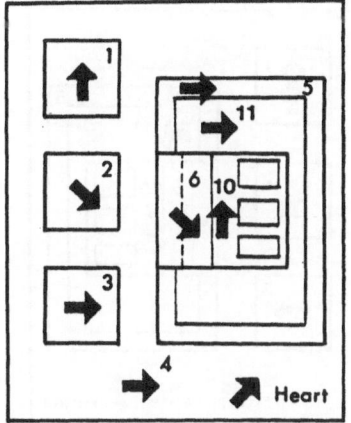

Figure 6   Selenium contents or concentrations in organs and
           tissues: comparison of simultaneous administration of
           methylmercury and selenite with selenite alone.
           Measurements were made as in Figure 5. 1. Maternal brain;
           2. Maternal liver; 3. Maternal kidney; 4. Maternal blood;
           5. Uterus; 6. Placenta; 10. Fetus; 11. Amniotic fluid.
           ↑ increased content or concentration; ↓ decreased
           content or concentration; → no change; ↘,↗ statistically
           non-significant decrease or increase.

brain retains much more mercury in the BMS group than in the
methylmercury group or in the coadministration group; thus, the
arrow is doubled for the maternal brain in Figure 5; and 2) the
similar reductions in the placental and fetal accumulation of
mercury occur in both the coadministration and BMS groups (Tables 2
and 4). Figures 6 and 7 show the changes in selenium concentrations:
1) as shown in Table 4, the increase in the maternal brain selenium
is similar to that observed for mercury (BMS > Hg+Se > Se); 2) the

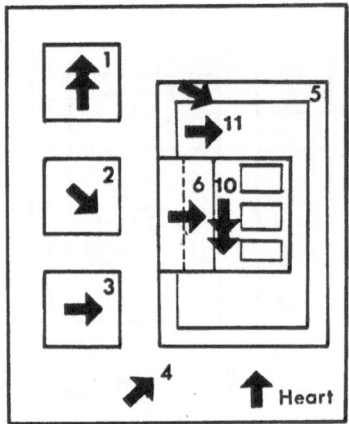

Figure 7   Selenium contents or concentrations in organs and
           tissues: comparison of bis(methylmercuric) selenide (BMS)
           administration with administration of methylmercury and
           selenite, or comparison of BMS with selenite alone.
           Measurements were made as in Figure 4.   Double arrows show
           increase or decrease in BMS group, compared with both
           simultaneous administration and selenite alone groups.
           Single arrows show increase or decrease of selenium
           concentration in BMS group, compared with selenite alone
           group.   1. Maternal brain; 2. Maternal liver; 3. Maternal
           kidney; 4. Maternal blood; 5. Uterus; 6. Placenta; 10.
           Fetus; 11. Amniotic fluid.

placental selenium content and concentration are similar in the
coadministration group, the BMS group, and the selenite alone group
(Table 4); and 3) fetal selenium accumulation is decreased in the
BMS group, and coadministration group, compared with the selenite
alone group (Tables 2 and 4).

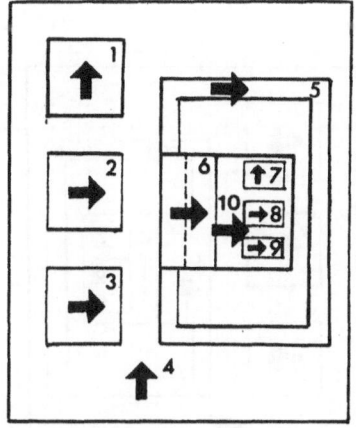

Figure 8   Total mercury contents or concentrations in organs and
           tissues: comparison of simultaneous administration of
           methylmercury and selenite with methylmercury alone.
           Chemicals were injected subcutaneously with various
           dose-combinations of methylmercury and selenite. Mice
           were killed 24 hours after injection. 1. Maternal brain;
           2. Maternal liver; 3. Maternal kidney; 4. Maternal blood;
           5. Uterus; 6. Placenta; 10. Fetus.
           ↑ increased content or concentration; ↓ decreased
           content or concentration; → no change.

        The mechanisms underlying the increase in fetal selenium
concentration in the coadministration group and the decrease in the
BMS group are of interest. Does coexisting methylmercury alter the
placental membrane to allow the passage of selenium but not
methylmercury or BMS ? We are now interested in how this finding
relates to the mechanism of the modification of methylmercury
toxicity by selenite.

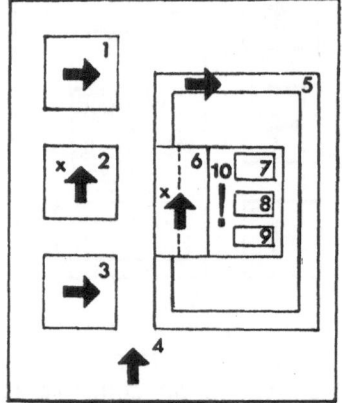

Figure 9   Inorganic mercury contents or concentrations in organs and
           tissues: comparison of simultaneous administration of
           methylmercury and selenite with methylmercury alone.
           Measurements were made as in Figure 8. X indicates
           increase of inorganic mercury concentrations only at a
           certain dose-combination. Exclamation mark indicates no
           detectable amount of inorganic mercury. 1. Maternal
           brain; 2. Maternal liver; 3. Maternal kidney; 4. Maternal
           blood; 5. Uterus; 6. Placenta; 10. Fetus.
           ↑ increased content or concentration; ↓ decreased content
           or concentration;
           → no change; ↘, ↗ statistically non-significant decrease
           or increase.

       Selenium modifies methylmercury toxicity at various
dose-combinations. In vitro formation of BMS in the soluble
fraction of mouse liver was reported to be dose-dependent, being
most favorable at $5 \times 10^{-5}M$ of both methylmercury and selenite;

Table 5 Mercury Contents 24 hours after Subcutaneous Injection of Methylmercury and Selenite to Pregnant Mice (percent of the dose; mean ± S.D.)[d]

MeHg-Se (μmol/kg)	Maternal					Placenta	Amniotic Membrane
	Brain	Liver	Spleen	Kidneys	Uterus		
1.5- 0	0.556+0.119	14.98+3.37	0.296+0.061	4.03+0.62	1.26+0.20	0.258+0.040	0.072+0.010
1.5- 1.5	0.710+0.111 *	17.06+2.34	0.422+0.242	3.34+0.32	1.48+0.16	0.233+0.045	0.052+0.010
1.5-15.0	0.835+0.076	14.93+0.93	0.303+0.043	2.50+0.34	1.08+0.17	0.215+0.027	0.055+0.005
15.0- 0	0.319+0.067 *	10.60+2.03	0.237+0.070	3.00+0.69	1.07+0.05	0.187+0.044	0.049+0.011
15.0- 1.5	0.564+0.135	11.03+3.29 *	0.234+0.083	3.11+0.54	1.12+0.35	0.235+0.060	0.070+0.011
15.0-15.0	0.728+0.160	16.28+2.62	0.251+0.059	3.73+0.18	1.35+0.18	0.212+0.018	0.065+0.014[a]
Factor							
MeHg	c	c	c	n.s.	n.s.	n.s.	n.s.
Se	c	n.s.	n.s.	n.s.	n.s.	n.s.	n.s.
Interaction	n.s.	b	n.s.	c	b	n.s.	c

*The difference between two means by the least significant differences method ($p < 0.05$).
[a]The number of samples was 3.
b or c; Significant ($p < 0.05$ or $p < 0.01$, by two-way analysis of variance).
[d]Satoh and Suzuki, 1979.

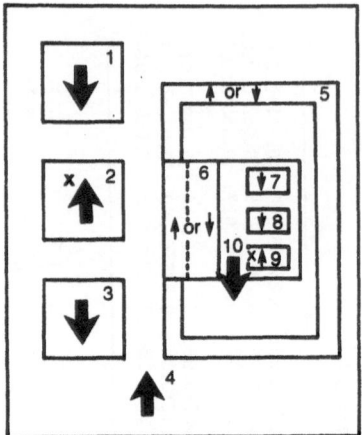

Figure 10   Total mercury concentrations in organs and tissues:
            comparison of simultaneous administration of mercuric
            chloride and selenite with mercuric chloride alone.
            Measurements were made as in Figure 8. X indicates
            increase observed at a certain dose-combination of
            $HgCl_2$ and selenite. 1. Maternal brain; 2. Maternal
            liver; 3. Maternal kidney; 4. Maternal blood; 5. Uterus;
            6. Placenta; 10. Fetus.

about 25 percent of the added methylmercury was recovered as BMS
(Naganuma et al., 1980). Therefore, if BMS formation is involved in
the modification of metabolism and toxicity of methylmercury, its
role would be one of a restrictive character. A variety of
dose-combinations of methylmercury and selenium need to be studied
to evaluate the full spectrum of interactions. In vivo modification
of methylmercury metabolism by selenite in pregnant mice also varies
according to the dose-combination (Satoh and Suzuki, 1979). Data
for various dose combinations of methylmercury and selenium are
shown in Tables 5, 6, and 7 and summarized in Figure 6. Among the

Table 6   Mercury Concentration in Maternal Blood and Amniotic Fluid
24 hours after Subcutaneous Injection of Methylmercury and
Selenite to Pregnant Mice (nmol/ml; mean ± S.D.)[c]

MeHg-Se (μmol/kg)	Whole Blood	Red Blood Cells	Plasma	Amniotic Fluid
1.5- 0	0.90±0.15	1.71±0.32	0.29±0.04	0.06±0.03
1.5- 1.5	0.75±0.10	1.33±0.26	0.32±0.05	0.04±0.02
1.5-15.0	1.18±0.08	2.38±0.19	0.28±0.01	0.03±0.01
15.0- 0	6.27±1.04	11.59±2.34	2.12±0.44	0.28±0.10
15.0- 1.5	7.96±1.06 *	15.43±2.89 *	2.42±0.37	0.27±0.06
15.0-15.0	10.04±1.37 *	20.65±2.78 *	2.18±0.42	0.45[a]
Factor				
MeHg[b]	b	b	b	
Se	b	b	n.s.	
Interaction	b	b	n.s.	

*The difference between means is significant by the least
significant difference method (p < 0.05).
[a]The number of samples was 2.
[b]Significant (p < 0.01, by two-way analysis of variance).
[c]Satoh and Suzuki, 1979.

combinations tested, the low dose-level of methylmercury (1.5
μmol/kg, subcutaneous) administered simultaneously with selenite
(1.5 or 15.0 μmol/kg, subcutaneous) produced an elevation only of
maternal brain mercury levels, compared with injections of
methylmercury alone (Table 5). The high-dose level of methylmercury
(15.0 μmol/kg, subcutaneous) administered with selenite (1.5 or 15.0
μmol/kg, subcutaneous) produced an elevation of mercury levels in
maternal blood (Table 6) and fetal brain (Table 7) in addition to
maternal brain (Table 5, Figure 8).

Inorganic mercury concentrations were also determined for
various dose combinations of methylmercury and selenite (Satoh and
Suzuki, unpublished). Data are not shown but are summarized in
Figure 9. Changes in inorganic mercury accumulation in maternal
liver and placenta (indicated with X) was observed only at a certain
dose-combination. The 15 μmol/kg methylmercury:15 μmol/kg selenite

combination produced significantly elevated concentrations of
inorganic mercury in maternal liver; the 15 μmol/kg methylmercury:
1.5 μmol/kg selenite dose produced a significant increase in mercury
concentration in placenta. Inorganic mercury accumulation in the
blood, especially in erythrocytes, was dependent on the dose of
selenite, and no inorganic mercury was detected in the fetal organs
(exclamation mark in Figure 9).

The modified mercury distribution after coadministration of
mercuric chloride and selenite in pregnant mice is shown in Tables
8, 9, 10 and 11, and is summarized in Figure 10. In this study, the
most interesting finding is a remarkable reduction of fetal mercury
accumulation with coadministration selenite as shown in Tables 10
and 11 (Satoh et al., 1981).

Thus, the effect of selenite in the placental transfer and
fetal accumulation of methylmercury can be summarized as follows:

1) Simultaneously-administered selenite does not enhance the
placental transfer and fetal accumulation of mercury (administered
as methylmercury). Mercury concentrations in the fetal brain,
however, are elevated by selenite;

2) Methylmercury, but not BMS, is easily transferred through
the placenta; and

3) Fetal organs and tissues in mice do not show appreciable
capacity to break down the C-Hg bond of methylmercury.

The effects of methylmercury on the placental transfer and
fetal accumulation of selenium are summarized as follows:

1) The fetal accumulation of selenium is enhanced by
administration of methylmercury; and

2) Selenium in the form of BMS is transferred less easily
through the placenta than is selenite.

MODIFICATION BY SELENITE OF THE DOSE-RESPONSE RELATIONSHIP OF
METHYLMERCURY IN MOUSE EMBRYOS AND FETUSES

Next, we should examine how selenium modifies the dose-response
relationship of methylmercury in the mouse embryo and fetus. The
embryo (or fetus) itself has been considered by some to be the
critical or target organ in methylmercury toxicity (Suzuki, 1979).
In selenium toxicity, the placenta is more susceptible than the
embryo as shown in our recent experiments (Yonemoto et al., 1980).
This placental damage due to selenite may account for the fetal
growth retardation at the dose utilized in a previous experiment
(Nobunaga et al., 1979).

Table 7 Mercury Contents in Fetal Organs and Fetus 24 hours after Injection of Methylmercury and Selenite to Pregnant Mice (percent of the dose; mean ± S.D.)[e]

MeHg-Se (μmol/kg)	Brain		Liver	Kidneys	Fetus[b]
1.5- 0	0.068±0.010	(1.05±0.14)[a]	0.139±0.037	0.0041±0.0016	1.33±0.16
1.5- 1.5	0.064±0.016	(0.82±0.19)	0.160±0.020	0.0052±0.0013	1.30±0.05
1.5-15.0	0.071±0.017	(0.79±0.15)	0.144±0.015	0.0062±0.0021	1.18±0.17
15.5- 0	0.045±0.012 *	(7.00±2.02) *	0.147±0.054	0.0066±0.0037	1.32±0.36
15.0- 1.5	0.088±0.024	(11.63±2.51)	0.177±0.056	0.0076±0.0022	1.31±0.46
15.0-15.0	0.073±0.007	(11.21±2.56)	0.176±0.024	0.0070±0.0011	1.37±0.15
Factor					
MeHg	n.s.	d	n.s.	c	n.s.
Se	c	c	n.s.	n.s.	n.s.
Interaction	c	c	n.s.	n.s.	n.s.

*The difference between means is significant by the least significant difference method (p < 0.05).
[a]The numerals in parentheses were concentrations of mercury in fetal brain (nmol/g).
[b]The numerals were average for individual fetus.
c or d; Significant (p < 0.05 or p < 0.01, by two-way analysis of variance).
[e]Satoh and Suzuki, 1979.

Table 8   Mercury Concentrations in Maternal Blood and Amniotic Fluid
24 hours after Subcutaneous Injection of Mercuric Mercury
and Selenite to Pregnant Mice (nmol/g; mean ± S.D.)[d]

Hg-Se (μmol/kg)	Maternal Blood	Amniotic Fluid
1.5- 0	1.3±0.3 *	0.008[a]
1.5- 1.3	1.8±0.7 *	0.006[a]
1.5-12.7	2.1±0.5 *	0.006[a]
15.0- 0	3.4±1.4 *	0.04±0.04
15.0- 1.3	8.7±2.0 * *	0.06±0.02
15.0-12.7	16.2±3.3	0.06±0.02
15.0-25.3	18.4±4.9[b]	--

Variables**		
Hg	c	
Se	c	
Interaction	c	

*The difference between two means is significant by the
least significant different method (p < 0.05).
**Variables in the analysis of variance.
[a]Amniotic fluid samples were unified for all the four
mice of group.
[b]All the mice of this group aborted before sacrifice;
therefore the data are not subjected to the statistical
analysis.
[c]Significant (p < 0.005, by two-way analysis of
variance).
[d]Satoh et al., 1981.
Number of mother mice in each group was 4.

        Theoretically, modification of the dose-response
relationship may occur as one of three types: in the first type, no
apparent change may be observed in the dose-response relationship
per se, but closer examination may reveal that the level of mercury
in the critical organ may be considerably altered by a simultaneous
administration of selenium; the second type is a parallel shift of
the line representing the relationship; the third type is a change
in the slope of that line.

Table 9   Mercury Contents in Maternal Organs 24 hours after Subcutaneous Injection of Mercuric Mercury and Selenite (percent of the dose; mean ± S.D.)[d]

Hg-Se (µmol/kg)	Brain	Liver	Spleen	Kidneys	Uterus
1.5- 0	0.09±0.01 *	7.8±0.7 *	0.22±0.04	11.4±0.8 *	1.5±0.21 *
1.5- 1.3	0.06±0.03 *	13.9±2.2 *	0.45±0.05	11.3±5.0 *	1.6±0.17 *
1.5-12.7	0.05±0.01	7.5±4.4	0.37±0.37	2.3±0.5	0.8±0.03
15.0- 0	0.03±0.01	5.8±1.9 *	0.21±0.16 *	8.2±3.1 *	0.8±0.14 *
15.0- 1.3	0.03±0.01	6.3±0.8 *	0.34±0.07 *	8.1±2.1 *	1.1±0.09 * *
15.0-12.7	0.02±0.005	12.6±3.4	1.08±0.42	2.8±0.5	0.6±0.06
15.0-25.3[a]	0.007±0.004	8.8±3.5	0.85±0.50	2.1±1.1	1.0±0.16
Variables[**]					
Hg	c	n.s.	n.s.	n.s.	c
Se	b	b	c	c	c
Interaction	n.s.	c	c	n.s.	b

*The difference between two means is significant by the least significant difference method (p < 0.05).
**Variables in the analysis of variance.
[a]All the mother mice aborted before sacrifice; therefore the data are not involved in the statistical analysis.
[b] or [c] Significant (p < 0.05   p < 0.005, by two-way analysis of variance).
[d]Satoh et al., 1981.

Table 10 Mercury Contents in Placenta, Amniotic Membrane and Fetus 24 hours after Mercuric Mercury and Selenite Injection (percent of the dose; mean ± S.D.)c

Hg-Se (μmol/kg)	Placenta		Amniotic Membrane		Fetus	
	As Litter	Individual	As Litter	Individual	As Litter	Individual
1.5- 0	6.2+1.3	0.56+0.09 *	4.2+0.5 *	0.38+0.05 *	0.32+0.11 *	0.03 +0.008
1.5- 1.3	6.4+1.0 *	0.96+0.15 *	5.9+1.1 *	0.90+0.25 *	0.17+0.03 *	0.03 +0.007 *
1.5-12.7	2.4+0.09	0.24+0.07 *	4.3+1.2	0.42+0.09	0.02+0.02	0.002+0.002 *
15.0- 0	1.7+0.3 *	0.23+0.09	1.6+0.5	0.20+0.04	0.28+0.08 *	0.03 +0.009
15.0- 1.3	2.7+0.3 *	0.26+0.06	2.1+0.4	0.20+0.05	0.45+0.06 *	0.04 +0.015 *
15.0-12.7	2.4+0.2	0.27+0.07	1.8+0.3	0.20+0.05	0.09+0.03	0.01 +0.005 *
Variables**						
Hg	b	b	b	b	n.s.	n.s.
Se	b	a	n.s.	n.s.	b	b
Interaction	b	a	n.s.	n.s.	b	b

*The difference between two means is significant by the least significant difference method (p < 0.05).
**Variables in the analysis of variance.
a or b Significant (p < 0.01 or p < 0.005, by two-way analysis of variance).
cSatoh et al., 1981.

Table 11 Mecury Contents in Fetal Organs 24 hours after Mercuric Mercury and Selenite Injection (percent of the dose; mean ± S.D.)[c]

Hg-Se (µmol/kg)	Brain	Liver	Kidneys
15.0- 0	0.008±0.002	0.034±0.006	0.002±0.001*
15.0- 1.3	0.007±0.003* *	0.038±0.004* *	0.005±0.002*
15.0-12.7	0.003±0.001	0.008±0.002	0.001±0.001
F-statistics	a	b	a

*The difference between two means is significant by the least significant difference method ($p < 0.05$).
[a] or [b]Significant ($p < 0.05$, $p < 0.005$, by one-way analysis of variance).

If the modification by selenite followed type 1, an increased toxicity would be accompanied by an elevation of mercury levels in the critical organ. Whilst the greater accumulation of methylmercury in fetal brain in response to the concurrent administration of selenite may indicate such a mechanism, the observations that the mercury concentrations in the fetus, placenta and uterus were unchanged or decreased, under such conditions suggest that the modification of the dose-response relationship follows a type 2 or type 3 format.

In mice fed methylmercury (15.9 or 31.9 nmol/g feed) and selenite (0 or 11.4 nmol/ml drinking water) for 30 days before mating, and through day 18 of gestation, the death rate of embryos and fetuses in each litter was compared with the mercury concentration in organs and tissues (Satoh and Suzuki, 1983). The early death rate (number of implantation sites and resorptions per total number of implants) demonstrated a significant correlation with either amniotic fluid or fetal brain mercury concentrations on day 18 of gestation. In both cases, the correlation coefficient was less than 0.5 - 0.6. In contrast, the total death rate (number of total embryonic and fetal death per total number of implants) was correlated with mercury concentrations in several organs, as shown in Table 12.

Table 12   Correlations of Total Death Rate with Mercury
            Concentrations in Organs[c]

Organ	Correlation Coefficient (r)
fetal liver	0.683[a]
amniotic fluid	0.841[a]
amniotic membrane	0.715[a]
maternal blood	0.782[a]
uterus	0.720[a]
maternal liver	0.528[b]
maternal brain	0.547[b]

[a]significant at $p < 0.01$.
[b]significant at $p < 0.05$.
[c]correlations were calculated for all animals
   including both the groups receiving methylmercury alone
   and those receiving methylmercury selenite simultaneously.

These correlations suggest that the mercury burden in the organs
and tissues (e.g., amniotic fluid an maternal blood) which most
directly support embryonic and fetal life is closely correlated with
the death rate of embryos and fetuses. Whatever the mechanism of
toxicity modification, the correlation remains between the organ
mercury concentration and the death rate, even in the group to which
selenium was administered simultaneousely. Correlation coefficients
were also calculated separately for the animal group receiving
selenite versus those not receiving selenite. In the latter group
(i.e., treated with methylmercury alone), all coefficients, except
that for fetal brain, became greater than those for the combined
groups. For animals receiving selenite and methylmercury
simultaneously, there was no significant correlation between total
fetal and embryonic death rates and the mercury concentrations in
maternal brain, maternal liver, uterus, amnionic membrane, or fetal
liver. However, a significant correlation remained between total
death rate and mercury concentration in maternal blood ($r = 0.941$,
$p < 0.05$) and in amnionic fluid ($r = 0.860$, $p < 0.05$). The
correlation of death rate with blood and amniotic fluid mercury
concentrations is most interesting, considering the close
relationship of these two tissues to the embryo and fetus.

Figure 11 shows the alterations by selenite in the dose-response
relationship, when total fetal and embryonic death rate is plotted
versus organ concentration of mercury. In both maternal blood and

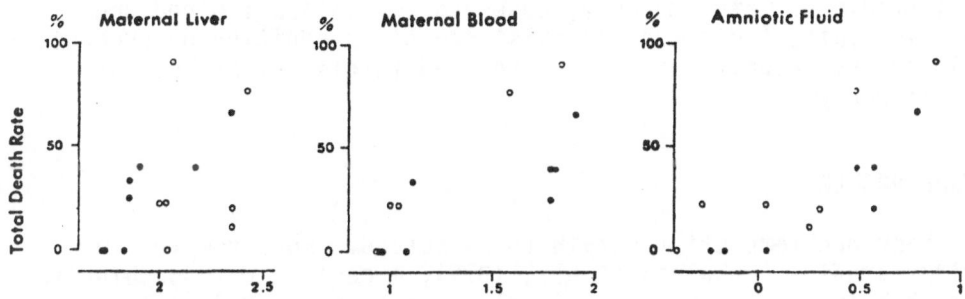

Figure 11 Modification by selenite of the dose-response relationship
of methylmercury toxicity in mouse embryos and fetuses.
The total death rate of embryos and fetuses per total
number of implants on day 18 of gestation versus log
organ mercury (as total) concentration on the same day.
o, selenium and methylmercury coadministered;
●, methylmercury alone. Mice were fed methylmercury
(15.9 or 31.9 nmol/g feed) and selenite via drinking
water (0 or 11.4 nmol/ml). Feeding period was from 30
before mating to day 18 of gestation.

amniotic fluid, the dose-response relationship has been modified
according to the type 2 or the type 3 pattern. However, as expected
from the loss of significant correlation, no definite pattern of
modification in the dose-response relationship is recognized in the
maternal liver.

These results may be interpreted as follows:

1) The absence of significant correlation between the early
death rate and organ mercury concentration may be explained by the
delay between the time when early death usually occurs and time of
mercury determination (on day 18 of gestation).

2) The mercury concentrations in fetal organs do not
necessarily represent those of the entire population of embryos and
fetuses at the critical period, because only surviving fetuses were
analysed for mercury. Thus, mercury concentration in maternal blood
or amniotic fluid may more closely represent fetal exposure to
methylmercury; these show a greater significance of correlation with
total death rate, both with and without coadministration of selenite.

3) The modification by selenite of the dose-response relationship of methylmercury, observed for maternal blood and amniotic fluid, indicates the existence of an additive or synergistic influence by selenite on the embryo- and fetolethal effects of methylmercury.

FUTURE PROBLEMS

Many problems still remain to be solved. For example, in earlier studies (Nobunaga et al., 1979), a certain dose-combination of methylmercury (31.9 nmol/g feed) and selenite (22.8 nmol/ml drinking water) was found to increase both the survival rate of embryos and fetuses and the prevalence of congenital anomalies. This finding could not be explained on the basis of data previously obtained, and this led to further experiments. Changes in the placental transfer of selenium in the form of BMS offer a possible explanation. Formation of BMS appears to depend on the dose of mercury and selenium; BMS also reduces the amount of accumulated selenium and its toxicity on the fetoplacental complex. This could explain the increased survival. Nevertheless, a different approach may be necessary to study the modification mechanism of methylmercury teratogenicity. After exposure to a high dose, most of the fetuses may show gross abnormalities. If the death occurs selectively in the animals with congenital anomalies, the increased survival would result in an apparent increase in the prevalence of congenital anomalies. Careful examination of dead embryos and fetuses may provide useful information.

ACKNOWLEDGEMENT

The author appreciates the valuable comments and advice of Drs. G. Ohi and N. Imura and also thanks his collaborators.

REFERENCES

Amin-Zaki, L., Elhassani, S., Majeed, M.A., Clarkson, T.W., Doherty, R.A. and Greenwood, M.R., 1974, Studies of infants postnatally exposed to methylmercury, J. Pediat. 85:81-84.
Amin-Zaki, L., Elhassani, S., Majeed, M.A., Clarkson, T.W., Doherty, R.A., Greenwood, M.R. and Giovanoli-Jakubczak, T., 1976, Perinatal methylmercury poisoning in Iraq, Am. J. Dis. Child, 130:1070-1076.
Amin-Zaki, L., Majeed, M.A., Clarkson, T.W. and Greenwood, M.R., 1978, Methylmercury poisoning in Iraqi children: Clinical observations over two years, Br. Med. J. 11:613-616.

Amin-Zaki, L., Majeed, M.A., Elhassani, S.B., Clarkson, T.W., Greenwood, M.R. and Doherty, R.A., 1979, Prenatal methylmercury poisoning, clinical observations over five years, Am. J. Dis. Child 133:172-177.

Bakir, F., Damluji, S.F., Amin-Zaki, L., Murtadha, M., Khalidi, A., Al-Rawi, N.Y., Tikriti, S., Dhahir, H.I., Clarkson, T.W., Smith, J.C. and Doherty, R.A., 1973, Methylmercury poisoning in Iraq, Science 181:230-241.

Barlow, S.M., McElhatton, P.R. and Sullivan, F.M., 1975, The relation between maternal restraint and food deprivation, plasma corticosterone, and induction of cleft palate in the offspring of mice, Teratology 12:97-104.

Beck, F., 1976, Comparative placental morphology and function, Environ. Health Perspect. 18:5-12.

Berlin, M., Carlson, J. and Norseth, T., 1975, Dose-dependence of methylmercury metabolism. A study of distribution: Biotransformation and excretion in the squirrel monkey, Arch. Environ. Health 30:307-313.

Bornhausen, M., Musch, H.R. and Greim, H., 1980, Operant behavior performance changes in rats after prenatal methylmercury exposure, Toxicol. Appl. Pharmacol. 56:305-310.

Brenner, R.P. and Snyder, R.D., 1980, Late EEG findings and clinical status after organic mercury poisoning, Arch. Neurol. 37:282-284.

Burton, G.V. and Meikle, A.W., 1980, Acute and chronic methylmercury poisoning impairs rat adrenal and testicular function, J. Toxicol. Environ. Health 6:597-606.

Calabrese, E.J., 1981, Nutrition and environmental health: The influence of nutritional status on pollutant toxicity and carcinogenicity, Vol. 2, in: "Minerals and Macronutrients", pp. 145-146, John Wiley and Sons, New York.

Casterline, J.L., Jr. and Williams, C.H., 1972, Elimination pattern of methylmercury from blood and brain of rats (dams and offspring) after delivery, following oral administration of its chloride salt during gestation, Bull. Environ. Contam. Toxicol. 7:292-295.

Chang, L.W. and Sprecher, J.A., 1976, Degenerative changes in the neonatal kidney following in utero exposure to methylmercury, Environ. Res. 11:392-406.

Choi, B.H., Lapham, L.W., Amin-Zaki, L. and Saleem, T., 1978, Abnormal neuronal migration, deranged cerebral cortical organization, and diffuse white matter astrocytosis of human fetal brain: A major effect of methylmercury poisoning in utero, J. Neuropathol. Exp. Neurol. 37:719-733.

Cortese, I., Cristino, R. and Cuomo, V., 1980, Behavioral effects induced by low doses of methylmercury in rats, Proceedings of the B.P.S. p. 168.

Engleson, G. and Herner, T., 1952., Alkylmercury poisoning, Acta Paediatr. 41:289-294.

Fujimoto, T., Fuyuta, M., Kiyofuji, E. and Hirata, S., 1979,
    Prevention by tiopronin (2-mercaptopropionyl glycine) of
    methylmercuric chloride-induced teratogenic and fetotoxic
    effects in mice, Teratology 20:297-302.
Fuyuta, M., Fujimoto, T. and Hirata, S., 1978, Embryotoxic effects
    of methylmercuric chloride administered to mice and rats during
    organogenesis, Teratology 18:353-366.
Fuyuta, M., Fujimoto, T. and Kiyofuji, E., 1979, Teratogenic effects
    of a single oral administration of methylmercuric chloride in
    mice, Acta Anat. 104:356-362.
Ganther, H.E., Goudie, C., Sunde, M.L., Kopecky, M.J., Wagner, P.,
    Oh, S-W. and Hoekstra, W.G., 1972, Selenium: Relation to
    decreased toxicity of methylmercury added to diets containing
    tuna, Science 175:1122-1124.
Greene, R.M. and Kochhar, D.M. (1975). Some aspects of
    corticosteroid-induced cleft palate: A review, Teratology
    11:47-56.
Harada, Y., 1968, Congenital (or fetal) Minamata disease, in:
    "Minimata Disease", Study group of Minimata Disease, pp.
    93-117, Kumamoto University, Japan.
Harada, M., 1978, Congenital Minamata disease: Intrauterine
    methylmercury poisoning, Teratology 18:285-288.
Harris, S.B., Wilson, J.G. and Printz, R.H., 1972, Embryotoxicity
    of methylmercury chloride in golden hamsters, Teratology
    6:139-142.
Hemm, R.D., Arslanoglou, L. and Pollock, J.J., 1977, Cleft palate
    following prenatal food restriction in mice: Association with
    elevated maternal corticosteroids, Teratology 15:243-248.
Iijima, S., Tohyama, C., Lu, C.C. and Matsumoto, N., 1978,
    Placental transfer and body distribution of methylmercury and
    selenium in pregnant mice, Toxicol. Appl. Pharmacol. 44:143-146.
Inoue, M., Hoshino, K. and Murakami, U., 1972, Effect of
    methylmercuric chloride on embryonic and fetal development in
    rats and mice, Ann. Rep. Res. Inst. Environ. Med. Nagoya Univ.
    19:69-74.
Ishihara, N. and Suzuki, T, 1976, Biotransformation of methylmercury
    in vitro, Tohoku J. Exp. Med. 120:361-363.
Iverson, F. and Hierlihy, S.L., 1974. Biotransformation of
    methylmercury in the guinea pig, Bull. Environ. Contam.
    Toxicol. 11:85-91.
Iwata, H., Okamoto, H. and Ohsawa, Y., 1973, Effect of selenium on
    methylmercury poisoning, Res. Commun. Chem. Pathol. Pharmacol.
    5:673-680.
Johnson, S.L. and Pond, W.G., 1974, Inorganic vs. organic Hg
    toxicity in growing rats: Protection by dietary Se but not Ze,
    Nutr. Rep. Int. 9:135-147.
Khera, K. and Tabacova, S., 1973, Effects of methylmercury chloride
    on the progeny of mice and rats treated before or during
    gestation, Food Cosmet. Toxicol. 11:245-254.

Lee, M., Chan, K.K.-S., Sairenji, E. and Niikuni, T., 1979, Effect
    of sodium selenite on methylmercury-induced cleft palate in the
    mouse, Environ. Res. 19:39-48.
Marsh, D.O., Myers, G.J., Clarkson, T.W., Amin-Zaki, L., Tikriti,
    S. and Majeed, M.A., 1980, Fetal methylmercury poisoning:
    Clinical and toxicological data on 29 cases, Ann. Neurol.
    7:348-353.
Matsumoto, H., Suzuki, A. and Morita, C., 1967, Preventive effect
    of penicillamine on the brain defect of fetal rat poisoned
    transplacentally with methylmercury, Life Sci. 6:2321-2326.
Moriyama, H., 1967, A study on the congenital Minamata Disease,
    Kumamoto Igakukai Zasshi 41:406-528 (in Japanese).
Mottet, N.K., 1974, Effects of chronic low-dose exposure of rat
    fetuses to methylmercury hydroxide, Teratology 10:173-190.
Musch, H.R., Bornhausen, M., Kriegel, H. and Greim, H., 1978,
    Methylmercury chloride induces learning deficits in prenatally
    treated rats, Arch. Toxicol. 40:103-108.
Naganuma, A. and Imura, N., 1980, Bis(methylmercuric) selenide as
    a reaction product from methylmercury and selenite in rabbit
    blood, Res. Commun. Chem. Pathol. Pharmacol. 27:163-173.
Naganuma, A., Kojima, Y. and Imura, N., 1980, Interaction of
    methylmercury and selenium in mouse: Formation and
    decomposition of bis(methylmercuric) selenide, Res. Commun.
    Chem. Pathol. Pharmacol. 30:301-316.
Nobunaga, T., Satoh, H. and Suzuki, T., 1979, Effects of sodium
    selenite on methylmercury embryotoxicity and teratogenicity in
    mice, Toxicol. Appl. Pharmacol 47:79-88.
Nolen, G.A., Buehler, E.V., Geil, R.G. and Goldenthal, E.I., 1972a,
    Effects of trisodium nitrilotriacetate on cadmium and
    methylmercury toxicity and teratogenicity in rats, Toxicol.
    Appl. Pharmacol. 23:222-237.
Nolen, G.A., Bohne, R.L. and Buehler, E.V., 1972b, Effects of
    trisodium nitrilotriacetate, trisodium citrate and trisodium
    nitriloacetate-ferric chloride mixture on cadmium and
    methylmercury toxicity and teratogenesis in rats, Toxicol.
    Appl. Pharmacol. 23:238-250.
Ohi, G., Seki, H., Maeda, H. and Yagyu, H., 1975a, Protective effect
    of selenite against methylmercury toxicity: Obervations
    concerning time, dose and route factors in the development of
    selenium attenuation, Ind. Health 13:93-99.
Ohi, G., Nishigaki, S., Seki, H., Tamura, Y., Maki, T., Maeda, H.,
    Ochiai, S., Yamada, H., Shimamura, Y. and Yagyu, H., 1975b,
    Interaction of dietary methylmercury and selenium on
    accumulation and retention of these substances in rat organs,
    Toxicol. Appl. Pharmacol. 32:527-533.
Ohi, G., Nishigaki, S., Seki, H., Tamura, Y., Maki, T., Konno, H.,
    Ochiai, S., Yamada, H., Shimamura, Y., Mizoguchi, I. and Yagyu,
    H., 1976, Efficacy of selenium in tuna and selenite in
    modifying methylmercury intoxication, Environ. Res. 12:49-58.

Olson, F.C. and Massaro, E.J., 1977, Effects of methylmercury on murine fetal amino acid uptake, protein synthesis and palate closure, Teratology 16:187-194.

Olson, F.C. and Massaro, E.J., 1980, Developmental pattern of cAMP, adenyl cyclase, and cAMP phosphodiesterase in the palate, lung, and liver of the fetal mouse: Alterations resulting from exposure to methylmercury at levels inhibiting palate closure, Teratology 22:155-166.

Omata, S., Sato, M., Sakimura, K. and Sugano, H., 1980, Time-dependent accumulation of inorganic mercury in subcellular fractions of kidney, liver, and brain of rats exposed to methylmercury, Arch. Toxicol. 44:231-241.

Potter, S. and Matrone, G., 1974, Effect of selenite on the toxicity of dietary methylmercury and mercuric chloride in rat, J. Nutr. 104:638-647.

Ramel, C., 1967, Genetic effects of organic mercury compounds, Hereditas 57:445-447.

Robbins, M.S., Hughes, J.A., Sparber, S.B. and Mannering, G.J., 1978, Delayed teratogenic effect of methylmercury on hepatic cytochrome p-450-dependent monooxygenase systems of rats, Life Sci. 22:287-294.

Satoh, H. and Suzuki, T., 1979, Effects of sodium selenite on methylmercury distribution in mice of late gestational period, Arch. Toxicol. 42:275-279.

Satoh, H. and Suzuki, T., 1983, Embryonic and fetal death after in utero methylmercury exposure and organ mercury concentration in mice, Ind. Health 21: (in press).

Satoh, H., Suzuki, T., Nobunaga, T., Naganuma, A. and Imura, N., 1981, Effects of sodium selenite on distribution and placental transfer of mercuric mercury in mice of late gestational period, J. Pharm. Dyn. 4:191-196.

Scharpf, L.G., Hill, I.D., Wright, P.L. and Keplinger, M.L., 1973, Teratology studies on methylmercury hydroxide and nitrilotriacetate sodium in rats, Nature (London) 241:461-463.

Snell, K., Ashby, S.L. and Barton, S.J., 1977, Disturbances of perinatal carbohydrate metabolism in rats exposed to methylmercury in utero, Toxicology 8:277-283.

Snyder, R.D., 1971, Congenital mercury poisoning, N. Engl. J. Med. 284:1014-1016.

Snyder, R.D. and Seelinger, D.F., 1976, Methylmercury poisoning. Clinical follow-up and sensory nerve conduction studies, J. Neurol. Neurosurg. Psychiatr. 39:701-704.

Spyker, J.M. and Smithberg, M., 1972. Effects of methylmercury on prenatal development in mice, Teratology 5:181-187.

Spyker, J.M., Sparber, S.B. and Goldberg, A.M., 1972, Subtle consequences of methylmercury exposure: Behavioral deviations in offspring of treated mothers, Science 177:621-623.

Stillings, B.R., Lagally, H., Bauersfeld, P. and Soares, J., 1974, Effect of cystine, selenium, and fish protein on the toxicity and metabolism of methylmercury in rats, Toxicol. Appl. Pharmacol. 30:243-254.

Stoewsand, G.S., Bache, C.A. and Lisk, D.J., 1974, Dietary selenium protection of methylmercury intoxication of Japanese quail, Bull. Environ. Contam. Toxicol. 11:152-156.

Su, M-Q. and Okita, G.T., 1976a, Embryocidal and teratogenic effects of methylmercury in mice, Toxicol. Appl. Pharmacol. 38:207-216.

Su, M-Q. and Okita, G.T., 1976b, Behavioral effects on the progeny of mice treated with methylmercury, Toxicol. Appl. Pharmacol. 38:195-205.

Suzuki, T., 1977, Metabolism of mercurial compounds, in: "Advances in Modern Toxicology, Vol. 2", in: "Toxicology of Trace Elements", R.A. Goyer and M.A. Mehlman, eds., pp. 1-39, John Wiley and Sons, New York.

Suzuki, T., 1979, Dose-effect and dose-response relationships of mercury and its derivatives, in: "The Biogeochemistry of Mercury in the Environment", J.O. Nriagu ed., pp. 399-431, Elsevier/North-Holland, Amsterdam.

Suzuki, T. and Shishido, S., 1976, A possible change of the critical concentration of methylmercury in the brain of mice: Observations by a quantitative assessment of early neurological signs, in: "Effects and Dose-Response Relationships of Toxic Metals", G. Nordberg, ed., pp. 283-289, Elsevier, Amsterdam.

Syverson, T.L.M., 1974, Biotransformation of Hg-203 labelled methylmercuric chloride in rat brain measured by specific determination of Hg^{2+}, Acta Pharmacol. Toxicol. 35:277-283.

Ware, R.A., Chang, L.W. and Burkholder, P.M., 1974, Ultrastructural evidence for foeta, liver injury induced by in utero exposure to small doses of methylmercury, Nature, (London) 251:236-237.

Yomamoto, R. and Suzuki, T., 1981, Demethylation of methylmercury by simultaneous administration of selenite in mice. Proceedings of the Fifty-fourth Annual Meeting of Japan Association of Industrial Health, Japan. J. Ind. Health 23:853.

Yamane, Y., Fukino, H., Aida, Y. and Imagawa, M., 1977, Studies on the mechanism of protective effects of selenium against the toxicity of methylmercury, Chem. Pharm. Bull. 25:2831-2837.

Yonemoto, J., Satoh, H., Himeno, S. and Suzuki, T., 1980, Acute toxicity of sodium selenite in mice of late gestational period, J. Toxicol. Sci. 5:252-253.

Yonemoto, J., Naganuma, A., Suzuki, T., and Imura, N., 1983, Effects of vitamin E, glutathione and methylmercury on distribution and placental transfer of selenium in mice. Chemosphere (in press).

SESSION 6.   POSTNATAL ASPECTS OF THE METABOLISM OF METALS

Chairpersons: *Harold H. Sandstead and Richard A. Doherty*

SPECIFIC FEATURES OF METAL ABSORPTION IN SUCKLING ANIMALS

Krista Kostial

Institute for Medical Research and Occupational Health
Zagreb, Yugoslavia

ABSTRACT

The results obtained in rats and other animal species show differences in the pharmacokinetics and toxicity of lead, cadmium, mercury and manganese between suckling and weaned animals. Most of these differences are the result of specific features of metal metabolism in neonates: higher gastrointestinal absorption and lack of metal-metal interaction; different organ distribution, especially higher brain retention and higher gut retention of some metals. A higher acute toxicity, particularly after oral administration, is also likely to be the result of specific metal metabolism in this age group. These results indicate that the neonatal age represents a period of high risk for metal exposure.

INTRODUCTION

There are several indications that the neonatal age might be a period at increased risk of toxic metal exposure (Nordberg et al., 1978). This statement is mostly based on results obtained in experimental animals, since for ethical reasons, investigations in human neonates are rather limited. However, data from accidental poisonings as well as some epidemiological results support the assumption of increased susceptibility to metal poisoning in the human neonatal age (Ziegler et al., 1978; McCabe, 1979; Amin-Zaki et al., 1981). The increased susceptibility is likely to be the result of increased metal accumulation in the body, i.e., higher absorption, slower elimination and different organ distribution (Kostial et al., 1978) which is highly undesirable at the time of intense organ growth and development. Higher gastrointestinal

absorption of toxic metals is most probably the main reason for
increased body burden of metals in the very young (Kostial et al.,
1979b). Metal absorption from the gastrointestinal tract in the
neonatal period is so different from that in adult life that it
deserves special attention, especially as the knowledge of the
process involved in the absorption and transport of trace elements
in the body is generally very incomplete.

In this presentation, I am going to point out some of the
specific features of metal absorption in neonates. I shall present
data on the pharmacokinetics and toxicity of lead, cadmium, mercury
and manganese in rats of different age (mostly published and some
unpublished) obtained in the laboratory for Mineral Metabolism of
the Institute for Medical Research and Occupational Health in
Zagreb. Results obtained by other authors in newborn rats and other
animal species will also be discussed.

METHODS

All experiments were performed on random-bred albino rats from
our own animal house aged 1-54 weeks. Sucklings in litters reduced
to six one day after birth were kept in individual cages with their
mothers. Weaned rats and older animals (females) were housed in
plastic cages in groups of 10 to 15 animals per cage. They were fed
stock laboratory diet (1.2 percent Ca and 0.8 percent P). The milk-
fed animals received cow's milk several days before the beginning of
the pharmacokinetic studies. Trace elements were added to cow's
milk in concentrations of 100 ppm Fe, 50 ppm Zn, 200 ppm Mn and 20
ppm Cu as chlorides with the exception of iron which was added as
sulphate.

In pharmacokinetic studies, ^{203}Pb, ^{115m}Cd, ^{203}Pb, ^{203}Hg
and ^{54}Mn were given orally to sucklings by the method of
artificial feeding (Kostial et al., 1967) and to older animals by
gastric intubation or parenterally (intraperitoneally and
exceptionally, by intravenous injection). The radioisotopes of
cadmium, mercury and manganeses were supplied by the Radiochemical
Centre, Amersham, England, and those of lead by the Gustaf Werner
Institute, Uppsala, Sweden. The radioisotopes of lead and manganese
were almost carrier-free. The specific activity of ^{115}Cd and
^{203}Hg was about 0.5 µCi/mg. The retention in the whole body was
determined in a two-crystal scintillation counter 6-7 days
(exceptionally, earlier or later) after the radioisotope
administration. In some experiments, the carcass (whole body after
removal of the total gastrointestinal tract), gut (total
gastrointestinal tract contents included) and brain retentions were
also determined. In some experiments, the gut was divided into six
parts: the stomach, the small intestine, subdivided into three
sections of similar length - upper, middle and lower, and the large

intestine, subdivided into the caecum and the rest of the large intestine. The radioactivity of each gut section and its contents was determined in an automatic gamma counter. All results were corrected for radioactive decay and geometry of the samples. The whole body, carcass, gut and brain retentions were expressed as percentages of the dose. The radioactivity of gut sections was expressed as percentage of the total radioactivity of the gastrointestinal tract.

The toxicity of cadmium, mercury and manganese chloride was determined in animals of three different age groups (2, 3, 6 weeks). Metal chlorides were administered orally by a stomach tube or intraperitoneally in a volume of 1 ml per 200 g body weight. Six dose levels were used for each age group. Each dose level was tested on six animals. The LD_{50} values were calculated by the method of moving averages (Thompson and Weil, 1952) eight days after a single administration. The experimental results are presented on Tables. Only essential data are included (arithmetic means and the number of animals in brackets). References, whenever available are given for the results where more details, including statistical treatment of data for each experiment, can be found.

RESULTS

Effect of Age on Metal Retention and Distribution

The whole body retention of metals after oral administration of ^{203}Pb, ^{115m}Cd, ^{203}Hg and ^{54}Mn is presented in Table 1. In sucklings (one week old), the retention is very high. The values for lead range from 60 to 80, for cadmium from 20 to 40, for mercury from 50 to 70 and for manganese from 40 to 70 percent of the oral dose. At the age when animals start consuming rat food (about two weeks of age), the gastrointestinal absorption of metals suddenly drops to only a few percent of the oral dose or even lower. In 30 to 54-week-old rats, the whole body retention values for lead, cadmium and mercury range from 0.3 to about 2 percent. Manganese retention values are even lower (0.1 - 0.2 percent). The trend of decreasing absorption with increasing age is noticeable also after weaning, but this gradual decrease in absorption is very different from the sudden drop which occurs at the time of weaning.

The whole body retention of metals after intraperitoneal administration of ^{203}Pb, ^{115m}Cd ^{203}Hg and ^{54}Mn is presented in Table 2. When omitting the gastrointestinal tract and processes related to metal absorption - by administering metals intraperitoneally, a decrease in metal absorption with increasing age is also noticeable. It is, however, gradual and unrelated to the time of weaning. This indicates that the processes related to

K. KOSTIAL

Table 1   Whole Body Retention of ^{203}Pb, ^{115m}Cd, ^{203}Hg and ^{54}Mn
after Oral Administration: Percent Dose

Age Weeks	^{203}Pb % (n)[b] Ref.[c]			^{115m}Cd % (n) Ref.[c]			^{203}Hg % (n) Ref.[c]			^{54}Mn % (n) Ref.[c]		
1	57	(17)[a]	3	27	(24)	10	68	(18)	2	55	(11)	20
1	82	(54)[a]	4	39	(12)	11	38	(23)	1	40	(18)	1
1	-			35	(18)	12	53	(17)	15	67	(12)	16
1	-			30	(53)	13	73	(48)	13	65	(9)	17
1	-			20	(11)	2	48	(18)	12	-		
1	-			-			56	(18)	16	-		
1	-			-			50	(7)	17	-		
3	2.3	(8)	5	0.9	(10)	10	-		-	0.2	(10)	20
6	0.4	(10)	6	0.5	(10)	10	0.9	(10)	16	0.1	(11)	1
6	1.1	(18)	7	1.8	(18)	12	0.6	(6)	18	0.2	(10)	16
6	0.7	(8)	7	1.5	(12)	13	0.3	(14)	13	-		
6	0.4	(20)	8	-			0.7	(22)	19	-		
6	0.9	(12)	9	-			-			-		
16	0.6	(8)	5	0.6	(12)	11	0.9	(11)	1	0.1	(15)	20
54	-			0.3	(10)	10	-			0.1	(13)	20
54	-			0.5	(9)	14	-			-		

[a]Values obtained 3-4 days; (others 6-7 days) after
administration.
[b](n) = number animals.
[c]References.

1. Kostial et al., 1978
2. Kostial et al., 1979b
3. Kostial et al., 1971a

4. Kostial et al., 1971b
5. Kostial et al., 1973
6. Kostial and Kello, 1979
7. Jugo et al., 1975b
8. Kello and Kostial, 1973
9. Dekanic et al., 1975
10. Kello and Kostial, 1977a

11. Kostial et al., 1979a
12. Kostial et al., 1981
13. Kostial et al., personal communication
14. Rabar and Kostial, 1981a
15. Kostial et al., 1980a
16. Kostial et al., 1980b
17. Rabar and Kostial, 1981b
18. Kostial et al., 1979c
19. Kostial et al., 1981a
20. Rabar, 1976

the gastrointestinal absorption of metals in sucklings are the main
reason for high absorption of metals in this age group.

Age also influences metal distribution in the body. In earlier
experiments, we found higher metal values in the blood of sucklings

Table 2 Whole Body Retention of ^{203}Pb, ^{115m}Cd, ^{203}Hg and ^{54}Mn after Intraperitoneal Administration: Percent Dose

Age Weeks	^{203}Pb % (n)[b]	Ref.[c]	^{115m}Cd % (n)	Ref.[c]	^{203}Hg % (n)	Ref.[c]	^{54}Mn % (n)	Ref.[c]
1	-		97 (22)	24	87 (9)	2	93 (7)	1
1	-		93 (12)	11	-		-	
1	-		85 (9)	2	-		-	
1	-		96 (9)	21	-		-	
2	80 (9)	21	-		78 (6)[a]	25	-	
2	83 (9)	22	-		-		-	
3	61 (8)	5	-		-		43 (9)	20
6	54 (8)	8	82 (9)	10	57 (6)	18	29 (10)	1
18	37 (8)	5	82 (9)	11	56 (6)[a]	25	40 (10)	20
18	39 (15)	23	83 (18)	21	-		-	
18	42 (15)	22	-		-		-	
18	44 (10)	21	-		-		-	
54	-		72 (10)	24	-		44 (9)	20

[a]Values obtained 6-7 days after i.v. (others i.p.) administration.
[b](n) = number animals.
[c]References.

1. Kostial et al., 1978	20. Rabar, 1976
2. Kostial et al., 1979b	21. Kello and Kostial, 1978
5. Kostial et al., 1973	22. Jugo et al., 1975a
8. Kello and Kostial, 1973	23. Momcilovic and Kostial, 1974
10. Kello and Kostial, 1977a	24. Kello and Kostial, 1977b
11. Kostial et al., 1979c	25. Jugo, 1976
18. Kostial et al., 1979c	26. Kello et al., 1979a

(2-3 times for Pb, Hg, Cd and 6 times for Mn). Highest differences were found in brain retention in sucklings as compared to older rats (8 times for Pb, 19 for Hg and 28 for Mn) after intraperitoneal or intravenous administration of radioisotopes (Kostial et al., 1978). We obtained similar results after oral administration of ^{115m}Cd and ^{203}Hg. The brain retention in sucklings was always much higher than in weaned animals (Table 3). We also found differences in gut retention of metals, but these results will be presented later on.

Table 3   Effect of Age on ^{115m}Cd and ^{203}Hg Retention in the
Brain after Oral Administration: Percent Dose[a]

Age weeks	^{115m}Cd %	(n)[b]	Ref.[c]	^{203}Hg %	(n)[b]	Ref.[c]
1	0.05	(9)	15	0.18	(7)	15
1	0.05	(53)	13	0.22	(48)	13
6	0.001	(12)	13	0.001	(14)	13

[a]Values obtained 6-7 days after administration.
[b](n) = number animals.
[c] See references, Table 1.

Similar results were obtained by other authors not only in rats, but also in other animal species. Higher gastrointestinal absorption of cadmium, lead and manganese was reported in suckling rats, guinea pigs, pigs and calves (Forbes and Reina, 1972; Carter et al., 1974; Sasser and Jarboe, 1977, 1980; Quaterman and Morrison, 1978; Cahill et al., 1980; Rehnberg et al., 1980). The absorption of some other elements like Zr, Nb, Ce, Sr, Ba, and Ra was also higher in sucklings of various animal species (Taylor et al., 1962; Inaba and Lengemann, 1972; Shiraishi and Ishikawa, 1972; Mraz and Eisele, 1977; Eisele et al., 1980). Higher absorption of essential trace elements is also known to occur at this age (Bremner and Mills, 1981).

Higher brain retention and slower elimination in suckling rats and mice have been reported by various authors for Hg, Cd, Pb and Mn (Miller et al., 1975; Thomas and Smith, 1979; Mykkanen et al., 1979; Deskin et al., 1980; Wong et al., 1980; Wong and Klaassen, 1980; Klein and Koch, 1981).

The Effect of Milk Diet and Trace Element Additives on Gastrointestinal Absorption of Metals

Since milk is the only food of the very young, we assumed that milk might be one of the reasons for high intestinal absorption in neonates. Indeed, older animals on milk diet had higher absorption values of all metals (Table 4) than animals on control diet (Table 1). However, the absorption of metals in milk-fed weaned rats was never as high as in sucklings. This indicates that milk diet cannot be the only cause of increased metal absorption in sucklings.

Table 4   Effect of Milk on Whole Body Retention of ^{203}Pb, ^{115m}Cd and ^{203}Hg after Oral Administration: Percent Dose

Age weeks	^{203}Pb % (n)[b]	Ref.[c]	^{115}Cd % (n)[b]	Ref.[c]	^{203}Hg % (n)[b]	Ref.[c]
1	70 (71)a		35 (118)a		55 (139)a	
3	-		17 (11)	10	-	
6	23 (24)	8	7 (10)	10	3 (21)	19
6	17 (8)	6	8 (18)	14	3 (6)	18
18	-		-		7 (11)	1
52	-		6 (8)	10	-	

[a]Approximate mean from Table 1.
[b](n) = number animals.
[c]See references, Table 1.

Higher absorption in older rats on milk diet was found for Hg, Cd, Ra, Ce, Pu and some other elements by several authors (Taylor et al., 1962; Inaba and Lengemann, 1972; Sikov and Mahlum, 1972; Engstrom and Nordberg, 1978; Landry et al., 1979).

We tried to reduce the high absorption of toxic metals by adding essential trace elements to milk. The concentration of essential trace elements in milk is relatively low and they are known to compete with toxic metals for the same sites in the absorption process.

We found that the absorption of metals in suckling rats cannot be decreased by the addition of iron to milk, while similar addition of iron successfully reduced lead, cadmium and mercury absorption in weaned rats (Kostial et al., 1980a). We tried to reduce absorption by means of several other trace element additives (Mn, Zn, Fe, Cu), single or combined but again were unsuccessful. The exception was the reduction in ^{54}Mn absorption in sucklings receiving stable manganese additives in milk (Table 5).

This indicates the existence of a homeostatic control of manganese at this age which, however, appears to be rather inadequate. Namely, a very high manganese concentration in milk, i.e., 200 ppm, decreases the retention of orally-administered ^{54}Mn only 10 times. Inadequate or non-existing homeostasis in the very young was confirmed by other studies, e.g., for calcium, (Kostial et al., 1967), zinc (Momcilovic, 1978), iron (Gruden, 1980), and zinc

Table 5   Effect of Trace Element Additives to Milk on Whole Body Retention of ^{115m}Cd, ^{203}Hg and ^{54}Mn after Oral Administration: Percent Dose[a]

Age weeks	TE ppm	^{115m}Cd % (n)[b]	^{203}Hg % (n)[b]	^{54}Mn % (n)[b]	Ref.[c]
1	-	28 (9)	56 (18)	67 (12)	16
1	-	17 (9)	50 (7)	65 (9)	17
1	100 Fe	31 (9)	58 (18)	62 (11)	16
1	200 Mn	22 (9)	42 (7)	7 (9)	17
1	200 Mn, 100 Fe	27 (9)	38 (7)	7 (9)	17
1	50 Zn	26 (9)	45 (7)	63 (9)	17
1	50 Zn, 100 Fe	23 (8)	47 (7)	61 (9)	17
1	200 Mn, 100 Fe 50 Zn, 20 Cu	31 (9)	45 (7)	5 (9)	17
6	-	7 (8)	7 (9)	19 (11)	16
6	100 Fe	3 (9)	2 (10)	2 (12)	16

[a]Values obtained 6-7 days after administration.
[b](n) = number animals.
[c]See references, Table 1.

and manganese (Kirchgessner et al., 1981) in suckling rats. It may therefore be considered as a general characteristic of metal metabolism in neonates as discussed elsewhere (Kostial et al., 1979b). Our data also indicate that there are differences in metal-metal interaction between sucklings and older rats.

The Effect of Age on Intestinal Retention of Metals

We determined the gut retention of metals after oral administration to elucidate better the mostly unknown mechanism of metal absorption in the neonatal period. We noticed great differences in the gut retention of some metals between sucklings and weaned rats. The high absorption of lead and manganese in sucklings was almost entirely related to high carcass retention (80 - 90 percent) and only a small fraction of the oral dose was retained in the gut (10 to 20 percent) (Kostial et al., 1971b; 1980b). The increased whole body retention of ^{115m}Cd and ^{203}Hg in sucklings showed a different body distribution. Carcass retention represented only 20-40 percent and gut retention 60-80 percent of the dose (Table 6). In weaned rats, this distribution changed and

Table 6   Carcass and Gut Retention of ^{115m}Cd and ^{203}Hg Six
Days after Oral Administration: Percent Dose

Age weeks	Number animals	C[a] %	G %	G/WB	Ref.[b]
		^{115m}Cd			
1	53	9	20	69	13
1	11	9	11	55	2
1	8	13	21	62	12
1	9	5	22	81	15
6	18	1.5	0.2	12	12
6	12	1.3	0.2	13	13
		^{203}Hg			
1	48	22	52	70	13
1	18	13	54	81	11
1	18	10	40	80	12
1	18	23	33	59	15
1	7	12	41	77	26
6	6	0.6	0.06	9	17
6	22	0.6	0.10	14	18
6	14	0.3	0.05	14	13

[a]C - whole body after removal of total
gastrointestinal tract; G - total gastrointestinal
tract, content included; WB - whole body = C+G.
[b]See references, Tables 1, 2.

most of the oral dose of cadmium and mercury (90 percent) was
retained in the carcass. Only a small fraction of about 10 percent
was retained in the gut.

Higher gut retention and longer residence time was found in
suckling rats, pigs and guinea pigs for several metals (Cd, Ce, Nb,
Hg) by various authors (Inaba and Lengemann, 1972; Mraz and Eisele,
1977; Sasser and Jarboe, 1977; 1980; Asokan and Tandon, 1981; Cain
and Webb, 1982).

We also tried to determine the site of cadmium and mercury
retention in the gastrointestinal tract of sucklings rats. The
results presented in Table 7 show that the site of mercury and
cadmium retention in the intestine is an age and element-specific
process. The highest ^{203}Hg and ^{115m}Cd radioactivity was located

Table 7   Retention of ^{203}Hg and ^{115m}Cd in the Intestinal Tract
          Six Days after Oral Administration

Compartment	Suckling		Weanlings	
	n = 48	^{203}Hg n = 14		
Stomach	1[a]	10[b]	18[a]	4[b]
SI upper	1	40	7	3
middle	12	49	10	4
lower	60	293	11	4
LI caecum	13	175	26	8
lower	14	106	28	16
	n = 53	^{115m}Cd n = 12		
Stomach	5[a]	13[b]	14[a]	3[b]
SI upper	22	88	34	14
middle	14	70	27	9
lower	39	268	17	6
LI caecum	8	108	3	1
lower	14	128	5	3

[a]Percent radioactivity of the total G.I. tract.
[b]Percent radioactivity of the total G.I. tract per mg
  of wet weight of tissue.
  SI = small intestine; LI = large intestine.
  Results partially presented (Kostial, 1982).

in the ileum (lower small intestine), regardless of whether the
results are expressed as percentage of the total gastrointestinal
retention or as percentage of the total gastrointestinal
radioactivity per gram of wet tissue. The ileum, however, was not
the main site of cadmium and mercury retention in weaned rats.

The Effect of Age on Acute Toxicity of Metals

Acute metal toxicity decreased with age (Table 8). This effect
was much more pronounced after oral than after intraperitoneal
administration. The effect was especially striking for cadmium
chloride. In suckling rats, the toxicity of cadmium after oral
administration was only slightly lower than after intraperitoneal
administration.

Table 8 Toxicity of Cadmium, Mercury and Manganese Eight Days
         after Single Oral or Intraperitoneal Administration (LD$_{50}$
         Values mg/kg)

Age weeks	CdCl$_2$ p.o.	i.p.	HgCl$_2$ p.o.	i.p.	MnCl$_2$ p.o.	i.p.
2	47[a]	11[b]	35[a]	2[c]	804[a]	84[c]
2	16[a]	8[b]	-	-		
3	240[b]	12[b]	105[a]	6[c]	1860[a]	123[c]
6	211[b]	9[b]	92[a]	4[c]	1712[a]	197[c]

[a]Kostial et al., 1978.
[b]Kostial et al., 1979a.
[c]Maljkovic, 1982.

The results also indicate that changes in the gastrointestinal
absorption of metals related to age are mainly responsible for
higher oral toxicity to metals in sucklings.

DISCUSSION

The intestinal absorption of metals may be considered to depend
on two separate steps: one is the uptake and binding to intestinal,
tissue, and the other is transported from the tissue to the
circulatory system. The first step in neonates, i.e., the mucosal
uptake from the lumen, could occur by pinocytosis. Whether there is
any mechanism for the pericellular transfer of metals through the so
called "tight junctions" in the intestinal wall is still uncertain
(Bremner and Mills, 1981). Pinocytosis, i.e., the absorption of
macromolecules (Lecce, 1972), lasts in sucklings only until "closure"
time of the intestinal mucosa at about the time of weaning. Heavy
metals could form insoluble colloids at intestinal pH, and as a
result, a nonspecific pinocytosis might occur. Since the carrier-
mediated part of the metal transport depends on the maturation
process - this might be an additional reason for different
metal-metal interactions in sucklings as compared to adults. In our
experiments, the ileum was the main site of intestinal cadmium and
mercury retention in sucklings but not in weaned rats. Similar
results were obtained by Gallagher and co-workers (Gallagher et al.,
1973) for iron. The role of the ileum could be explained by the
morphology of the lining epithelium which is characterized by the
presence of pinocytotic vacuoles. However, differences in the site
of cadmium and mercury retention in the ileum of suckling rats

(Kostial, 1982) indicate that a cation-specific process might be involved in metal absorption in neonates even before the "closure" of the intestine.

The effect of milk diet could be explained in several ways: by the presence of milk binding-ligands - as found for zinc by Duncan and Hurley (1978); by higher fat content which increases metal absorption - as found for lead by Barltrop and Khoo (1979); by the presence of lactose which facilitates intestinal absorption of metals - as found for lead by Bushnell and DeLuca (1981); by the lower level of trace elements as assumed by Kello and Kostial (1977a) and Engstrom and Nordberg (1978); by an increase in absorption efficiency known to occur when liquid diets are given; by abrasive action of solid food (Bremner and Mills, 1981); etc.

Differences in metal distribution in relation to age could be attributed to the immaturity of certain organs, i.e., differences in brain retention to the immaturity of the blood-brain barrier. It is known that the neurotoxic effects are most sensitive in the perinatal organism, i.e., at the time when blood-brain barrier permeability enhances the action of several metals.

Differences in metal metabolism between sucklings and adults could be due to metal-binding ligands. Considerable effort is now being expanded on the study of the role of metallothionein and its involvement in the metabolism of essential and non-essential elements. The wide distribution of metallothionein in animal tissue, and the fact that several metals induce its synthesis, indicate a fundamental role of this protein in metal metabolism (Bremner and Mills, 1981). Metallothioneins were found to be higher in newborn than in older rats (Bell, 1980; Asokan and Tandon, 1981; Bakka and Webb, 1981). The intestinal copper complex and the hepatic zinc-thionein complex of the neonatal rat are supposed to provide immediately available - high-affinity binding sites for foreign cations such as cadmium and mercury (Webb and Cain, 1982). However, it was also found that metallothioneins do not play a major role in tissue distribution and retention of cadmium (Johnson and Foulkes, 1980; Wong and Klaassen, 1980) and that metallothioneins in the intestinal mucosa do not serve as a determinant of cadmium absorption (Kello et al., 1979a). According to Sasser and Jarboe (1977), much of the cadmium retained in the intestine of the newborn is bound to a copper complex. Cain and Webb (1982) assume that this is also true for mercury in neonates. The intestinal copper complex, however, does not bind lead (Cain and Webb, 1982). This is in agreement with our results that the high absorption of lead in suckling rats is almost entirely due to increased body retention without an increased gut retention (Kostial et al., 1971b). The higher retention of some metals in the gut might be a "protective mechanism" which prevents higher body accumulation of metals in the neonatal age. However, there are several other factors which should

be considered. Although the half-life of cadmium and mercury in
the gut of neonates is relatively short (Kostial et al., 1979b), a
part of this fraction is transferred to other parts of the body and
increases the already high body burden of metals in other organs.
High accumulation of metals (cadmium) in the gut might cause
depressed intestinal activity, cytotoxicity and enteropathy
(Richardson and Fox, 1974; Sasser and Jarboe, 1977). The gut
retention of toxic metals might also influence the intestinal
transport of essential elements causing deficiencies which are
highly undesirable in the immature. The high oral toxicity of
metals (especially cadmium) in neonates also indicates that the high
gut retention of metals at this age might not necessarily be a
protective mechanism.

It might be concluded that the results obtained by us and other
authors show age-related differences in the pharmacokinetics and
toxicity of several metals. Most of these differences are the
result of specific features of metal metabolism in the neonatal
period. Specific features of metal absorption are characterized by
higher gastrointestinal absorption, lack of metal-metal interaction
and higher gut retention of some metals. Different body distribution
is characterized by markedly higher brain retention in sucklings -
which might be the cause of neurotoxic effects of metals in this age
group. The higher acute toxicity of metals is most probably also
the result of specific metal metabolism in this age group. On the
basis of these findings, it seems reasonable to conclude that the
neonatal age represents a period of high risk for metal exposure.

ACKNOWLEDGEMENTS

My thanks are due to the scientific and technical staff of the
Laboratory for Mineral Metabolism of the Institute for Medical
Research and Occupational Health in Zagreb for their help and
enthusiasm in carrying out these investigations. My special thanks
are due to Mrs. M. Horvat for her valuable help in preparing this
manuscript.

This work was partly supported by a research grant from the
Scientific Council of Croatia and the Environmental Protection
Agency, USA.

REFERENCES

Amin-Zaki, L., Majeed, M.A., Greenwood, M.R., Elhassani, S.B.,
     Clarkson, T.W. and Doherty, R.A., 1981, Methylmercury poisoning
     in the Iraqi suckling infant: A longitudinal study over five
     years, J. Appl. Toxicol. 1:210-214.

Asokan, P. and Tandon, S.K., 1981, Effect of cadmium on hepatic metallothionein level in early development of the rat., Environ. Res. 24:201-206.

Bakka, A. and Webb, M., 1981, Metabolism of zinc and copper in the neonate: changes in concentrations and contents of thionein-bound Zn and Cu with age in the livers of the newborn of various mammalian species, Biochem. Pharmacol. 30:721-726.

Barltrop, D. and Khoo, H.E., 1979, The influence of dietary minerals and fat on the absorption of lead, Sci. Total Environ. 6:265.

Bell, J.U., 1980, Induction of hepatic metallothionein in the immature rat following administration of cadmium, Toxicol. Appl. Pharmacol. 54:148-155.

Bremner, I. and Mills, C.F., 1981, Absorption, transport and tissue storage of essential trace elements, Phil. Trans. R. Soc. Lond. B294:75.

Bushnell, P.J. and DeLuca, H.F., 1981, Lactose facilitates the intestinal absorption of lead in weanling rats, Science 211:61-63.

Cahill, D.F., Bercegeay, M.S., Haggerty, R.C., Gerding, J.E. and Gray, L.E., 1980, Age-related retention and distribution of ingested Mn_3O_4 in the rat, Toxicol. Appl. Pharmacol. 53:83-91.

Cain, K. and Webb, M., 1982, Metallothionein and its relationship to the toxicity of cadmium and other metals in the young, in: "Proceedings of the Symposium on the Health Evaluation of Heavy Metals in Infant Formula and Junior Food", Berlin, 1981, (in press), Springer Verlag, Berlin.

Carter, C.J., Miller, W.F., Neathery, M.W., Gentry, R.P., Stake, P.E. and Blackman, D.M., 1974, Manganese metabolism with oral and intravenous [54]Mn in young calves as influenced by supplemental manganese, J. Anim. Sci. 38:1284.

Dekanic, D., Maljkovic, T. and Kostial, K., 1975, Tetracyclines and lead metabolism in rats, Arch. Toxicol. 33:169.

Deskin, R. Bursian, S.J. and Edens, F.W., 1980, Neurochemical alterations induced by manganese chloride in neonatal rats, Neurotoxicol. 2:65.

Duncan, J.R. and Hurley, L.S., 1978, Intestinal absorption of zinc: a role for a zinc-binding ligand in milk, Am. J. Physiol. 235:556.

Eisele, G.R., Mraz, F.R., Woody, M.C., 1980, Gastrointestinal uptake of [144]Ce in the neonatal mouse, rat and pig, Health Phys. 39:185-192.

Engstrom, B. and Nordberg, G., 1978, Effects of milk diet on gastrointestinal absorption of cadmium in adult mice, Toxicol. 9:195.

Forbes, G.B. and Reina, J.C., 1972, Effect of age on gastrointestinal absorption (Fe, Sr, Pb) in the rat, J. Nutr. 102:647-652.

Gallagher, N.D., Mason, R. and Foley, K.E., 1973, Mechanism of iron absorption and transport in neonatal rat intestine, Gastroenterology 64:438-444.

Gruden, N., 1980, Body retention and tissue distribution of ^{59}Fe and ^{54}Mn in newborn rats fed iron-supplemented cow's milk, Reprod. Nutr. Develop. 20(5A):1539.

Inaba, J. and Lengemann, F.W., 1972, Intestinal uptake and whole body retention of ^{141}Ce by suckling rats, Health Phys. 22:169-175.

Johnson, D.R. and Foulkes, E.C., 1980, On the proposed role of metallothionein in the transport of cadmium, Environ. Res. 21:360-365.

Jugo, S., 1976, Retention and distribution of ^{203}HgCl$_2$ in suckling and adult rats, Health Phys. 30:240-241.

Jugo, S., Maljkovic, T. and Kostial, K., 1975a, The effect of chelating agents on lead excretion in rats in relation to age, Environ. Res. 10:271.

Jugo, S., Maljkovic, T. and Kostial, K., 1975b, Influence of chelating agents on the gastrointestinal absorption of lead, Toxicol. Appl. Pharmacol. 34:359-263.

Kello, D. and Kostial, K., 1973, The effect of milk on lead metabolism in rats, Environ. Res. 6:355.

Kello, D. and Kostial, K., 1977a, Influence of age and milk diet on cadmium absorption from the gut, Toxicol. Appl. Pharmacol. 40:277-282.

Kello, D. and Kostial, K., 1977b, Influence of age on whole body retention and distribution in suckling and adult rats, Environ. Res. 14:92-98.

Kello, D. and Kostial, K., 1978, Lead and cadmium in hair as an indicator of body burden in rats of different age, Bull. Environ. Contam. Toxicol. 20:618-623.

Kello, D., Dekanic, D., Kostial, K., 1979a, Influence on sex and dietary calcium on intestinal cadmium absorption in rats, Arch. Environ. Health 34:30-33.

Kello, D., Sugawara, N., Voner, C. and Foulkes, E.C., 1979b, On the role of metallothionein in cadmium absorption by rat jejunum in situ, Toxicol. 14:199-208.

Kirchgessner, M., Weigand, E. and Schwarz, F.J., 1981, Absorption of zinc and manganese in relation to age, in: "Trace Elements in Man and Animals", J. McHowell, J.J. Ganthorne, and C.L. White, eds., p. 125, Australian Academy of Science, Camberra, Perth.

Klein, A.W. and Koch, T.R., 1981, Lead accumulation in brain, blood and liver after low dosing in neonatal rats, Arch. Toxicol. 47:257.

Kostial, K., 1982, The absorption of heavy metals by the growing organism - experimental experience with animals, in: "Proceedings of the Symposium on Health Evaluation of Heavy Metals in Infant Formula and Junior Food", Berlin 1981, (in press) Springer Verlag, Berlin.

Kostial, K. and Kello, D., 1979, Bioavailability of lead in rats
     fed "human" diets, Bull. Environ. Contam. Toxicol. 21:312-314.

Kostial, K., Simonovic, I. and Pisonic, M., 1967, Effect of calcium
     phosphate on gastrointestinal absorption of strontium and
     calcium in newborn rats, Nature, London 215:1181-1182.

Kostial, K., Simonovic, I. and Pisonic, M., 1971a, Lead absorption
     from the intestine in newborn rats, Nature, London 233:561-564.

Kostial, K., Simonovic, I. and Pisonic, M., 1971b, Reduction of lead
     absorption from the intestine in newborn rats, Environ. Res.
     4:360.

Kostial, K., Kello, D. and Harrison, G.E., 1973, Comparative
     metabolism of lead and calcium in young and adult rats, Int.
     Arch. Arbeitsmed. 31:179.

Kostial, K., Rabar, I., Blanusa, M. and Landeka, M., 1979a,
     Influence of age on heavy metal absorption, Proc. Nutr. Soc.
     38:251-256.

Kostial, K., Rabar, Ciganovic, M. and Simonovic, I., 1979b, Effect
     of milk on mercury absorption and gut retention in rats, Bull.
     Environ. Contam. Toxicol. 23:566-571.

Kostial, K., Rabar, I., Blanusa, M. and Ciganovic, M., 1980a, The
     influence of trace elements on cadmium and mercury absorption
     in sucklings, Bull. Environ. Contam. Toxicol. 23:566-571.

Kostial, K., Rabar, I., Blanusa, M. and Simonovic, I., 1980b, The
     effect of iron additive to milk on cadmium, mercury and
     manganese absorption in rats, Environ. Res. 22:40-45.

Kostial, K., Blanusa, M., Rabar, I. and Simonovic, I., 1981a, More
     data on mercury absorption in relation to dietary treatment in
     rats, Toxicol. Lett. 7:201.

Kostial, K., Simonovic, I., Rabar, I. and Landeka, M., 1981b, Effect
     of rat's diet on ^{85}Sr, ^{115m}Cd and ^{203}Hg absorption in
     suckling rats, Environ. Res. 25:281-285.

Kostial, K., Kello, D., Jugo, S., Rabar, I and Maljkovic, T, 1978,
     The influence of age on metal metabolism and toxicity, Environ.
     Health Perspect. 25:81-86.

Kostial, K., Kello, D., Blanusa, M., Maljkovic, T. and Rabar, I.,
     1979, Influence of some factors on cadmium pharmacokinetics and
     toxicity, Environ. Health Perspect. 28:89-95.

Landry, T.D., Doherty, R.A. and Gates, A.H., 1979, Effects of three
     diets on mercury excretion after methylmercury administration,
     Bull. Environ. Contam. Toxicol. 2:151-158.

Lecce, J.G., 1972, Selective absorption of macromolecules into
     intestinal epithelium and blood by neonatal mice, J. Nutr.
     102:69-76.

Maljkovic, T., 1982, Effect of coal gasifier ash on the toxicity of
     some metals, Ph.D. Thesis, University of Zagreb, Zagreb.

McCabe, E.B., 1979, Age and sensitivity to lead toxicity: A review,
     Environ. Health Perspect. 29:29-33.

Miller, S.T., Cotzias, G.C. and Evert, H.A., 1975, Control of tissue
     manganese; initial absence and sudden emergence of excretion in
     the neonatal mouse, Am. J. Physiol. 229:1080-1084.

Momcilovic, B., 1978, Effect of zinc added to milk on ^{65}Zn absorption in newborn rats, Period. Biol. 80:141.

Momcilovic, B. and Kostial, K, 1974, Kinetics of lead retention and distribution in suckling and adult rats, Environ. Res. 80:214.

Mraz, F.R. and Eisele, G.R., 1977, Gastrointestinal absorption of ^{95}Nb by rats of different ages, Radiat. Res. 69:591.

Mykkanen, H.M., Dickerson, J.W.T. and M.C. Lancaster, 1979, Effect of age on the tissue distribution of lead in the rat, Toxicol. Appl. Pharmacol. 51:447-454.

Nordberg, G.F., Fowler, B.A., Friberg, L., Jernelov, A., Nelson, N., Piscator, M., Sanstead, H., Vostal, J. and Vouk, V.B., 1978, Factors influencing metabolism and toxicity of metals: a consensus report, Environ. Health Perspect. 25:3-41.

Quaterman, J. and Morrison, E., 1978, The effect of age on the absorption and excretion of lead, Environ. Res. 17:78-83.

Rabar, I., 1976, Effect of some factors on manganese metabolism in rats, M. Sc. Thesis, University of Zagreb, Zagreb.

Rabar, I., and Kostial, K., 1981a, Bioavailability of cadmium in rats fed various diets, Arch. Toxicol. 47:63.

Rabar, I. and Kostial, K., 1981b, Failure of trace element to decrease cadmium, mercury and manganese absorption in suckling rats, in: Proceedings in Life Science: "Industrial and Environmental Xenobiotics - Metabolism and Pharmacokinetics of Organic Chemicals and Metals", I. Gut, ed., p. 45, Springer Verlag, Berlin.

Rehnberg, G.L., Hein, J.F., Carter, S.D. and Laskey, J.W., 1980, Chronic manganese accumulation and distribution, J. Toxicol. Environ. Health 6:217-226.

Richardson, M.E. and Fox, M.R.S., 1974, Dietary cadmium and enteropathy in the Japanese quail - histochemical and ultrastructural studies, Lab. Invest. 31:722-731.

Sasser, L.B. and Jarboe, G.E., 1977, Intestinal absorption and retention of cadmium in neonatal rat, Toxicol. Appl. Pharmacol. 41:423-431.

Sasser, L.B. and Jarboe, G.E., 1980, Intestinal absorption and retention of cadmium in neonatal pigs compared to rats and guinea pigs, J. Nutr. 110:1641-1647.

Shiraishi, Y. and Ishikawa, R., 1972, Absorption and retention of ^{144}Ce abnd ^{95}Zr - ^{95}Nb in newborn, juvenile and adult rats, Health Phys. 22:373-378.

Sikov, M.R. and Mahlum, D.D., 1972, Plutonium in the developing animal, Health Phys. 22:707-712.

Taylor, D.M., Bligh, P.H. and Duggan, M.H., 1962, The absorption of calcium and radium from the gastronintestinal tract of the rat, Biochem. J. 83:25-29.

Thomas, D.J. and Smith, C., 1979, Distribution and excretion of mercuric chloride in neonatal rats, Toxicol. Appl. Pharmacol. 48:42-43.

Thompson, W.P. and Weil, C.S., 1952, Tables for convenient
     calculation of median effective dose (LD_{50} or ED_{50}) and
     instructions in their use, Biometrics 8:249.
Webb, M. and Cain, K., 1982, Functions of metallothionein, Biochem.
     Pharmacol. 31:137.
Wong, L. and Klaassen, C., 1980, Tissue distribution and retention
     of cadmium in rats during postnatal development: minimal role
     of hepatic metallothionein, Toxicol. Appl. Pharmacol.
     53:343-353.
Wong, K.L., Cachia, R. and Klaassen, C., 1980, Comparison of the
     toxicity and tissue distribution of cadmium in newborn and
     adult rats after repeated administration, Toxicol. Appl.
     Pharmacol. 56:317-325.
Ziegler, E.E., Edward, B.B., Jensen, R.L., Mahaffey, K.R. and Fomon,
     S.J., 1978, Absorption and retention of lead by infants,
     Pediat. Res. 12:29-34.

ARE DEVELOPMENTAL CHANGES IN METHYLMERCURY METABOLISM AND EXCRETION

MEDIATED BY THE INTESTINAL MICROFLORA?

Ian R. Rowland[1], Roy D. Robinson[2], Richard A. Doherty[2]
and Timothy D. Landry[3]

[1]British Industrial Biological Research Association
 Carshalton, Surrey, United Kingdom
[2]Environmental Health Sciences Center
 University of Rochester School of Medicine
 Rochester, New York
[3]Dow Chemical Company
 Midland, Michigan

ABSTRACT

Methylmercury, unlike mercuric mercury, is rapidly and almost completely absorbed from the mammalian gut, hence the body burden of mercury after exposure to methylmercury is related to the rate of mercury excretion. By comparison to adult mice, sucking mice excrete very little mercury after methylmercury exposure until the 16th-18th postnatal days, when there is an abrupt increase in fecal mercury excretion coinciding with the time of weaning. Several explanations of this developmental change in mercury elimination can be proposed, including an increase in biliary secretion of mercury compounds at weaning, changes in binding of mercury to gut contents or changes in the rate of demethylation of methylmercury by the intestinal microflora. It is probable that more than one of these factors are responsible but evidence is presented here to support the view that bacterial demethylation plays an important role. It is known that the majority of mercury in feces, after methylmercury exposure of adult animals, is in the mercuric form and that there is an increase in the amount of mercuric mercury in young mice at weaning when the rate of mercury elimination increases. The major changes in intestinal flora which occur during weaning are reflected in an increase in the ability of the gut contents of weaned mice to

demethylate methylmercury in vitro. Similarly, feces from neonatal
and preweaned human infants show negligible rates of methylmercury
demethylation in vitro by comparison to weaned infants and adults.
Further evidence for the implication of the gut flora in determining
rates of mercury excretion has been obtained by modification of the
gut flora by diet and antibiotics. We conclude that the conversion
of methylmercury to the poorly absorbed mercuric mercury by the
intestinal flora is a major factor determining excretion rate and
therefore body burden of mercury after methylmercury exposure.

INTRODUCTION

        The absorption and accumulation of many toxic metals are known
to change with the age of the animal and particularly significant
differences have been observed between neonatal and adult stages in
body burden and tissue concentrations of mercury, manganese, cadmium
and lead (Kostial et al., 1978; Jugo, 1976). In the immediate
postnatal period, a time characterised by marked changes in organ
function and development, mammals including humans appear to be more
susceptible to the toxic effects of metals, especially those
affecting behaviour, than when mature (Task Group on Metal
Interaction, 1978; Hastings et al., 1977; Mei and Okita, 1976;
Clarkson et al., 1981). The differences in metabolism and toxicity
of metals in neonates and adults may be due to a variety of
physiological factors, but the high intestinal absorption rate in
sucking animals, which appears to be non-specific and unable to
distinguish essential from toxic metals, is probably one of the most
important (Kostial et al., 1978; Forbes and Reina, 1972).

        Methylmercury is unusual among toxic metal compounds in being
rapidly and almost completely absorbed by the gut in adults as well
as infants (Miettinen, 1973; Walsh, 1982). Consequently, the
cumulative body burden of mercury after exposure to methylmercury is
determined not only by the duration and quantity of methylmercury
intake, but also by the rate of elimination of mercury by excretion,
the main route of which is via the feces.

        Dramatic differences have been found in the rate of excretion
of mercury in neonatal and weaned mice (Figure 1). When suckling
mice were given an oral dose of methylmercuric chloride, they
absorbed and retained the majority of the dose with a half-time of
mercury elimination greater than 100 days (Doherty and Gates,
1973). Older mice, given a similar dose of the organomercurial
excreted mercury much more rapidly (half time of mercury
elimination, approximately 6 days). This developmental change in
the rate of mercury excretion occurred abruptly at the 16-18th
postnatal days, coinciding with the time of weaning to a pelleted
rodent diet.

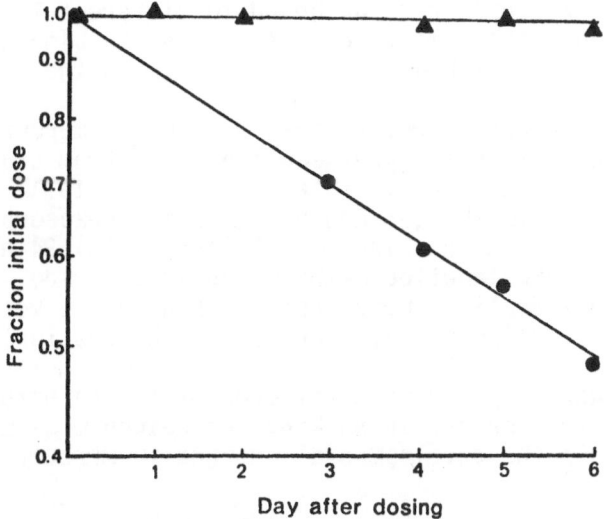

Figure 1   Body burden (fraction of initial dose) in groups of male
mice given a single oral dose of [203]Hg-labeled
methylmercuric chloride (0.4 mg Hg/kg). The body burden
was determined by whole body gamma counting. Dose given
at 2 days of age (▲) or 24 days of age (●).

POSSIBLE MECHANISMS RESPONSIBLE FOR DEVELOPMENTAL CHANGES IN RATE OF
MERCURY EXCRETION

1.   An increase in the Biliary Secretion of Mercury Compounds
     Coincident with Weaning

     In the adult rat after the almost complete absorption of an oral
dose of methylmercury, a proportion (0.5-3 percent in 2 hours) is
excreted in the bile. The majority (60-80 percent) of the mercury
in bile is found as methylmercury-glutathione complex, with about 20
percent apparently bound to a protein. A small proportion (4-5
percent) was found as protein-bound inorganic mercury (Ohsawa and
Magos, 1974; Norseth, 1973a; Klaassen, 1975; Norseth and Clarkson,
1971; Refsvik and Norseth, 1975). The methylmercury-glutathione
complex, or complexes derived from it by the action of pancreatic
enzymes (Hirata and Takahashi, 1981), is largely reabsorbed,
resulting in an enterophepatic circulation of mercury. Ballatori
and Clarkson (1982) have recently shown that pre-weanling rats
secrete much less methylmercury in bile than weaned animals. The
rate of secretion of mercury increases as the ability of the animal
to secrete glutathione in bile develops, eventually reaching the
adult level at 4 weeks of age. Biliary excretion of methylmercury
by mice has received little attention although Norseth (1973b) has

shown that mercury appears to be bound to different ligands in mouse and rat bile, and that time-dependent changes in binding of mercury in the bile are more marked in the mouse than in the rat.

There is evidence, however, that some methylmercury is deposited in the gut in the pre-weanling mouse from studies using a non-absorbable polythiol resin (Clarkson et al., 1971) which traps mercury secreted into the gut and prevents its reabsorption. When such a resin was fed to sucking mice (10 days old) 24 hours after a single dose of radio-labelled methylmercuric chloride, the body burden of mercury declined more rapidly than in pre-weanling mice not given the resin (Robinson, unpublished observation).

Thus, it would appear that differences in the extent of biliary excretion of methylmercury in sucking and weaned mice may only partially explain the developmental changes in mercury excretion.

2.   Changes in Binding of Mercury to Gut Contents

If mercury were more strongly bound to the gut contents of the weaned mice, then it would be expected that the fecal excretion would be higher in those animals than in pre-weaned mice. This possibility has not been explored in relation to the developmental changes, but in a study of factors responsible for the large diet-related differences in mercury excretion, we were unable to obtain any correlation of mercury excretion rate with concentrations of protein-bound or free sulphydryl groups in the small intestinal or caecum (Rowland et al., unpublished observations).

3.   Changes in Rate of Demethylation of Methylmercury

Mercuric mercury compounds, unlike methylmercury, are very poorly absorbed from the adult intestinal tract (Miettinen, 1973), so it is reasonable to postulate that, after an oral dose of methylmercury, any mercuric mercury deposited in the gut by demethylation would be excreted with the feces and not reabsorbed. The developmental changes in mercury elimination could then be explained by a low rate of demethylation of methylmercury in sucking animals which increases after weaning. Furthermore, under such conditions, the higher rate of absorption of metals by the sucking animal (see above) would ensure that any small amount of inorganic mercury produced by demethylation would be absorbed more quickly than in the adult.

There is a considerable amount of evidence to support the hypothesis that demethylation is a critical event affecting methylmercury elimination. It is known that the majority of mercury in feces after exposure of animals to methylmercury is in the mercuric form (Norseth and Clarkson, 1970; Rowland et al., 1980, Landry et al., 1979). It is also apparent that in the mouse, the formation of mercuric mercury after methylmercury exposure was much higher in 20-day-old animals than in pre-weanling animals of 4 or 10 days of age (Figure 2). Furthermore, when the 20-day-old animals were weaned (at 18 days), there was an increase in the amount of mercuric mercury formed which coincided with the abrupt change in rate of elimination of mercury (Figure 1). It should also be noted that the majority of the mercuric mercury in the 20-day-old mice was found in the feces (Figure 2).

SITES OF DEMETHYLATION OF METHYLMERCURY

There have been no systematic studies of the sites of methylmercury metabolism in mammalian tissues, although the liver has been suggested as a potential site of biotransformation (Norseth and Clarkson, 1970). However, the role of the intestinal microflora in biotransformation of methylmercury has received much attention and there is good evidence that it is a major site of demethylation. For example, Rowland et al. (1978) demonstrated a rapid rate of methylmercury metabolism by preparations of rat fecal and small intestinal contents and by cultures of bacteria from human feces.

The implication of the gut flora in demethylation of methylmercury provides an explanation for the developmental increase in methylmercury excretion since it can be postulated that changes in the composition of the microflora during development result in modification of the demethylating activity.

In the sucking mouse, the first organisms to colonize the gut are the lactobacilli and anaerobic streptococci which reach 10^9 cells/g feces. Other streptococci and enterobacteria are also found in similar numbers at around the twelfth postnatal day, but at the time of weaning, the latter groups diminish in number and an extremely heterogenous population of obligately anaerobic bacteria appear, including Fusobacterium and Eubacterium spp. and bacterioides (Schaedler, 1973). Similar dramatic changes in the gut microflora occur in the developing human infant. In the breast-fed baby, the fecal flora is dominated by bifidobacteria with bacteroides, enterobacteria and streptococci isolated less frequently and in lower numbers (Bullen et al., 1977; Tomkins et al., 1981). On weaning, the number of bacteroides in feces increases and clostridia are consistently isolated. These developmental changes in composition of gut flora are likely to engender great changes in metabolic activity in the gut, since relatively minor alterations in flora induced by dietary modifications in adult animals result in major alterations in enzyme activity (Wise et al., 1982).

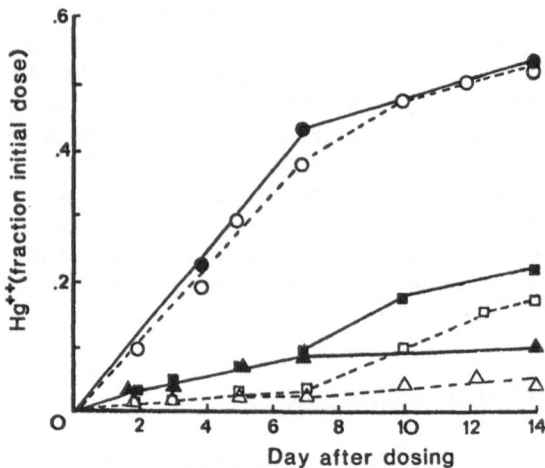

Figure 2 Formation of inorganic (mercuric) mercury after oral admini-
          stration of methylmercuric chloride (0.45 mg Hg/kg) to mice
          aged 4 (▲), 10 (■), or 20 (●) days. Cumulative total
          inorganic mercury (benzene non-extractable) was determined
          in whole body plus excreta. Cumulative fecal excretion of
          inorganic mercury (mean of two cages of mice each) of mice
          aged 4, (△), 10 (□), or 20 (○) days.

IN VITRO DEMETHYLATION STUDIES

To determine the capacity of the gut flora to demethylate
methylmercury, suspensions of cecal or colon contents from mice of
different ages were incubated under anaerobic conditions at 37°C with
^{203}Hg-labelled methylmercuric chloride in a medium buffered at pH
7.0 (Rowland et al., 1978). Samples of the incubation mixture were
removed at various times and the form of mercury present analyzed by
the benzene extraction method of Cappon and Smith (1977). Benzene-
extractable radioactivity was termed methylmercury and the benzene
non-extractable fraction termed inorganic or mercuric mercury.

When incubated with cecal contents from adult mice (3 months
old), methylmercuric chloride was rapidly demethylated and in 8
hours, 50 percent of the mercury in the incubation mixture was in the
inorganic form (Figure 3). Sterilization of the cecal preparation,
by filtration through a membrane filter or by antibiotics, completely
inhibited demethylation, indicating that bacteria were responsible
(Figure 3). Colon contents from 20-day-old (weaned) mice
demethylated methylmercuric chloride at rates similar to those in
adult animals, but colon contents from sucking mice (10 days old)
demethylated very slowly (Table 1).

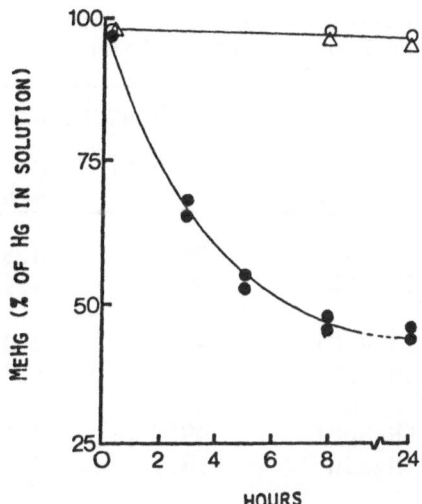

Figure 3   Rate of demethylation of [203]Hg-labelled methylmercuric
           chloride by cecal contents from adult mice (●) and the
           effect of sterilization of the cecal contents by antibiotics
           (○) or by passage through a 0.45 μm pore size, membrane
           filter (△). Cecal contents from 10 mice were pooled and
           suspended (0.1 g/ml) in medium (pH 7.0). Results of
           duplicate incubations are shown.

     Incubations of gut contents with methylmercury glutathione
(Ch$_3$HgGSH) were included, since this is the form of the
organomercurical which is initially excreted in bile. Clearly,
however, the intestinal bacteria from both the 10-day and 20-day-old
mice treated the mercurial in a similar fashion to methylmercury
chloride.

     These data correlate with the low rate of inorganic mercury
production in vivo by neonatal mice and the higher demethylation
rate seen in 24-day-old animals (Figure 2).

     To determine whether human infants showed similar age-related
changes in methylmercury demethylating activity in the gut, we
incubated freshly-collected cecal samples from babies, infants and
adults with radio-labelled methylmercury, as described above. Due
to the small number of samples, the data can only be considered
preliminary, but it can be seen that as with the neonatal mice,
fecal preparations from neonatal humans were unable to demethylate
methylmercury, nor could milk-fed, non-weaned infants (Table 2).
Upon weaning, however, the capacity to demethylate methylmercury
developed rapidly, the rate of demethylation being similar to that
seen in adults, although there was clearly a considerable variability
of demethylating activity after weaning.

Table 1   In Vitro Demethylation of ^{203}Hg-labelled Methylmercury by
         Cecal and Colon Contents of Sucking and Weaned Mice

Age of mice	Forms of Mercury	Benzene Extractable Hg		
		% Total ^{203}Hg in Solution at		
		0 hrs	24 hrs	48 hrs
10 days (sucking)	CH$_3$HgCl	98.1	93.5	91.7
	CH$_3$GSH	95.5	94.9	92.6
20 days (weaned)	CH$_3$HgCl	97.7	49.9	48.0
	CH$_3$GSH	97.8	45.9	42.3
Control (no gut contents)	CH$_3$HgCl	98.4	97.7	97.9
	CH$_3$GSH	98.1	97.7	47.4

Colon contents were suspended (10 percent w/v) in culture
medium (pH 7.0) and incubated under anaerobic conditions
with CH$_3$HgCl (0.5 µg/ml) at 37°C. At the times shown,
samples were removed and subjected to benzene extraction as
described by Cappon and Smith (1977). Values shown are the
results of single incubation from the pooled colon contents
of at least 6 mice.

The in vitro data indicate that the human neonate and infant
are unable to demethylate methylmercury in the gut, which, coupled
with a reduced biliary excretion rate, suggest that they excrete
methylmercury very slowly. Thus, their risk from methylmercury
accumulated in utero, or by sucking or other routes, may be greater
than expected under the assumption that their excretion rates are
similar to that of adults.

EFFECT OF MODIFICATION OF FLORA BY DIET AND ANTIBIOTICS ON
METHYLMERCURY ELIMINATION

The significance of the intestinal demethylation of
methylmercury to the tissue concentrations and toxicity of mercury
in the intact animal has been assessed by modifying the flora using
diet and antibiotics. We have previously shown that the feeding of
different diets markedly affects rate of excretion of mercury after
methylmercury exposure (Landry et al., 1979).

The developmental changes in gut flora seen on weaning can be
considered as a response to a major change in diet, from milk to a
solid, more complex diet. In theory, therefore, it should be

Table 2   In Vitro Demethylation of Methylmercury by Bacteria from Human Feces

Age	Sex	Diet	% Organic Hg after 24 hr Incubation
2 days	M or F	Breast milk and/or Formula milk	96.8* (SD 1.62)
4.5 months	M	Formula milk	90.0
8 months	F	Solid	28.9
10 months	M	Whole milk	87.8
4.5 years	F	Solid	18.0
33 years	M	Solid	62.0

Feces, collected as soon as possible after evacuation, were suspended (10 percent w/v) in culture medium (pH 7.0) and incubated under anaerobic conditions with $CH_3{}^{203}HgCl$ (0.5 g/ml) at 37°C.   After 24 hours, the incubation mixtures were extracted with benzene as described by Cappon and Smith (1977).
*Mean of 8 samples.

possible to modify the gut flora by dietary changes so that it becomes similar to that of the pre-weaning animal. Adult mice (3-months-old) changed from a pelleted rodent diet (Agway RMH 3000) to evaporated whole milk, showed marked qualitative and quantitative alterations in gut flora after only 10 days on the new diet (Table 3).

Although the milk diet did not induce a cecal flora identical to that of sucking mice, the ability of the flora to demethylate methylmercury in vitro was negligible by comparison to that of mice fed the pelleted rodent diet; after incubation of the cecal contents with ^{203}Hg-labelled methylmercuric chloride for 20 hours, the percent of mercury in solution in the organic form was 91 percent for the milk-fed mice and only 25 percent for the mice given the pelleted diet. Consumption of the evaporated milk diet also had a marked influence on the rate of whole body elimination of mercury after a single oral dose of methylmercuric chloride, increasing the half-time of elimination to 18.0 days, in comparison to 10.5 days for mice given the pelleted rodent diet (Figure 4; Landry et al., 1979).

Table 3   Effect of Diet on Mouse Cecal Microflora

Bacterial Group	Log_{10} Range of Viable Count	
	RMH 3000	Milk
Anaerobes	9.1 - 9.5	10.7 - 10.9
Lactobacilli	7.6 - 8.0	7.3 - 9.0
Streptococci	4.6 - 5.5	6.7 - 7.8
Enterobacteria	2.0 - 3.9	5.3 - 7.6
Staphylococci	3.0 - 3.7	3.8 - 5.2

Mice were fed either RMH 3000 or evaporated whole milk for 10 days and their cecal microflora analysed as described by Veilleux and Rowland (1981).

Furthermore, when the intestinal flora was eliminated by antibiotics (streptomycin, bacitracin and neomycin, 1 mg/day), thus completely inhibiting microbial demethylation in the gut, the rate of elimination of mercury was decreased still further and was similar in milk-fed and RMH 3000-fed mice (Figure 4). The rate of excretion of mercury in feces reflected the body burden data, the excretion rates being highest in feces from animals fed the pelleted diet and lowest in the animal given antibiotics (Figure 5). These data are consistent with the theory that the rate of intestinal demethylation of methylmercury is a major factor governing the rate of elimination of mercury. The lower rates of whole body elimination of mercury, in milk-fed mice and in those given antibiotics, resulted in higher tissue concentrations of mercury (Figure 6). For example, the mercury concentrations in brain and blood of milk-fed mice was increased by 21 percent and 38 percent, respectively, over the concentrations in RMH 3000-fed animals. Treatment of the RMH 3000-fed mice with antibiotics increased the mercury concentration in brain by 25 percent, in the liver by 66 percent, and in blood by 110 percent; the concentration in the kidney was not significantly affected.

Rowland et al. (1980) demonstrated the significance for methylmercury toxicity of the elimination of the gut flora in the rat. The incidence and severity of the clinical signs of neurotoxicity and of pathological damage to the cerebellum after methylmercury administration were much greater in rats given antibiotics (hence having a low rate of demethylation in the

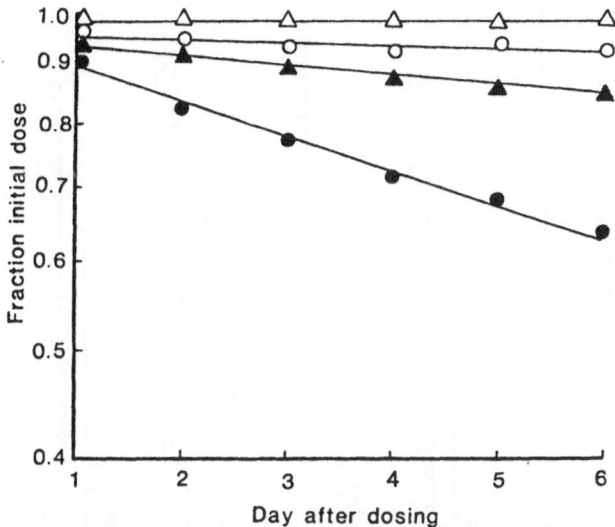

Figure 4   Body burden (fraction of initial dose) in female mice
(3-months-old) given a single oral dose of methylmercuric
chloride (0.5 mg Hg/kg).   Values shown are the means for 4
animals.   Mice were started on the milk diet and/or
antibiotics 7 days before dosing with methylmercury.   RMH
3000 fed (●); RMH 3000 + antibiotics (○); evaporated
whole milk fed (▲); evaporated whole milk + antibiotics
(△).

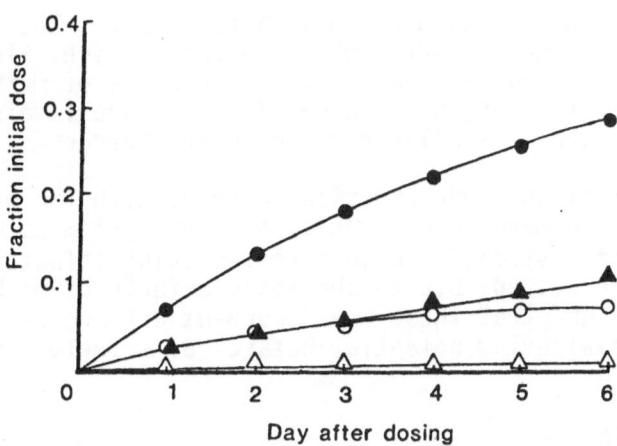

Figure 5   Cumulative fecal excretion of mercury in mice fed different
diets and given a single oral dose of methylmercuric
chloride (0.5 mg Hg/kg).   RMH 3000 (●); RMH 3000 +
antibiotics (○); milk (▲); milk + antibiotics (△).

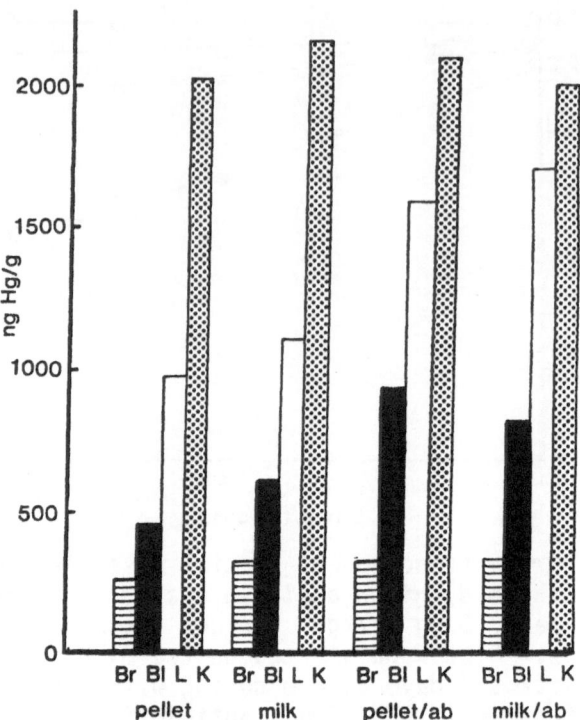

Figure 6   Tissue concentrations of mercury in mice given a single
           oral dose of methylmercuric chloride (0.4 mg/kg). Brain
           (Br); blood (Bl); liver (L); kidney (K).

intestine) than in rats with a conventional flora. The evidence
described above suggests that sucking infants, which, like
antibiotic-treated animals, have negligible rates of methylmercury
demethylation in the gut, would have higher tissue levels of mercury
than adults exposed to similar doses of methylmercury.

     The higher tissue concentrations coupled with the high
sensitivity of the developing central nervous system to damage by
neurotoxic agents, strongly suggest that sucking infants are
potentially more susceptible to the toxic effects of methylmercury
than are adults and that these age-dependent effects should be
considered in evaluating potential hazards of methylmercury exposure.

ACKNOWLEDGEMENTS

     We thank Donna Oberst and Frederick Genett for their excellent
technical assistance and NIEHS for financial support (NIEHS ES
01247, ES 1248, US/DOE EY 76C023490).

REFERENCES

Ballatori, N. and Clarkson, T.W., 1982, Developmental changes in the biliary excretion of methylmercury and glutathione, Science 261:61-63.

Bullen, C.L., Tearle, P.V. and Stewart, M.G., 1977, The effect of "humanized" milks and supplemented breast feeding on the focal flora of infants, J. Med. Microbiol. 10:403-413.

Cappon, C.J. and Smith, J.C., 1977, Gas chromatographic determination of inorganic mercury and organomercurials in biological materials, Anal. Chem. 49:365-369.

Clarkson, T.W., Small, H. and Norseth, T., 1971, The effect of a thiol containing resin on the gastro-intestinal absorption and fecal excretion of methylmercury compounds in experimental animals, Fed. Proc. 30:543.

Clarkson, T.W., Cox, C., Marsh, D.O., Myers, G.J., Al-Tikriti,S.J., Amin-Zaki, L. and Dabbagh, A.R., 1981, in: "Measurement of Risks", G.G. Berg and H.D. Mallie, eds., p.111-130, Plenum Press, New York.

Doherty, R.A. and Gates, A.H., 1973, Epidemic methylmercury poisoning: Application of a mouse model, Pediat. Res. 7:319.

Forbes, G.B. and Reina, J.C., 1972, Effect of age on gastro-intestinal absorption of Fe, Sr, and Pb in the rat, J. Nutr. 102:747-652.

Hastings, L., Cooper, G.P., Bornschein, R.L. and Michaelson, I.A., 1977, Behavioural effects of low level neonatal lead exposure, Pharmacol. Biochem. Behav. 7:37-42.

Hirata, E. and Takahashi, H., 1981, Degradation of methylmercury glutathione by the pancreatic enzymes in bile, Toxicol. Appl. Pharmacol. 58:483-491.

Jugo, S., 1976, Retention and distribution of $^{203}HgCl_2$ in suckling and adult rats, Health Phys. 30:240-241.

Klaassen, C.D., 1975, Biliary excretion of mercury compounds, Toxicol. Appl. Pharmacol. 33:356-365.

Kostial, K., Kello, D., Jugo, S., Rabar, I. and Maljkovic, T., 1978, Influence of age on metal metabolism and toxicity, Environ. Hlth. Perspect. 25:81-86.

Landry, T.D., Doherty, R.A. and Gates, A.H., 1979, Effects of three diets on mercury excretion after methylmercury administration, Bull. Environ. Contam. Toxicol. 22:151-158.

Mei, Q.S. and Okita, G.T., 1976, Behavioural effects on the progeny of mice treated with methylmercury, Toxicol. Appl. Pharmacol. 38:106-205.

Miettinen, J.K., 1973, Absorption and elimination of dietary mercury (Hg^{2+}) and methylmercury in man, in: "Mercury, Mercurials and Mercaptans", M.W. Miller and T.W. Clarkson, eds., p. 233-243, Charles C. Thomas, Springfield, IL.

Norseth, T., 1973a, Biliary excretion and intestinal reabsorption of mercury in the rat after injection of methylmercuric chloride, Acta Pharm. Toxicol. 33:280-288.

Norseth, T., 1973b, Biliary complexes of methylmercury, a possible role in organ distribution, in: "Mercury, Mercurials and Mercaptans", M.W. Miller and T.W. Clarkson, eds., p. 264-276, Charles C. Thomas, Springfield, IL.

Norseth, T. and Clarkson, T.W., 1970, Studies on the biotransformation of ^{203}Hg-labelled methylmercuric chloride in rats, Arch. Environ. Hlth. 21:717-727.

Norseth, T. and Clarkson, T.W., 1971, Intestinal transport of ^{203}Hg-labelled methylmercuric chloride, Arch. Environ. Hlth. 22:568-577.

Ohsawa, M. and Magos, L., 1974, The chemical form of methylmercury complex in the bile of the rat, Biochem. Pharmacol. 23:1903-1905.

Refsvik, T. and Norseth, T., 1975, Methylmercuric compounds in the bile, Acta Pharmacol. Toxicol. 36:67-78.

Rowland, I.R., Davies, M.J. and Grasso, P., 1978, Metabolism of methylmercuric chloride by the gastro-intestinal flora of the rat, Xenobiotica 8:37-43.

Rowland, I.R., Davies, M.J. and Evans, J.G., 1980, Tissue content of mercury in rats given methylmercuric chloride orally: influence of intestinal flora, Arch. Environ. Hlth. 35:155-160.

Schaedler, R.W., 1973, The relationship between the host and its intestinal microflora, Proc. Nutr. Soc. 32:41-47.

Task Group on Metal Interaction, 1978, Factors influencing metabolism and toxicity of metals: a consensus report, Environ. Hlth. Perspect. 25:3-41.

Tomkins, A.M., Bradley, A.K., Oswald, S. and Drasar, B.S., 1981, Diet and the fecal microflora of infants, children and adults in rural Nigeria and urban U.K., J. Hyg. Camb. 86:285-293.

Veilleux, B.G. and Rowland, I.R., 1981, Simulation of the rat intestinal ecosystem using a two-stage continuous culture system, J. Gen. Microbiol. 123:103-115.

Walsh, C.T., 1982, The influence of age on the gastrointestinal absorption of mercuric chloride and methylmercury chloride in the rat, Environ. Res. 27:412-420.

Wise, A., Mallett, A.K. and Rowland, I.R., 1982, Dietary fibre, bacterial metabolism and toxicity of nitrate in the rat. Xenobiotica, 12:111-118.

TRACE ELEMENT ABSORPTION IN INFANTS: POTENTIALS AND LIMITATIONS

Bo Lonnerdal and Carl L. Keen

Department of Nutrition
University of California
Davis, California

ABSTRACT

Bioavailability of trace elements from infant formulas is generally considered to be lower than that from human milk. Therefore, formulas are usually supplemented with trace elements in excess of concentrations normally found in human milk. Failure to provide adequate levels of the elements in the formula can result in deficiency states. Clinical cases of iron, zinc and copper deficiency during infancy due in part to consumption of formulas providing inadequate amounts of the elements have been reported. Caution should be taken when supplementing formulas, since excess amounts of one element can interfere with the absorption of another element. Formulas have been found to have widely varying trace element ratios, and the potential for interactions between Fe/Mn, Fe/Zn and Zn/Cu are discussed. To minimize the need for supplementing large amounts of an element, new modes of supplementation, including chelating agents as well as trace element binding proteins (such as lactoferrin for iron), which yield a high bioavailability, are necessary. Data from experiments using novel ligands are discussed.

INTRODUCTION

The importance of adequate nutrition during infancy is well recognized. This early period of an individual's life encompasses rapid growth and development. As a result, suboptimal intake of an essential nutrient(s) during this time period can have severe and pronounced effects on the infant's health and well-being. Despite the recognition of the essentiality of trace elements during this

759

period of development, deficiency cases of iron, copper or zinc are
frequently reported in infants and young children. The etiology of
the deficiency states can be separated into two broad classes: 1)
those which are due to a genetic error of metabolism and 2) those
which are the result of an insufficient or imbalanced dietary intake
of the element. Representative of the first class of deficiency
states would be the genetic disorders in humans - acrodermatitis
enteropathica, and Menkes' disease. The phenotypic expression of
acrodermatitis enteropathica mimics severe dietary zinc deficiency
while the phenotypic expression of Menkes' disease is analogous to
the signs of dietary copper deficiency. Both of these genetic
disorders, if untreated, can be lethal. The second class of
deficiency states can be subclassified into three categories: a)
dietary insufficiency due to a lack of the nutrient (primary
deficiency); b) the element is present in the diet at a
concentration that would normally be considered adequate, but other
factors in the diet restrict its bioavailability to the infant
(conditioned deficiency); and c) the level in the diet and its
bioavailability would normally be considered adequate but due to a
disease state (in particular those accompanied by diarrhea), the
nutrient uptake is still suboptimal (disease-induced deficiency).

In this paper, we will consider primarily the etiology of the
second class of deficiencies with particular reference to those
which occur as a result of primary deficiency or inadequate
bioavailability of the element. The conditioned deficiencies will
be discussed with emphasis on 1) differences in bioavailability due
to molecular localization of the elements from food normally
ingested during infancy (breast milk, cow milk, formula) and 2) on
potential deficiency induced by the excess ingestion of a nutrient
which will inhibit the absorption and/or utilization of another
nutrient. With this second type of interaction, a nutrient which is
fed at what normally would be considered a non-toxic level, may
actually have a toxicological effect through the induction of a
deficiency of another nutrient.

IRON NUTRITION

Without question, the trace element deficiency most commonly
recognized during infancy is that of iron. The incidence of
hemoglobin values lower than normal (<10.5-11.0) in infants iron-
responsive anemia in infants and young children has been reported to
be as high as 32 to 76 percent (Simmons and Gurney, 1982). The
nutritional explanation for this anemia is that while the term
infant is born with high tissue stores of iron, during the period of
rapid growth when the infant has a high requirement for the element,
the infant usually consumes milk and formulas which are low in iron.
Thus, when the iron stores of the infant are exhausted, the synthesis
of hemoglobin is compromised. Although the iron concentration of

breast milk and cow milk is similar (0.2 to 0.5 µg/l) (Lonnerdal et al., 1981a) (Figure 1), breast-fed infants do not develop iron deficiency anemia (defined by at least two criteria) as quickly as infants fed cow milk (Saarinen, 1978). The difference in onset and incidence of anemia has been suggested to be due primarily to a difference in the bioavailability of iron in these fluids, although this difference can be exacerbated by increased occult blood loss in infants fed cow milk. The bioavailability of iron from breast milk has been reported to be 50 percent or higher when using a radioisotope-labelling technique using an extrinsic tag (Saarinen et al., 1977; McMillan et al., 1977). Similar values are obtained when using an indirect method of calculating iron absorption by increases in total body content of iron (Saarinen and Siimes, 1979; Garry et al., 1981). In contrast to the high bioavailability of human milk iron, iron absorption in infants fed cow milk has been found to be around 10 percent. In our opinion, part of this difference in iron bioavailability is due to a difference in the localization of the element in these two fluids. In human milk, a significant part of iron (approximately 30 percent) is bound to lactoferrin, a protein which is present in very low concentration in cow milk. The remainder of the iron is bound to fat (~30 percent) and to low molecular weight compounds (~30 percent) (Fransson and Lonnerdal, 1980). In contrast, iron in cow milk is primarily bound to casein (~70 percent) and the remainder to fat (~15 percent) and whey (~10 percent) (Lonnerdal et al., 1981b). We have recently shown that iron bound to lactoferrin provided in a milk diet is highly

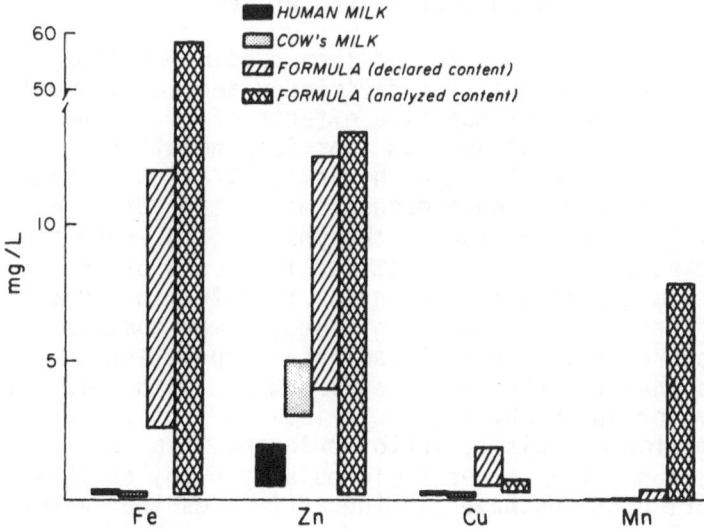

Figure 1   Trace element concentrations in human milk, cow milk and infant formula.

bioavailable when using animal models (Fransson et al., 1981). The bioavailability of iron bound to casein is not known; however, it can be postulated that, due to the high proportion of casein in cow milk, which is poorly digested and absorbed (Fomon, 1974), the element which is reported to be bound to casein would not be highly bioavailable, based on its association constant (Hegenauer et al., 1979). Therefore, the observed difference in bioavailability of iron from human and cow milk may be due in part to a combination of binding of iron to lactoferrin in human milk and the binding of iron to casein in cow milk. A facilitated uptake of iron from lactoferrin is supported by Cox et al. (1979).

Iron Supplementation: Benefits and Hazards

To compensate for the low bioavailability of iron in cow milk, formulas based on this fluid are supplemented with iron as ferrous sulphate. The level of supplementation used is generally stated to be 6 to 12 mg/l, although analyzed levels as high as 50 mg/l have been found for some formulas (Lonnerdal et al., 1981c) (Figure 1). The bioavailability of iron from the supplemented formulas has been reported to range from 4 to 10 percent (Saarinen et al., 1977), a fact which sometimes has been used by others to support the theory that iron absorption and retention by the infant from breast milk is always superior to that from formula. However, due to the level of supplementation, the net uptake of iron from the supplemented formula will exceed that from breast milk. Thus, the prevalence of iron deficiency in infants fed iron-supplemented formula is low (Saarinen, 1978). The localization of the supplemented iron in the milk formulas has not been well characterized.

While the supposed benefit of iron supplementation, that of reducing the prevalence of iron deficiency anemia, is well recognized, the potential negative effects of iron supplementation have received less attention. One possible negative effect of iron supplementation is that through the administration of high levels of the element, the host defense mechanisms of the infant may be compromised. This compromise is thought to occur when the level of iron supplementation is sufficient, or in excess of the amount needed, to saturate lactoferrin and/or transferrin. Under normal conditions, these two iron-binding proteins may compete for iron with siderophores released from bacterial populations. These siderophores chelate iron in the environment to increase its availability for uptake by the bacteria. As iron can be a limiting nutrient for microorganisms, lactoferrin and transferrin (if unsaturated) can act to prevent microbial growth, as these iron-transport proteins have binding affinities that allow them to withhold iron from the bacterial siderophores. Evidence that such a process may be occurring can be derived from several reports that have documented an increase in infections in children suffering from protein-energy malnutrition, following supplementation with iron. Several excellent reviews related to this topic have been published (Beisel, 1982; Bullen et al., 1978; Chandra et al., 1977). It should be emphasized that those studies showing a negative effect of iron supplementation on immunity have primarily dealt with children suffering from protein-energy malnutrition. Whether a similar negative effect of iron supplements occurs in well-nourished children is not known.

A second potential negative impact of iron supplementation is that high levels of this element may interfere with the absorption of other trace elements which have similar physico-chemical properties such as valency, orbital shells, coordination number, etc. Two essential elements which a have been shown to be affected by supplemental iron at the site of absorption are zinc and manganese. Direct competitive interaction of zinc and iron has been demonstrated in intestinal segments of rats in vivo and in vitro (Forth and Rummel, 1973). In the murine model system, a change in the iron:zinc molar ratio from 2.5:1 to 10:1 in the perfusate resulted in an inhibition of zinc absorption (Hamilton et al., 1978). Solomons and Jacob (1981) have reported that in human adults, changing the iron:zinc ratio from 1:1 to 3:1 can substantially inhibit zinc uptake. This effect, however, was observed only when the iron and zinc were given in salt forms. Thus, heme-iron and protein-bound zinc were not found to interact. In contrast to the observation of an interaction between iron and zinc in the above studies, others have found, in short-term experiments, that fortification of milk with iron has little effect on the uptake of zinc in rats (Momcilovic and Kello, 1977; Gruden and Momcilovic, 1979). We have also found that supplementation of milk with iron from an initial level of 1 mg/l to 6 mg/l, a level of supplementation recommended by the American Academy of Pediatrics for infant formulas (Committee on Nutrition of the American Academy of Pediatrics, 1976), has no effect on the zinc levels in tissues analyzed, even after feeding the respective diets for four weeks, while tissue iron levels were significantly affected (Fransson et al., 1982). A possible explanation for the different results in the above experiments is that while relative levels (molar ratio) of iron to zinc can be similar among studies, the absolute amount fed can differ considerably. Thus, in the report of Solomons and Jacob (1981), the concentration of iron in the fluid provided to the subjects (Coca Cola) ranged from 250 to 750 mg/l, while in the studies in which no interaction was observed, the levels ranged from 1 to 25 mg/l in the milk formulas. A delineation of an absolute level of iron needed for interference with zinc absorption, and whether there are developmental changes in the level, needs to be determined. These questions are of particular concern, as some infant formulas have iron added up to a final concentration of 50 mg/l, while zinc is found at a concentration of 0.5 to 5 mg/l (Lonnerdal et al., 1981a) (Figure 2). These concentrations of iron

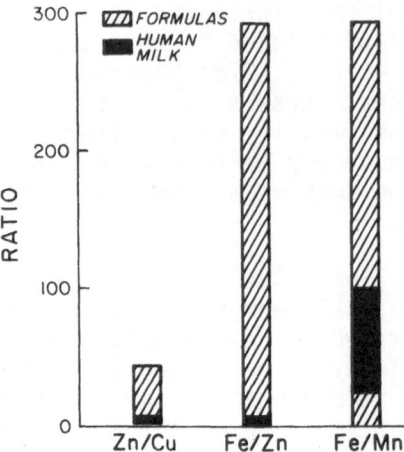

Figure 2   Ratios of zinc, copper, iron and manganese in formula and
human milk.

and zinc yield ratios from 10:1 to 100:1, greatly exceeding those
ratios in studies where an interaction has been found. An
explanation for the varying results reported is that the fluids
used, Coca Cola and milk, have chemical properties which exert
different effects on absorption with regard to iron and zinc (e.g.,
pH, phosphate content).

        In contrast to the lack of an effect of moderate iron
supplementation on zinc absorption from milk formulas, there is a
pronounced effect of the iron supplementation on manganese
absorption and/or retention.

        We have examined the effect of iron supplementation on tissue
magnanese levels using the weanling mouse as a model. Animals were
fed a cow milk diet with no added iron (1 mg/l) or a diet which was
supplemented with iron as iron chloride (6 mg/l) for four weeks. As
anticipated, supplemented mice had higher tissue iron levels than
those in control tissues. Thus, presumably the supplemented animal
has an improved iron status and the desired effect is achieved. An
effect of the supplementation, however, which may not have been
beneficial to the animal, is that tissue manganese levels were
considerably lower in supplemented mice than in controls. The same
result was obtained whether iron was supplemented as a salt or bound
to a protein (lactoferrin) (Fransson et al., 1982). An antagonistic
effect of iron-supplement milk on intestinal uptake of manganese has
also been reported by others (Gruden, 1979; Momcilovic, 1979). This
negative impact of iron supplementation on tissue manganese levels
in young mice should be of concern with regard to infant nutrition.

While some infant formulas are supplemented with manganese, the levels vary considerably (Figures 1 and 2). While we recognize that the functional significance of reductions in tissue manganese levels in infants is not known, we believe that this is an area of research which should receive more attention, due to the routine use of iron supplementation. There are reports by Dupont et al. (1977) and Papavasiliou et al. (1979) showing that some children and adults who have seizure disorders can have suboptimal manganese status. This emphasizes the importance of elucidating the impact of reduced tissue manganese levels due to iron supplementation, as reduced manganese availability at the neuronal level could contribute to a biochemical lesion that with epileptogenic lesions might increase the likelihood of seizure activity.

In the above section, we have discussed the possibility of inducing a manganese deficiency by excess iron supplementation. The converse, that of inducing manganese toxicity by excess manganese supplementation of a formula which is low in iron should also be considered. Chandra and Shukla (1976) have shown that the susceptibility to manganese toxicity in young rats is enchanced in cases of iron deficiency. This phenomenon should also be studied in sucking animals, particularly since in very young animals, it appears that excretion of manganese is very limited, and that increased dietary intake of the element results in high tissue levels (Hurley, 1982). We have found that some infant formulas contain manganese levels that are more than 1000-fold higher than in human milk (Figures 1 and 2). We are currently investigating the bioavailability of manganese in these formulas and its effect on iron bioavailability.

ZINC NUTRITION

Another element which has been frequently reported to be suboptimal or deficient in infants and young children is zinc. The potential severity of zinc deficiency during infancy may be best illustrated by the genetic disorder acrodermatitis enteropathica. The phenotypic expression of the disorder includes eczematoid skin lesions, alopecia, diarrhea and immune dysfunction. The disorder is often precipitated by the changing of the infant's diet from breast milk to formula. It was recognized by Moynahan (1974) that this disorder is characterized by abnormal zinc transport across the intestine and can be treated by oral zinc supplementation. Despite the fact that formula (or cow milk) may contain as much or more zinc as that found in breast milk, the infant with acrodermatitis enteropathica will develop signs of zinc deficiency. Due to this observation, it was hypothesized that the localization of zinc and the resultant bioavailability of it are different between these two fluids (Eckhert et al., 1977). A difference in molecular localization of the element between human and cow milk has since been documented. In human milk, a significant amount of zinc has been shown to be bound to citrate, while in cow milk, little zinc is bound to this ligand (Lonnerdal et al., 1980). As it is known that zinc bound to citrate is easily absorbed (Vohra and Kratzer, 1966) this may account for some of the difference in bioavailability observed. Similar to iron, an additional factor that may be responsible for this difference in bioavailability of zinc is the high casein content of cow milk relative to breast milk (> 10:1). In cow milk, a very large part of zinc (~80 percent) is bound to casein (Lonnerdal and Forsum, 1979). As the casein can form curds in the stomach of the infant which may be poorly digested, zinc bound to casein may have low bioavailability. In contrast to cow milk, the major zinc-binding protein in human milk is serum albumin (Lonnerdal et al., 1982a).

Another compound that has been implicated in the zinc absorption process is picolinic acid (pyridine-2-carboxylic acid). Evans and Johnson (1980a) reported the characterization and quantitation of picolinic acid in human milk and postulated that is is an important zinc-binding ligand in human milk. The identification of the LMW ligand binding zinc in milk as picolinic acid has been questioned, partly because of the methodology employed in its isolation and subsequent quantitation (Hurley and Lonnerdal, 1982). However, another laboratory, using the same technique as Evans et al. (1980a), reported that the LMW zinc complex in human milk is zinc citrate (Martin et al., 1981), in agreement with the findings of Lonnerdal et al. (1980), using the borohydride-treated columns. It has also been demonstrated that picolinic acid added to human milk ultrafiltrate does not elute at the same position as the LMW zinc complex of human milk (Hurley and Lonnerdal, 1982). Picolinic acid is present in milk, but the amount estimated by Evans et al. (1980a)(308 μM) seems to be too high by a large factor. Rebello et al. (1982), using high pressure liquid chromatography (HPLC), have reported the concentration of picolinic acid in human milk to be < 3.7 μM. May et al. (1982) showed by computer calculation that, when using the picolinic concentration found by Rebello et al. (1982), citrate would be the major low molecular weight ligand for zinc in human milk, although these authors question if citrate directly would improve zinc absorption. However, Arver (1982) who has reported that citrate binds zinc in both human milk and prostatic fluid has argued that citrate may be crucial for zinc delivery to other proteins. The observation by Blakeborough et al. (1981) that at pH 4.5, similar to the pH of the gastrointestinal tract of the infant, citrate binds zinc in human milk suggests that citrate may have a functional role in the intestine of the infant.

Perhaps due to the recognition that acrodermatitis enteropathica is a disorder of zinc metabolism, several case reports of infants with clinical signs similar to those seen for the symptomatic

acrodermatitis enteropathica patient have been presented in the last
few years. In most instances, the milk that these infants consumed
has been shown to be deficient in zinc. These findings have been
observed in both formula-fed infants and breast-fed infants (Aggett
et al., 1980; Morishima et al., 1981). That zinc nutriture can be a
problem in some infants, even though overt skin lesions are not
present, has also been demonstrated. Walravens and Hambidge (1976)
have shown that formula-fed infants can have a growth spurt when
given supplemental zinc. Similar observations have been made in
pre-school children (Hambidge et al., 1976). The observation that
the zinc status in formula-fed infants was lower than that in
breast-fed infants was surprising, as the level of zinc in the
formula was higher than that commonly reported for breast milk
(Figure 1). It has subsequently been found that zinc from human
milk has a bioavailability which exceeds that from formula (Hambidge
et al., 1979), even for the infant not suffering from acrodermatitis
enteropathica. Plasma zinc levels in infants fed breast milk were
found to be higher than those in infants fed cow milk or formula. A
similar finding of zinc bioavailibilty being higher in human milk
compared to formula and cow milk has also been reported in adults
(Casey et al., 1981).

     Due to the recognition of the low bioavailability of zinc from
cow milk and formula, it is recommended by the American Academy of
Pediatrics that zinc be supplemented to formula to a level of 5.8
mg/l (> 3 times higher than that in human milk). However, even with
this high level of zinc supplementation, the serum zinc level in
formula-fed infants is still lower than that in breast-fed infants
(Hambidge et al., 1979).

     The physiological importance of the differences in zinc status
in infants fed cow milk compared to those fed breast milk, besides
the slight difference in growth, is not known. A potential problem
is that the infant may be compromised with respect to its ability to
respond to stress and trauma. Zinc deficiency has been shown to be
a serious clinical problem in some children recovering from protein
calorie malnutrition. In particular, these children, upon
refeeding, may have difficulties in depositing lean tissue mass and
may have severe thymic atrophy. Both of these problems are
responsive to zinc therapy (Golden and Golden, 1981).

Zinc Supplementation

     While the potential benefits of zinc supplementation of formula
are evident from the above, a potential negative effect of excess
zinc supplementation is that zinc at high levels can inhibit the
absorption and/or retention of copper, an element which has similar
physico-chemical properties (Hill, 1976; Matrone, 1974). High levels
of dietary zinc have been reported to reduce copper absorption in

the adult human (Prasad et al., 1978; Greger et al., 1978), although it is not known if such an effect occurs in the infant. The induction of copper deficiency could result in arterial wall damage both through decreased connective tissue cross-linking (Rucker and Tinker, 1977) and by perturbation in serum cholesterol profile (Allen and Klevay, 1980; Lonnerdal et al., 1982b). The zinc to copper ratio in foods has been proposed by Klevay (1975) to be a potential risk factor in cardiovascular disease originating during early childhood. In particular, this author has suggested that the difference in zinc/copper ratio in human milk compared to cow milk or formula may be of sufficient magnitude to induce a copper deficiency state, causing an increased susceptibility of the formula-fed infant to future cardiovascular disease.

It is now generally accepted that the zinc/copper ratio in foods is of most importance when the absolute level of one of the elements is marginal or low. This may be a particular problem in the formula which is fortified with zinc but not with copper. We have found that some formulas have a very high ratio of zinc/copper (>10:1) where the copper level is quite low (Figures 1 and 2). There have been case reports of premature infants fed these formulas and developing copper deficiency. Common signs of copper deficiency in infants include anemia, leukopenia, neutropenia and a high incidence of bone fractures. While the primary cause of this deficiency has been attributed to a lack of copper in the diet (Tanaka et al., 1980), the deficiency may have been exacerbated by excess zinc in the formula.

A NEED FOR MAXIMUM LEVELS OF TRACE ELEMENT SUPPLEMENTATION

From the above comments, it should be evident that maximum as well as minimum levels for trace element concentrations in infant formula should be followed. However, while minimum levels of iron, zinc, copper and manganese have been recommended by the Committee on Nutrition of the American Academy of Pediatrics (1976), only iron has had a maximum level recommended (17.5 mg/l or 2.5 mg/100 Kcal, assuming a caloric density of 700 Kcal/l). We believe that this level may be higher than is necessary, since very little beneficial effect on the infant's iron status has been reported when the recommended level of 6 mg/l is increased to 12 mg/l. Assuming that no substantial beneficial effect is obtained by exceeding 12 mg/l (1.8 mg/100 Kcal) and that 4 percent of this amount is absorbed by the infant, this will mean that 0.48 mg/l will be absorbed. A comparable value for breast milk is 0.3 mg of iron/l and absorption of ~50 percent, i.e. 0.15 mg/l. Thus, a 40-fold higher iron concentration will yield a 3-fold higher absorption, at a level not yet demonstrated to have any negative effects.

Extrapolating from the above, 40-fold higher levels of zinc, copper and manganese in formula than in breast milk may serve as guidelines for maxima. The concentration of zinc in breast milk is 1 mg/l, i.e. 40 mg/l (or 5.7 mg/100 Kcal) will be a maximum in formula. The concentration of copper is around 0.2 mg/l, i.e. 8 mg/l or 1.1 mg/100 Kcal and for manganese, a level of 5 μg/l, i.e. 200 μg/l or 28.6 μg/100 Kcal.

However, it should be noted, that it is assumed that the absorption values for these elements are similar to those for iron, and that a similar difference exists between formula and breast milk. Data are not yet available in the literature.

We also would like to emphasize that we think it is important not to increase the level of one of these nutrients too much without increasing the levels of the others, since it is known that these elements may compete with each other at the level of absorption. Thus, a reasonable constant <u>ratio</u> of these trace minerals to each other should be maintained.

POTENTIALS FOR NEW MODES OF SUPPLEMENTATION OF THE INFANT

From the previous sections, it is apparent that the infant may be in a precarious situation with regard to trace element nutrition. Some of these infants, who have genetic disorders of trace element metabolism, are relatively easy to identify. While these infants are certainly dramatic representations of the effects of a trace element deficiency during infancy, they may be only the tip of an iceberg representing a population which may be undernourished with regard to these essential nutrients (Figure 3). Presumably, due to the characterization of the signs of these genetic diseases, infants with severe dietary insufficiencies of trace elements are also being recognized. Mild deficiencies, as evidenced by slight anemia and retarded growth, are sometimes more difficult to diagnose, although current data would suggest that the population of infants in these groups may be larger than normally appreciated. Finally, perhaps the largest population of infants is those in whom trace element status is adequate under normal conditions but is inadequate if the infant is presented with a challenge from the environment. This may include recovery from a traumatic injury, surgery or infections.

It is evident from the above that supplementation of the infant with some of the essential trace elements is required under current feeding practices. For the breast-fed infant, there are two possible modes of supplementation: 1) giving the supplement directly to the infant; and 2) supplementation of the mother with high levels of minerals, such that her milk is "enriched" with

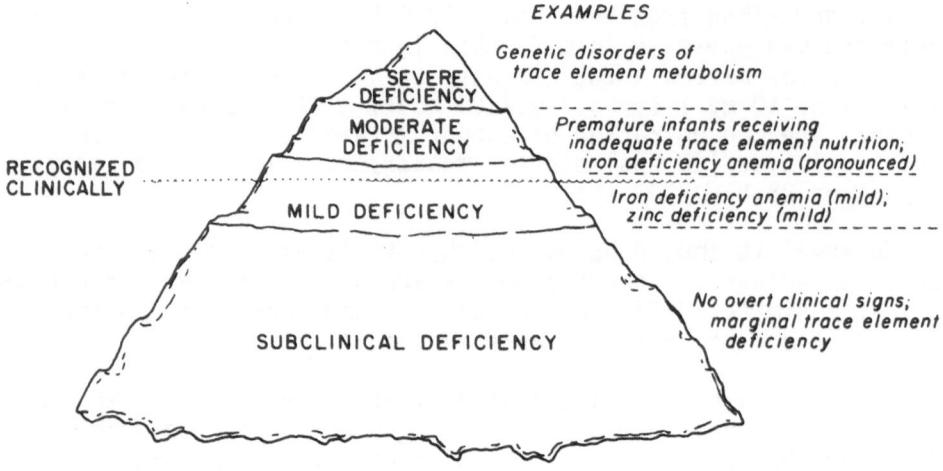

Figure 3 Trace element deficiency in infants.

regard to the element under consideration. While dietary survey
studies have not found a pronounced effect of supplements on human
milk trace element composition (Lonnerdal et al., 1981a), studies
with experimental animals, using high levels of mineral
supplementation, have shown that levels of the element in maternal
milk can be increased above normal, and furthermore that these
increases are reflected in the suckling's tissues (Keen et al.,
1980; Anaokar and Garry, 1981). We have found in our studies that
this is true for both iron and copper. These elements, when
supplemented to the dam in the form of a chelate to nitrilotriacetic
acid (NTA) given in the water, significantly increased milk iron and
copper levels and this increase was reflected in the sucking rat
pups. A similar finding was reported by Anaokar and Garry (1981),
although the mode of iron supplementation to the rat dam was through
the addition of iron sulphate to a solid diet. Which mode of
supplementation is the most efficacious is an important question
that needs to be resolved. In contrast to the effects of iron and
copper supplementation, we did not find zinc supplementation to the
dam to result in increased milk zinc concentration. Others have
found that zinc supplementation of the rat results in increased milk
zinc concentration (Evans and Johnson, 1980b). However, the level
of zinc in the basal diet was marginal in this study, therefore the
findings on zinc supplementation may have actually been due to the
correction of the marginal zinc diet. It is known that the
consumption of a zinc-deficient diet can result in a low milk zinc
concentration (Mutch and Hurley, 1974). The effects of maternal
manganese supplementation on milk manganese conentration have not
been investigated.

As discussed above, one of the issues in supplementing formula-fed infants is that care should be taken not to supplement at a level which would have toxicological consequences, while on the other hand, one wishes to ensure that the infant has an optimal intake and retention of the element. One way of meeting these two criteria can be through the design of vehicles of supplementation which would yield a bioavailability superior to that of the inorganic salts presently used.

As the levels of supplementation which have been used in the studies where a very high increase in milk trace element concentration above normal was found, it is important to check for potential negative effects of the supplementation on both the mother and the infant, prior to attempting similar studies in humans. This may be of particular concern with regard to what was previously discussed about iron supplementation and incidence of infections (Keen et al., 1982). Supplementation of the infant directly, offers the advantage of knowing that the supplement is being ingested by the infant, a situation which is not guaranteed when supplementation is via the mother. Obvious hazards of direct supplementation include: 1) potential interference with normal host-defense mechanisms; and 2) over-supplementation of one element at a level which interferes with the metabolism of another.

One of the major problems, as discussed above, is the design of an infant formula which contains the nutrient in question in amounts sufficient to meet the need of the infant, while at the same time at a level which will not interfere with the absorption of another required nutrient. One of the more promising areas of research in this area is the identification of the optimal vehicles for delivering the element(s). Ligands, such as nitrilotriacetic acid (discussed above), EDTA, and lactobionate, are among the vehicles presently being tested as potential replacements for providing the elements in the inorganic salt form. The use of these different ligands is in part based on the theory that they will donate the element to different compounds in the formula which may have varying bioavailability (Hegenauer et al., 1979). Identification of "optimum" chelates would allow supplementation of the formula with a minimum of the nutrient in question. An alternative to the use of low molecular weight chelates for the supplementation of an element would be to use proteins which can bind the elements and deliver them to selective receptor sites in the intestine. To date, this area has received little attention with the possible exception of the use of lactoferrin as a mode of iron supplementation, as it not only has specific receptor sites in the intestine (Cox et al., 1979), but it also has potent antimicrobial properties which could be a benefit to the infant. Although the concentration of lactoferrin in cow milk is low, it is feasible to isolate this protein in large amounts due to the very high quantities of whey produced in cheese manufacturing. Analogous proteins for the delivery of zinc, copper and manganese have not been identified.

In summary, while a critical need of the infant for the
nutrients iron, zinc, copper and manganese during development has
been appreciated for along time, the diet of the infant can often be
less than optimal with regard to the intake of these nutrients.
While the effects of consuming a diet with inadequate levels of the
nutrients are straightforward and well documented (except for
manganese), potential deleterious effects of consumption of a diet
with excess levels of one of the elements is less appreciated.
These effects should be a focus for future research in the area of
pediatric nutrition. An additional area which warrants considerable
efforts is the design of optimum vehicles for the delivery of the
elements to the infant.

REFERENCES

Aggett, P.J., Atherton, D.J., More, J., Davey, J., Delves, H.T. and
    Harries, J.T., 1980, Symptomatic zinc delivery in a breast-fed
    preterm infant, Arch. Dis. Child. 55:547-550.
Allen, K.G.D. and Klevay, L.M., 1980, Hyperlipoproteinemia in rats
    due to copper deficiency, Nutr. Rep. Int. 22:295-299.
Anaokar, S.G. and Garry, P.J., 1981, Effects of maternal iron
    nutrition during lactation on milk iron and rat neonatal iron
    status, Am. J. Clin. Nutr. 34:1505-1512.
Arver, S., 1982, Zinc and zinc ligands in human seminal plasma.
    III. The principal low molecular weight ligand in prostatic
    secretion and seminal plasma, Acta Physiol. Scand. 116:67-73.
Beisel, W.R., 1982, Single nutrients and immunity, Am. J. Clin.
    Nutr. 35:417-468.
Blakeborough, P., Salter, D.N. and Gurr, W.I., 1981, Zinc binding in
    human and cow's milk, Proc. XII Int. Cong. Nutr. No. 957.
Bullen, J.J., Rogers, M.J. and Griffiths, E., 1978, Role of iron in
    bacterial infection, Curr. Top. Microbiol. Immunol. 80:1-30.
Casey, C.E., Walravens, P.A. and Hambidge, K.M., 1981, Availability
    of zinc: loading tests with human milk, cow's milk and infant
    formulas, Pediatrics 68:394-396.
Chandra, S.V. and Shukla, G.S., 1976, Role of iron deficiency in
    inducing susceptibility to manganese toxicity, Arch. Toxicol.
    35:319-323.
Chandra, R.K., Au, B., Woodford, G. and Hyam, P., 1977, Iron status,
    immune resonse and susceptibility to infection, in: "Iron
    Metabolism", H. Kies, ed., pp. 249-268, Elsevier/Excerpta
    Medica, North-Holland, Amsterdam.
Committee on Nutrition of the American Academy of Pediatrics, 1976,
    Iron supplementation for infants, Pediatrics 58:757-760.
Cox, T.M., Mazurier, J., Spik, G., Montreuil, J. and Peters, T.J.,
    1979, Iron-binding proteins and influx of iron across the
    duodenal brush border, Biochim. Biophys. Acta 588:120-128.
Dupont, T., Harpur, E.R., Skoryna, S.C. and Tanaka, Y., 1977,
    Manganese: its neurological and teratological significance in
    man, Biochemistry 10:11.

Eckhert, C., Sloan, M., Duncan, J.R. and Hurley, L.S., 1977, Zinc
    binding: a difference between human and bovine milk, Science
    195:789-790.
Evans, G.W. and Johnson, P.E., 1980a, Characterization and
    quantitation of a zinc binding ligand in human milk, Pediatr.
    Res. 14:876-880.
Evans, G.W. and Johnson, P.E., 1980b, Zinc concentration of liver
    and kidneys from rat pups nursing dams fed supplemental zinc
    dipicolinate or zinc acetate, J. Nutr. 110:2121-2124.
Fomon, S.J., 1974, "Infant Nutrition", W.B. Saunders Co.,
    Philadelphia.
Forth, W. and Rummel, W., 1973, Iron absorption, Physiol. Rev.
    53:724-792.
Fransson, G.-B. and Lonnerdal, B., 1980, Iron in human milk, J.
    Pediatr. 96:380-384.
Fransson, G.-B., Keen, C.L. and Lonnerdal, B., 1982, Iron
    supplementation of milk through iron-lactoferrin: Effect on
    tissue iron and manganese, Fed. Proc. 41:778.
Fransson, G.-B., Lonnerdal, B., Keen, C.L., Ersson, B.,
    Thoren-Tholling, K. and Hambraeus, L., 1981, Lactoferrin and
    iron absorption. Proceedings of XII International Congress of
    Nutrition, No. 822.
Garry, P.J., Owen, G.M., Hooper, E.M. and Gilbert, B.A., 1981, Iron
    absorption from human milk and formula with and without iron
    supplementation, Pediatr. Res. 15:822-828.
Golden, M.N.H. and Golden, B.E., 1981, Trace elements - potential
    importance in human nutrition with particular reference to zinc
    and vanadium, Br. Med. Bull. 37:31-36.
Greger, J.L., Zaikis, S.C., Abernathy, R.P., Bennett, O.A. and
    Hoffman, J., 1978, Zinc, nitrogen, copper, iron and manganese
    balance in adolescent females fed two levels of zinc, N. Nutr.
    108:1449-1456.
Gruden, N., 1979, Transduodenal iron transport in rats fed milk diet
    supplemented with iron and/or manganese, Nutr. Rep. Int.
    19:69-74.
Gruden, N. and Momcilovic, B., 1979, ^{65}Zn transport in the duodenum
    and jejunum of rats fed milk enriched with iron, Nutr. Rep.
    Int. 19:483-489.
Hambidge, K.M., Walravens, P.A., Brown, R.A., Webster, J., White, S.,
    Anthony, M. and Roth, M.L., 1976, Zinc nutrition of preschool
    children of the Denver Head Start Program, Am. J. Clin. Nutr.
    29:734-738.
Hambidge, K.M., Walravens, P.A., Casey, C.A., Brown, R.A. and Bender,
    C., 1979, Plasma zinc concentrations of breast-fed infants, J.
    Pediatr. 94:607-608.
Hamilton, D.L., Bellamy, J.E.C., Valberg, J.D. and Valberg, L.S.,
    1978, Zinc, cadmium and iron interaction during intestinal
    absorption in iron-deficient mice, Can. J. Physiol. Pharmacol.
    56:384-389.

Hegenauer, J., Saltman, P., Ludwig, D., Ripley, L. and Ley, A., 1979,
    Iron-supplemented cow milk. Identification and spectral
    properties of iron bound to casein micelles, J. Agric. Food
    Chem. 27:1294-1301.
Hill, C.H., 1976, Mineral interrelationships, in: "Trace Elements in
    Human Health and Disease", Vol. II, A.S. Prasad and D. Oberleas,
    eds., p. 281, Academic Press, New York.
Hurley, L.S., 1982, Manganese, in: "Present Knowledge in Nutrition",
    R. Olson, ed., The Nutrition Foundation, Washington, D.C., in
    press.
Hurley, L.S. and Lonnerdal, B., 1982, Zinc binding in human milk:
    Citrate versus picolinate, Nutr. Rev. 40:65-71.
Keen, C.L., Lonnerdal, B., Sloan, M.V. and Hurley, L.S., 1980, Effect
    of dietary iron, copper, and zinc chelates of nitrilotriacetic
    acid (NTA) on trace metal concentrations in rat milk and
    maternal and pup tissues, J. Nutr. 110:897-906.
Keen, C.L., Lonnerdal, B. and Hurley, L.S., 1982, Increased milk iron
    by dietary supplementation-entirely beneficial , Am. J. Clin.
    Nutr. 35:627-628.
Klevay, L.M., 1975, Coronary heart disease: The zinc/copper
    hypothesis, Am. J. Clin. Nutr. 28:764-774.
Lonnerdal, B. and Forsum E., 1979, Casein content of human milk,
    Proceedings of Third European Nutrition Conference, 239.
Lonnerdal, B., Stanislowski, A.G. and Hurley, L.S., 1980, Isolation
    of a low molecular weight zinc binding ligand from human milk,
    J. Inorg. Biochem. 12:71-78.
Lonnerdal, B., Keen, C.L. and Hurley, L.S., 1981a, Iron, copper, zinc
    and manganese in milk, Ann. Rev. Nutr. 1:149-174.
Lonnerdal, B., Keen, C.L. and Hurley, L.S., 1981b, Trace elements in
    milk from various species, in: "Trace Element Metabolism in Man
    and Animals (TEMA-4)", McC.J. Howell, J.M. Gawthorne, C.L.
    White, eds., p. 249, Australian Academy of Science, Canberra.
Lonnerdal, B., Keen, C.L., Ohtake, M. and Tamura, T., 1981c, Trace
    element and mineral content of infant formulas, Am. J. Clin.
    Nutr. 34:640-.
Lonnerdal, B., Hoffman, B. and Hurley, L.S., 1982a, Zinc and copper-
    binding proteins in human milk, Am. J. Clin. Nutr. 35:1170-1176.
Lonnerdal, B., Keen, C.L., Reinstein, N. and Hurley, L.S., 1982b,
    Effects of varying dietary zinc and copper levels during
    pregnancy in the rat, Am. J. Clin. Nutr. 35:850.
Martin, M.T., Licklider, K.F., Brushmiller, J.G. and Jacobs, F.A.,
    1981, Detection of low molecular weight copper (II) and zinc
    (II) binding ligands in ultrafiltered milks - the citrate
    connection, J. Inorg. Biochem. 15:55-66.
Matrone, G., 1974, Chemical parameters in trace-element antagonism,
    in: "Trace Element Metabolism in Animals (TEMA-2)", W.G.
    Hoekstra, J.W. Suttie, H.E. Ganther and W. Mertz, eds., p. 91,
    University Park Press, Baltimore.
May, P.M., Smith, G.L. and Williams, D.R., 1982, Computer calculation
    of zinc (II) complex distribution in milk, J. Nutr.
    112:1990-1993.

McMillan, J.A., Oski, F.A., Lourie, G., Tomarelli, R.M. and Landaw, S.A., 1977, Iron absorption from human milk, simulated human milk, and proprietary formulas, Pediatrics 60:896-900.

Momcilovic, B., 1979, Experimental design for the study of dietary interactions in infant rat nutrition, Period. Biol. 81:559-565.

Momcilovic, B. and Kello, D., 1977, The effect of milk enriched with iron on ^{65}Zn absorption, Nutr. Rep. Int. 15:651-657.

Morishima, T., Yagi, S. and Takemura, T., 1981, An aquired form of acrodermatitis enteropathica due to long term lactose-free milk alimentation, in: "Trace Element Metabolism in Man and Animals (TEMA-4)", McC.J. Howell, J.M. Gawthorne, C.L. White, eds., p. 487, Australian Academy of Science, Canberra.

Moynahan, E.J., 1974, Acrodermatitis enteropathica: a lethal inherited human zinc-deficiency disorder, Lancet ii:399.

Mutch, P.B. and Hurley, L.S., 1974, Effect of zinc deficiency during lactation on postnatal growth and development of rats, J. Nutr. 104:828-842.

Papavasiliou, P.S., Kuth, H., Miller, S.T., Rosal, V., Wang, Y.Y. and Aronson, R.B., 1979, Seizure disorders and trace metals: Manganese tissue levels in treated epileptics, Neurology 29:1466-1473.

Prasad, A.S., Brewer, G.J., Schoomaker, E.G. and Rabbani, P., 1978, Hypocupremia induced by zinc therapy in adults, J. Am. Med. Assoc. 240:2166-2168.

Rebello, T., Lonnerdal, B. and Hurley, L.S., 1982, Picolinic acid in milk, pancreatic juice, and intestine: Inadequate for role in zinc absorption, Am. J. Clin. Nutr. 35:1-5.

Rucker, R.B. and Tinker, D., 1977, Structure and metabolism of arterial elastin, Int. Rev. Exp. Pathol. 17:1-42.

Saarinen, U.M., 1978, Need for iron supplementation in infants on prolonged breast feeding, J. Pediatr. 93:177-180.

Saarinen, U.M. and Siimes, M.A., 1979, Iron absorption from breast milk, cow's milk and iron-supplemented formula: An opportunistic use of changes in total body iron determined hy hemoglobin, ferritin and body weight in 132 infants, Pediatr. Res. 13:143-147.

Saarinen, U.M., Siimes, M.A. and Dallman, P.R., 1977, Iron absorption in infants: High bioavailability of breast milk iron as indicated by the extrinsic tag method of iron absorption and by the concentration of serum ferritin, J. Pediatr. 91:36-38.

Simmons, W.K. and Gurney, J.M., 1982, Nutritional anemia in the English-speaking Caribbean and Suriname, Am. J. Clin. Nutr. 35:327-337.

Solomons, N.W. and Jacob, R.A., 1981, Studies on the bioavailability of zinc in humans: effect of heme and nonheme iron on the absorption of zinc, Am. J. Clin. Nutr. 34:475-482.

Tanaka, Y., Hatano, S., Nishi, Y. and Usui, T., 1980, Nutritional copper deficiency in a Japanese infant on formula, J. Pediatr. 96:255-256.

Vohra, P. and Kratzer, F.H., 1966, Influence of various phosphates
    and other complexing agents on the availability of zinc for
    turkey poults, J. Nutr. 89:106-112.
Walravens, P.A. and Hambidge, K.M., 1976, Growth of infants fed a
    zinc supplemented formula, Am. J. Clin. Nutr. 29:1114-1121.

DIFFERENCES IN EXPOSURE AND METABOLIC RESPONSE OF INFANTS AND ADULTS TO LEAD, CADMIUM AND ZINC

Kathryn R. Mahaffey

Division of Nutrition, Food and Drug Administration
Department of Health and Human Services
Cincinnati, Ohio

ABSTRACT

Substantial differences exist between infants and adults in their exposures to lead, camium and zinc and in the sources of these exposures. In addition, metabolic responses of infants and children to environmental levels of these metals are different from those of adults. The toxicity of lead and cadmium to all age groups has been recognized for a number of years. Nonindustrial lead toxicity occurs principally among young children, whereas the toxic effects of cadmium in bone and kidney are throught to be manifested only after decades of exposure have produced a substantial body burden of cadium. In contrast, zinc deficiency has been reported to occur among infants and children far more commonly than has zinc toxicity. Despite differences in the likelihood that modern human populations will develop toxicity or deficiency of these metals, several general physiological and behavioral characteristics converge to modify metal exposure during infancy and early childhood.

EXPOSURE DURING INFANCY AND EARLY CHILDHOOD

The various sources of environmental exposure to lead (Mahaffey, 1978), cadmium (Nriagu, 1982), and zinc (Hambidge, 1981) are reviewed elsewhere. Pediatric exposure to metals differs from exposure of adults. Infants and very young children can greatly increase their ingestion of metals through pica and mouthing of objects. Mouthing of hands and objects is considered to be normal in infants, and nearly all infants under one year of age exhibit this behavior. In a survey of children 12 to 72 months of age, Barltrop (1966) reported that 78 percent mouthed objects and 35 percent ingested the objects. Pica, defined as the habitual ingestion of nonfood substances, occurs among young children; depending on the type of objects ingested, e.g., paint, colored newspapers or magazines, pica can greatly increase the intake of lead and occasionally cadmium.

Among children, acute lead intoxication is characterized by pronounced central nervous system (CNS) damage in which cerebral edema, coma and convulsions occur; in the most severe cases, death results (Lin-Fu, 1980). Acute oral exposure to cadmium can cause acute gastrointestinal poisoning manifested by vomiting, diarrhea and crampy abdominal pain of sudden onset (Chisolm, 1980). Symptoms of poisoning due to ingestion of high levels of zinc are described as nausea, vomiting, abdominal cramps, diarrhea and fever (Li and Vallee, 1980).

Because of the high concentration of lead and, under some circumstances, cadmium in sources such as paint or urban street dirt, consumption of only small quantities may produce toxicity. In contrast, modest elevations in the concentration of lead or cadmium in food and beverages can have toxicologic significance because of the relatively large quantities of fluid and food consumed. For example, infants living in an area with acidic water and water-supply pipes or lead-lined water-storage cisterns received most of their lead exposure from water used to dilute powdered infant formula or other beverages such as juice (Sherlock et al., 1982).

In the absence of metabolic abnormalities, zinc deficiency in infants is secondary to low levels of zinc in food, poor bioavail-ability of dietary zinc, and a high requirement for zinc for growth. The relative importance of these factors is not fully understood.

CONTRAST BETWEEN INFANTS AND ADULTS IN LEVELS OF CADMIUM, LEAD AND ZINC EXPOSURE

Exposure from Dust and Dirt

Under specific environmental conditions, an individual source of metals may dominate all other sources contributing to exposure. Clinically evident, severe poisonings among children due to high-lead dirt are secondary to sporadic ingestion of these sources via pica or mouthing of hands and objects. However, discussion of severe pediatric lead toxicity is outside the scope of this paper.

Increased exposure to cadmium and lead through mouthing of hands and objects is common among infants and young children. Estimates of the quantities of lead transferred to the child via the hands have been published. Sayre et al. (1974) reported an increase in the amount of lead on children's hands when the amount of lead in household dust increased. Lepow et al. (1974) found that mean lead concentrations of 2400 µg/g of dirt could be removed from the hands of young children living in environments where outdoor dirt averaged 1200 ppm lead and indoor dust averaged 11,000 ppm lead. Each cleaning of the children's hands removed approximately 25-30 µg lead. The children who were subjects in this study had blood lead concentrations between 40 and 120 µg/100 ml for a period of 6 to 24 months. Duggan and Williams (1977) estimated that a young child has a typical daily intake intake of between 20 and 200 µg of lead from street dust, with an average of approximately 50 µg. This type of transfer is not limited to very young children. For example, Roels et al. (1980), in a study of subjects whose mean age was 11 years, reported that blood lead levels were approximately 10 µg/100 ml when the amount of lead on the hand was less than 20 µg. When lead on the hand was 480 µg/hand, mean blood lead concentrations were greater than 28 µg/100 ml. If the sources of lead (e.g., yellow-pigmented paints, colored newsprint, dirt or dust from specific industries) contain cadmium as well as lead, transfer of cadmium to the infant or young child via the hands would also be.expected to occur.

Young infants can have metal exposure secondary to parental occupation. Transfer of lead across the placenta has been recognized for a number of years (Cantarow and Trumper, 1944; Barltrop, 1969). Typically, blood levels of newborn infants are very similar to or slightly lower than those of the mother (Haas et al., 1972; Gershanik et al., 1974; Clark, 1977; Lauwerys et al., 1978; Alexander and Delves, 1981). The adverse effects of high levels of in utero lead exposure have been recognized for centuries. During the past few decades lead exposure has been brought under a degree of control; evaluation of the effects of current levels of lead exposure on infant development is the subject of several longitudinal studies not yet completed. Some information in the routes of transfer of lead from the workplace to pregnant women and infants exists. Ryu et al. (1978) presented a case report of a newborn infant with a substantially elevated body burden of lead whose mother had been employed in a lead storage battery plant until 7 weeks before delivery. Follow-up of blood lead levels until the infant was 9 months of age indicated that the infant's blood lead concentrations decreaed during that time. The investigators noted that in the absence of important postnatal exposure to lead, an infant exposed prenatally can reduce its body burden of lead relative to body mass. However, other infants, whose parents continued to have occupational exposure to lead, acquired a substantial amount of lead in the home secondary to transfer on the parent's clothing or person (Fomon, 1978). These patterns of increased lead exposure were observed when either the mother or father was employed in a lead industry.

Several additional epidemiological investigations of infants and older children also demonstrate transfer of lead from the

parent's workplace to the home. Baker et al. (1977) reported an
outbreak of lead toxicity among children whose fathers were employed
in a secondary lead smelter. The children's blood lead levels were
related closely to their fathers' blood lead concentrations and
duration of employment. The apparent vehicle of exposure was lead
dust carried home on work clothing. Transfer of lead from the
workplace into the home is not limited to situations in which
workers bring their work clothing home. In a study population of
children ages 12 to 83 months, Morton et al. (1982), using
case-control techniques, determined that the mean blood lead levels
of children whose parents were lead workers were significantly
greater than those of children whose parents were not employed in a
lead-related industry. Detailed analysis of lead exposure indicated
that the workers' personal hygiene habits, as well as the level of
lead exposure in the workplace, were associated with the children's
blood lead levels.

        Soil and dirt contain substantial quantities of zinc; however,
many soils, particularly clays, act as a resin to decrease the
bioavailability or biotoxicity of zinc (Nriagu, 1980). Soils and
dirt may also be heavily contaminated with cadmium, particularly
secondary to industrial cadmium sources (Nriagu, 1982).

Exposure from Air, Food and Water

        In addition to exposures secondary to increased contact with
dust and dirt, metabolic differences of infants and young children
also contribute to higher intakes of metals from air and diets in
comparison with adults. Young children, particularly infants under
2 years of age, consume higher doses (per kg body weight) of lead,
cadmium and zinc from air, water and food secondary to a higher basal
metabolic rate, greater physical activity and growth. Even if the
same concentrations of metal are present, more of the metal is
ingested or inhaled because of the infant's higher requirement for
calories, fluid and air. Decreases in mean caloric consumption on a
body weight basis for selected time periods between birth and 44
years are shown in Table 1. These data are based on results of
metabolic studies (Fomon, 1974) and dietary surveys conducted in the
United States during the 1970s (United States National Center for
Health Statistics, 1977, 1979, 1981).

        Diet is the predominant source of intake of lead, cadmium and
zinc for infants, toddlers and adults if air, water and dust are not
unusually contaminated with these metals. Total food intake differs
with age (Table 2) as do types of foods consumed. Based upon dietary
survey data, the Food and Drug Administration (FDA) has conducted
the Total Diet Studies for both infants and toddlers and for adults
for a number of years. Data in Table 3 illustrate specific food
groups and their patterns of consumption by infants, toddlers and

Table 1   Body Weight and Caloric Intake of Infants, Children, and
          Adults[a]

Age	Body Weight kg	Mean Caloric Intake	
		Total	Per kg Body Weight
Birth	3.2	405	115
6 Months	7.5	760	100
2 Years	12.4	1488	104
18 Years			
Male	69	2949	40
Female	57	1739	30
Adult[b]			
Male	79	2646	33
Female	67	1579	24

[a]Sources of data: Mean caloric intakes during first 6
months of life based on data from Fomon (1974). All
other data, United States National Center for Health
Statistics (1977, 1979, 1981).
[b]Ages 25-44 years,

adults. Details of the dietary survey data used to establish these
food patterns are described in the FDA Compliance Program
Evaluations for Fiscal Years 1975 through 1979 (Food and Drug
Administration, 1979a,b; 1980a,b,c,d; 1981a,b,; 1982a,b) and by
Duggan and McFarland (1967).

It is essential to note two important limitations of the data.
First, the adult diet is based on food intake of 15- to 20-year-old
males consuming an average of approximately 3000 g of food and
beverages per day. Dietary intake of a number of nutrients (e.g.,
zinc) and toxicants (e.g., lead) are higher than those ingested by
the general population having lower caloric intakes. Second, as
increased application of contamination control techniques in the
laboratory and the general environment has occurred, estimated
quantities of lead and cadmium present in the diet have decreased
(Kolbye et al., 1974; Mahaffey et al., 1975; Satzger et al., 1982).
These changes resulting from contamination control appear to have
far less impact on zinc analyses because of the higher levels of
zinc present in foods.

Table 2   Food Intakes for 6-Month-Old Infants, 2-Year-Old Toddlers, and 15-20-Year Old Adult Males[a]

	Infant	Toddler	Adult
Total, g/day	1387	1549	2976
Average body weight, kg	8.2	13.7	69.1
Relative food intake, g food/kg body weight	169	113	43
Ratio of relative food intake to relative adult food intake	3.9	2.6	1.0

[a]Sources of data: Food and Drug Administration (1979a,b).

        With recognition of these limitations, the following estimates of dietary lead and cadmium intake are reported for the purpose of contrasting levels of intake relative to body size for infants and adults. As shown by data presented in Table 4, total lead intake increases with age, but lead intake from diet decreases with age when calculated on a body weight basis. Total dietary zinc and cadmium intakes increase with age, as does overall food intake, but decrease on a body weight basis when the intakes of 2-year-old toddlers are contrasted with those of adults (Table 4).

Lead

        Additional estimates of lead intake at different ages illustrate the same pattern shown by the Total Diet Study program. Lead intakes from diet at different ages have been estimated by using data on lead concentration in foods and survey data on reported food intake (Beloian, 1982; Beloian and McDowell, 1982; Nutrition Foundation, 1982). These reports have illustrated the extent to which infants and young children have higher dietary lead intakes relative to body weight than do adults even if the concentrations of lead present in the foods consumed are the same. For example, the Nutrition Foundation report (1982), using data from four dietary surveys, indicated that mean daily dietary lead intake increased from 20-46 μg for 0- to 6-month infants to 60-73 μg for 48- to 60-month-old children, but on a body weight basis, intake decreased from 3.6-7.9 μg/kg body weight in the 0- to 6-month age group to 3.9-4.2 μg/kg body weight in the 48- to 60-month age group. The Nutrition Foundation report (1982) indicated that 1-year-old children consumed

Table 3   FDA Total Diet Studies: Percent Distribution by Food Groups
for Diets of Infants, Toddlers, and Young Adult Males

	Food Group	Infants	Toddlers	Adults
I	Drinking water	16.7	22.2	23.1
II	Milk[a]	45.6	33.0	25.4
III	Other Dairy and Dairy Substitutes	10.0	4.6	Included in II
IV	Meat, Fish and Poultry	3.5	8.1	9.1
V	Grain and Cereal Products	2.8	7.4	14.2
VI	Potatoes	0.5	1.8	6.0
VII	Vegetables	7.1	4.8	8.4
VIII	Fruit and Fruit Juices	9.8	9.5	8.6
IX	Fats and Oils	0.5	0.9	2.4
X	Sugars and Adjuncts	0.9	1.9	2.8
XI	Beverages	2.6	5.8	Included in I
	Total in grams	1387	1549	2976

[a]Includes infant formula.

an average of 61 μg lead/day (5.4 μg/kg body weight/day) based on
Canadian dietary survey data. In contrast, adults 40 through 64
years of age ingested approximately 40-100 percent more lead (89
μg/day for females and 113 μg/day for males); however, their intake
on a body weight basis was approximately one-fourth as high (1.4 and
1.6 μg/kg body weight/day for females and males, respectively).
Beloian (1982) calculated simlar age-related decreases in dietary
lead intakes on a body weight basis (Table 5) for children.
McDowell and Beloian (Food and Drug Administration, personal
communication, 1982) calculated lead intakes for 4918 males and
females 18-54 years of age; mean lead intake was estimated as 1.5 ±
0.6 (SD) μg/kg body weight and increased to 2.4 μg/kg body weight at
the 90th percentile of food intake. All data were calculated based
on mean lead concentrations found in foods. The 90th percentile

Table 4   Average Daily Dietary Intake of Metals by Infants, Toddlers, and Adults[a]

	Lead, µg		Cadmium, µg		Zinc, mg	
	Total	Per kg Body Weight	Total	Per kg Body Weight	Total	Per kg Body Weight
	25.2	3.1	5.9	0.72	4.94	0.60
Toddlers	35.8	2.6	10.9	0.79	8.79	0.64
Adults	95.1	1.4	30.9	0.45	16.78	0.24

[a]Source of data: Food and Drug Administration (1981a,b).

Table 5   Calculated Dietary Lead Intake for Children Ages Birth to 5 Years: United States, 1973-1978[a]

Age Group	Sample Size	Mean	SD	Daily Mean Lead Intake			
				50 Pctl.	90 Pctl.	95 Pctl.	99 Pctl.
Daily Mean Lead Intakes (mg)[b] and Increasing Mean Lead Intake by Percentiles							
0-5 Months	67	15	12	11	31	36	55
6-23 Months	264	59	25	54	89	110	140
2-5 Years	873	82	28	79	120	130	170
Daily Mean Lead Exposure (µg/kg body weight)[b] and Increasing Rate of Lead Exposure by Percentiles							
0-5 Months	67	2.7	2.0	2.5	5.4	6.8	7.3
6-23 Months	264	6.1	2.4	5.8	9.1	10.0	12.0
2-5 Years	873	5.6	2.3	5.3	8.5	9.6	12.0

[a]Source of data: Beloian (1982).
[b]Dietary lead intakes for each infant or child were based on mean concentrations of lead present in foods during the period 1973-1978.

intakes reflect differences in the amount of food consumed rather than the concentration of lead present in the food. The Nutrition Foundation report noted that the pattern of foods consumed at the 90th percentile intake is similar to the pattern at the 50th percentile; however, the quantities of individual foods consumed were larger.

Origins of dietary lead are multiple, but lead-soldered side-seam cans are an important source. The Nutrition Foundation report (1982) indicated that at the 50th percentile of dietary lead intake 13-22 percent of the lead came from cans; at the 90th percentile, the contribution from cans ranged from 20 to 40 percent. The percentage of dietary lead derived from cans differs in countries where infants are breast fed or where infant formula is stored in non-lead-soldered cans. Most pureed foods, intended primarily for infants and very young children, are packaged in glass rather than lead-soldered side-seam cans. Metal-packaged canned foods, intended primarly for non-infant food markets, are increasingly being packaged in electrically welded cans rather than lead-soldered cans. Because of the reduced concentration of lead in infant foods in recent years (Table 6), dietary lead intake for children 0-5 months old has been markedly reduced (Table 7). However, dietary lead intakes of children over 6 months of age remain higher than those of adults on a body weight basis.

Cadmium

Sources of dietary cadmium include industrial pollution, use of industrial sewage slude on crop lands as a fertilizer, other fertilizers, water runoff from cadmium industries (e.g., electroplating, producers of pigments, manufacturers of plastic stabilizers), and atmospheric deposition (Nriagu, 1982). Table 8 shows the total dietary cadmium intake from food and beverages for infants, toddlers, and adults. During Fiscal Years 1975 through 1979, no temporal trend in dietary cadmium intake for a specific age group was observed in these data. Kaferstein and Muller (1981) reported that dietary cadmium intakes of infants between the ninth and twelfth months of life were slightly more than 70 µg per week (10 µg/day) if the water was not unusually contaminated with cadmium.

Zinc

Results of the Total Diet Study (Table 9) indicate that there has been relatively little change in dietary zinc during Fiscal Years 1975 through 1979. Although these levels of intake meet the United States National Research Council's recommendations for dietary zinc intake (Food and Nutrition Board, 1980), there has been a question of the bioavailability of zinc in dairy products and some

Table 6   Lead Levels (ppm) in Foods for Infants: United States, 1971-1981

Type of Food	1971-75	1976-77	1979-80	1980-81
Pureed infant foods	0.15[a]	0.05[b]	0.03	0.03[c]
Infant juices[d]	0.30[e,f]	0.45[b]	0.15	0.02[c]
Infant formula	0.10[g,h]	0.55[h,i]	0.02[h]	0.02[h,j]
Evaporated milk	0.52[h]	0.10[h,k]	0.08[h]	0.07[h,l]

[a]Infant Food Manufacturers (IFM), 11/14/75, concerning 1974 pack.
[b]Internal FDA memorandum, 11/14/77.
[c]IFM Report 12/7/81.
[d]Packed in glass (1979).
[e]IFM Report to FAO/WHO for 1972 and 1973 packs.
[f]FDA, FY-74 Survey, 1973 pack.
[g]IFM 1/24/75, Lead Intake of U.S. Infants.
[h]Concentrate, not "as consumed".
[i]FDA, FY-76 Survey, Infant Formulas.
[j]Infant Formula Council, 8/12/81.
[k]Evaporated Milk Association (EMA), 6/23/77; final lead concentration depends on lead level in water used to dilute concentrate.
[l]EMA, 1/27/82.

Table 7   Daily Mean Lead Intake for Baseline 1973-1978 and Calendar Year 1980 and Reduction in Daily Intake Between the Two Years[a]

Age Group	Daily Mean Lead Intake, 1973-1978	1980	Reduction, %, 1973-1978 to 1980
0-5 Months	15	8	47
6-23 Months	59	55	7
2-5 Years	82	82	0

[a]Source of data: Beloian and McDowell (1982).

Table 8   Total Daily Cadmium Intake from Food and Beverages (µg/Day)[a]

	FY-75	FY-76	FY-77	FY-78	FY-79
Infant	5	12	6	6	4
Toddler	11	14	8	11	9
Adult	34	33	37	31	33

[a]Source of data: Food and Drug Administration (1979a,b; 1980a,b,c,d; 1981a,b; 1982a,b).

infant formulas. Casey et al. (1981) demonstrated that the increase in plasma zinc level was substantially greater among adult female subjects given zinc with human milk than with a comparable amount of zinc in cow's milk or infant formulas. The basis for greater bioavailability of zinc from human milk has been reviewed by Hurley and Lonnerdal (1982), and enhancement of bioavailability in human milk was attributed to a low molecular weight zinc-binding ligand. Interaction with metals may also influence the quantities of zinc needed in the diet (Lonnerdal, this volume).

ABSORPTION

Early infancy is characterized by patterns of gastrointestinal absorption that differ from those of mature animals. The young of a species absorb substantially higher percentages of ingested metals than do mature animals (Kostial, this volume). Neonates also absorb immunoglobulins and other complex macromolecules for a short period of time after birth (Lecce, 1972). The length of this period varies with the species (Kraehenbuhl and Campiche, 1969; Rothberg, 1969), and in humans the enhanced absorption of macromolecules rapidly diminishes. However, absorption of lead and cadmium remains substantially higher during infancy and very early childhood compared with that of adults; in contrast, absorption of zinc does not appear to be greatly enhanced in the young infant and child (Table 10).

Lead

A number of studies with experimental animals have demonstrated higher absorption and retention of lead by suckling animals (Forbes and Reina, 1972; Kostial et al., 1974). Age substantially influences the absorption of lead by human subjects as well. Infants and young children absorb substantially more lead than do adults (Alexander et al., 1974; Ziegler et al., 1978). Adults typically absorb 5-10 percent of their dietary lead intake; in contrast, infants and very

Table 9   Total Daily Zinc Intake from Food and Beverages (mg/Day)[a]

	FY-75	FY-76	FY-77	FY-78	FY-79
Infant	5.3	8.2	4.3	4.9	5.4
Toddler	8.3	9.5	7.8	8.8	8.3
Adult	18.4	19.1	18.0	16.8	17.8

[a]Source of data: Food and Drug Administration (1979a,b;
1980a,b,c,d; 1981a,b; 1982a,b).

young children absorb in excess of 40 percent and retain over 30
percent when the dietary lead intake exceeds 5 µg/kg body weight/
day. The age at which patterns of absorption of ingested lead
approach the adult levels is not known. Ziegler et al. (1978) found
that infants between the ages of 14 and 746 days did not show age-
related differences in the percentage of lead absorbed or retained.
Data from long-term balance studies in 11- to 13-year-old children
indicated that the percentage of lead absorption resembled that of
young children more than that of adults (Macy, 1946); however,
because of limitations in the type of analytical techniques available
at that time, these data must be regarded as only semiquantitative.

Cadmium

As with lead, infants and young children absorb a substantially
higher percentage of ingested cadmium than do adults. Sasser and
Jarboe (1977) reported that 2-hour-old rat pups absorbed
approximately 6 times as much cadmium as did one-day-old rat pups.
In these very young animals, cadmium retention time in the
gastrointestinal tract was greatly prolonged. Similarly, elevated
cadmium absorption in young animals has been reported and studied
extensively (Kostial et al., 1979). Although the absorption of
ingested cadmium varies with dietary conditions (Hietanen, 1982),
adult humans typically absorb less than 10 percent of intake. A
range of values has been reported for adult human subjects. An
average of 6 percent with a range of 4.7 to 7.0 percent was reported
by Rahola et al. (1972, cited in Travis and Haddock, 1980) in a study
involving five adult male volunteers. In contrast, absorption of
cadmium by children from early infancy through 8 years of age
averaged 55 percent (Alexander et al., 1974).

Table 10   Gastrointestinal Absorption of Dietary Lead, Cadmium and Zinc for Infants and Children Contrasted with Adults

Metal	Mean Absorption	
	Infants and Children	Adults
Lead	$42^a, 53^c$	$5-10^b$
Cadmium	55^c	$<10^d$
Zinc	18^c	30^e

[a]Ziegler et al. (1978) for infants ages 14 to 746 days.
[b]Summary of balance data reviewed by Mahaffey (1978).
[c]Alexander et al. (1974) for children <8 years old.
[d]World Health Organization (1980).
[e]Walravens (1980).

Zinc

Comparably increased absorption of zinc during the neonatal period does not appear to occur. Alexander et al. (1974) found that the percentage absorption of dietary zinc among infants and young children was similar to that of adults. Balance studies in preterm infants have indicated that the immature fetal intestine is unable to absorb sufficient zinc, resulting in a negative balance for up to 60 days after birth (Dauncey et al., 1977). It is not entirely clear whether or not the relatively poor absorption of dietary zinc by infants is secondary to the limited bioavailability of zinc in formulas.

TISSUE DISTRIBUTION OF METALS

In addition to a higher dietary intake on a body weight basis and a higher percentage absorption of ingested lead and cadmium from the gastrointestinal tract, the young have a different pattern of tissue metal retention than do adults. In evaluations of data on concentrations of metals in tissues of young animals, increases in total body size and age-associated changes in rate of growth or various body organs must be considered. Although organ weights of individuals vary greatly at birth, the average brain weight is approximately 10.5 percent of the body weight (Sunderman and Baerner, 1949). Brain weight is approximately 8-9 percent of body weight at 6 months and 2 years of age. Adult brain weight shows greater variability because of substantial differences in body size of adults, but averages 1.4-2.2 percent of the body weight

(Sunderman and Baerner, 1949). In contrast, although the kidney increases in size with age, the combined weight of left and right kidneys is rather consistently 0.3-0.4 percent of body weight in the absence of gross pathology.

Lead

Kostial et al. (1974) and Jugo (1980) reported that young animals retained a higher percentage of lead administered intraperitoneally or intravenously. The increase in retention of lead is reflected by its rapid clearance from blood to other tissues. Bone uptake of ^{203}Pb administered intraperitonealy was greater in suckling rats than in mature rats (Momcilovic and Kostial, 1974). In addition, Willes et al. (1977) reported that after oral administration of a single dose of ^{210}Pb(NO$_3$)$_2$, infant and juvenile monkeys had higher ^{210}Pb bone:blood ratios than did adult monkeys.

In the young, the brain seems especially vulnerable to accumulation of lead. Goldstein and Diamond (1974) found that in 1-month-old rats there was a linear relationship between the intravenous dose of lead and the amount of lead present in the blood and brain 24 hours later. They observed that the ratio of brain lead to blood lead was constant over a 1000-fold range of lead doses, and that even with an intravenous dose of 1 µg the brain accumulated lead, demonstrating an extremely low threshold in transfer of lead to the brain in animals of this age. Although lead readily entered the brain from blood, it was not as readily removed. One week after lead administration, blood lead levels were 1/7th of the initial values; however, during the same period there was no significant change in brain lead.

In experiments in which lead was fed to young and adult animals, differences in tissue accumulation occurred. Compared with adult animals, the young accumulate lead in tissues readily. For example, under circumstances where rat dams had a higher lead intake than the pups, the concentration of lead in the brains of the dams was lower than that in the brains of the pups (Goldstein and Diamond, 1974). Mykkanen et al. (1979) established that concentrations of lead in blood, kidney, liver, and brain in young rats were related to total lead intake; however, the dose-response curve was markedly different. One-week-old pups had blood lead concentrations similar to those of the dam despite the fact that maternal milk contained only 1/1000 the concentration of lead present in the maternal diet. When young animals were given the same concentration of lead as the dam, the young animals' blood lead levels were several-fold higher than those of the dam.

Because differences in food intake were a factor in the

increased tissue retention reported by others, as a part of our
activities during the past 3 years we have evaluated the effects of
age on tissue lead distribution in studies with rats. In the first
experiments, a constant concentration of lead (200 ppm in water) was
given to young adults (weighing approximately 80 g at the start of
the experiment) for 7 weeks. As the animals grew, lead dosage on a
body weight basis decreased even though the concentration of lead in
water remained unchanged. Older animals had consistently lower
exposures to lead at the same concentration of lead in water. In a
second experiment, comparable dosage on a body weight basis (mg
lead/kg/week) for young and adult animals was achieved by varying
the concentration of lead in water. Under both sets of experimental
conditions young animals retained a greater percentage of lead in
brain, kidney, and femur. When blood lead concentrations were
plotted against tissue lead levels, the slopes of the regression
line were significantly higher for young rats than they were for
adult rats, indicating that tissue lead levels rose faster than
blood lead concentrations in contrast to adult animals (Mahaffey,
1983).

     A question of substantial interest when setting limits on
environmental exposure of infants and toddlers to lead has been the
relationship between environmental exposure to lead (external dose)
and blood lead level (internal dose). Before publication of results
from the Glasgow Duplicate Diet Study (Department of the Environment,
1982), the best available estimates for infants were based on
interpretation of information obtained with adult subjects. For
example, the expert committee retained by the Nutrition Foundation
has evaluated numerous sources of data and estimated the dose-
response curve in adults. Details of the methods used to establish
the association between blood lead level and environmental exposure
to lead are presented in the Nutrition Foundation Expert Advisory
Committee (1982). Figure 1 is based on that committee's evaluation
of the data for adult subjects and indicates that the increase in
blood lead concentration is curvilinear with lead intakes up to 2500
µg/day. Results of the Glasgow Duplicate Diet Study (Department of
the Environment, 1982) shown in Figure 2 indicated that 4-month-old
infants had dietary lead intakes ranging from approximately 0.04 to
3.4 mg lead/week (approximately 6 to 486 µg lead/day). Analyses of
the data indicated that the blood lead concentrations associated with
dietary lead intake (mostly secondary to lead contamination of the
water supply) were more accurately predicted by equations based on a
curvilinear rather than a linear association between dietary lead
intake and blood lead. Although for both infants and adults a
curvilinear curve best predicted blood lead from dietary lead,
infants had far higher blood lead levels than would adults exposed to
the same external dose of lead. If the animal data are applicable to
human infants, brain lead retention would rise even more rapidly than
blood lead levels. Change in CNS function in young humans are
considered to be the critical effect of lead.

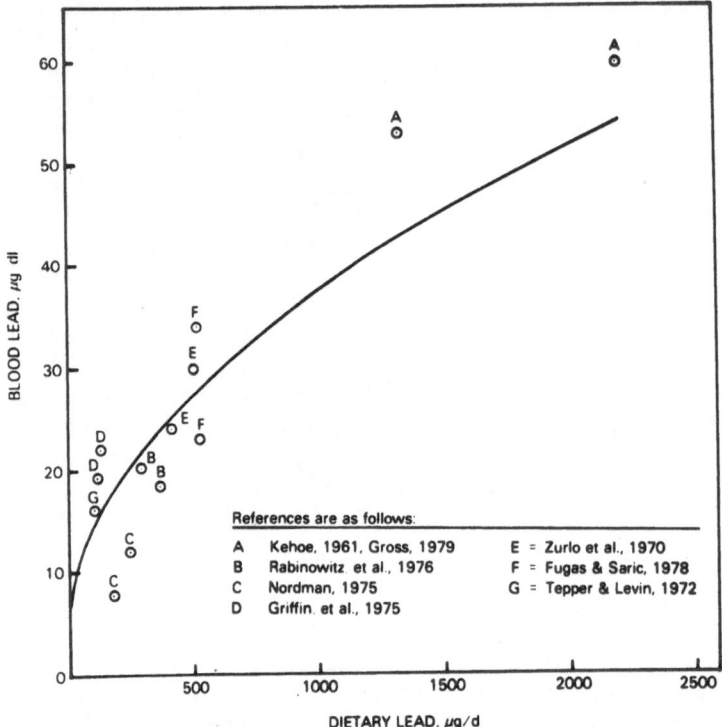

Figure 1   The relationship of dietary lead intake in adults to blood
lead concentrations.   Nutrition Foundation Expert Advisory
Committee, 1982.

Data from the Glasgow study demonstrated that the lead intakes
of breast-fed infants were lower than those of bottle-fed infants
under circumstances in which the water used to prepare the formula
was extensively contaminated with lead.   However, there is an
interesting contrast between formula-fed and breast-fed infants.
Although the intercept of the regression line was 3 times lower for
the breast-fed infants than the bottle-fed infants, the slope of the
regression line for blood lead plotted against dietary lead was
greater for breast-fed infants.   This may indicate that the lead in
human milk was more bioavailable than lead in cow's milk or that the
relationship between blood lead and dietary lead intake was
curvilinear.

Cadmium

Concentrations of cadmium in the newborn are quite low.   The
body burden of cadium is accumulated beginning early in life.
Information for specific tissues on the accumulation patterns of

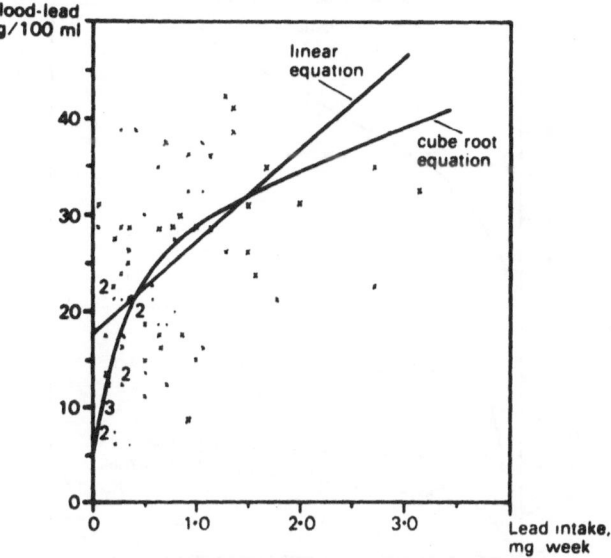

Figure 2   Blood lead concentration versus weekly lead intake for
           bottle-fed infants. Dietary lead intakes ranged from
           approximatly 6 to 486 μg per day. The cube root equation
           was reported to fit the data more precisely than the
           linear equation at the lower range of dietary intakes
           identified in this investigation. The Glasgow Duplicate
           Diet Study (1979/1980), Department of the Environment
           (1982).

orally administered cadmium over a prolonged time period is quite
limited. Sabbioni et al. (1978) reported results of a 2-year
feeding study in which rats were fed 61 ppb cadmium (50 ppb cadmium
in water as cadmium chloride and 11 ppb cadmium in food). Data
presented in Figure 3 demonstrate that during the first 100 days
there was an initial rapid increase in the cadmium concentrations in
kidney, intestine, liver, pancreas, spleen, lung, and testes. The
increase in organ cadmium content would be especially demonstrated
if total cadmium accumulation was calculated, because the total
accumulation would reflect the increase in size of organs as well as
increased cadmium concentration during this period of rapid growth.
After the first 100 days of cadmium administration, cadmium
concentration continued to increase in kidney, spleen, lung, and
testes; however, intestine, liver, and pancreas accumulated only
minimal amounts after the first 100 days. Cadmium concentrations in
brain were lower than in any other tissue measured and showed very
limited increases. Subcellular distributions of [109]Cd in kidney,
liver, intestine, and pancrease were similar and did not change to
an appreciable extent with age during the 800-day course of the

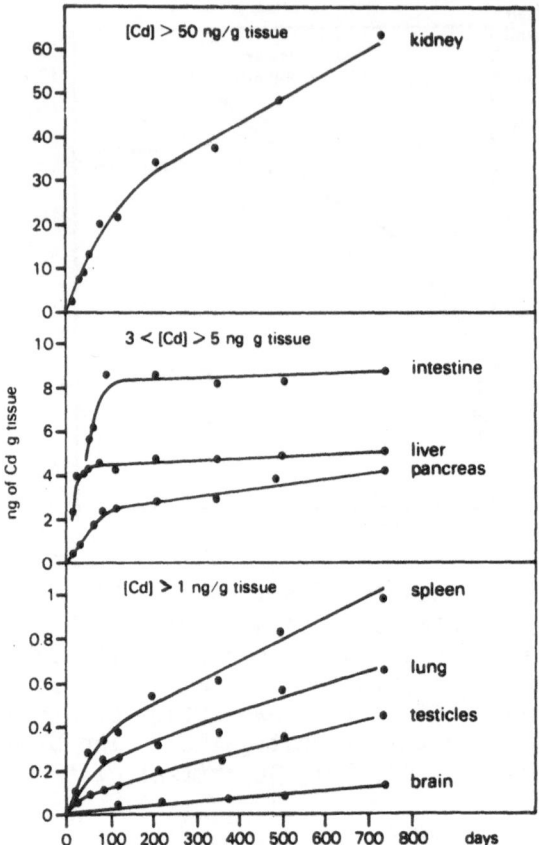

Figure 3 Cadmium accumulation patterns in different tissues of rats
          sacrificed at various times during a period of exposure to
          61 ppb cadmium. Accumulation patterns are based on uptake
          of [109]Cd during the experimental period. Animals
          weighed 150-170 g at the start of the experiment:
          accordingly, total cadmium concentrations are higher than
          those shown in this figure because of the presence of
          cadmium in organs at the start of the experimental
          period. Sabbioni et al. (1978). Reprinted with
          permission of Elsevier Scientific Publishing Company.

study. Henke et al. (1970), using neutron activation analysis,
determined cadmium concentrations in liver and kidney of 41 human
subjects. Cadmium was detectable in newborn infants and the
concentrations increased 200-fold during the first 3 years of life
(Figure 4). The total increase in renal cadmium was even greater
than is shown by the concentration data because of increasing
weights of the kidneys and liver between birth and 3 years of age.

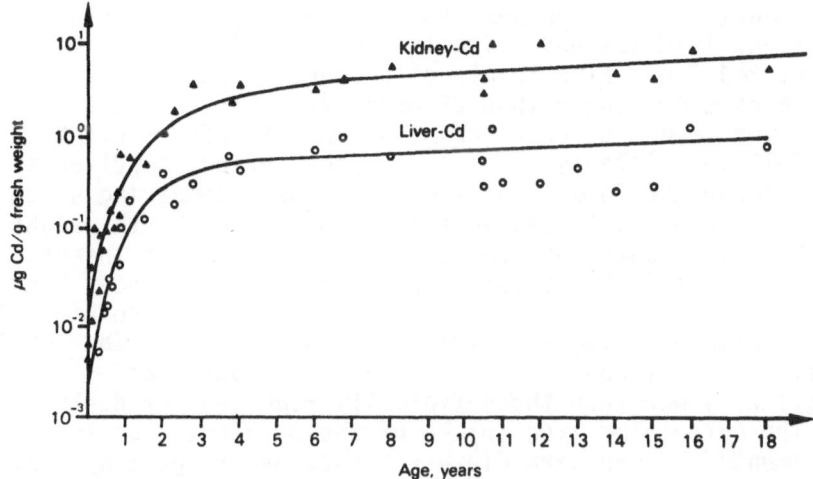

Figure 4   Cadmium concentrations in kidney and liver of human
            subjects determined by neutron activation analysis. Henke
            et al. (1970). Reprinted with permission of Springer-
            Verlag, New York.

Median cadmium concentrations of renal cortex have been reported to
be 900 (Livingston, 1972) and 725 (Schroeder and Balassa, 1961)
times higher in adults than in infants.

    The human brain appears to exhibit a substantially attenuated
accumulation of cadium in contrast to other organs. In an extensive
summary of published data on concentrations of camium in human
tissues, Cherry (1982) noted that brain cadmium levels in adults are
usually not increased greatly even in workers heavily exposed to
cadmium. Unfortunately, there seem to be few data on brain cadmium
concentrations of human infants; most samples have been obtained
from persons aged 7 years or older. However, Suzuki et al. (1979)
reported that cadmium concentrations in the brain of postnatal humans
(ages 0, 1, 3, 5, 7, 8, 11, 17, 20 and 37 years) were substantially
higher than those in tissue of fetal origin. Because of the effects
of other metals on development of the CNS and the relatively greater
transfer of metals into the immature CNS, uptake of cadium into the
infant's brain is a subject of importance.

Zinc

    Tissue zinc levels in infants appear to decline during the early
postnatal period. Dauncey et al. (1977) have shown that preterm
infants were in negative zinc balance because they could not reabsorb

even the amounts of zinc present in pancreatic and intestinal secretions and in discarded epithelial cells. McIntosh et al. (1974) reported femur zinc levels of preterm infants dying after either 8-14 days or longer than 28 days after birth; the quantities of zinc in the femurs of both groups of infants were lower than those of full-term infants. The longer the infants survived after birth, the lower the femur zinc stores became. Comparing serum zinc levels of 27 preterm infants, 24 full-term but low birth weight (i.e., <2500 g) infants, and 38 full-term birth weight infants, Gibson and DeWolfe (1981) found no significant differences between sexes or among the three groups. Serum zinc levels were highest at birth and declined during the first 3 months of life. The levels then remained fairly constant between 3 and 6 months at concentrations lower than those typically reported for North American adults. The calculated zinc intake of these infants was less than that recommended by Canadian Dietary Standards, suggesting that the decline may be secondary to an inadequate intake of zinc (Gibson and DeWolfe, 1981).

EFFECTS OF CHANGING TISSUE METAL CONCENTRATIONS IN INFANTS AND YOUNG CHILDREN

Because of age-associated differences in tissue metal concentrations accompanying exposures to a specific environmental level of a metal, data comparing biological effects at comparable tissue levels of the metal are somewhat difficult to identify. These data have been reviewed elsewhere for lead (Mahaffey, 1983) and demonstrate that infants and young children show greater effects of lead at similar exposures when compared with adults. It has been observed that children have a greater inhibition of hematopoiesis at a particular blood lead concentration. For children under 12 years of age, the no-response level for free erythrocyte protoporphyrin (FEP) appears to be lower than 10 μg lead/100 ml whole blood (Cavalleri et al., 1981). Among adults, FEP increases when blood lead levels exceed 10 μg/100 ml in females (Stuik, 1974; Torimuri and Kawai, 1981) and 30 μg/100 ml in males (Stuik, 1974).

Currently, the most sensitive lead-associated change thought to reflect impaired hormonal function of the kidney is reduction of plasma levels of 1,25-dihydroxyvitamin D. This vitamin D metabolite, which is formed in the kidney, is active in stimulating gastrointestinal absorption of calcium and phosphorus. Children having highly elevated body burdens of lead, consistent with a blood lead level >60 μg/100 ml, had severely reduced levels of 1,25-dihydroxyvitamine D_3 (Rosen et al., 1980). Because of the health effects associated with this degree of elevation in the body lead burden, the children underwent chelation therapy with ethylenediaminetetraacetic acid. The therapy decreased the blood lead levels and increased the plasma 1,25-dihydroxyvitamin D_3 to concentrations observed among control subjects. It is possible that this change reflects a different rate of destruction of 1,25-dihydroxyvitamin D3 or formation of another metabolite rather than reduced renal formation of 1,25-dihydroxyvitamin D3. Reduced plasma 1,25-dihydroxyvitamine D3 levels have been observed in lead-fed rats (Smith et al., 1981).

Reduction in plasma 1,25-dihydroxyvitamin D3 occurs over a wide range of blood lead levels in children under 5 years of age (Figure 5). Regression analysis of data associating blood lead concentration with plasma 1,25-dihydroxyvitamin D3 levels in young children has demonstrated a strong negative correlation (r = -0.88) over the observed range of blood lead levels, 12 to 120 µg/100 ml (Mahaffey et al., 1982). In contrast, Landrigan et al. (1981) found no alteration in mean plasma 1,25-dihydroxyvitamin D3 concentrations among adult workers with prolonged lead exposure. In addition to age of the subjects, concurrent exposure to cadmium and silica may have played a role in the absence of response among the adults.

A detailed review of age-related effects of lead on the CNS is published elsewhere (Mahaffey, 1983). Many of the CNS effects of lead are related to delays in development and accordingly are age-dependent. Extensive clinical experience has established the susceptibility of the infant and young child to CNS damage after exposure to high doses of lead. Age-related responsiveness has been demonstrated in the sense that to induce severe CNS lesions, rodents must be exposed to lead prenatally or during the suckling period (Krigman et al., 1974; Goldstein and Diamond, 1974). As more has become known about the range of CNS effects caused by lead, the question of sensitivity of the developmental process to lower levels of exposure to lead has been addressed. Several investigators have reported delays in synaptogenesis (McCauley et al., 1979) and delayed attainment of mature levels of lipid characteristic of the myelination process (Stephens and Garber, 1981) among animals exposed to levels of lead not resulting in overt toxicity. Fox (1979) observed that when neonatal rats were exposed to lead via the dams' milk from parturition to weaning the lead-exposed group exhibited delayed maturation, altered developmental patterns, and long-term disturbances of CNS function.

Cadmium

By comparison with lead, relatively little is known about effects of low-dose cadmium exposure on the young animal in contrast to the adult. Krigman et al. (1979) reported that cadmium will induce vasculopathy in suckling rats but not in weanling rats. Rats exposed to cadmium prenatally and through the suckling period showed a decrease in spontaneous locomotor activity, but no differences could be demonstrated in their capacities in either acquisition or

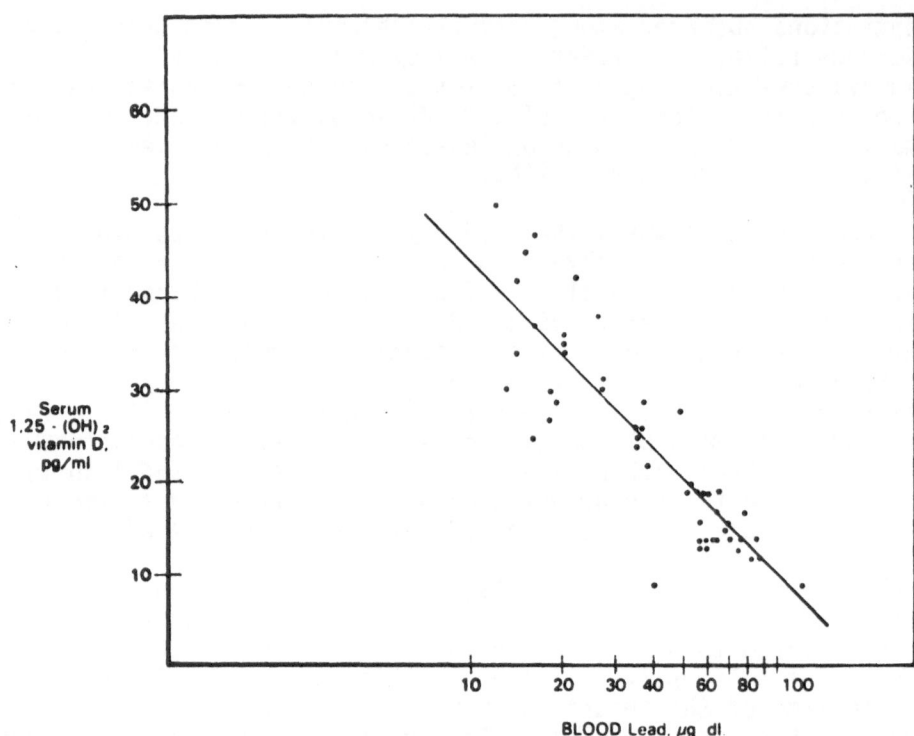

Figure 5   Association between blood lead concentration and serum
1,25-dihydroxyvitamin D among children ages 2 to 3 years.
Mahaffey et al. (1982).

reversal of a discrimination task (Hastings et al., 1978). Karp and
Robertson (1982) noted that information on biochemical abnormalities
associated with increased cadmium ingestion is completely lacking
for human infants and few data are available for experimental
animals. Cadmium exposure is known to substantially alter tissue
levels of a number of nutritionally required metals (Mahaffey et
al., 1981, and references cited therein).

Zinc

Zinc is a required nutrient and is necessary for nucleic acid
metabolism, protein synthesis, and cell (Gordon et al., 1981;
Hambidge, 1981) and membrane integrity (Bettger and O'Dell, 1981).
During infancy, requirements for this nutrient are high. Impairment
of cell-mediated immune response in human infants has been shown by
Weston et al. (1977). Behavioral abnormalities are prominent in
severe zinc deficiency (Walravens et al., 1978) and may also occur

in less severe cases of zinc depletion. Irritability, lethargy, and
depression have been described even at an early stage in the clinical
course (Hambidge, 1981).

CONCLUSIONS

Exposures to lead and cadmium are greater relative to body
weight for infants and very young children compared with adults.
Because of the diversity of sources of lead and cadmium, there are
wide variations in total exposures to these metals. At relatively
low exposure to lead and cadmium, diet can be a major source of
these metals. As the dose-response relationship between
environmental exposure and health effects has been elucidated,
progressively lower levels of lead and cadmium have been identified
as important, particularly among infants and very young children.
Zinc intake during infancy and the infants' requirement for the metal
in growth and development result in a general clinical picture quite
different from that of lead and cadmium.

REFERENCES

Alexander, F.W. and Delves, H.T., 1981, Blood lead levels during
    pregnancy, Int. Arch. Occup. Environ. Health 48:35-39.
Alexander, F.W., Clayton, B.E. and Delves, H.T., 1974, Mineral and
    trace-metal balances in children receiving normal and synthetic
    diets, Q. J. Med. 43:89-111.
Baker, E.L., Folland, D.S., Taylor, T.A., Frank, M., Peterson, W.,
    Lovejoy, G., Cox, D., Housworth, J. and Landrigan, P.J., 1977,
    Lead poisoning in children of lead workers. Home contamination
    with industrial dust, N. Engl. J. Med. 296:260-261.
Barltrop, D., 1966, The prevalence of pica, Am. J. Dis. Child.
    112:116-123.
Barltrop, D., 1969, Transfer of lead to the human foetus, in:
    "Mineral Metabolism in Paediatrics", D. Barltrop and W.L.
    Burland, eds., pp. 135-151, Blackwell Scientific Publication,
    Inc., Oxford.
Beloian, A., 1982, Use of a food consumption model to estimate human
    contaminant intake, Environ. Monit. Assessment 2:115-127.
Beloian, A. and McDowell, M., 1982, Estimates of lead intakes among
    children up to 5 years of age, 1973-1978 and 1980, Food and Drug
    Administration, Washington, D.C.
Bettger, W.J. and O'Dell, B.L., 1981, A critical physiological role:
    zinc in the structure and function of membranes, Life Sci.
    28:1425-1438.
Cantarow, A. and Trumper, M., 1944, "Lead Poisoning", p. 143,
    Williams and Wilkins Co., Baltimore.
Casey, C.W., Walravens, P.A. and Hambidge, K.M., 1981, Availability
    of zinc: Loading tests with human milk, cow's milk, and infant
    formula, Pediatrics 68:394-396.

Cavalleri, A., Baruffini, A., Minoia, C. and Bianco, L., 1981,
    Biological response of children to low levels of inorganic
    lead, Environ. Res. 25:415-423.
Cherry, W.H., 1982, Distribution of cadmium in human tissues, in:
    "Cadmium in the Environment. Part II. Health Effects", J.O.
    Nriagu, ed., pp. 72-483, John Wiley and Sons, New York.
Chisolm, J.J. Jr., 1980, Poisonings from heavy metals (mercury,
    lead, and cadmium), Pediatr. Ann. 9:458-468.
Clark, A.R.L., 1977, Placental transfer of lead and its effects on
    the newborn, Postgrad. Med. J. 53:674-678.
Dauncey, M.J., Shaw, J.C.L. and Urman, A.J., 1977, The absorption
    and retention of magnesium, zinc and copper by low birth weight
    infants fed pasteurized milk, Pediatr. Res. 11:991-997.
Department of the Environment, 1982, The Glasgow Duplicate Diet
    Study (1979/80), A joint study for the Department of the
    Environment and the Ministry of Agriculture, Fisheries and
    Food. Control Directorate on Environmental Pollution.
    Pollution Report No. 11, Her Majesty's Stationery Office,
    London.
Duggan, M.J. and Williams, S., 1977, Lead-in-dust in city streets,
    Sci. Total Environ. 7:91-97.
Duggan, R.E. and McFarland, F.J., 1967, Residues in food and feed.
    Assessments include raw food and feed commodities, market
    basket items prepared for consumption, meat samples taken at
    slaughter, Pestic. Monit. J. 1:1-5.
Fomon, S.J., 1974, "Infant Nutrition," (2nd ed.), W.B. Saunders
    Company, Philadelphia/London.
Fomon, S.J., 1978, Progress Report, Food and Drug Administration
    Contract Number 223-75-2238, Washington, D.C.
Food and Drug Administration, 1979a, Compliance Program Evaluation,
    FY-75 Total Diet Studies - Adult (7320.08), United States
    Department of Health, Education, and Welfare, Washington, D.C.
Food and Drug Administration, 1979b, Compliance Program Evaluation,
    FY-75 Total Diet Studies - Infant and Toddler (7320.33), United
    States Department of Health, Education, and Welfare, Washington,
    D.C.
Food and Drug Administration, 1980a, Compliance Program Report of
    Findings, FY-76 Total Diet Studies - Adult (7320.57), United
    States Department of Health, Education, and Welfare, Washington,
    D.C.
Food and Drug Administration, 1980b, Compliance Program Report of
    Findings, FY-76 Total Diet Studies - Infant and Toddler
    (7320.58), United States Department of Health, Education, and
    Welfare, Washington, D.C.
Food and Drug Administration, 1980c, Compliance Program Report of
    Findings, FY-77 Total Diet Studies - Adult (7320.73), United
    States Department of Health, Education and Welfare, Washington,
    D.C.

Food and Drug Administration, 1980d, Compliance Program Report of
    Findings, FY-77 Total Diet Studies - Infants and Toddlers
    (7320.74), United States Department of Health, Education,
    Welfare, Washington, D.C.
Food and Drug Administration, 1981a, Compliance Program Report of
    Findings, FY-78 Total Diet Studies - Adult (7305.003), United
    States Department of Health and Human Services, Washington, D.C.
Food and Drug Administration, 1981b, Compliance Program Report of
    Findings, FY-78 Total Diet Studies - Infants and Toddlers,
    (7305.002), United States Department of Health and Human
    Services, Washington, D.C.
Food and Drug Administration, 1982a, Compliance Program Report of
    Findings, FY-79 Total Diet Studies - Adult (7305.002). United
    States Department of Health and Human Services, Washington, D.C.
Food and Drug Administration, 1982b, Compliance Program Report of
    Findings, FY-79 Total Diet Studies - Infants and Toddlers
    (7305.002). United States Department of Health and Human
    Services, Washington, D.C.
Food and Nutrition Board, National Academy of Sciences - National
    Research Council, 1980, Recommended Dietary Allowances, Edn. 9,
    National Academy of Sciences Press, Washington, D.C.
Forbes, G.B. and Reina, J.C., 1972, Effect of age on gastrointestinal
    absorption (Fe, Sr, Pb) in the rat, J. Nutr. 102:647-652.
Fox, D.A., 1979, Physiological and neurobehavioral alterations during
    development in lead exposed rats, Neurobehavioral Toxicol.
    1:193-206.
Fugas, M. and Saric, M., 1978, Health Study of Lead-Exposed
    Population, International Lead Zinc Research Organization
    Project LH-171, New York, cited in Nutrition Foundation Expert
    Advisory Commission Report, 1982.
Gershanik, J.J., Brooks, G.G. and Little, J.A., 1974, Blood lead
    values in pregnant women and their offspring, Am. J. Obstet.
    Gynecol. 119:508-511.
Gibson, R.S. and DeWolfe, M.S., 1981, Changes in serum zinc
    concentrations of some Canadian full term and low birthweight
    infants from birth to six months, Acta Pediatr. Scand.
    70:497-500.
Goldstein, G.W. and Diamond, I., 1974, Metabolic basis of lead
    encephalopathy, Res. Publ. Assoc. Nerv. Ment. Dis. 53:393-304.
Gordon, E.F., Gordon, R.C. and Passal, D.B., 1981, Zinc metabolism:
    Basic, clinical, and behavioral aspects, J. Pediatr. 93:341-349.
Griffin, T.B., Coulson, F., Goldberg, L., Wills, H. and Russell,
    J.C., 1975, Clinical studies of men continuously exposed to
    airborne particulate lead, in: "Lead Environmental Quality and
    Safety, Suppl. Vol. 2", F. Coulston, and F. Korte, eds., George
    Thieme Publishers, Stuttgart, cited in Nutrition Foundation
    Expert Advisory Committee Report, 1982.
Gross, S., 1979, Oral and Inhalation Lead Exposure in Human Subjects,
    Lead Industries Association, New York, cited in Nutrition
    Foundation Expert Advisory Committee Report, 1982.

Haas, T., Wieck, A.G., Schaller, K.H., Mache, K. and Valentin, H.,
    1972, Die usuelle Bleibelastung bei Neugeburenen und ihren
    Muttern, Zentralbl. Bakteriol. Orig. B 155:341-349.
Hambidge, K.M., 1981, Zinc deficiency in man: Origins and effects,
    Philos. Trans. R. Soc. London Ser. B 294:129-144.
Hastings, L., Choudhury, H., Petering, H.G. and Cooper, G.P., 1978,
    Behavioral and biochemical effects of low level prenatal
    cadmium exposure in rats. Bull. Environ. Contam. Toxicol.
    20:96-101.
Henke, G., Sachs, H.W. and Bohn, G., 1970, Cadmium-bestimmungen in
    Leber und Nieren von Kindern und Jugendlichen durch
    Neutronaktivierunganalyse, Arch. Toxicol. 26:8-16.
Hietanen, E., 1982, Gastrointestinal absorption of cadmium, in:
    "Cadmium in the Environment, Part II, Health Effects", J.O.
    Nriagu, ed., pp. 55-68, John Wiley and Sons, New York.
Hurley, L.S. and Lonnerdal, B., 1982, Zinc binding in human milk:
    Citrate versus picolinate, Nutr. Rev. 40:65-71.
Jugo, S., 1980, Chelatable fraction of ^{203}Pb in blood of young and
    adult rats, Environ. Res. 21:336-342.
Kaferstein, F.K. and Muller, J., 1981, Schwermetalle in
    Sauglingsnahrung (Heavy Metals in the Infant Diet), Dietrich
    Reimer Verlag, Berlin.
Kaferstein, F.K. and Mueller, J., 1981, Schwermetalle in
    Sauglingsnahrung (Heavy Metals in the Infant Diet), Dietrich
    Reimer Verlag, Berlin.
Karp, W.B. and Robertson, A.F., 1982, Cadmium, the placenta, and the
    infant, in: "Cadmium in the Environment. Part II. Health
    Effects", J.O. Nriagu, ed., pp. 729-742, John Wiley and Sons,
    New York.
Kehoe, R.A., 1961, The metabolism of lead in man in health and
    disease. I. The normal metabolism of lead, J.R. Inst. Public
    Health, 24:81-97, cited in Nutrition Foundation Expert Advisory
    Committee Report, 1982.
Kolbye, A.C., Mahaffey, K.R., Fiorino, J.A., Corneliussen, P.E. and
    Jelinek, C.F., 1974, Food exposure to lead, Environ. Health
    Perspect. 7:65-74.
Kostial, K., Maljkovic, T. and Jugo, S., 1974, Lead acetate toxicity
    in rats in relation to age and sex, Arch. Toxicol. 31:265-269.
Kostial, K., Kello, D., Blanusa, M., Maljkovic, T. and Rabar, I.,
    1979, Influence of some factors on cadmium pharmacokinetics and
    toxicity, Environ. Health Perspect. 28:89-95.
Kraehenbuhl, J.P. and Campiche, M.A., 1969, Early stages of
    intestinal absorption of specific antibodies in the newborn, J.
    Cell Biol. 42:345-365.
Krigman, M.R., Druse, M.J., Traylor, T.D., Wilson, M.H., Nowell, L.R.
    and Hogan, E.L., 1974, Lead encephalopathy in the developing
    rat: Effects on cortical ontogenesis, J. Neuropathol. Exp.
    Neurol. 33:671-686.
Krigman, R.R., Bouldin, T.W., Bagnell, C.R. and Rhyne, J., 1979,
    Heavy metal vasculopathy in the neonatal rat, J. Neuropathol.
    Exp. Neurol. 39:80a.

Landrigan, P.J., Albrecht, W.N., Watanabe, A. and Lee, S., 1981, National Institute of Occupational Safety and Health Report, 1976, HETA 80-116, December, Cincinnati, Ohio.

Lauwerys, R., Buchet, J.P., Roels, H. and Hubermont, G., 1978, Placental transfer of lead, mercury cadmium and carbon monoxide in women: I. Comparison of the frequency distributions of the biological indices in maternal and umbilical cord blood, Environ. Res. 15:278-289.

Lecce, J.G., 1972, Selective absorption of macromolecules into intestinal epithelium and blood by neonatal mice, J. Nutr. 102:69-76.

Lepow, K.L., Bruckman, L., Rubin, R.A., Markowitz, S., Gillette, M. and Kapish, J., 1974, Role of airborne lead in increased body burden of lead in Hartford children, Environ. Health Perspect. 7:99-102.

Li, T.-K. and Vallee, B.L., 1980, The biochemical and nutritional roles of other trace elements, in: "Modern Nutrition in Health and Disease", 6th ed., R.S. Goodhart and M.E. Shila, eds., p. 428, Lea and Febiger, Philadelphia.

Lin-Fu, J.S., 1980, Lead poisoning and undue lead exposure in children: History and current status, in: "Low Level Lead Exposure: The Clinical Implications of Current Research", H.H. Needleman, ed., pp. 5-16, Raven Press, New York.

Livingston, H.D., 1972, Measurement and distribution of zinc, cadmium and mercury in human kidney tissue, Clin. Chem. 18:67-72.

Macy, I.G., 1946, "Nutrition and Chemical Growth in Childhood, Vol. II, Original Data", Charles Thomas, Springfield, Illinois.

Mahaffey, K.R., 1978, Environmental exposure to lead, in: "The Biogeochemistry of Lead", J.O. Nriagu, ed., pp. 1-36, Elsevier/ North-Holland Biomedical Press, Amsterdam.

Mahaffey, K.R., 1983, Absorption of lead by infants and young children, in: "Symposium on Health Evaluation of Heavy Metals in Infant Formula and Junior Foods", Springer-Verlag, Berlin (in press).

Mahaffey, K.R., Corneliussen, P.E., Jelinek, C.F. and Fiorino, J.A., 1975, Heavy metal exposure from foods, Environ. Health Perspect. 12:63-69.

Mahaffey, K.R., Capar, S.G., Gladen, B.C. and Fowler, B.A., 1981, Concurrent exposure to lead, cadmium, and arsenic. Effects on toxicity and tissue metal concentrations in the rat, J. Lab. Clin Med. 98:485-481.

Mahaffey, K.R., Rosen, J.F., Chesney, R.W., Peeler, J.T., Smith, C.N. and DeLuca, H.F., 1982, Association between age, blood lead concentration, and serum 1,25-dihydroxycholecalciferol levels among children, Am. J. Clin. Nutr. 35:1327-1331.

McCauley, P.T., Bull, R.J. and Luttenhoff, S.D., 1979, Association of alterations in energy metabolism with lead-induced delays in rat cerebral cortical development, Neuropharmacology, 18:93-101.

McIntosh, N., Shaw, J.C.L. and Toghizadeh, A., 1974, Direct evidence for calcium and trace element deficits in the skeleton of preterm infants, Pediatr. Res. 8:896.

Momcilovic, B. and Kostial, K., 1974, Kinetics of lead retention and distribution in suckling and adult rats, Environ. Res. 8:214-220.

Morton, D.E., Saah, A.J., Silberg, S.L., Owens, W.L., Roberts, M.A. and Saah, M.D., 1982, Lead absorption in children of employees in a lead-related industry, Am. J. Epidemiol. 115:549-555.

Mykkanen, H.M., Dickerson, J.W.T. and Lancaster, N.C., 1979, Effect of age on the tissue distribution of lead in the rat, Toxicol. Appl. Pharmacol. 51:447-454.

Nordman, C.H., 1975, "Environmental Lead Exposure in Finland, A Study of Selected Population Groups", Doctoral Thesis, University of Helsinki, cited in Nutrition Foundation Expert Advisory Committee Report, 1982.

Nriagu, J.O., 1980, "Zinc in the Environment, Part I: Ecological Cycling", John Wiley and Sons, New York.

Nriagu, J.O., 1982, "Cadmium in the Environment, Parts I and II", John Wiley and Sons, New York.

Nutrition Foundation Expert Advisory Committee, 1982, Assessment of the Safety of Lead and Lead Salts in Food, The Nutrition Foundation, Inc., Washington, D.C.

Rabinowitz, M., Wetherell, G.W. and Kopple, J.D., 1976, Kinetic analysis of lead metabolism in human health, J. Clin. Invest. 58:260-270, cited in Nutrition Foundation Expert Advisory Committee Report, 1982.

Rahola, T., Aaron, R. and Miettinen, J.K., 1972, Half-time studies of mercury and cadmium by whole-body counting; assessment of radioactive contaminants in man, International Atomic Energy Agency-SM-150-13, cited in Travis and Haddock, 1980.

Roels, H.A., Bucket, J.-P., Lauwerys, R.R., Bruaux, P., Claeys-Thoreau, F., Lafontaine, A. and Verduyn, G., 1980, Exposure to lead by the oral and the pulmonary routes of children living in the vicinity of a primary lead smelter, Environ. Res. 22:81-94.

Rosen, J.F., Chesney, R.W., Hamstra, A., DeLuca, H.F. and Mahaffey, K.R., 1980, Reductions in 1,25-dihydroxyvitamin D in children with increased lead absorption, N. Engl. J. Med. 302:1128-1131.

Rothberg, R.M., 1969, Immunoglobulin and specific antibody synthesis during the first weeks of life in premature infants, J. Pediatr. 75:391-399.

Ryu, J.E., Ziegler, E.E. and Fomon, S.J., 1978, Maternal lead exposure and blood concentration in infancy, J. Pediatr. 93:476-478.

Sabbioni, E., Marafante, E., Amantini, L., Ubertalli, L. and Pietra, R., 1978, Cadmium toxicity studies under long term-low level (LLE) conditions, Sci. Total Environ. 10:135-161.

Sasser, L.B. and Jarboe, G.E., 1977, Intestinal absorption and retention of cadmium in neonatal rat, Toxicol. Appl. Pharmacol. 41:423-431.

Satzger, R.D., Clow, C.S., Bonnin, E. and Fricke, F.L., 1982, Determination of background levels of lead and cadmium in raw agricultural crops by using differential pulse anodic stripping voltammetry, J. Assoc. Off. Anal. Chem. 65:987-991.

Sayre, J.W., Charney, E., Vostal, J. and Piers, J.B., 1974, House and hand dust as a potential source of childhood lead exposure, Am. J. Dis. Child. 127:167-170.

Schroeder, H.A. and Balassa, J.J., 1961, Abnormal trace metals in man: Cadmium, J. Chron. Dis. 14:236-254.

Sherlock, J., Smart, G., Forbes, G.I., Moore, M.R., Patterson, W.J., Richards, W.N. and Wilson, T.S., 1982, Assessment of lead intakes and dose-response for a population in Ayr exposed to a plumbosoluent water supply, Human Toxicol. 1:115-122.

Smith, C.M., DeLuca, H.F., Tanaka, Y. and Mahaffey, K.R., 1981, Effect of lead ingestion on function of vitamin D and its metabolites, J. Nutr. 111:1321-1329.

Stephens, M.C.G. and Garber, G.B., 1981, Development of glycolipids and gangliosides in lead-treated neonatal rats, Toxicol. Lett. 77:373-378.

Stuik, E.J., 1974, Biological response of male and female volunteers to inorganic lead, Int. Arch. Arbeitmed. 33:83-97.

Sunderman, F.W. and Baerner, F., 1949, "Normal Values in Clinical Chemistry", W.B. Saunders Company, Philadelphia.

Suzuki, K., Esashi, T., Suzue, R., Nishimura, H. and Matsumoto, H., 1979, Tissue concentrations of cadmium, lead and chromium in Japanese ranging from the fetus to elder subjects, Toxicol. Lett. 4:481-484.

Tepper, L.B. and Levin, L.S., 1972, "A Survey of Air and Pollution Lead Levels in Selected American Communities", Final Report (EPA Contract PH 22-68-28) cited in Nutrition Foundation Expert Advisory Committee Report, 1982.

Torimuri, H. and Kawai, M., 1981, Free erythrocyte protoporphyrin (FEP) in a general population, workers exposed to low-level lead, and organic-solvent workers, Environ. Res. 25:310-316.

Travis, C.C. and Haddock, A.G., 1980, Interpretation of the observed age-dependency of cadmium burdens in man, Environ. Res. 22:46-60.

United States National Center for Health Statistics, 1977, Dietary Intake Findings: United States, 1971-974, United States Department of Health, Education, and Welfare. Number HRA 77-1647, Series 11, No. 202, National Center for Health Statistics, Hyattsville, Maryland.

United States National Center for Health Statistics, Growth Norms, Adapted from Hamill, P.V.V., Drizd, T.A., Johnson, C.L., Reed, R.B., Roche, A.F. and Moore, W.M., 1979, Physical growth: National Center for Health Statistics Percentiles, Am. J. Clin. Nutr. 32:607-629.

United States National Center for Health Statistics, 1981, Height
    and Weight of Adults Ages 18-74 Years by Socioeconomic and
    Geographic Variables: United States, DHHS Publication No.
    (PHS) 81-1674, Series 11, No. 224, National Center for Health
    Statistics, Hyattsville, Maryland.
Walravens, P.A., 1980, Nutritional importance of copper and zinc in
    neonates and infants, Clin. Chem. 26:185-189.
Walravens, P.A., van Doornick, W.J. and Hambidge, K.M., 1978, Metals
    and mental function, J. Pediatr. 93:535-541.
Weston, W.L., Huff, J.C., Humbert, J.R., Hambidge, K.M., Neldner,
    K.H.and Walravens, P.A., 1977, Zinc correction of defective
    chemotaxis in acrodermatitis enteropathica, Arch. Dermatol.
    113:422-425.
Willes, R.F., Lok, E. and Truelove, J.F., 1977, Retention and tissue
    distribution of $^{210}Pb(NO_3)_2$ administered orally to infant
    and adult monkeys, J. Toxicol. Environ. Health, 3:395-406.
World Health Organization, 1980, Recommended Health-Based Limits in
    Occupational Exposure to Heavy Metals, World Health Organization
    (Technical Report Series No. 647), Geneva.
Ziegler, E.E., Edwards, B.B., Jensen, R.L., Mahaffey, K.R. and Fomon,
    S.J., 1978, Absorption and retention of lead by infants,
    Pediatr. Res. 12:29-34.
Zurlo, N., Griffini, A.M. and Vigliani, E.C., 1970, The content of
    lead in blood and urine of adults living in Milan, not
    occupationally exposed to lead, Am. Ind. Hyg. Assoc. J.
    31:92-95, cited in Nutrition Foundation Expert Advisory
    Committee Report, 1982.

SPECIAL TOPIC PAPERS

THE INTERNATIONAL PROGRAMME ON CHEMICAL SAFETY IN RELATION TO

REPRODUCTIVE AND DEVELOPMENTAL TOXICOLOGY

Michel Mercier and Jiri Parizek

International Programme on Chemical Safety
WHO, Geneva, Switzerland

The International Programme on Chemical Safety, the IPCS, which
is a joint venture of the United States Environment Programme, the
International Labour Organization, and the World Health Organization
is completing the second year of its operational existence.

The priorities of the Programme include several for which your
meeting is of particular interest such as the evaluation of the risk
from exposure to chemicals as well as promotion and improvement of
related methodology.

IPCS documents, aiming at evaluation of health risks, have to
take into account all the well established and relevant scientific
facts and principles. Some chemicals can have direct detrimental
effects on gonads and reproduction. Furthermore, it is known that
exposure to certain chemicals during specific critical periods of
development can result in developmental deviations and for this
reason the IPCS documents concerned with the evaluation of the
health risks of a particular chemical or class of chemicals always
include an assessment of the teratogenic potential of the chemical.
Assessment of the effects on the embryo and the fetus and of all
their possible manifestations during intrauterine and postnatal life
is of course one of the important components of developmental
toxicology.

Evaluation of the health risks of exposures to chemicals has to
include considerations not only of the critical periods of
development, but also of the fact that subjects of certain age can
belong to a critical segment of population, e.g., due to special
characteristics of exposure (for instance, the amount and type of
food consumed per kg body weight), differences in rate of

809

absorption from the gastrointestinal tract in individuals of different ages, differences in body distribution, metabolism and excretion of chemicals, or age-dependent changes in the characteristics of target tissues resulting in differences in sensitivity to toxic substances, in repair processes, and so on.

The assessment of risks of reproductive failure or developmental deviation associated with exposure to certain chemicals as well as identification of segments of the population at special risk due to age-dependent characteristics, deserve special methodological consideration.

For this reason the IPCS has given a high priority to the critical assessment of the methods available for the integrated evaluation of risks for progeny associated with prenatal exposure to chemicals. A relevant IPCS Working Group was one of the first to be established when developing the methodology component of the IPCS in 1981 and it is expected that an IPCS monograph will be produced next year containing a critical evaluation of the predictive power of methods in this area with a review of the scientific background available for further possible improvements.

Another related study has been conducted by SGOMSEC (Scientific Group on Methodologies for the Safety Evaluation of Chemicals), a scientific group co-sponsored by SCOPE/ICSU, WHO and UNEP. Within IPCS, this group convened a scientific meeting in 1981 to consider methods for assessing the effects of chemicals on reproductive functions and a joint report prepared on the basis of this seminar will be published this year, together with more than 20 individual contributions prepared by the participants.

In 1981, WHO co-sponsored a symposium on the evaluation of heavy metals in infant formulae and junior food and as a follow-up of this symposium, IPCS is now considering the convening of a special task group addressing the problem of assessing the health risks connected with exposure to chemicals during early postnatal life.

These are only a few examples of the present activities and interests of IPCS directly related to this meeting. The IPCS will certainly follow the results of this meeting with a great interest and hope for future cooperation.

QUALITY CONTROL IN LABORATORIES TESTING FOR ENVIRONMENTAL POLLUTION*

Lars Friberg

Department of Environmental Hygiene
National Institute of Environmental Medicine
Karolinska Institute, Stockholm, Sweden

INTRODUCTION

To evaluate experimental and epidemiological data, the quality of the data must meet certain requirements. This is true for effects parameters as well as for dose estimates. A complete treatment of the subject related to quality control in the assessment of environmental pollution is very extensive and impossible to set forth in a brief presentation such as this. Therefore, I will limit discussion to quality control aspects for analysis of two trace metals, lead and cadmium, in blood and kidney. The presentation will be based primarily on results from a global UNEP/WHO project on assessment of exposure to lead and cadmium through biological monitoring. This project which was recently concluded was coordinated by the Karolinska Institute (Department of Environmetal Hygiene) and the National (Swedish) Institute of Environmental Medicine (Vahter, 1982; Friberg and Vahter, 1983). The project was carried out within the framework of UNEP's Global Environmental Monitoring System (GEMS) and was initiated in 1978 on the basis of recommendations from a UNEP/WHO meeting of a Government Expert Group on Health-related Monitoring.

---

* Presented at Caracas.

One objective of the project was to carry out pilot studies of selected segments of the population in a number of countries taking into consideration differences in climate and development. The countries included in the project were: Belgium, India, Israel, Japan, Mexico, People's Republic of China, Peru, Sweden (ex officio), USA and Yugoslavia. To make possible intercountry comparisons of data, one occupational group, teachers, were chosen for the analysis of lead and cadmium in blood. Cases of sudden unexpected death were used for analysis of cadmium in kidney cortex. Two hundred teachers and approximately fifty autopsy cases from one metropolitan area of each country were included in the project.

PREVIOUS STUDIES

There are a large number of reports in the literature on "normal" levels of lead and cadmium in the blood of non-occupationally exposed persons. Unfortunately, most of these published reports lack quality control data which makes valid international comparison of the exposure to lead and cadmium based on blood level impossible. A review of published data showed that mean concentrations of lead in blood in the general population are in the order of 40-50 µg Pb/100ml and those for cadmium 2-5 µg Cd/100 ml or even higher. Such values are in accordance with a corresponding lack of quality control data. The literature also contains several reports on intra- and interlaboratory comparison studies which clearly emphasize the urgent need for quality control programs. Two examples will serve to illustrate this point. Berlin et al. (1973) sent three samples of blood to 22 different laboratories for analysis. For one of the samples the blood lead level reported ranged from 14 to 86 µg Pb/100 ml, for another sample from 21 to 117 µg Pb/100 ml and for a third sample from 12 to 74 µg Pb/100 ml. In another study (Lerner, 1975) blood obtained from a single person was divided into 35 separate samples and sent to a well recognized laboratory over a period of 9 months together with other samples. A considerable variation in lead levels was reported with a mean of 19 µg Pb/100 ml blood and a standard deviation of 5.7 µg Pb/100 ml. The values reported ranged from 12 to 42 µg Pb/100 ml blood.

Based on this knowledge, it was considered a necessary and important part of the project to include a program for rigid quality control in connection with sampling, storage, transport and analysis of tissues and body fluids. The participating institutions agreed that the actual monitoring of teachers' samples should not be embarked upon until the laboratories involved had completed the training phase of the project satisfactorily. A close collaboration was established with an ongoing monitoring program for lead in blood within the Common Market (Berlin, 1982; Vahter, 1982).

METHODS

Analytical Procedures

The purpose of the project was not to standardize analytical procedures. Indeed, it was recommended that each participating laboratory use methods of its own choice, providing they produced results meeting the quality assurance criteria. Advice was to be given, however, on suitable methods particularly in cases where the use of new analytical activities was started.

For blood analysis, the participating laboratories as a rule used atomic absorption spectrophotometry (AAS) with background correction. For lead in blood, three laboratories used the Delves Cup technique (Delves, 1970; Ediger and Coleman, 1972) modified according to Lind (personal communication). Seven laboratories used electrothermal atomization (ETA), originally reported by Matousek and Stevens (1971). Three used the method by Fernandez (1975) and four the method by Stoeppler and Brandt (1980), in most cases modified according to Lind (personal communication).

For cadmium in kidney cortex all laboratories used flame AAS. Five used dry ashing pretreatment and four used wet digestion pretreatment.

Quality control samples

Quality control samples for analysis of lead and cadmium in blood consisted of hemolyzed cow blood containing EDTA and sterilized by gamma irradiation. The samples were spiked with lead and cadmium. For quality control analysis of cadmium in kidney cortex, samples of freeze-dried horse kidney cortex were provided. Horse kidneys were used since horses accumulate cadmium in the kidney cortex with age to an even greater extent than humans. The US National Bureau of Standards (NBS) have certified samples of bovine liver available for cadmium analysis. However, there is only one concentration available and this concentration is too low to be of any real value for kidney cortex analysis. It is necessary that approximately the same concentration of a specific element be analyzed in the EQC samples as is present in the actual monitoring samples. Both the blood and kidney samples could be stored frozen for extended periods of time without any change in metal concentration. The quality control (QC) samples were sent airfreight frozen and in special containers to the participating laboratores and were received by the laboratories in good condition.

Most laboratories received twelve sets of QC samples, each set consisting of six samples. The results from each laboratory were evaluated statistically in order to decide whether to accept or

reject the laboratory's current performance. The main purpose of
the procedure was to prevent systematic errors in the range of values
likely to occur. Blood samples delivered to the laboratories were
spiked with between 10-40 μg Pb/100 ml in the case of lead, and
between 0.1-1.5 μg Cd/100 ml for cadmium. Cadmium in kidney cortex
samples usually varied between 50-400 mg Cd/kg dry weight.

Statistical evaluation

A regression line of the reported versus "true" values was
calculated. In this way it was possible to obtain an average of the
laboratories' current performance and to establish an acceptance
criterion based on the extent to which the regression line was
allowed to deviate from the ideal y=x; of course certain deviation
from the ideal had to be accepted. The following limits for maximum
allowable deviation (MAD-lines) from the regression line y=x were
employed. Naturally this line may be varied ad libitum for other
projects.

For lead in blood (μg/100 ml)	$y = x \pm (0.1x + 20)$
for cadmium in blood (μg/100 ml)	$y = x \pm (0.1x + 1)$
for cadmium in kidney cortex (mg/kg dry weight)	$y = x \pm (0.15x)$

I will not discuss the statistical analysis in detail but refer
to the original reports (Vahter, 1982; Friberg and Vahter, 1983).
In order to ascertain with a certain power, in this particular case
80 percent, that the "true" regression line representing the
laboratories' performance does not fall outside the MAD-lines, the
calculated regression line must conform to stricter criteria.
Therefore, so-called acceptance lines were calculated, based on
among other factors the number of EQC samples analyzed. Figure 1
displays a hypothetical result showing the regression line based on
six reported values as well as acceptability lines and MAD-lines.

In Figure 2 results are shown for one laboratory on three
different occasions. During period A and period B the data deviate
markedly from the acceptability lines while for period C the
regression line falls within the acceptability lines.

In order to obtain a quantitative estimate to allow easy
comparison of results from different QC runs, ratios were constructed
based on the principles depicted in Figure 3. The difference between
the function values at each evaluation point and the "true" values
(the value shown on the regression line y=x) were divided by the
accepted deviation at the evaluation points. The calculations can
be expressed as:

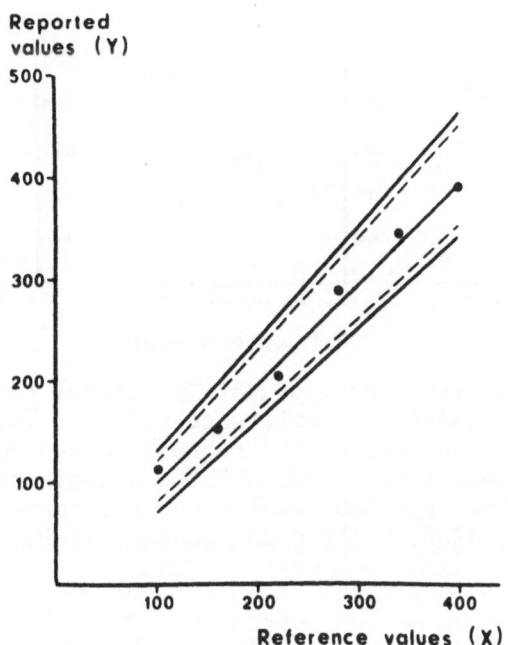

Figure 1   Regression line based on six reported values.   Solid lines
           indicate the MAD-lines and dotted lines the acceptance
           lines (Vahter, 1982; Friberg and Vahter, 1983).

$$\frac{a_1}{b_1} \text{ and } \frac{a_2}{b_2}$$

where a_1 and a_2 in Figure 3 indicate the differences between the
end points of the calculated regression line and the "true" values,
and b_1 and b_2 indicate the accepted deviation from the "true"
value (differences between the acceptance lines and the "true"
values).

     In Figure 3, A shows an accepted QC run, although the
calculated regression line is just contiguous with acceptance at the
upper evaluation point.   B shows a rejected QC run with a ratio of
6.7 at the lower evaluation point.

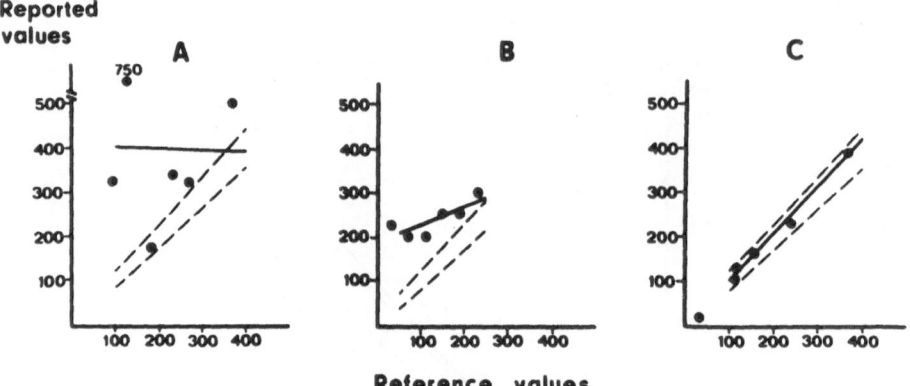

Figure 2   Diagrams with reported quality control results (µg Pb/1)
plotted against the reference values. The solid line
indicates the calculated regression and dotted lines
(acceptance lines) indicate the acceptance interval. A
and B show rejected results and C accepted results
(Vahter, 1982; Friberg and Vahter, 1983).

RESULTS FROM QUALITY CONTROL STUDIES

        Calculated ratios are displayed in bar diagrams, which simplify
the tracing of changes in performance for the different laboratories
during the training phase of the project (Figures 4 and 5). The
left bar in each pair of bars represents the outcome at the lower
evaluation point and the right bar the outcome at the upper
evaluation point. Positive bars indicate that reported values were
high, negative bars that reported values were low in relation to the
calculated ideal values. The dotted lines represent the acceptance
interval.

        As can be seen from the figures, gross difference from expected
values (assuming accurate analysis) were found for several of the
laboratories during the early part of the training phase.
Obviously, the fact that a laboratory performs well in the analysis
of one metal is no guarantee that this holds true for other metals.
The results also show that there was a defininte improvement over
time and by the end of the study all laboratories performed
satisfactory analyses. Results indicate, however, the necessity for
not only a limited number of quality control analysis but for
quality control analysis on a continuous basis.

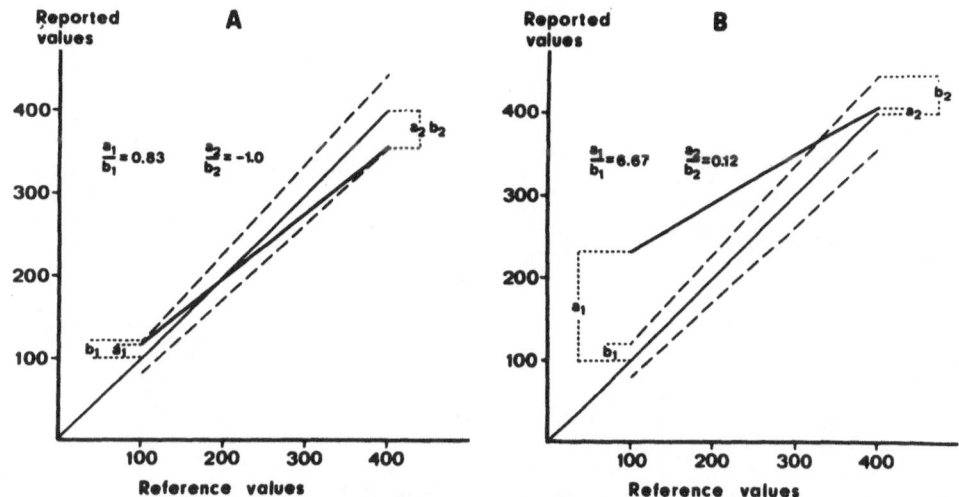

Figure 3   Illustrations of the procedure used for the calculation of
            ratios between obtained deviation from the reference value
            and the accepted deviation at the preset evaluation points
            (100 and 400 µg Pb/1). For explanation, see text. A
            gives an example of an accepted QC run and B of a rejected
            QC run (Vahter, 1982; Friberg and Vahter, 1983).

        Figures 6 and 7 show the results of the quality control analysis
during the actual monitoring of teachers' blood. In this particular
case we have pooled the data from five separate quality control runs
which means that in most cases the evaluation is based on thirty
samples for each laboratory. As can be seen, all laboratories met
the criteria for acceptance.

        In addition to the quality control program reported here,
duplicate analysis of a number of samples analyzed in Japan, Mexico
and Peru was carried out. Figure 8 shows the results of the
comparison on lead analyses performed in Mexico City and at our
laboratory in Sweden. As can be seen, agreement is reasonably
good. Good agreement was also reported for duplicate analyses
carried out in Japan, or Peru and Sweden.

        Generally, analyses of cadmium in horse kidney cortex
constituted no problem, mainly because concentrations of cadmium in
these samples were high. With very few exceptions the QC analyses
were acceptable according to established critera. The data are
given in detail in Vahter (1982).

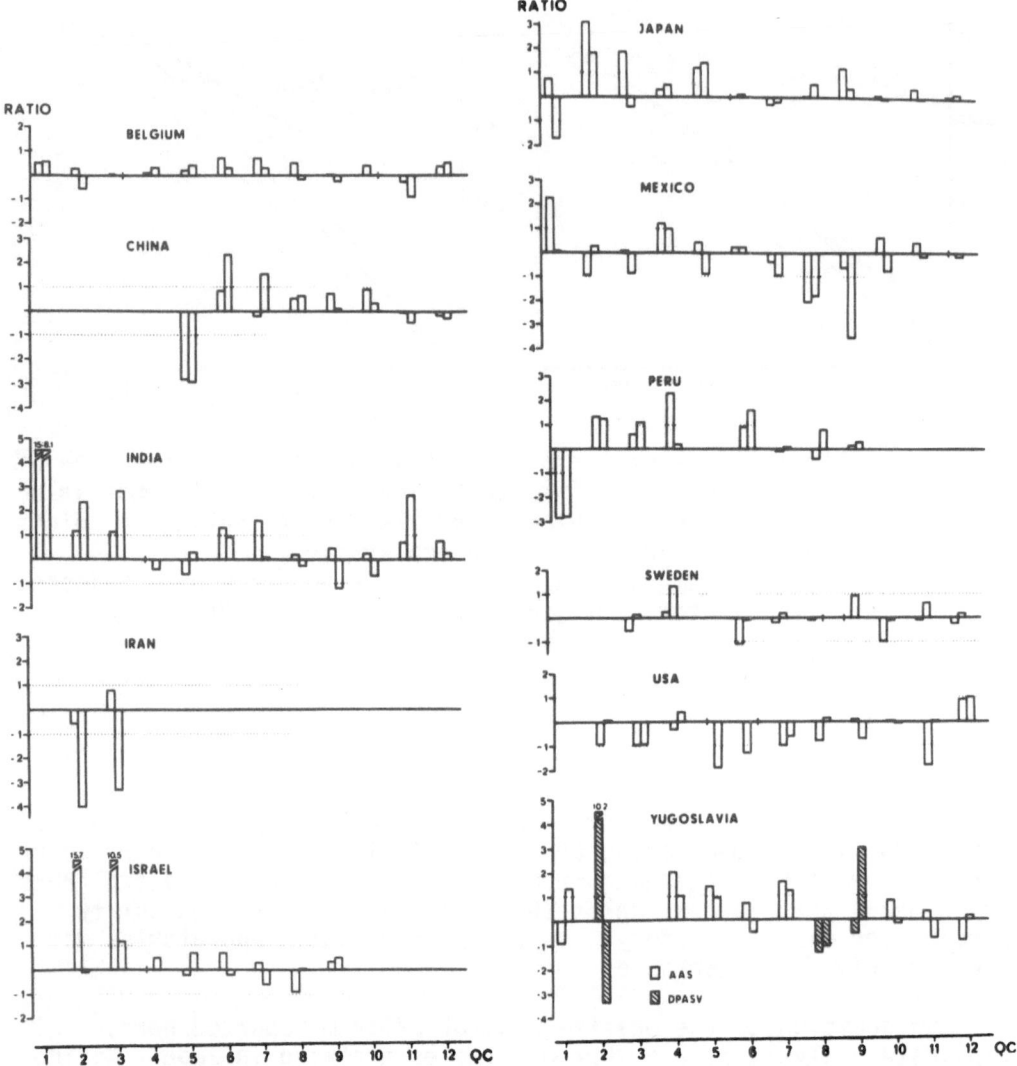

Figure 4   Results of analysis of lead in blood for quality control
runs 1-12 (training phase) expressed as ratios between
obtained and accepted deviations from "true" values
(reference values).   The QC runs are presented in the
order they have been analyzed.   For further explanation,
see text.   Dotted lines represent the acceptance interval
(Vahter, 1982).

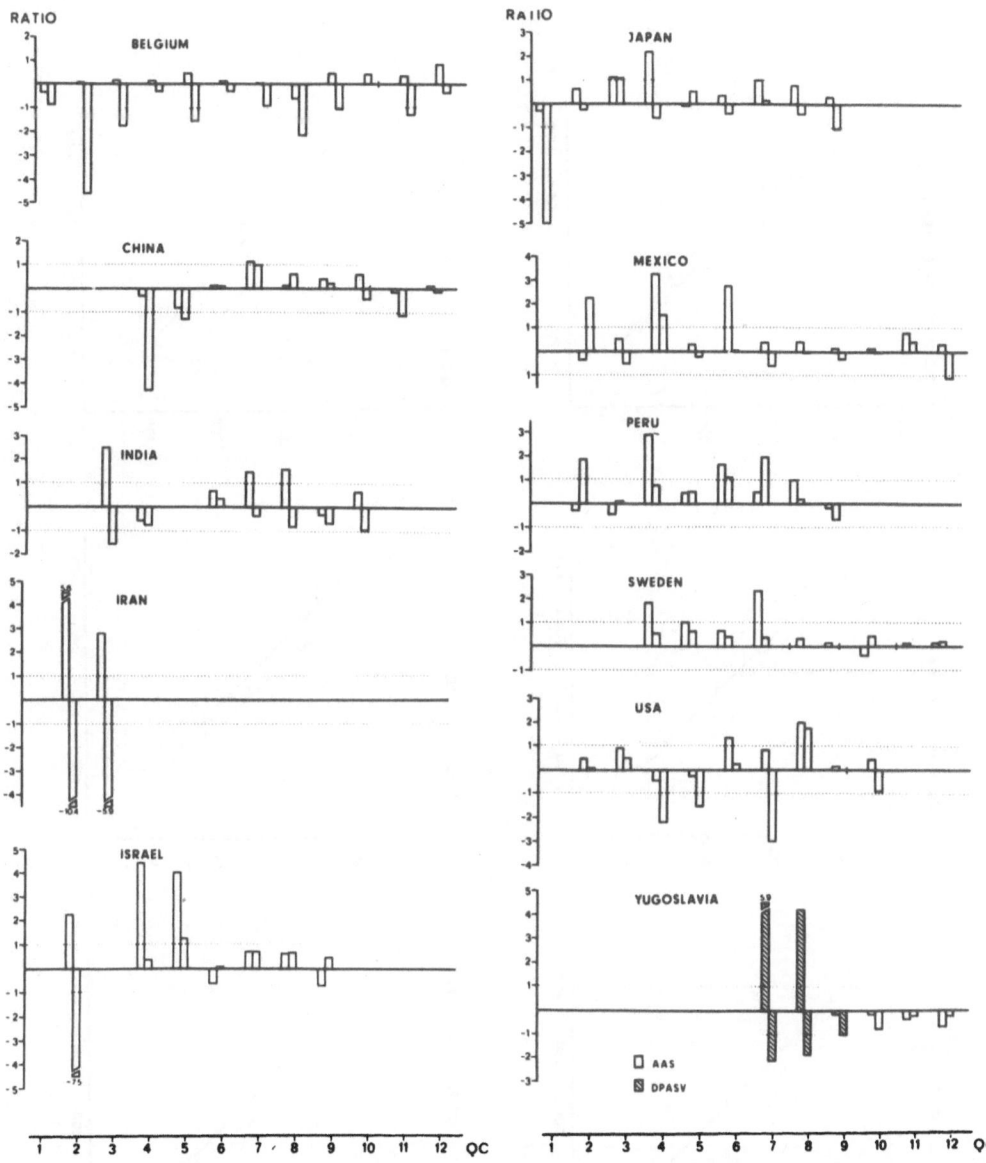

Figure 5 Results of analysis of cadmium in blood for quality
         control runs 1-12 (training phase) expressed as ratios
         between obtained and accepted deviations from "true"
         values (reference values). The QC runs are presented in
         the order they have been analyzed. For further
         explanation, see text. Dotted lines represent the
         acceptance interval (Vahter, 1982).

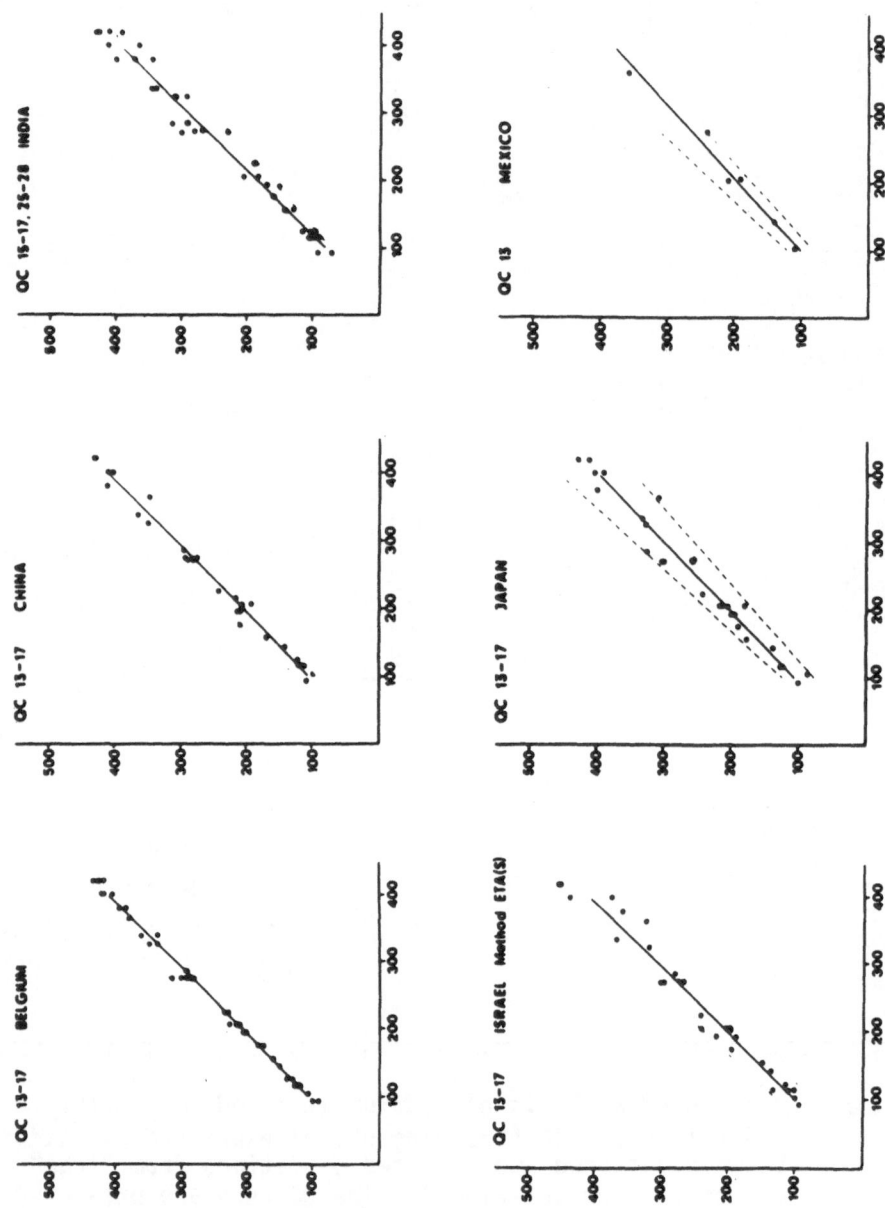

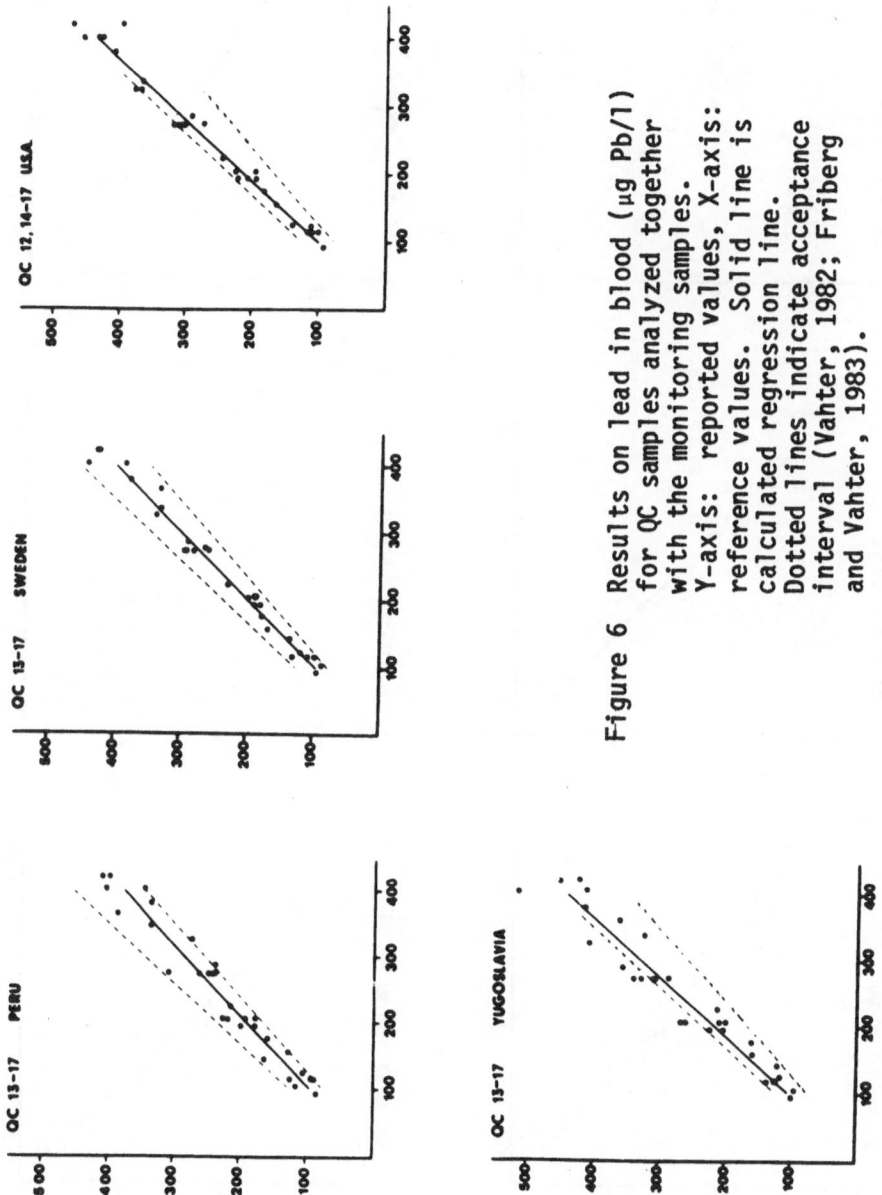

Figure 6 Results on lead in blood (μg Pb/l) for QC samples analyzed together with the monitoring samples. Y-axis: reference values, X-axis: reported values. Solid line is calculated regression line. Dotted lines indicate acceptance interval (Vahter, 1982; Friberg and Vahter, 1983).

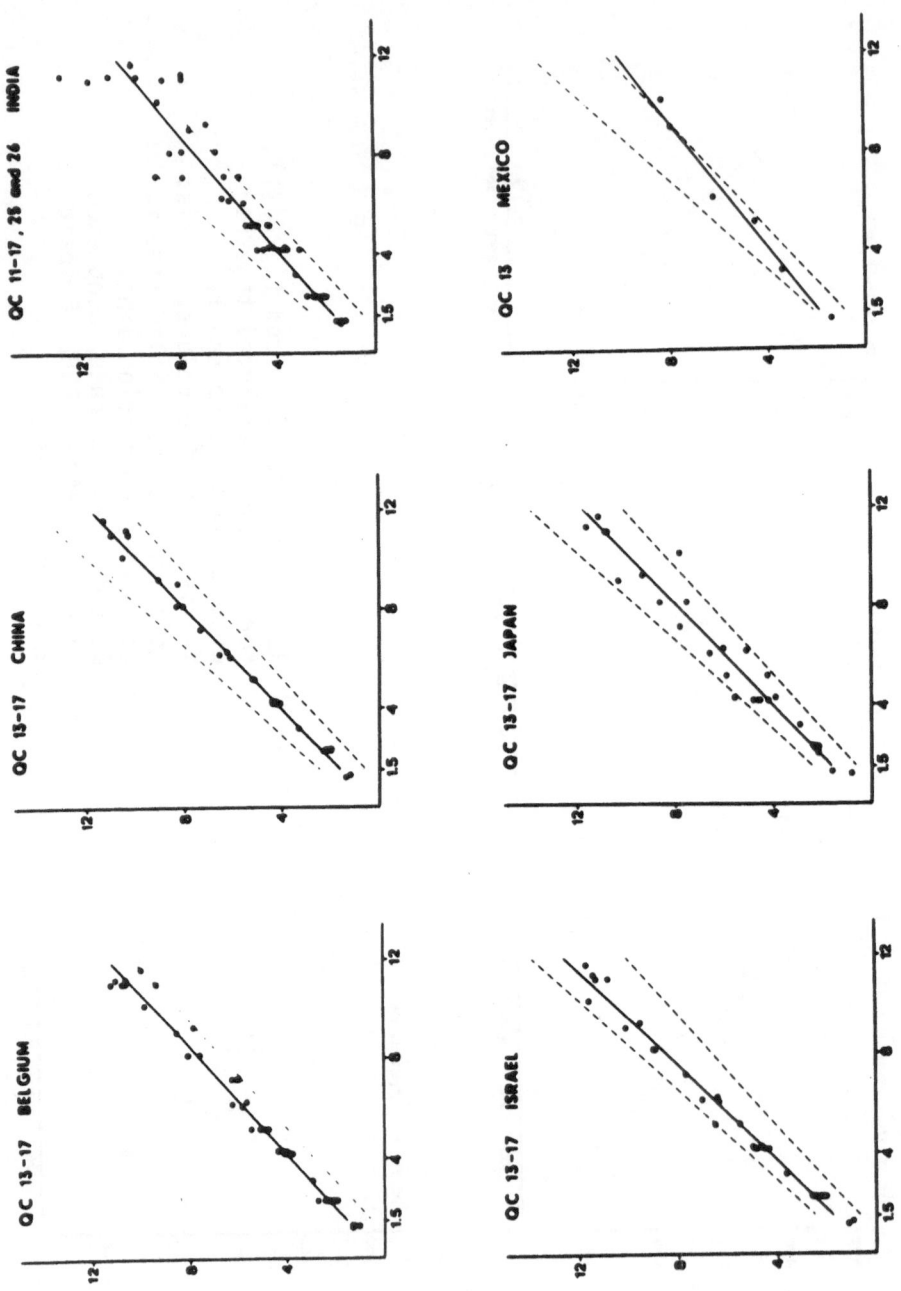

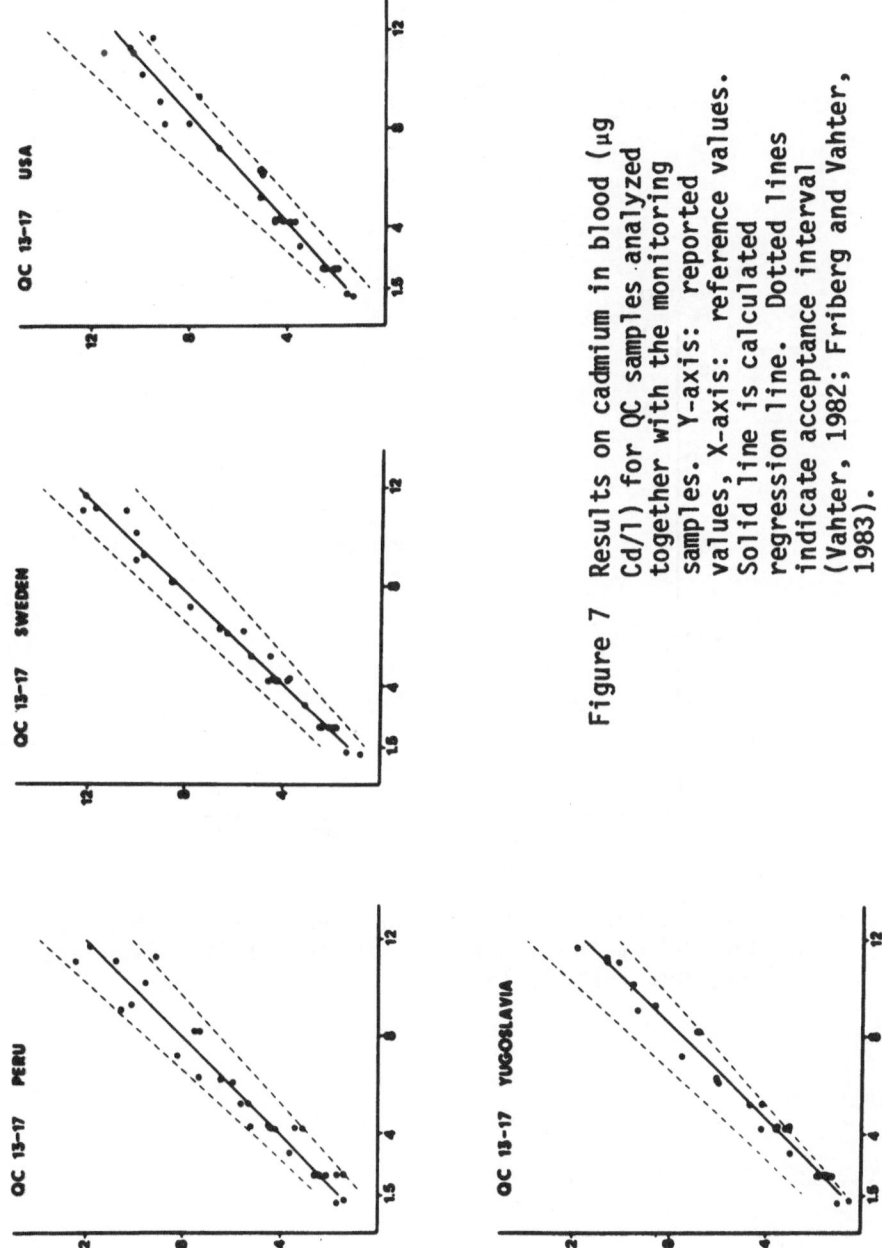

Figure 7 Results on cadmium in blood (μg Cd/l) for QC samples analyzed together with the monitoring samples. Y-axis: reported values. X-axis: reference values. Solid line is calculated regression line. Dotted lines indicate acceptance interval (Vahter, 1982; Friberg and Vahter, 1983).

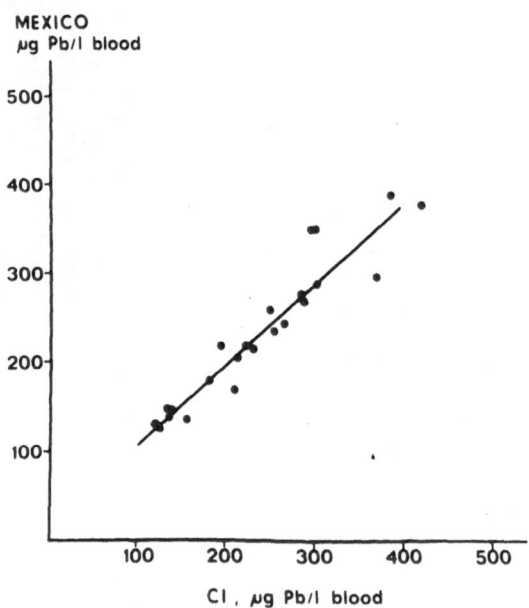

Figure 8   Comparison between results on lead in blood obtained in
Sweden and at the laboratory in Mexico City (Vahter, 1982;
Friberg and Vahter, 1983).

PREANALYTICAL QUALITY CONTROL

An important part of any quality control program is preanalytical quality control. There are many possibilities for the contamination of biological samples, e.g., the use of unsuitable blood collecting vials and contaminated anticoagulants. Contamination may also originate from skin which is not properly cleaned and from contaminated cleaning solutions. To avoid such problems as far as possible, evacuated blood collection tubes (Venoject) containing heparin from the same batch were provided by our laboratory; the metal content in a suitable number of tubes from each batch had been previously controlled. It was recommended that prior to collecting blood, the skin should be carefully washed and then cleaned with disposable napkins, saturated with 70 percent isopropyl alcohol. We provided the laboratories with special napkins. Written instructions on how to collect the samples were also provided. During a meeting in Stockholm the procedures to be used were demonstrated. After collection of the blood samples, the blood from each tube was transferred to three 5 ml polypropylene tubes; these tubes were also provided by us.

To avoid significant contamination and also to obtain standardized tissue samples, all participating laboratories received a film depicting procedures for the collection of kidney cortex samples at autopsies. This film was produced by WHO/IAEA in relation to the project "WHO/IAEA Joint Research Programme on Trace Elements in Cardiovascular Diseases (Autopsy Studies)" (Masironi and Parr, 1979).

MONITORING RESULTS

Results from the actual monitoring of blood and kidney samples are presented in detail in the UNEP/WHO report (Vahter, 1982). Figures 9 and 10 give an overview of the results of the blood analyses and in Figure 11 some of the data on cadmium and kidney cortex are reported.

The results indicate that large differences occur between countries. There are also differences related to sex and smoking habits. For example, for cadmium in blood, smoking habit is obviously the most important factor. It is beyond the scope of this presentation to discuss the health implications of the results or possible reasons for the differences found. This is discussed in the original report. Furthermore, the UNEP/WHO has started a program for an evaluation of the reasons for the differences.

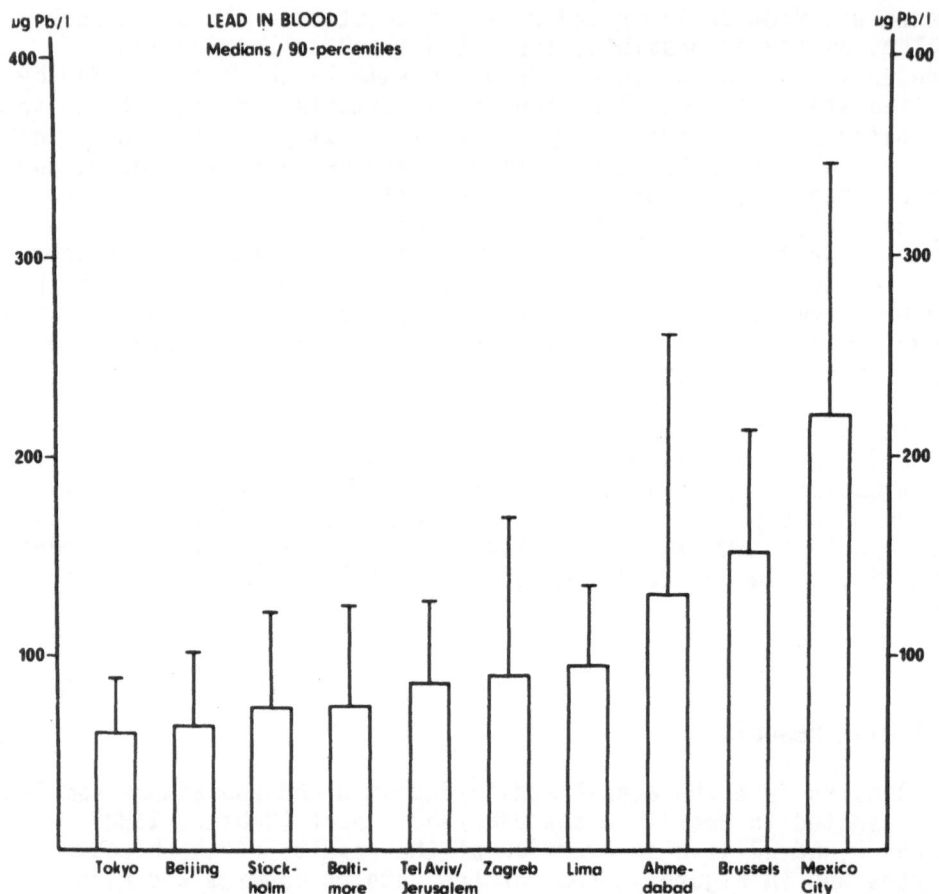

Figure 9   An overview of the results of blood analyzed for lead in
            actual monitoring in cities throughout the world. The
            height of each column is the median blood lead
            concentration and the bar is the upper 90 percentile.
            The data are taken from a UNEP/WHO Report (Vahter, 1982).

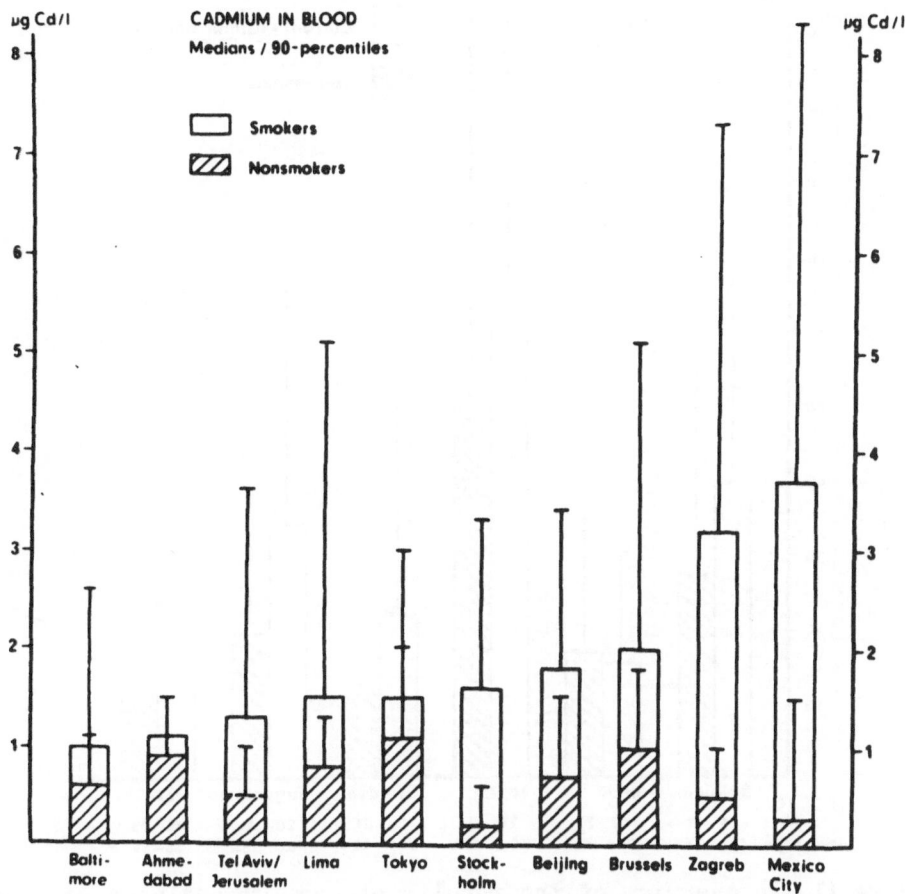

Figure 10 An overview of the results of blood analyzed for cadmium
in actual monitoring in cities throughout the world. The
heights of the columns are the median blood cadmium
concentrations for smokers (open and nonsmokers (hatched
areas). The horizontal bar is the upper 90 percentile.
The data are taken from a UNEP/WHO Report (Vahter, 1982).

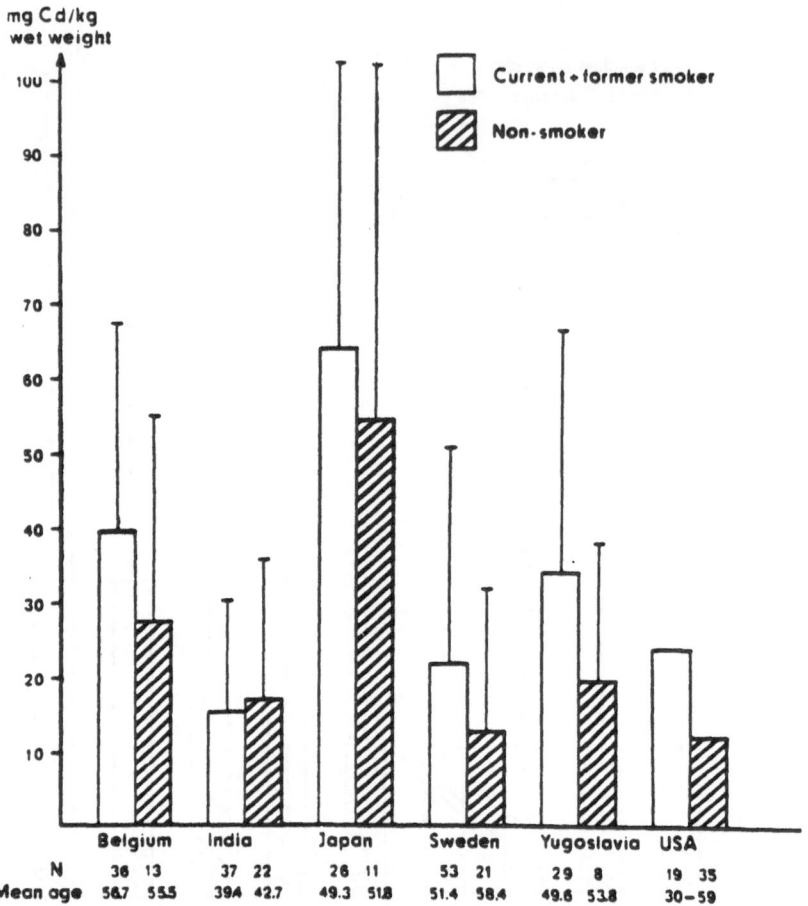

Figure 11 An overview of the results of cadmium analyses of kidney
cortex in autopsy samples taken in different countries
throughout the world. The column height is the median
value and the horizontal bar is the 90 percentile. The
open columns are samples from current plus from
nonsmokers. The total number of samples from each
country and the mean ages are indicated by the figures
beneath the horizontal axis. The data are taken from a
UNEP/WHO Report (Vahter, 1982).

REFERENCES

Berlin, A., 1982, Assessment of exposure to lead of the general population in the European Community through biological monitoring. Presented at the Workshop on Integrated Exposure Assessment Monitoring, Environ. Monit. Assess. 2:225-231.

Berlin, A., Del Castilho, P. and Smeets, J., 1973, European intercomparison programmes, in: "Proceedings of the International Symposium, Environmental Health Aspects of Lead", Amsterdam, 2-6 October, 1972, pp. 1033-1046.

Delves, H.T., 1970, A micro-sampling method for rapid determination of lead in blood by atomic absorption spectrophotometry, Analyst 95:431-438.

Ediger, R.D. and Coleman, R.L., 1972, A modified Delves cup atomic absorption procedure for determination of lead in blood, At. Absorpt. Newsl. 11:33-36.

Fernandez, F.J., 1975, Micromethod for lead determination in whole blood by atomic absorption, with use of the graphite furnace, Clin. Chem. 21:558-561.

Friberg, L. and Vahter, M., 1983, Assessment of exposure to lead and cadmium through biological monitoring. Results of a UNEP/WHO global study, Environ. Res. 30: (in press).

Lerner, S., 1975, Blood lead analysis - precision and stability, J. Occup. Med. 17:153-154.

Masironi, R. and Parr, R.M., 1979, Collection and trace element analysis of post-mortem human samples: The WHO/IAEA Research Programme on Trace Elements in Cardiovascular Diseases, in: "The Use of Biological Specimens for the Assessment of Human Exposure to Environmental Pollutants", A. Berlin, A.H. Wolff and Y. Hasagawa, eds., pp. 275-294, Martinus Nijhoff Publishers, The Hague.

Matousek, J.P. and Stevens, B.J., 1971, Biological application of the carbon rod atomizer in atomic absorption spectroscopy, Clin. Chem. 17:363-368.

Stoeppler, M. and Brandt, K., 1980, Contributions to automated trace analysis. Part V. Determination of cadmium in whole blood and urine by electrothermal atomic-absorption spectrophotometry, Fresenius Z. Anal. Chem. 300:372-380.

Vahter, M., ed., 1982, "Assessment of Human Exposure to Lead and Cadmium through Biological Monitoring". Prepared for United Nations Environmental Programme and WHO. National Swedish Institute of Enviromental Medicine and Karolinska Institute (Department of Enviromental Hygiene), Stockholm.

PARTICIPANTS

Nazzareno Ballatori
University of Rochester
Rochester, New York

Maths Berlin
University of Lund
Lund, Sweden

George Berg
University of Rochester
Rochester, New York

Maryka Bhattacharyya
Argonne National Laboratory
Argonne, Illinois

Philip J. Bushnell
New York University
New York, New York

Elsa Cernichiari
University of Rochester
Rochester, New York

J.J. Chisolm
Department of Pediatrics
Johns Hopkins University
Baltimore, Maryland

M. George Cherian
University of Western Ontario
London, Ontario, Canada

Ben Choi
University of California
Irvine Medical Center
Orange, California

Thomas W. Clarkson
University of Rochester
Rochester, New York

Bengt R.G. Danielsson
University of Uppsala
Uppsala, Sweden

Lennert Dencker
University of Uppsala
Uppsala, Sweden

Richard A. Doherty
University of Rochester
Rochester, New York

Virgil Ferm
Dartmouth Medical School
Hanover, New Hampshire

Bruce A. Fowler
National Institute of
Environmental Health Science
Research Triangle Park,
North Carolina

Lars Friberg
The Karolinska Institute
Stockholm, Sweden

Arthur Furst
3736 La Celle Ct.
Palo Alto, California

Helene Gardner
University of Rochester
Rochester, New York

Allen Gates
University of Rochester
Rochester, New York

Steven Gilbert
Health and Welfare Canada
Ottawa, Ontario, Canada

William Hart
Eastman Kodak Company
Rochester, New York

Kari Hemminki
Institute of Occupational Health
Helsinki, Finland

Robert Infurna
University of Rochester
Rochester, New York

Bruce Kelman
Battelle Pacific Laboratories
Richland, Washington

Robert Kilpper
Xerox Corporation
Rochester, New York

Curtis Klaassen
University of Kansas Medical Center
Kansas City, Kansas

Elzbieta Komsta-Szumska
National Research Council
Ottawa, Ontario, Canada

Nellie Laughlin
University of Wisconsin
Madison, Wisconsin

Insu Lee
National Institute of Environmental
Health Sciences
Research Triangle Park,
North Carolina

Alain Leonard
C.E.N. - S.C.K.
Mol, Belgium

Bo Lonnerdal
University of California
Davis, California

Arthur Levin
Hoffman - LaRoche
Nutley, New Jersey

E.M.K. Lui
University of Western Ontario
London, Ontario, Canada

Laszlo Magos
Medical Research Council
Carshalton, England

Katherine Mahaffey
Food and Drug Administration
Cincinnati, Ohio

Donald Mattison
NICHD, National Institutes
of Health
Bethesda, Maryland

Myron Mehlman
Mobil Oil Corporation
Princeton, New Jersey

Robert Mermelstein
Xerox Corporation
Rochester, New York

Richard Miller
University of Rochester
Rochester, New York

N. Karle Mottet
University of Washington
Seattle, Washington

Norton Nelson
New York University
New York, New York

Wendy Ng
University of Rochester
Rochester, New York

Gunnar Nordberg
University of Umea
Umea, Sweden

Magnus Piscator
University of Pittsburgh
Pittsburgh, Pennsylvania

Jiri Parizek
World Health Organization
Geneva, Switzerland

Deborah Rice
Health and Welfare Canada
Ottawa, Ontario, Canada

David Richardson
Eastman Kodak Company
Rochester, New York

Roy Robinson
University of Rochester
Rochester, New York

Patricia Rodier
University of Rochester
Rochester, New York

Ian Rowland
BIBRA
Carshalton, England

Lonnie Russell
Southern Illinois University
Carbondale, Illinois

Polly R. Sager
University of Rochester
Rochester, New York

Harold Sandstead
U.S. Department of Agriculture
Grand Forks, North Dakota

Zahir A. Shaikh
University of Rochester
Rochester, New York

Jerry Stara
EACO - Cincinnati
Cincinnati, Ohio

J.H.J. Copius Peereboom-Stegeman
Laboratory for Cell Biology
Amsterdam, Netherlands

F. William Sunderman, Jr.
University of Connecticut
Farmington, Connecticut

Tsuguyoshi Suzuki
University of Tokyo
Tokyo, Japan

Helen Tryphonas
Health and Welfare Canada
Ottawa, Ontario, Canada

Tore Syversen
University of Trondheim
Trondheim, Norway

Rosalind Volpe
International Lead Zinc
Research Organization
New York, New York

J.J. Vostal
General Motors
Warren, Michigan

Michael Webb
Medical Research Council
Carshalton, England

Patrick Weir
University of Rochester
Rochester, New York

Mariann Wide
University of Uppsala
Uppsala, Sweden

AUTHOR INDEX

835

837